INGENIX.
Physician Solutions

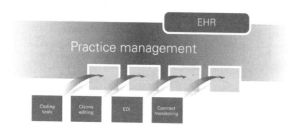

FOR PRICING DETAILS

Visit **www.ingenix.com/physicians**

Call toll-free **1.800.765.6704** and mention source code **FB11F**

Have a Fully Integrated Practice.

More companies rely on our medical coding expertise than anyone in the industry. That first-hand knowledge of all the stakeholders gives us unique insight, and we use it to create integrated information, technology and consulting solutions that address the range of financial and clinical challenges practices face.

← Payers – Connect with thousands of payers to verify eligibility and manage referral requirements, remittances and claims

← Clinical partners – Work with real-time clinical data from labs, pharmacies, radiologists, hospitals and other key partners

← Patients – Automate your appointment confirms, electronic statements, collect payments online, letters and inbound patient calls

Powerful solutions that work as one.

Start with your practice management platform or ours. Then plug in the powerful applications you need to enhance care or optimize your revenue cycle.

- **Electronic health records (EHR).**
  Low-cost, web-based EHR that puts your practice and your patients first. Ingenix CareTracker integrates with all the operational functions of the practice, improves quality and reduces costs

- **Practice management.**
  Next-generation, web-based practice management with today's financial and administrative productivity. Our automated billing process electronically connects to more than 1,000 national insurance plans and submits your claims for you, overnight

- **Coding tools.**
  The industry's broadest and most preferred coding tools. Our ever-evolving coding solutions are available in multiple formats to meet your needs

- **Claims editing.**
  Powerful claims software that leverages our information and your rules. The industry's average resubmission cost is $25 per claim—our solutions help you get paid faster

- **Electronic data interchange (EDI).**
  The way to navigate EDI your way, through clearinghouse connections, direct connections or both. Our connectivity solutions are HIPAA compliant, easy-to-use, efficient and affordable

- **Contract monitoring.**
  Organizing and managing your payer agreements for automated reimbursement and compliance. If your total claims value is underpaid by 5%, you're losing about a day's worth of earnings every month

Ingenix | Information is the Lifeblood of Health Care | Call toll-free 1.800.765.6704.

www.shopingenix.com

INGENIX
2011 Essential Coding Resources

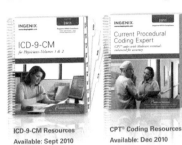

ICD-9-CM Resources	CPT® Coding Resources	HCPCS Resources
Available: Sept 2010	Available: Dec 2010	Available: Dec 2010

SAVE UP TO 20%
with source code FB11D

Visit www.shopingenix.com and enter the source code to save 20%.

Call toll-free **1.800.INGENIX (464.3649)**, option 1 and save 15%.

2011 Essential Coding Resources

Looks can be deceiving. Competitors attempt to imitate Ingenix code books because interpreting coding and reimbursement rules correctly and understanding the professional workflow is what we've helped coding professionals do successfully for over 25 years. Count on Ingenix to deliver accurate information, familiar features, industry-leading content, and innovative additions that help you improve coding practices, comply with HIPAA code set regulations, and realize proper reimbursement.

← A professional team's expertise
← Trusted and proven ICD-9-CM, CPT® and HCPCS coding resources
← Industry-leading content
← More value, competitive prices

Key Features and Benefits

Select from a range of formats for your ICD-9-CM, CPT,® and HCPCS coding resources to fit your individual preferences, skill level, business needs, and budget—you can trust your resource to be accurate and complimentary to your daily work when it's under an Ingenix cover.

2011 ICD-9-CM
Physician, Hospital, Home Health, and Skilled Nursing (with Inpatient Rehabilitation and Hospices) editions available

- New Look! Modified font and more vibrant colors increase readability
- New! Highlighted coding informational notes
- New! Snap-in tab dividers (*Expert* spiral editions only)
- More official coding tips and ICD-10 Spotlight codes
- Hallmark additional digit required symbols, intuitive color-coded symbols and alerts, QuickFlip™ color bleed tabs, dictionary headers, and symbol keys

2011 Current Procedural Coding Expert
- Code "Resequencing" identification
- Interventional radiology guidance section
- Reimbursement and mid-year changes information not found in the American Medical Association's CPT® code books
- Easy-to-navigate design
- Comprehensive and up-to-date listings with an extensive, user-friendly index
- PQRI icons and appendix

2011 HCPCS Level II Expert
- Comprehensive code updates for accurate reporting of supplies and services in physician, hospital outpatient, and ASC settings
- User-friendly format and expanded index to ease code look-up
- Important coding indicators and icons, PQRI icons, detailed illustrations, glossary of terms, and special MUEs

---

Ingenix | Information is the Lifeblood of Health Care | Call toll-free 1.800.INGENIX (464.3649), option 1.

100% Money Back Guarantee If our merchandise ever fails to meet your expectations, please contact our Customer Service Department toll-free at 1.800.INGENIX (464.3649), option 1, for an immediate response. Software: Credit will be granted for unopened packages only.

Also available from your medical bookstore or distributor. CPT is a registered trademark of the American Medical Association.   FB11D

# INGENIX®

Coders' Desk Reference *for* HCPCS

2011

Notice

Coders' Desk Reference for HCPCS was conceived to be an authoritative source of information about coding and reimbursement issues. Every effort has been made to verify accuracy, and information is believed reliable at the time of publication. Absolute accuracy cannot be guaranteed, however. This publication is made available with the understanding that the publisher is not engaged in rendering legal or other services requiring a professional license. Please address questions regarding this product to the Ingenix customer service department at 1.800.INGENIX (464.3649), option 1 or e-mail us at customerservice@ingenix.com.

Our Commitment to Accuracy

Ingenix is committed to producing accurate and reliable materials. To report corrections, please visit www.ingenixonline.com/accuracy or email accuracy@ingenix.com. You can also reach customer service by calling 1.800.INGENIX (464.3649), option 1.

Copyright

Copyright 2010 Ingenix

All rights reserved. No part of this publication may be reproduced or transmitted in any form or by any means, electronic or mechanical, including photocopy, recording, or storage in a database or retrieval system, without the prior written permission of the publisher.

Made in the USA.
ISBN 978-1-60151-417-2

Acknowledgments

The following staff contributed to the development and/or production of this book:

Julie Orton Van, CPC, CPC-P, *Product Manager*
Karen Schmidt, BSN, *Technical Director*
Stacy Perry, *Manager, Desktop Publishing*
Lisa Singley, *Project Manager*
Wendy Gabbert, CPC, CPC-H, *Clinical/Technical Editor*
Angela Galaviz, BSBM, CPC-H, *Clinical/Technical Editor*
Regina Magnani, RHIT, *Clinical/Technical Editor*
Tracy Betzler, *Desktop Publishing Specialist*
Hope M. Dunn, *Desktop Publishing Specialist*
Kimberli Turner, *Editor*

Clinical/Technical Editors

Wendy Gabbert, CPC, CPC-H
Ms. Gabbert has more than 25 years of experience in the health care field. She has extensive background in CPT/HCPCS and ICD-9-CM coding. She served several years as a coding consultant. Her areas of expertise include physician and hospital CPT coding assessments, chargemaster reviews, and the outpatient prospective payment system (OPPS). She is a member of the American Academy of Professional Coders and American College of Medical Coding Specialists.

Angela Galaviz, BSBM, CPC-H
Ms. Galaviz has more than 15 years of experience in the health care industry in patient accounting. Her areas of expertise include facility revenue cycle management, Medicare billing and coverage, chargemaster, and the outpatient prospective payment system (OPPS). She is an active member of the Healthcare Financial Management Association (HFMA).

Regina Magnani, RHIT
Ms. Magnani has more than 30 years of experience in the health care industry in both health information management and patient financial services. Her areas of expertise include facility revenue cycle management, patient financial services, CPT/HCPCS and ICD-9-CM coding, the outpatient prospective payment system (OPPS), and chargemaster development and maintenance. She is an active member of the Healthcare Financial Management Association (HFMA), the American Health Information Management Association (AHIMA), and the American Association of Healthcare Administrative Management (AAHAM).

Contents

Introduction to HCPCS iii
   Coding Systems iii

Using Modifiers 1
   Ambulance Modifiers 1
   HCPCS Level II Modifiers 1

Documentation Standards 13
   Medical Records Documentation for
      Providers 13
   General DME Documentation
      Standards 13
   Documentation for DMEPOS
      Suppliers 14

Durable Medical Equipment, Prosthetics,
Orthotics, and Supplies (DMEPOS) 17
   The DMEPOS Industry 17
   Special Federal and Third-Party Payer
      Definitions 17
   Accreditation 19

Durable Medical Equipment, Prosthetics,
Orthotics, and Supplies and the Office of
Inspector General 23

General Billing, Claims, and Coverage
Issues 27
   ASC X12N 837 (Version 4010)
      Professional Claim Format 27
   Provider Taxonomy Codes 27
   Medical Necessity and DMEPOS 27
   Certificates of Medical Necessity 28
   DMEPOS Prior Authorizations/Advance
      Determination of Medicare
      Coverage 32
   Local Coverage Determination (LCD) ... 32
   Medicare Program Requirements 33
   Mandatory Provider and Supplier Claim
      Submission 33
   Electronic DMEPOS Claims 34
   Signature on File (SOF) Requirements . 35
   Beneficiary Right to Itemized
      Statements 35
   Private Contracting or Opting Out 36
   Medicare Secondary Payer Policies and
      DMEPOS 37
   Medicare Coverage for Beneficiaries in
      State or Local Custody Under a Penal
      Authority 39
   DMEPOS Claims Jurisdictions 39

Medicare and DME MAC Claims
     Denials 40
The Advance Beneficiary Notice (ABN) of
     Noncoverage 41
Equipment and Service Upgrades 41
Duplicate Claim Denials 43
The Purchase and Rental of DMEPOS
     Items 43
DMEPOS Repairs and Maintenance 45

Appeals, Grievances, and Sanctions 49
   Medicare Appeals 49
   LCD (Local Coverage Determination)
      Appeals (Reconsiderations) 51
   Third-Party Payer Appeals 52
   Third-Party Payer Sanctions 53

Fraud, Abuse, and Compliance 55
   Introduction 55
   Definitions of Fraud and Abuse 55
   Definition of Compliance 56
   Criminal and Civil Statutes 56
   Federal Fraud and Abuse Investigative
      Programs 57
   Medicare Integrity Program 57
   Physician Order Fraud 59
   Realigning Internal Operations 60
   The OIG's Compliance Program
      Guidance for the DMEPOS
      Industry 61
   Lines of Communication 61
   Anti-Kickback and Self-Referral
      Concerns 62
   Auditing and Monitoring 62
   Whistleblowers 63
   Billing Companies: OIG Guidelines 63
   Fraud and Abuse by Medicare Patients .. 64

The Health Insurance Portability and
Accountability Act (HIPAA) of 1996 67
   HIPAA Administrative Simplification 67

Reimbursement Guidelines 71
   DMEPOS Utilization and Authorization 71
   PPS and Consolidated Billing 72
   Financial Management Guidelines 73
   Financial Formulas 73
   Conducting Cost and Reimbursement
      Analyses 74
   DMEPOS Cost Study 74

Glossary 77

Medicare Guidelines for Selected Topics 99
Diabetic Supplies and Services 99
Dressings 102
Drugs, Biologicals, and
    Radiopharmaceuticals 103
Enteral Nutrition 106
Hospital Beds 107
Infusion Pumps, External; Equipment
    and Supplies 109
Lens 113
Ostomy Devices and Supplies 114
Oxygen (O2) and O2 Equipment 114
Parenteral Nutrition 116
Pressure Reducing Support Surfaces:
    Groups I, II, and III 118
Prosthetic and Orthotic Devices 123
Transcutaneous Electrical Nerve
    Stimulation 127
Urological Supplies 128
Wheelchairs and Power Mobility
    Devices 131

Medicare Noncovered Codes 133

HCPCS Lay Descriptions 139

Introduction to HCPCS

Coding is a complicated business. It is not enough to have current copies of the *International Classification of Diseases, Ninth Edition, Clinical Modification* (ICD-9-CM), *Physicians Current Procedural Terminology, Fourth Edition* (CPT®), and Healthcare Common Procedure Coding System (HCPCS Level II) books. Medical coders also need dictionaries and specialty texts if they are to accurately translate physicians' operative reports or patient charts into reimbursement codes.

That's why Ingenix has developed the *Coders' Desk Reference* series—to provide a one-stop resource with answers to a wide variety of coding questions. We polled the medical reimbursement community and our technical staff to determine the issues causing bottlenecks in a coder's workload.

We found that experienced coders are frustrated by limited definitions accompanying many CPT, ICD-9-CM, and HCPCS Level II codes. Beginning coders need guidelines on the use of ICD-9-CM, CPT, and HCPCS codes and basic information about medical and reimbursement issues. Everyone requires up-to-date information about the anticipated changes to these coding systems.

Coders' Desk Reference for HCPCS answers the questions of both experienced and novice medical coders concerning medical supplies and equipment, as well as select services provided on an outpatient basis. It is a compendium of answers to a wide variety of coding questions and an introduction to new systems in coding structures. In order to code accurately, you must first have an understanding of the coding systems.

Coding Systems

Coding is the means by which providers and suppliers communicate their services with Medicare, Medicaid, third-party payers, and managed care organizations (MCOs). The correct use and reporting of modifiers and codes have become the defining elements in the reimbursement process for medical and surgical services, including services and items of durable medical equipment, prosthetics, orthotics, and supplies (DMEPOS). Assignment of the appropriate codes and adequate medical record documentation are necessary to avoid or minimize risk of fraud and abuse charges.

ICD-9-CM Diagnosis Coding

Diagnostic statements contained within medical records and other medical documentation are assigned codes from the ICD-9-CM. The correct use and reporting of ICD-9-CM codes is an important facet of the reimbursement process.

Diagnosis codes establish the necessity for which medical and surgical services, procedures, and DMEPOS items are furnished. Coding with ICD-9-CM is mandatory for all Medicare claims, Medicaid claims, third-party payer claims, and most MCO claims. In rare instances, claims for services or procedures submitted to self-funded insurance pools and workers' compensation carriers do not require ICD-9-CM codes, but do require a clearly descriptive diagnostic statement.

When reporting the appropriate diagnosis codes on claims for services, procedures, and DMEPOS items furnished to patients, ICD-9-CM diagnosis codes, CPT codes, and HCPCS Level II codes must be linked to identify the reason each service or procedure is rendered.

Providers and suppliers nationwide have discovered that many payers, including Medicare and Medicaid programs, will deny or delay claims because of incorrect or inappropriate ICD-9-CM code assignments. Many providers and suppliers have experienced these costly denials and delays. Following are some of the problem areas identified by payers in the use of ICD-9-CM codes:

- Invalid ICD-9-CM codes used
- ICD-9-CM codes not reported to the highest level of specificity (e.g., four-digit and five-digit codes must be reported if appropriate)
- Additional digits, particularly zeroes, added to valid three-digit or four-digit ICD-9-CM codes to make them five-digit codes. This invalidates the ICD-9-CM codes
- No medical record or supplier documentation given to support the use of a particular ICD-9-CM code
- ICD-9-CM code reported does not match the sex of the patient
- ICD-9-CM code reported does not adequately support the service billed, or is not a diagnosis code recognized under medical necessity policy for the service reported

CPT Codes (HCPCS Level I)

CPT is a standardized system of five-digit codes and descriptive terms developed, maintained, and copyrighted by the American Medical Association (AMA). Updated quarterly, CPT codes communicate to payers, and in some instances other providers and even patients, the procedures and services performed during a medical encounter.

CPT codes are the most widely accepted procedure codes for reporting medical services performed by physicians and facilities for many outpatient services. Considered HCPCS Level I codes, Medicare and Medicaid carriers are required to use CPT codes on health care claims, as designated in The Health Insurance Portability and Accountability Act of 1996 (HIPAA). An example of a CPT code follows:

30115   Excision, nasal polyp(s), extensive

Codes are grouped by body system, site, and/or type of procedure or service. They compose a nationally recognized system of codes that describe various services and procedures, including the following:

- Evaluation and management
- Anesthesia
- Surgery
- Radiology
- Laboratory and pathology
- Medicine

HCPCS Level II Codes

HCPCS is an acronym (pronounced "hick-picks") for the Healthcare Common Procedure Coding System. This coding system presents national codes used to report supplies and equipment, as well as select services provided on an outpatient basis. HCPCS codes are published by CMS and updated quarterly. These codes can be obtained through the federal government and through publishers such as Ingenix, which produces a complete annual and updateable edition of the HCPCS Level II codes.

HCPCS Level II codes may be used throughout the United States in all Medicare regions. They consist of one alpha character (A through V) followed by four digits. For example:

J7308   Aminolevulinic acid HCL for topical administration, 20%, single unit dosage form (354 mg)

L4350   Ankle control orthotic, stirrup style, rigid, includes any type interface, prefabricated, includes fitting and adjustment

HCPCS Level II codes describe:

- DME equipment, devices, accessories, supplies, and repairs; prosthetics; orthotics; medical and surgical supplies
- Medications
- Provider services
- Temporary Medicare codes (most commonly found in the Q codes)
- Other disparate items and services, such as ambulance services
- Temporary national codes (non-Medicare) (S codes)

The majority of services and procedures performed are reported with CPT codes. However, because the CPT coding system does not describe specific drugs, durable medical equipment (DME), prosthetics, orthotics, supplies, and certain other services, the HCPCS Level II coding system must be used.

CPT and HCPCS Level II codes are designated code sets for use in electronic HIPAA complaint transactions. CPT codes are widely accepted by third-party payers with minimal problems. HIPAA covered entities are by law required to accept HCPCS Level II codes. However, providers may encounter problems with some HCPCS Level II codes. For example, Medicare does not accept HCPCS Level II codes that begin with an S and many third-party payers do not accept codes that begin with a G.

Payers who accept HCPCS Level II codes require the code that most accurately describes the item provided. For example, a Medicare patient is given a physician's order for a gastrostomy tube. Durable medical equipment Medicare administrative contractors (DME MAC) instructs providers to report HCPCS code B4087 Gastrostomy/jejunostomy tube, standard, any material, any type, each. If this patient had been a non-Medicare beneficiary covered by a plan that did not accept HCPCS Level II codes, the CPT code 99070 Supplies and materials (except spectacles), provided over and above those usually included with the office visit or other services rendered (list drugs, trays, supplies, or materials provided), would be reported with a description of the gastrostomy tube.

Keeping Current in Coding

The various coding systems change quarterly. To correctly report and be reimbursed for DMEPOS services and items, providers and suppliers must keep up-to-date with respect to these changes. Additionally, to maintain compliance in reporting services and items furnished to patients—especially

Medicare and state Medicaid patients—providers and suppliers are required to report the most current codes and be knowledgeable about appropriate code reporting.

Some of the changes these coding systems undergo include:

- Code and modifier additions
- Code and modifier deletions
- Revisions of code and modifier descriptions
- Changes in grammar
- Parenthetical and instructional note changes
- Guideline changes
- Index entry changes

Providers and suppliers can choose from a variety of coding resources and educational seminars to keep up-to-date on quarterly changes. Providers and suppliers of DMEPOS should attend, at a minimum, an annual Medicare update for correct coding and billing procedures. This will help ensure compliance with federal standards.

HCPCS Level II Lay Descriptions

HCPCS Level II lay descriptions are written by Ingenix technical staff for people with medical training. They may not offer the details office personnel need to choose a code based on the contents of an operative report or patient's chart. Ordered numerically, each HCPCS Level II code is followed by a detailed description of the procedure that code represents.

Coders' Desk Reference for HCPCS was developed to help providers comply with the emerging standards by which DMEPOS supplies, medications, provider services, temporary Medicare codes, and other disparate items and services are coded, reported, and paid. Remember that Coders' Desk Reference for HCPCS is a medical reference and, as such, it is inappropriate to use this manual to select medical treatment.

The dental (D) codes are not included in the official 2011 HCPCS Level II code set. The American Dental Association (ADA) holds the copyright on those codes and instructed CMS to remove them. As a result, Ingenix has removed them from this product; however, Ingenix has additional resources available for customers requiring the dental codes. Please go to www.ShopIngenix.com or call 1.800.INGENIX (464.3649).

Using Modifiers

The HCPCS Level II codes are alphanumeric codes developed by CMS as a complementary coding system to the AMA's CPT codes. HCPCS Level II codes describe procedures, services, and supplies not found in the CPT® manual.

Similar to the CPT coding system, HCPCS Level II codes contain modifiers that serve to further define services and items without changing the basic meaning of the HCPCS Level II code with which they are reported.

It is important to note that HCPCS Level II modifiers may be used in conjunction with CPT codes, such as 69436 LT Tympanostomy (requiring insertion of ventilating tube), general anesthesia, left ear. Likewise, CPT modifiers can be used when reporting HCPCS Level II codes, such as L4396 50 Ankle contracture splint, bilateral (this scenario can also be reported with modifiers RT and LT, depending on the third-party payer's protocol). In some cases, a report may be required to accompany the claim to support the need for a particular modifier's use, especially in cases when the presence of a modifier causes suspension of the claim for manual review and pricing.

Ambulance Modifiers

For ambulance services modifiers, there are single alpha characters with distinct definitions that are paired together to form a two-character modifier. The first character indicates the origination of the patient (e.g., private residence, physician office, etc.) and the second character indicates the destination of the patient (e.g., hospital, skilled nursing facility, etc.). When reporting ambulance services, the name of the hospital or facility should be included on the claim. If reporting the scene of an accident or acute event (character S) as the origin of the patient, a written description of the actual location of the scene or event must be included with the claim.

Ambulance modifiers must be reported as two characters. The first character represents the origin and the second character represents the destination. For example, an ambulance transport from an accident scene to an acute care hospital would have modifier SH appended to the ambulance HCPCS code.

Ambulance Modifier Listing

D   Diagnostic or therapeutic site other than "P" or "H" when these are used as origin codes

E   Residential domiciliary, custodial facility (other than 1819 facility)

G   Hospital-based ESRD facility

H   Hospital

I   Site of transfer (for example, airport or helicopter pad) between modes of ambulance transport

J   Freestanding ESRD facility

N   Skilled nursing facility

P   Physician's office

R   Residence

S   Scene of accident or acute event

X   Intermediate stop at physician's office on way to hospital (destination code only). Note: Modifier X can only be used as a designation code in the second position of a modifier

HCPCS Level II Modifiers

Alphabetical Listing

A1   Dressing for one wound
A2   Dressing for two wounds
A3   Dressing for three wounds
A4   Dressing for four wounds
A5   Dressing for five wounds
A6   Dressing for six wounds
A7   Dressing for seven wounds
A8   Dressing for eight wounds
A9   Dressing for nine or more wounds
AA   Anesthesia performed personally by anesthesiologist

- CPT codes approved for use with modifier AA are 00100–01999.

- If an anesthetist assists the physician in the care of a single patient, the service is considered personally performed by the physician. The anesthesiologist should report this service with modifier AA and the appropriate CPT code from series 00100–01999.

- Modifier AA affects Medicare payment.

AD   Medical supervision by a physician; more than four concurrent anesthesia procedures

- Modifier AD affects Medicare payment as a distinct fee schedule amount exists.
- AE Registered dietitian
- AF Specialty physician
- AG Primary physician
- AH Clinical psychologist
- AI Principal physician of record
- AJ Clinical social worker
  - Medicare limits allowable to 75 percent of the physician fee schedule.
- AK Nonparticipating physician
- AM Physician, team member service
  - The physician member of a team is required to perform one out of every three visits made by a team member.
  - Modifier AM should be used to indicate a team member visit was performed by the physician.
  - Team member visits will be denied if only one person rendering services is billing for team services, as this is inappropriate billing practice.
  - Modifier AM has no effect on payment.
- AP Determination of refractive state was not performed in the course of diagnostic ophthalmological examination
  - Modifier AP has no effect on payment.
- AQ Physician providing a service in an unlisted health professional shortage area (HPSA)
- AR Physician scarcity area
- AS PA, nurse practitioner, or clinical nurse specialist services for assistant-at-surgery
- AT Acute treatment
  - This modifier should be used when reporting services 98940, 98941, or 98942.
  - Modifier AT has no effect on payment for Medicare and many third-party carrier claims.
- AU Item furnished in conjunction with a urological, ostomy, or tracheostomy supply
- AV Item furnished in conjunction with a prosthetic device, prosthetic, or orthotic
- AW Item furnished in conjunction with a surgical dressing
- AX Item furnished in conjunction with dialysis services
- AY Item or service furnished to an ESRD patient that is not for the treatment of ESRD
- AZ Physician providing a service in a dental health professional shortage area for the purpose of an electronic health record incentive payment
- BA Item furnished in conjunction with parenteral enteral nutrition (PEN) services
- BL Special acquisition of blood and blood products
- BO Orally administered nutrition, not by feeding tube
- BP The beneficiary has been informed of the purchase and rental options and has elected to purchase the item
- BR The beneficiary has been informed of the purchase and rental options and has elected to rent the item
- BU The beneficiary has been informed of the purchase and rental options and after 30 days has not informed the supplier of his/her decision
- CA Procedure payable only in the inpatient setting when performed emergently on an outpatient who expires prior to admission
- CB Service ordered by a renal dialysis facility (RDF) physician as part of the ESRD beneficiary's dialysis benefit, is not part of the composite rate, and is separately reimbursable
- CC Procedure code change
  - Modifier CC is used by the carrier when the procedure code submitted had to be changed for administrative reasons or because an incorrect code was filed.
  - Payment rule: Payment determination will be based on the new code used by the contractor carrier/fiscal intermediary.
  - Modifier CC has no effect on payment.
- CD AMCC test has been ordered by an ESRD facility or MCP physician that is part of the composite rate and is not separately billable
- CE AMCC test has been ordered by an ESRD facility or MCP physician that is separately reimbursable based on medical necessity
- CF AMCC test has been ordered by an ESRD facility or MCP physician that is not part of the composite rate and is separately billable
- CG Policy criteria applied
- CR Catastrophe/disaster related
- CS Item or service related, in whole or in part, to an illness, injury, or condition that was caused by or exacerbated by the effects, direct or indirect, of the 2010 oil spill in the gulf of Mexico, including but not limited to subsequent clean up activities
- DA Oral health assessment by a licensed health professional other than a dentist
- E1 Upper left, eyelid
- E2 Lower left, eyelid
- E3 Upper right, eyelid
- E4 Lower right, eyelid

Using Modifiers

EA Erythropoetic stimulating agent (ESA) administered to treat anemia due to anticancer chemotherapy

EB Erythropoetic stimulating agent (ESA) administered to treat anemia due to anticancer radiotherapy

EC Erythropoetic stimulating agent (ESA) administered to treat anemia not due to anticancer radiotherapy or anticancer chemotherapy

- Report modifiers EA, EB, and EC when ESA is administered to a patient who is not ESRD or who is not on maintenance dialysis. Report these modifiers with HCPCS Level II codes J0881 and J0885 only.

ED Hematocrit level has exceeded 39% (or hemoglobin level has exceeded 13.0 g/dl) for three or more consecutive billing cycles immediately prior to and including the current cycle

EE Hematocrit level has not exceeded 39% (or hemoglobin level has not exceeded 13.0 g/dl) for three or more consecutive billing cycles immediately prior to and including the current cycle

- Report modifier ED or EE on claims for EPO for ESRD patients receiving dialysis in renal dialysis facilities. Claims reporting no modifier or both modifiers will be returned to the provider for correction.

EJ Subsequent claims for a defined course of therapy (e.g., EPO, sodium hyaluronate)

EM Emergency reserve supply (for ESRD benefit only)

EP Service provided as part of Medicaid Early Periodic Screening Diagnosis and Treatment (EPSDT) program

ET Emergency services

- This modifier should be applied to report dental procedures performed in emergency situations.

EY No physician or other licensed health care provider order for this item or service

F1 Left hand, second digit
F2 Left hand, third digit
F3 Left hand, fourth digit
F4 Left hand, fifth digit
F5 Right hand, thumb
F6 Right hand, second digit
F7 Right hand, third digit
F8 Right hand, fourth digit
F9 Right hand, fifth digit
FA Left hand, thumb

FB Item provided without cost to provider, supplier or practitioner, or full credit received for replaced device (examples, but not limited to, covered under warranty, replaced due to defect, free samples)

- Modifier FB is used to indicate a device used in a procedure was provided without cost.
- Report modifier FB with the procedure.

FC Partial credit received for replaced device

- Report modifier FC when a credit greater than or equal to 50 percent and less than 100 percent has been given for a replaced device.
- Report modifier FC with the procedure.

FP Service provided as part of family planning program

G1 Most recent URR reading of less than 60

- URR is the urea reduction ratio, a calculation that demonstrates the effectiveness of renal dialysis.

G2 Most recent URR reading of 60 to 64.9
G3 Most recent URR reading of 65 to 69.9
G4 Most recent URR reading of 70 to 74.9
G5 Most recent URR reading of 75 or greater
G6 ESRD patient for whom less than six dialysis sessions have been provided in a month

- The Balanced Budget Act (BBA) of 1997 requires CMS to develop and implement a method to measure and report on the quality of dialysis services.
- ESRD facilities must use modifiers to reflect the most recent urea reduction ratio (URR), along with CPT code 90999 *Unlisted dialysis procedure inpatient or outpatient*, on all claims filed to Medicare for hemodialysis. Consequently, it will be necessary for ESRD facilities to also report a HCPCS code with the dialysis revenue code (0820, 0821, and 0829). ESRD facilities (both hospital-based and free-standing) should report CPT code 90999 and one of the G modifiers as appropriate, on all claims filed for hemodialysis services. This information will provide data to CMS regarding the adequacy of hemodialysis for quality improvement initiatives. ESRD facilities must monitor hemodialysis adequacy monthly for all facility patients. Home hemodialysis patients may be monitored less frequently, but not less often than quarterly.
- Because CMS will be profiling facilities based on the URR ranges reported, CMS is recommending dialysis facilities to use a

standardized methodology for drawing the pre- and postdialysis blood urea nitrogen (BUN) samples that are used in the calculation of the URR. Facilities may use the slow flow/stop pump or blood reinfusing sampling techniques.

G7 Pregnancy resulted from rape or incest, or pregnancy certified by physician as life threatening

- This modifier is appended to the CPT procedure code for abortion services and indicates that the pregnancy resulted from rape or incest, or that the physician considers the pregnancy to be life threatening to the mother.
- Reporting this modifier on a claim communicates to the contractor that the physician certifies that the abortion meets Medicare's coverage policy. Medicare will cover an abortion when:
  - the pregnancy is the result of an act of rape or incest
  - the woman suffers from a physical disorder, physical injury, or physical illness, including a life-endangering physical condition caused by or arising from the pregnancy itself, that would, as certified by a physician, place the woman in danger of death unless an abortion is performed
- Claims submitted with modifier G7 for abortion services may be subject to postpayment review by the contractor.
- Third-party payers, other than Medicare, may not accept this modifier. Individual payers should be queried for claim submission requirements.

G8 Monitored anesthesia care (MAC) for deep complex, complicated or markedly invasive surgical procedure

G9 Monitored anesthesia care for patient who has a history of severe cardio-pulmonary condition

GA Waiver of liability statement issued as required by payer policy, individual case

- This modifier indicates that the provider or supplier has a required signed advance beneficiary notice (ABN) retained in the patient's chart.
- The purpose of the waiver of liability is to ensure that the provider will be paid for the services performed, and to protect the beneficiary from receiving unnecessary services. Providers who acquire a waiver of liability for a covered service should use modifier GA directly following a procedure code to indicate that a beneficiary has signed a waiver of liability form. The provider should keep the form on file. No other statement regarding the waiver of liability is required when modifier GA is used. Modifier GA at the end of a procedure code is sufficient evidence that the beneficiary has signed an advance notice. If the beneficiary subsequently requests a review of the denial, Medicare will request the provider or supplier to forward a copy of the notice for their files.

- An advanced notice may be applied to an extended course of treatment provided the notice identifies each service for which Medicare is likely to deny payment. A separate notice is required, however, if additional services for which Medicare is likely to deny payment are furnished later in the course of treatment.
- Medicare will deny payment for services reported with modifier GA. The beneficiary can appeal the denial.

GB Claim being resubmitted for payment because it is no longer covered under a global payment demonstration

GC This service has been performed in part by a resident under the direction of a teaching physician

- When a teaching physician's services are billed using this modifier, the teaching physician is certifying that he or she was present during the key portion of the service and was immediately available during the other portions of the service.
- When an anesthesiologist uses modifier QK for two to four medically directed procedures, he or she would not also append modifier GC to the anesthesia code. Only modifier QK is used.
- When there is a one-on-one situation with a resident and a teaching anesthesiologist (teaching setting), the anesthesiologist would append modifier GC only.
- Modifiers QK and GC are never used together.
- Modifier GC has no effect on payment.

GD Units of service exceeds medically unlikely edit value and represents reasonable and necessary services

GE This service has been performed by a resident without the presence of a teaching physician under the primary care exemption

- This modifier identifies services being billed under the primary care exception to the guideline for governing presence

Using Modifiers

during the key portion of a service by the teaching physician.
- Modifier GE has no effect on payment.

GF Nonphysician (e.g., nurse practitioner (NP), certified registered nurse anesthetist (CRNA), certified registered nurse (CRN), clinical nurse specialist (CNS), physician assistant (PA)) services in a critical access hospital

GG Performance and payment of a screening mammogram and diagnostic mammogram on the same patient, same day
- Report modifier GG when the radiologist who interprets a screening mammography orders and interprets additional films based on the results of the screening mammogram while the beneficiary is still at the facility for the screening exam. When this occurs, Medicare will pay for both the screening and diagnostic mammograms.

GH Diagnostic mammogram converted from screening mammogram on same day
- Report modifier GH when the radiologist's interpretation results in additional films and no additional payment is requested. When this modifier is reported, Medicare pays only for the diagnostic mammogram.
- The radiologist is considered the ordering physician in this situation and must furnish his or her national provider identifier (NPI) for Medicare claims. Diagnostic mammography claims submitted to Medicare without the ordering physician's NPI will be denied and returned as unprocessable.

GJ Opt out physician or practitioner emergency or urgent service
- Use this modifier for claims submitted to Medicare for services rendered by an opt out provider who has not signed a private contract with the Medicare patient requiring emergent or urgent medical care.
- The provider may not charge the Medicare beneficiary more than what a nonparticipating provider would be permitted to charge, and must submit the claim to Medicare on the beneficiary's behalf.
- If modifier GJ is not reported on the claim for emergency or urgent care rendered to a Medicare beneficiary by the opt out provider, the claim will be denied and returned as unprocessable.

GK Reasonable and necessary item/service associated with GA or GZ modifier

GL Medically unnecessary upgrade provided instead of nonupgraded item. No charge. No advance beneficiary notice (ABN).

GM Multiple patients on one ambulance trip

GN Service delivered under an outpatient speech-language pathology plan of care

GO Service delivered under an outpatient occupational therapy plan of care

GP Service delivered under an outpatient physical therapy plan of care

GQ Via asynchronous telecommunications system

GR This service was performed in whole or in part by a resident in a department of veteran's affairs medical center or clinic, supervised in accordance with VA policy

GS Dosage of EPO or darbepoetin alfa has been reduced and maintained in response to hematocrit or hemoglobin level

GT Via interactive audio and video telecommunication systems

GU Waiver of liability statement issued as required by payer policy, routine notice

GV Attending physician not employed or paid under arrangement by the patient's hospice provider

GW Service not related to hospice patient's terminal condition

GX Notice of liability issued, voluntary under payer policy
- Use this modifier when the provider has a signed voluntary advance beneficiary notice (ABN) in the patient's chart.
- This should be used if the provider wants a patient's statement of liability for services that are excluded by statute.
- Services with modifier GX will be denied.

GY Item or service statutorily excluded, does not meet the definition of any Medicare benefit or for non-Medicare insurers, is not a contract benefit

GZ Item or service expected to be denied as not reasonable and necessary

H9 Court-ordered
HA Child/adolescent program
HB Adult program, non-geriatric
HC Adult program, geriatric
HD Pregnant/parenting women's program
HE Mental health program
HF Substance abuse program
HG Opioid addiction treatment program
HH Integrated mental health substance abuse program

HI	Integrated mental health and mental retardation/developmental disabilities program		K1	Lower extremity prosthesis functional level-1: has the ability or potential to use a prosthesis for transfers or ambulation on level surfaces at fixed cadence. Typical of the limited and unlimited household ambulator
HJ	Employee assistance program			
HK	Specialized mental health programs for high-risk populations			
HL	Intern		K2	Lower extremity prosthesis functional level-2: has the ability or potential for ambulation with the ability to traverse low level environmental barriers such as curbs, stairs or uneven surfaces. Typical of limited community ambulator
HM	Less than bachelor degree level			
HN	Bachelors degree level			
HO	Masters degree level			
HP	Doctoral level			
HQ	Group setting		K3	Lower extremity prosthesis functional level-3: has the ability or potential for ambulation with variable cadence. Typical of community ambulator who has the ability to traverse most environmental barriers and may have vocational, therapeutic or exercise activity that demands prosthetic utilization beyond simple locomotion
HR	Family/couple with client present			
HS	Family/couple without client present			
HT	Multi-disciplinary team			
HU	Funded by child welfare agency			
HV	Funded state addictions agency			
HW	Funded by state mental health agency		K4	Lower extremity prosthesis functional level-4: has the ability or potential for prosthetic ambulation that exceeds the basic ambulation skills, exhibiting high impact, stress or energy levels, typical of the prosthetic demands of the child, active adult, or athlete
HX	Funded by county/local agency			
HY	Funded by juvenile justice agency			
HZ	Funded by criminal justice agency			
J1	Competitive acquisition program (CAP) no-pay submission for a prescription number			
J2	Competitive acquisition program (CAP), restocking of emergency drugs after emergency administration		KA	Add-on option/accessory for wheelchair
			KB	Beneficiary requested upgrade for ABN, more than 4 modifiers identified on claim
J3	Competitive acquisition program (CAP), drug not available through CAP as written, reimbursed under average sales price methodology		KC	Replacement of special power wheelchair interface
			KD	Drug or biological infused through DME
			KE	Bid under round one of the DMEPOS competitive bidding program for use with noncompetitive bid base equipment
J4	DMEPOS item subject to DMEPOS competitive bidding program that is furnished by a hospital upon discharge			
			KF	Item designated by FDA as Class III device
JA	Administered intravenously		KG	DMEPOS item subject to DMEPOS competitive bidding program number 1
JB	Administered subcutaneously			
	• Report modifier JA or JB to indicate the route of administration when erythropoiesis-stimulating agents (ESA), such as epoetin alfa and darbepoetin alfa, are reported. When both methods of administration are used, such as in a renal dialysis facility, report separate lines to identify the number of administrations provided using each method.		KH	DMEPOS item, initial claim, purchase or first month rental
				• DMEPOS is the acronym for durable medical equipment, prosthetics, orthotics, and supplies.
				• Report with modifier RR for rented DME.
			KI	DMEPOS item, second or third month rental
				• Report with modifier RR for rented DME.
JC	Skin substitute used as a graft		KJ	DMEPOS item, parenteral enteral nutrition (PEN) pump or capped rental, months four to 15
JD	Skin substitute not used as a graft			
JW	Drug amount discarded/not administered to any patient			
			KK	DMEPOS item subject to DMEPOS competitive bidding program number 2
K0	Lower extremity prosthesis functional level- 0; does not have the ability or potential to ambulate or transfer safely with or without assistance and a prosthesis does not enhance their quality of life or mobility		KL	DMEPOS item delivered via mail
			KM	Replacement of facial prosthesis including new impression/moulage

Using Modifiers

KN Replacement of facial prosthesis using previous master model
KO Single drug unit dose formulation
KP First drug of a multiple drug unit dose formulation
KQ Second or subsequent drug of a multiple drug unit formulation
KR Rental item–billing for partial month
KS Glucose monitor supply for diabetic beneficiary not treated with insulin using previous master model
KT Beneficiary resides in a competitive bidding area and travels outside that competitive bidding area and receives a competitive bid item
KU DMEPOS item subject to DMEPOS competitive bidding program number 3
KV DMEPOS item subject to DMEPOS competitive bidding program that is furnished as part of a professional service
KW DMEPOS item subject to DMEPOS competitive bidding program number 4
KX Requirements specified in the medical policy have been met
KY DMEPOS item subject to DMEPOS competitive bidding program number 5
KZ New coverage not implemented by managed care
LC Left circumflex coronary artery;
LD Left anterior descending coronary artery

- Modifiers LC, LD, and RC are used when more than one intervention is required on a major vessel and its branches. CPT codes describe codes for coronary angioplasty, atherectomy, and stent procedures in terms of the "initial" vessel and a "subsequent" vessel.
- Modifiers LC, LD, and RC will be used to indicate the specific vessel involved in the procedure and should be used when one of the following procedures is reported:

  92980 Transcatheter placement of an intracoronary stent(s), percutaneous, with or without other therapeutic intervention, any method; single vessel

  92981 each additional vessel (add-on code)

  92982 Percutaneous transluminal coronary balloon angioplasty; single vessel

  92984 each additional vessel (add-on code)

  92995 Percutaneous transluminal coronary atherectomy, by mechanical or other method, with or without balloon angioplasty; single vessel

  92996 each additional vessel (add-on code)

- Note: Do not bill additional vessel codes without first billing the single vessel code.
- There are three procedures (stent, balloon angioplasty, and atherectomy). Each procedure has two codes: a single vessel code and an additional vessel code. The single-vessel code is only used the first time that intervention is used during the interventional session. If the intervention is performed on more than one vessel, the additional vessel code should be used. The following are examples of the proper way to code the vessels:

  92980 RC, 92981 LC, 92981 LD
  92980 RC, 92982 LC*, 92995 LD*
  92982 RC, 92984 LC, 92984 LD
  92995 RC, 92996 LC, 92996 LD
  92995 RC, 92996 LC, 92982 LD*

- Procedure codes 92982 and 92995 cannot be billed separately from procedure code 92980 when provided on the same vessel. Procedure code 92982 cannot be billed separately from procedure code 92995 when performed on the same vessel. According to the CCI, modifier 59 does not need to be included with these procedures.

LL Lease/rental (use the LL modifier when DME equipment rental is to be applied against the purchase price)
LR Laboratory round trip
LS FDA-monitored intraocular lens implant
LT Left side

- This modifier indicates the side of the body on which a procedure is performed. It does not indicate a bilateral procedure.
- Modifiers LT and RT have no effect on payment; however, failure to use when appropriate could result in delay or denial (or partial denial) of the claim.

M2 Medicare secondary payer (MSP)
MS Six-month maintenance and servicing fee for reasonable and necessary parts and labor, which are not covered under any manufacturer or supplier warranty
NB Nebulizer system, any type, FDA-cleared for use with specific drug

Using Modifiers

NR New when rented (use the NR modifier when DME which was new at the time of rental is subsequently purchased)

NU New equipment

P1 Anesthesia physical status—Normal, healthy patient

P2 Anesthesia physical status—Patient with mild, systemic disease

P3 Anesthesia physical status—Patient with severe, systemic disease

P4 Anesthesia physical status—Patient with severe, systemic disease that is a constant threat to life

P5 Anesthesia physical status—Moribund patient who is not expected to survive without the operation

P6 Anesthesia physical status—Declared brain-dead patient whose organs are being removed for donor purposes

PA Surgical or other invasive procedure on wrong body part
- Medicare will not pay for surgery performed on the wrong patient or wrong body part, or an incorrect procedure performed on a patient. All payments for these mistakenly performed procedures and any related services will be denied.
- For outpatient services, one of the three modifiers (PA, PB, or PC) should be appended to line items related to the surgical error.

PB Surgical or other invasive procedure on wrong patient
- Medicare will not pay for surgery performed on the wrong patient or wrong body part, or an incorrect procedure performed on a patient. All payments for these mistakenly performed procedures and any related services will be denied.
- For outpatient services, one of the three modifiers (PA, PB, or PC) should be appended to line items related to the surgical error.

PC Wrong surgery or other invasive procedure on patient
- Medicare will not pay for surgery performed on the wrong patient or wrong body part, or an incorrect procedure performed on a patient. All payments for these mistakenly performed procedures and any related services will be denied.
- For outpatient services, one of the three modifiers (PA, PB, or PC) should be appended to line items related to the surgical error.

PI Positron Emission Tomography (PET) or PET/Computed Tomography (CT) to inform the initial treatment strategy of tumors that are biopsy proven or strongly suspected of being cancerous based on other diagnostic testing, once per cancer diagnosis

PL Progressive additional lenses

PS Positron Emission Tomography (PET) or PET/Computed Tomography (CT) to inform the subsequent treatment strategy of cancerous tumor when the beneficiary's treating physician determines that the PET study is needed to inform subsequent anti-tumor strategy

PT Colorectal cancer screening test; converted to diagnostic test or other procedure

Q0 Investigational clinical service provided in a clinical research study that is in an approved clinical research study

Q1 Routine clinical service provided in a clinical research study that is in an approved clinical research study

Q2 HCFA/ORD demonstration project procedure/service

Q3 Live kidney donor surgery and related services
- Use modifier Q3 to identify postoperative live kidney donor services that are reimbursed at 100 percent of the Medicare fee schedule amount.

Q4 Service for ordering/referring physician qualifies as a service exemption
- Use this modifier when the ordering or referring provider has a financial relationship with the entity performing the service, and for which the service qualifies as one of the service-related exemptions.

Q5 Service performed by a substitute physician under a reciprocal billing arrangement
- Modifier Q5 is to be applied to the end of a procedure code to indicate that the service was provided by a substitute physician. The regular physician should keep a record on file of each service provided by the substitute physician, associated with the substitute physician's UPIN, and make this record available to Medicare upon request.
- This modifier has no effect on payment.

Q6 Service furnished by a locum tenens physician
- Locum tenens physicians generally have no practice of their own; they usually move from area to area as needed. The patient's regular physician may submit a claim and receive Medicare Part B payment for a covered and medically necessary visit of a locum tenens physician who is not an

Using Modifiers

employee of the regular physician and whose services for patients of the regular physician are not restricted to the regular physician's office. The locum tenens physician should not provide the visit services to Medicare patients for a continuous period of longer than 60 days.

- This modifier has no effect on payment.

Q7, Q8, and Q9—Foot care

- Documentation of the systemic conditions and class findings must be in the patient's record. The record must be maintained in the physician's office and available for medical review by the carrier. Documentation should indicate the course of treatment and length of treatment for infectious conditions. Documentation should include the affected toe, including the clinical evidence of mycosis, the manner in which and to what extent the nail was debrided, and the antifungal agent used in the office note/progress note.
- A description of the qualifying symptoms should be documented
- Ambulatory patients must exhibit a marked limitation in ambulation, pain, or secondary infection resulting from the thickening and dystrophy.
- Non-ambulatory patients must suffer from pain or secondary infection resulting from the thickening and dystrophy of the infected nail plate.
- Routine foot care is excluded from Medicare coverage.
- General diagnosis such as ASHD, circulatory problems, vascular disease, and venous insufficiency are not sufficient to permit payment for routine foot care.

Q7 One Class A finding
- Class A findings: Nontraumatic amputation of foot or integral skeletal portions thereof.
- This modifier was established to allow the provider to report class findings without having to write a narrative description on the claim form or submit additional documentation with the claim. This modifier should be used in conjunction with foot care procedures (e.g., 11720, 11721) to indicate the severity of the patient's systemic condition and justify the medical necessity of a procedure that is usually denied as routine.

Q8 Two Class B findings
- Class B findings:
  - absent posterior tibial pulse
  - absent dorsalis pedis pulse
  - advance trophic changes such as (three required):
    - hair growth (decrease or absence)
    - nail changes (thickening)
    - pigmentary changes (discoloration)
    - skin texture (thin, shiny)
    - skin color (rubor or redness)
- This modifier was established to allow the provider to report class findings without having to write a narrative description on the claim form or submit additional documentation with the claim. This modifier should be used with foot care procedures (e.g., 11720, 11721) to indicate the severity of the patient's systemic condition and to justify the medical necessity of a procedure that is usually denied as routine.

Q9 One Class B and two Class C findings
- Class C findings:
  - claudication
  - temperature changes (e.g., cold feet)
  - edema
  - paresthesia
  - burning
- This modifier was established to allow the provider to report class findings without having to write a narrative description on the claim form or submit additional documentation with the claim. This modifier should be used in conjunction with foot care procedures (e.g., 11720, 11721) to indicate the severity of the patient's systemic condition and to justify the medical necessity of a procedure that is usually denied as routine.

QC Single channel monitoring

QD Recording and storage in solid state memory by a digital recorder
- This modifier has no effect on payment.

QE Prescribed amount of oxygen is less than one liter per minute (LPM)

QF Prescribed amount of oxygen exceeds four liters per minute (LPM) and portable oxygen is prescribed

QG Prescribed amount of oxygen is greater than four liters per minute (LPM)

QH Oxygen conserving device is being used with an oxygen delivery system

QJ Services/items provided to a prisoner or patient in state or local custody, however the state or local government, as applicable, meets the requirements in 42 CFR 411.4 (B)

QL Patient pronounced dead after ambulance called
QM Ambulance service provided under arrangement by a provider of services
- Modifiers QM and QN should be used when a patient has an inpatient status at one hospital and is transferred to another hospital or facility for tests or treatment and then is returned to the first hospital.
- This modifier is valid for Medicare; however, the service would be denied under Medicare Part B since it is considered a Medicare Part A expense.

QN Ambulance service furnished directly by a provider of services
- Modifiers QM and QN should be used when a patient has an inpatient status at one hospital and is transferred to another hospital or facility for tests or treatment, and then is returned to the first hospital.
- This modifier is valid for Medicare; however, the service would be denied under Medicare Part B since it is considered a Medicare Part A expense.

QP Documentation is on file showing that the laboratory test(s) was ordered individually or ordered as a CPT-recognized panel other than automated profile codes 80002-80019, G0058, G0059, and G0060
- Sufficient documentation would be the requisition form showing that the physician had individually ordered tests either by code or the corresponding code definition.
- The individual tests that constitute an organ or disease related CPT panel do not need to be ordered individually in order for the laboratory to use modifier QP. The laboratory may bill using the CPT code for organ or disease oriented panel with modifier QP when the physician orders the components of the panel.
- CMS does not require laboratories to use this modifier, but some contractors (fiscal intermediary or carrier) strongly advise its use.

QS Monitored anesthesia care services
- Monitored anesthesia care (MAC) services will be closely watched to ensure medical necessity is documented. ICD-9-CM codes should accurately describe the condition requiring MAC anesthesia. CMS collects data for MAC, even though it is paid the same as general anesthesia. The anesthesiologist or CRNA monitors the patient's vital signs, furnishes the preanesthesia exam, prescribes the necessary anesthesia care, administers medications, and furnishes required postoperative anesthesia care.

QT Recording and storage on tape by an analog tape recorder
- This modifier has no effect on payment.

QW CLIA waived test

QX CRNA service: with medical direction by a physician
- Payment rule: Limits payment to 55 percent of the amount that would have been allowed if personally performed by a physician or nonsupervised CRNA.

QY Medical direction of one certified registered nurse anesthetist (CRNA) by an anesthesiologist

QZ CRNA service: without medical direction by a physician
- Payment rule: No effect on payment. Payment would be equal to the amount that would have been allowed if personally performed by a physician.

RA Replacement of a DME, orthotic or prosthetic item

RB Replacement of a part of DME, orthotic or prosthetic item furnished as part of a repair

RC Right coronary artery

RD Drug provided to beneficiary, but not administered "incident-to"

RE Furnished in full compliance with FDA-mandated risk evaluation and mitigation strategy (REMS)

RR Rental (use the RR modifier when DME is to be rented)
- Use this modifier in conjunction with the appropriate "rental" modifiers KH, KI, and KJ.
- Modifier RR is placed directly after the HCPCS Level II code for the DME followed by the appropriate rental modifier as above.

RT Right side (used to identify procedures performed on the right side of the body)
- There are many procedure codes that require a physician to indicate the side of the body on which a procedure was performed by using modifiers RT and LT.
- When billing for a separately identifiable/unrelated surgical procedure performed during the postoperative period of another surgical procedure, procedure code modifiers RT (right) and LT (left) must be indicated on the claim as appropriate. In addition, modifier 79 (unrelated procedure or service by the same physician during the

Using Modifiers

postoperative period) must be submitted on the subsequent claim.
- This modifier indicates the side of the body on which a procedure is performed. It does not indicate a bilateral procedure.
- Modifiers LT and RT have no effect on payment; however, failure to use when appropriate could result in delay or denial (or partial denial) of the claim.

SA Nurse practitioner rendering service in collaboration with a physician
SB Nurse midwife
SC Medically necessary service or supply
SD Services provided by registered nurse with specialized, highly technical home infusion training
SE State and/or federally-funded programs/services
SF Second opinion ordered by a professional review organization (PRO) per section 9401, p.l. 99-272 (100% reimbursement—no Medicare deductible or coinsurance)
- Use this modifier when the second opinion is ordered or requested by QIO.
- For Medicare beneficiaries, when this modifier is reported the service is eligible for 100 percent reimbursement. The usual deductible and/or coinsurance amounts are not applied.

SG Ambulatory surgery center (ASC) facility service
- This modifier is no longer required on Medicare claims. Physician and nonphysician practitioner fees must be billed on a separate claim form from the ASC facility fees.

SH Second concurrently administered infusion therapy
SJ Third or more concurrently administered infusion therapy
SK Member of high risk population (use only with codes for immunization)
SL State supplied vaccine
SM Second surgical opinion
SN Third surgical opinion
SQ Item ordered by home health
SS Home infusion services provided in the infusion suite of the IV therapy provider
ST Related to trauma or injury
SU Procedure performed in physician's office (to denote use of facility and equipment)
SV Pharmaceuticals delivered to patient's home but not utilized

SW Services provided by a certified diabetic educator
SY Persons who are in close contact with member of high-risk population (use only with codes for immunization)
T1 Left foot, second digit
T2 Left foot, third digit
T3 Left foot, fourth digit
T4 Left foot, fifth digit
T5 Right foot, great toe
T6 Right foot, second digit
T7 Right foot, third digit
T8 Right foot, fourth digit
T9 Right foot, fifth digit
TA Left foot, great toe
TC Technical component. Under certain circumstances, a charge may be made for the technical component alone. Under these circumstances, the technical component charge is identified by adding modifier TC to the usual procedure number. Technical component charges are institutional charges and not billed separately by physicians. However, portable x-ray suppliers only bill for technical component and should utilize modifier TC. The charge data from portable x-ray suppliers will then be used to build customary and prevailing profiles.
- There are stand-alone procedure codes that describe technical component only codes (e.g., staff and equipment costs) of diagnostic tests. They also identify procedures that are covered only as diagnostic tests and, therefore, do not have a related professional component. Do not use modifier TC on these codes. Technical component services only are institutional and should not be billed separately by the physicians. However, portable x-ray suppliers only bill for the technical component and should use modifier TC.

TD RN
TE LPN/IVN
TF Intermediate level of care
TG Complex/high tech level of care
TH Obstetrical treatment/services, prenatal or postpartum
TJ Program group, child and/or adolescent
TK Extra patient or passenger, non-ambulance
TL Early intervention/individualized family service plan (IFSP)
TM Individualized education program (IEP)
TN Rural/outside providers' customary service area

TP	Medical transport, unloaded vehicle	UA	Medicaid level of care 10, as defined by each state
TQ	Basic life support by volunteer ambulance provider	UB	Medicaid level of care 11, as defined by each state
TR	School-based individualized education program (IEP) services provided outside the public school district responsible for the student	UC	Medicaid level of care 12, as defined by each state
		UD	Medicaid level of care 13, as defined by each state
TS	Follow-up service	UE	Used durable medical equipment
TT	Individualized service provided to more than one patient in same setting		• Use this modifier when the used equipment is purchased by a beneficiary.
TU	Special payment rate, overtime	UF	Services provided in the morning
TV	Special payment rates, holidays/weekends	UG	Services provided in the afternoon
TW	Back-up equipment	UH	Services provided in the evening
U1	Medicaid level of care 1, as defined by each state	UJ	Services provided at night
U2	Medicaid level of care 2, as defined by each state	UK	Services provided on behalf of the client to someone other than the client (collateral relationship)
U3	Medicaid level of care 3, as defined by each state	UN	Two patients served
U4	Medicaid level of care 4, as defined by each state	UP	Three patients served
		UQ	Four patients served
U5	Medicaid level of care 5, as defined by each state	UR	Five patients served
		US	Six or more patients served
U6	Medicaid level of care 6, as defined by each state	V5	Vascular catheter (alone or with any other vascular access)
U7	Medicaid level of care 7, as defined by each state	V6	Arteriovenous graft (or other vascular access not including a vascular catheter)
U8	Medicaid level of care 8, as defined by each state	V7	Arteriovenous fistula only (in use with 2 needles)
U9	Medicaid level of care 9, as defined by each state	V8	Infection present
		V9	No infection present
		VP	Aphakic patient

Documentation Standards

Medical Records Documentation for Providers

Documentation in the medical record must contain information justifying hospitalization, an observation stay, an encounter or visit, or services provided for a patient. It must indicate that services are provided using current medical knowledge and treatment for the condition or injury, and that the services are medically necessary. In addition, the documentation must stand up to the scrutiny of others.

To meet the requirements of medical necessity for all health care services reported to the Medicare program, the patient's medical record must reflect the nature and extent of the diagnosis or injury, with clear documentation of the following patient-specific facts:

- Physical examination findings
- Diagnostic tests/analyses results
- Relation of diagnosis to the DMEPOS item
- Complicating comorbidities
- Physical functional abilities and/or limitations (ability to ambulate or transfer, amount of time needed to be spent in a bed, extent of use of a wheelchair, types/frequencies of activities recommended for outside the home, etc.)
- Duration of the diagnosis (acute, acute but refractory to treatment, chronic)
- Overall expected course/prognosis
- Rehabilitation potentials

In most instances, an evaluation and management (E/M) service is rendered before or during the same session that an order for DMEPOS is given. Requirements for the correct reporting of E/M services are beyond the scope of this publication; however, in addition to the criteria listed above for medical record documentation, an appropriate patient history must be obtained.

In general, the following three criteria (known as key elements of E/M documentation) should appear in the patient's medical record to correctly report an E/M service:

- Patient history
- Physical examination
- Level of medical decision-making

This is a requirement under both the American Medical Association's (AMA) and the Centers of Medicare and Medicaid Services' (CMS) guidelines.

Providers who dispense DMEPOS should take note that during audits of E/M services, a prevalent finding is the lack of review of systems information. This is an integral part of the patient's history. The absence or inadequate documentation of this part of the patient's history will cause an auditor to downgrade the original level of E/M, resulting in an overpayment situation in which the provider will have to refund the reimbursement difference to the payer or the patient.

Providers may receive requests from DMEPOS suppliers for copies of patient medical records that support the medical necessity of the provider's order. This is generally in response to a direct demand made upon the supplier from the Medicare contractor to substantiate the need for DMEPOS items. Providers should respond promptly to any requests made by the DMEPOS supplier for additional information. Suppliers do report certain difficulties in obtaining copies of medical records from provider offices.

General DME Documentation Standards

The following documentation is necessary for DMEPOS items regardless of the payer:

- The provider should sign and date an order for the DMEPOS item.
- If the treating provider is also supplying the item, the clinical notes should substantiate the need for the item.
- The diagnosis establishing the medical necessity for the item must be documented in the medical record.
- If the medical necessity for the item, as determined by the payer, cannot be established due to the nature of the patient's condition,

injury, or illness, then the patient must sign a waiver before receiving the item. For Medicare patients, this waiver is called the advance beneficiary notice (ABN). This document must be kept on file in case the Medicare contractor, Medicaid agency, third-party payer, or managed care plan requests proof of the advance notice.

- It is recommended that the provider keep a copy of the Certificate of Medical Necessity (CMN) in the patient's medical record. An order or CMN on its own will not justify medical necessity even if the physician signs it.

- If a DME Information Form (DIF) is used instead or in conjunction with the CME, a copy of the DIF should be kept in the patient's medical record. In some cases, the DIF replaces the CMN for certain DME supplies. The DIF must be signed by the supplier. The DIF contains much of the same information and does not require a narrative description of the equipment, cost, or a physician signature. *See the section below for more information on DIFs.*

- Provider records must substantiate the information and answers contained in the CMN.

Documentation for DMEPOS Suppliers

Suppliers are required to have the following information on file before submitting a claim to the Durable medical equipment Medicare administrative contractor (DME MAC):

- Dispensing order
- Certificate of medical necessity (CMN) if applicable
- DME MAC information form (DIF) if applicable
- Patient's diagnosis from the provider
- Information for the use of specific modifiers required in certain DME program safeguard contractors' (PSC) policies
- Attestation statements required in certain DME PSC policies

Suppliers must keep documentation on file for seven years.

Suppliers are required to maintain proof of delivery in their files and it must be available to the DME PSC on request. If this information is not provided, claims will be denied and the supplier will have to refund the payment amount. Suppliers who consistently do not provide documentation to support services may be referred to the Office of Inspector General (OIG) for imposition of sanctions.

The three methods of delivery are:

- Delivering directly to the beneficiary or authorized representative
- Utilizing a delivery/shipping service to deliver items
- Delivery of items to a nursing facility on behalf of the beneficiary

Suppliers have the responsibility to ensure that coverage criteria are met before providing an item, or they risk having payment for the claim rejected. The supplier is liable for the dollar amount involved unless an appropriate ABN has been obtained. This is a CMS directive to all DMEPOS suppliers, one that is routinely scrutinized during supplier audits.

Provider Orders for DMEPOS

Provider orders for DMEPOS usually take the form of clinical record or progress note annotations, or they can take the form of separate, individual orders. These separate orders can be written on:

- Prescription forms
- Internally generated practice DMEPOS order forms
- Forms supplied by the third-party payer for DMEPOS authorization and reimbursement

In any case, a copy of the order may have to accompany the claim to the payer (if a paper claim) or must be retained on file (if an electronic claim).

For DMEPOS items billed to third-party payers, the provider must have documentation that adequately demonstrates the medical necessity of the item. This is true for any medical service. This information must be a permanent part of the patient's medical record, as should the original order for the DMEPOS item. An order or CMN on its own will not justify medical necessity even if the physician signs it.

In many instances, an entry made directly into the clinical record notes or progress notes can aptly serve as the provider order for the DMEPOS item, especially in situations where the DMEPOS supplier and the health care provider are one and the same. In these cases, the medical record entry must be complete and disclose all of the same information necessary for separate provider order documents.

Any detailed written order must contain:

- Patient's name; insured's name
- Other patient identifying information (third-party payer ID number, patient's social security number, date of birth, patient's address and telephone number)
- DMEPOS item ordered with full description

- DMEPOS options or features that will be billed separately or that may require an upgraded HCPCS Level II code — if these codes are recognized by the payer — for the item
- Expected duration of use of the DMEPOS item; prognosis as it is known at the time of the DMEPOS order
- Patient's diagnosis, including ICD-9-CM code and narrative description
- Provider's signature and date
- State date of DMEPOS order

Orders for supplies to be used on a continuing or periodic basis must contain information about the quantities of the supplies needed, frequency of change (for dressings, pads, and so on), and expected duration of use.]

If the DMEPOS item is a drug, the order must specify the name of the drug, concentration (if applicable), dosage, frequency of administration, and duration of infusion (if applicable).

Someone other than the physician may complete the detailed description of the item. However, the treating physician must review the detailed description and personally sign and date the order to indicate agreement.

The *Medicare Program Integrity Manual*, Pub. 100-08, chapter 5, section 5.1.1.1, advises that except as noted below, suppliers may dispense most items of DMEPOS based on a verbal order. This verbal dispensing order must include:

- A description of the item
- The patient's name
- The physician's name
- The start date of the order

Suppliers must maintain written documentation of the verbal order and this documentation must be available to Medicare upon request. For items that are dispensed based on a verbal order, the supplier must obtain a written order that meets the requirements of this section.

Verbal orders are unacceptable for certain DME billable to Medicare. A written order prior to delivery is required for:

- Pressure reducing pads
- Mattress overlays, mattresses, and beds
- Seat lift mechanisms
- TENS units
- Power operated vehicles

- Other items as denoted by contractor local or regional coverage decisions

For these items, the supplier must have received a written order that has been both signed and dated by the treating physician before dispensing the item.

If replacement supplies are needed for the use of purchased DMEPOS, the provider must specify on the prescription, or on the CMN, the type of supplies needed and the frequency with which they must be replaced, used, or consumed. "As needed" or "PRN" statements are not acceptable.

A new order is required when:

- There is a change in the order for the accessory, supply, drug, or item
- An item is replaced
- There is a change in the supplier
- The documentation section of a particular medical policy may require a new order on a regular basis (even if there is no change in the order)

For items that require a CMN, and for accessories, supplies, and drugs related to an item requiring a CMN, the CMN may serve as the written order IF the narrative description of the item is detailed enough. This applies to both hard copy and electronic orders and CMNs.

Separate Physician and Provider Orders

Suppliers of DMEPOS must conform to the demands of their participating contracts with the various third-party payers. DMEPOS items require an official order signed and dated by the ordering provider. The order must detail the patient's identifying information, including but not limited to a description of the DMEPOS item and the reason the patient requires the DMEPOS prescription. The provider's signature may or may not be a stamp facsimile or other substitute; some payers require an original signature. A faxed copy of the original order is usually sufficient for suppliers to fill the DMEPOS order and submit their claim for the item furnished.

However, in the case of illegible or faded faxed copies of DMEPOS orders, suppliers should insist on the original order being mailed or delivered by courier in prompt fashion. When the payer requires special forms (supplied by the payer) to be completed before the authorization, dispensation, and reimbursement of the DMEPOS item, these forms are generally viewed as a substitution for the provider order. The forms are usually supplied in duplicate or triplicate so the physician or provider has an immediate copy; the copy must become a permanent part of the patient's medical record.

Durable Medical Equipment, Prosthetics, Orthotics, and Supplies (DMEPOS)

The DMEPOS Industry

Wheelchairs, artificial limbs, braces, surgical dressings, and medications are all examples of durable medical equipment, prosthetics, orthotics, and supplies, known by the acronyms DME and POS, or simply DMEPOS.

The DMEPOS industry includes manufacturers, pharmaceutical companies, medical equipment and supply companies (suppliers and vendors), and providers. Entities peripheral to the DMEPOS industry, but having direct impact on its operations, include the Food and Drug Administration (FDA), which approves the use of medical devices and pharmaceuticals in the United States, and federal and state health care programs such as Medicare and Medicaid, which provide DMEPOS coverage and/or reimbursement for millions of beneficiaries. Other third-party payers, various preferred provider organizations (PPOs), workers' compensation carriers, and managed care organizations (MCOs) also influence the DMEPOS industry.

Health insurance benefits for DMEPOS, in general, are entangled in a mesh of rules and regulations governing coverage and reimbursement. The Centers for Medicare and Medicaid Services (CMS) is the federal agency that runs the Medicare program and oversees the Medicaid program. CMS has strict criteria that must be met by both suppliers and providers of DMEPOS, as well as numerous rules and regulations covering every aspect of the DMEPOS reimbursement process. These include coding, claims preparation, provider and supplier certifications, options for equipment rental and purchase, and a host of other billing directives. CMS's model of DMEPOS reimbursement, viewed as generally effective even if somewhat cumbersome, has inspired a number of third-party payers to pattern their own reimbursement protocol after it to some degree. While a state Medicaid program has some degree of flexibility, many will follow the Medicare program guidelines.

Special Federal and Third-Party Payer Definitions

For federally funded health care programs, such as Medicare and the Children's Health Insurance Program (CHIP), and for programs that are partially funded by the federal government, such as state Medicaid programs, there are strict definitions of what constitutes DMEPOS. A number of commercial insurance plans also follow this same framework, or a similar one, constructed around the prescription, dispensation, reporting, and reimbursement of DMEPOS.

Defining DME

According to CMS, DME must meet specific criteria to be eligible for coverage. These criteria are shown here in the form of questions. The provider or supplier must be able to answer yes to all of these questions for the equipment or device to be recognized as eligible for reimbursement under the Medicare program:

- **Can the medical equipment withstand repeated use?** Medicare Fact: Many items, though durable in nature, such as braces (orthoses) and prostheses, are not considered DME. These items fall into different categories of DMEPOS classifications. Medical supplies such as incontinent pads, catheters, bandages, stockings, irrigating kits, sheets, and bags are expendable in nature and do not qualify as DME.

- **Is the medical equipment primarily and customarily used for medical purposes?** Medicare Fact: Certain types of medical equipment are considered "presumptively medical," meaning the sole purpose of the equipment is to provide medical benefits to the patient. A variety of devices and equipment fall into this category, including hospital beds, respirators, nebulizers, commodes, traction devices, and oxygen tents. Other types of medical equipment are considered "presumptively nonmedical," meaning that the devices and equipment are not only used for medical benefits, but also for purposes of personal comfort, ambient control, environmental enhancement, or convenience. For example, an air conditioner might yield certain medical benefits to a patient recuperating from a cardiac event. The air conditioner will lower the room temperature, which may in turn assist the patient with fluid retention by minimizing fluid loss. However, because the primary and customary use of the air conditioner is not for the purpose of body fluid maintenance, it is not considered DME and payment will not be made for this equipment under the Medicare program.

- **Is the medical equipment not of use to a person without illness or injury or in need of improvement of a malformed body part?** Medicare Fact: An order or CMN on its own will not justify medical necessity even if the physician signs it. There must be documentation in the patient's medical record to substantiate the medical necessity for the item.

- **Is the medical equipment appropriate for home use?** Medicare Fact: For a patient's DME rental or purchase to be eligible for coverage under this criterion, the patient's home must be a personal dwelling or apartment, a relative's home, a home for the aged, or some other type of institution fulfilling the domiciliary needs of the patient. However, it cannot be a skilled nursing facility or a hospital.

An answer of no to any of the preceding questions could render the DME as ineligible for Medicare coverage.

The Medicare Program Integrity Manual, Pub. 100-08, chapter 5, section 5.1, further clarifies that a rental start date may coincide with the patient's discharge date from a facility that is not the patient's home.

Orthotic and prosthetic devices are not subject to the home use requirement for coverage and payment purposes.

Special exceptions can be made by the Medicare program, some state Medicaid programs, and other third-party payers even when the DME equipment or device does not meet the accepted definition of DME by specifically contradicting two of the criteria: (1) the equipment or devices are not primarily and customarily used for medical purposes, and/or (2) the equipment or devices can be used in the absence of illness, injury, or deformity. A DMEPOS item, described by one or both of these contradicting criteria, may be eligible for Medicare coverage if the therapeutic purpose is clearly distinguished, such as in the use of a heat lamp where the medical need for heat therapy has been established. The fact that the patient's course of treatment is under the supervision of the physician must also be in evidence.

Defining Prostheses

Prosthetic devices, as recognized by CMS and many third-party payers, are those devices that replace all or part of an internal body organ, or replace all or part of the function of a permanently inoperative or malfunctioning internal body organ. This category of devices includes:

- Artificial limbs
- Breast and eye prostheses
- Maxillofacial devices
- Joint implants
- Devices that replace all or part of the ear or nose
- Ostomy and colostomy bags
- Irrigation and flushing equipment directly related to ostomy/colostomy care

An example of a prosthesis is a urinary collection and retention system that replaces the function of the bladder in cases of permanent urinary incontinence. Replacement of a prosthetic device may be covered, but only when the replacement is required because of a change in the beneficiary's physical condition. Adjustments to an artificial limb or other prosthetic device required by wear or by a change in the beneficiary's physical condition may be likewise covered when ordered by a physician.

While parenteral and enteral nutrition (PEN) is covered by the Medicare program in many instances, there is a disparity between information in the Code of Federal Regulations (CFR) and information provided by the durable medical equipment Medicare administrative contractors (DME MAC) in the classification of PEN as a prosthetic. The CFR, in Chapter 42, Section 414.202, states that PEN and related accouterments are not considered to be prosthetic, while the DMERC supplier manuals list these items as general prosthetics. The *Publications*

100 likewise details PEN as covered under the prosthetic device benefit. The conditions for coverage are not affected by this classification disparity. PEN is covered for patients who, due to chronic illness or injury, cannot take in sustenance through oral feeding and/or who have a permanently inoperative internal body organ or function and must receive life-sustaining nutrients via parenteral or enteral means.

Defining Orthoses

An orthosis or orthotic device is used for the correction or prevention of skeletal deformities. This includes braces for the neck, shoulder and arm, forearm, wrist and hand, hip, leg, ankle, and foot, as well as spinal or back devices. If there is a change in the beneficiary's physical condition that requires replacements and adjustments, those may also be covered. However, according to CMS, to be classified as an orthotic, the brace must be a rigid or semi-rigid device used for supporting a weak or deformed body member, or for restricting or eliminating motion in a diseased or injured part of the body.

Orthoses can be classified as prefabricated or custom fabricated. A prefabricated orthosis is typically manufactured and sold without specific patient data, or in other words, without the patient's personal measurements and orthotic requirements. These devices and appliances can usually be bent, trimmed, and molded many times (with or without heat) to meet specific patient physical and therapeutic needs. An orthosis that is assembled at the point of service from prefabricated component parts is still considered to be a prefabricated orthosis.

A custom fabricated orthosis is one that has been made by following a specific patient's physical measurements and therapeutic requirements. These devices and appliances require more than bending, trimming, or simple molding to properly fit the specific patient. The creation of custom fabricated orthoses involves a significant amount of detailed work, such as building each orthotic device from component materials of plastic, metal, and fabrics. A molded-to-patient, custom, fabricated orthosis is one in which an impression of the patient's body part is taken and the resultant impression cast is used to construct the orthosis.

Defining Supplies

Within the DMEPOS industry, a supply is an item or accessory needed for the effective use of a DME, prosthetic or orthotic device, or appliance. Such supplies include those drugs and biologicals that must be placed directly into equipment to achieve the therapeutic benefit of the DME or to ensure the proper functioning of the equipment. An example of this is the use of heparin within a home dialysis system. To be eligible for coverage by Medicare, Medicaid, and third-party payers, supplies must be medically necessary and must be prescribed by the treating provider. Supplies eligible for reimbursement by these programs and payers are typically not those bought off the shelf or over the counter at local drug stores and grocery stores, with the exception of recent additions to the list of covered supplies for a patient's home use, such as supplies needed with a glucometer for the monitoring of diabetes mellitus.

Medical supplies are considered to be part of a provider's practice expense, and payment for many supplies by the Medicare program and most state Medicaid programs is included in the practice expense portion of the payment or fee schedule amount reimbursed to the provider for the primary medical or surgical service. The supplies are considered incidental to the primary medical or surgical service. Other third-party payers follow the definition of billable medical and surgical supplies found in the CPT book, which is stated in CPT guidelines as "supplies and materials provided by the physician (e.g., sterile trays/drugs), over and above those usually included with the office visit or other services rendered." Many payers require the use of the only CPT code used to report medical and surgical supplies, which is 99070 Supplies and materials (except spectacles) provided by the physician over and above those usually included with the office visit or other services rendered (list drugs, trays, supplies, or materials provided). Because this CPT code is general in its description, additional documentation or a special notation in the appropriate field for electronic claims is needed to describe the specific supply being reported.

Health care facilities must follow federal guidelines for each type of facility (hospital inpatient, hospital outpatient, ASC, skilled nursing facility, etc.) when reporting supplies to Medicare for separate payment.

Accreditation

The Medicare Modernization Act of 2003 (MMA) mandates that the Secretary of Health and Human Services establish and implement quality standards for suppliers of DMEPOS. All suppliers that furnish items or services listed below must comply with the quality standards in order to receive Medicare Part B payments and to retain a supplier billing number. Suppliers of the following items or services must be accredited:

- DME
- Medical supplies
- Home dialysis supplies and equipment

- Therapeutic shoes
- Parenteral and enteral nutrient, equipment, and supplies
- Transfusion medicine
- Prosthetic devices, prosthetics, and orthotics

Suppliers of the following Items are not included:

- Medical supplies furnished by home health agencies
- Drugs used in DME, such as inhalation drugs and drugs infused with a DME pump
- Other Part B drugs, such as immunosuppressive drugs and antiemetic drugs

The Medicare Improvements for Patients and Providers Act of 2008 (MIPPA) requires all DMEPOS suppliers to meet quality standards for Medicare accreditation by September 30, 2009. Certain professionals and persons do not have to meet this deadline unless quality standards are developed specifically for these professionals and persons. CMS will work in collaboration with the medical and professional groups to develop specific quality standards. Providers and suppliers exempt from the September 30, 2009 deadline are:

- Physicians (as defined in Section 1861(r) of the Act)
- Physician assistants
- Nurse practitioners
- Physical therapists
- Occupational therapists
- Speech-language pathologists
- Clinical nurse specialists
- Certified registered nurse anesthetists
- Certified nurse-midwives
- Clinical social workers
- Clinical psychologists
- Registered dietitians
- Nutritional professionals

The Patient Protection and Affordable Care Act, Public Law 111-148, exempts a pharmacy from accreditation if it meets all of the following criteria:

- Total billings by the pharmacy for DMEPOS are less than 5 percent of total pharmacy sales.
- The pharmacy has been enrolled as a supplier of durable medical equipment, prosthetics, orthotics, and supplies, and has been issued a provider number for at least five years.
- No final adverse action has been imposed on the pharmacy in the past five years.
- The pharmacy submits an attestation, as determined by CMS, that the pharmacy meets the first three criteria.
- The pharmacy agrees to submit materials as requested during the course of an audit conducted on a random sample of pharmacies selected annually.

Existing DMEPOS suppliers, except identified exempt professionals, that are enrolled in the Medicare program must obtain and submit proof of accreditation to the National Supplier Clearinghouse (NSC).

New suppliers, except those currently exempt, submitting an enrollment application to the NSC must be accredited prior to submitting the application.

All DME suppliers must comply with the quality standards in order to retain their Medicare supplier number and to receive Medicare payment. The quality standards are comprised of two parts. The first part is supplier business services and covers the following areas:

- Administration
- Financial management
- Human resource management
- Consumer services
- Performance management
- Information management
- Product safety

The second part of the quality standards includes general product services, such as preparation, delivery and setup, training, and follow-up. Detailed standards are included for respiratory equipment, supplies, and services; manual wheelchairs, power mobility devices, including complex rehabilitative wheelchairs, and assistive technology; custom-fabricated and custom-fitted orthoses, external breast prostheses, therapeutic shoes and inserts, and their accessories and supplies; and custom-made somatic, ocular, and facial prostheses. A list of accrediting organizations and detailed quality standards are available at: http://www.cms.gov/MedicareProviderSupEnroll/07_DMEPOSAccreditation.asp#TopOfPage.

DME Competitive Bidding Program

Section 302 of the Medicare Prescription Drug, Improvement, and Modernization Act of 2003 (MMA) (Pub. L. 108-173) requires Medicare to replace the current durable medical equipment (DME) payment methodology for certain items with a competitive acquisition process to improve the effectiveness of its methodology for setting DME

Durable Medical Equipment, Prosthetics, Orthotics, and Supplies (DMEPOS)

payment amounts. This new bidding process will establish payment amounts for certain durable medical equipment, enteral nutrition, and off-the-shelf orthotics. Competitive bidding provides a way to harness marketplace dynamics to create incentives for suppliers to provide high-quality items and services efficiently and at reasonable cost. The Medicare DME competitive bidding program has five objectives:

- To use competitive bidding for DME and to use this to determine appropriate prices for categories of DME covered by Medicare Part B
- To protect beneficiary access to high-quality DME throughout the program
- To reduce the amount Medicare pays for DMEPOS and bring the reimbursement amount more in line with that of a competitive market
- To limit the burden on beneficiaries by reducing their out-of-pocket expenses
- To mitigate proliferation of use of certain items of DMEPOS by contracting with suppliers who engage in a business model that is beneficial for the program and for Medicare beneficiaries

CMS has awarded a contract to the durable medical equipment, prosthetics, orthotics, and supplies (DMEPOS) competitive bidding implementation contractor (CBIC), Palmetto GBA, LLC, of Columbia, S.C.

Palmetto GBA will conduct certain functions related to the Medicare DMEPOS competitive bidding program, such as preparing the request for bids (RFB), performing bid evaluations, selecting qualified suppliers, and setting payments for all competitive bidding areas. In addition, Palmetto will be responsible for overseeing an education program for beneficiaries, suppliers, and referral agents. Palmetto will also help CMS and its contractors monitor program effectiveness, access, and quality.

DME in a designated competitive bidding area must be supplied by a Medicare-contracted supplier in order to bill Medicare for specifically identified DME. Restrictions will be based upon ZIP codes where beneficiaries receiving these items maintain their permanent residence. All suppliers of competitively bid DME must bill the DME MAC for these specified items.

The competitive bidding items will be identified by HCPCS codes. General categories of items include:

- Oxygen supplies and equipment
- Standard power wheelchairs, scooters, and related accessories
- Complex rehabilitative power wheelchairs and related accessories (Group 2)
- Mail-order replacement diabetic supplies
- Enteral nutrients, equipment and supplies
- CPAP, RADs, and related supplies and accessories
- Hospital beds and related accessories
- Walkers and related accessories
- Support surfaces (Group 2 mattresses and overlays) in Miami

MIPPA designated the metropolitan statistical areas (MSA) for the round 1 rebid of the competitive bidding program. These are the same MSAs selected for the initial round 1 in 2007 except for Puerto Rico, which is excluded from the round 1 rebid.

The round 1 rebid will affect the following MSAs:

- Cincinnati – Middletown (Ohio, Kentucky, and Indiana)
- Cleveland – Elyria – Mentor (Ohio)
- Charlotte – Gastonia – Concord (North Carolina and South Carolina)
- Dallas – Fort Worth – Arlington (Texas)
- Kansas City (Missouri and Kansas)
- Miami – Fort Lauderdale – Pompano Beach (Florida)
- Orlando (Florida)
- Pittsburgh (Pennsylvania)
- Riverside – San Bernardino – Ontario (California)

After many delays, the DME competitive bidding program is scheduled to begin January 1, 2011.

For additional information see http://www.cms.gov/DMEPOSCompetitiveBid/01_overview.asp#TopOfPage.

Durable Medical Equipment, Prosthetics, Orthotics, and Supplies and the Office of Inspector General

The Office of Inspector General (OIG) Work Plan formulated September 2010 and published October 2010 explains ongoing assignments from years past and the planned assignments for 2011 with respect to the programs and operations of the Department of Health and Human Services (HHS). The entire Work Plan for FY 2011 is available for viewing at http://www.oig.hhs.gov/publications/workplan/2011/FY11_WorkPlan-All.pdf or you may obtain a copy by calling the OIG's Office of External Affairs at 202.619.1343. To report possible instances of waste, fraud, or abuse, you may file a report with the OIG Hotline at 800.447.8477 or go to HHSTips@oig.hhs.gov.

Beneficiaries Receiving Various Types of DME

The OIG will continue its review of Part B payments to DME suppliers of power mobility devices, hospital beds and accessories, oxygen concentrators, and enteral/parenteral nutrition. The Social Security Act (SSA) section 1862(a)(1)(A) provides that CMS pay for items and supplies when they are reasonable and necessary. Prior OIG reviews have shown that Medicare has made payments for DME not ordered by physicians, not delivered to the beneficiaries, or not needed by the beneficiaries. The OIG will select suppliers in various geographic areas that have a high volume of claims with reimbursement to determine if payments were made appropriately.

Medicare Payments for Claims with Modifiers

The OIG continues to review Medicare payments to DME suppliers who have submitted claims with modifiers. Section 1833(e) of the SSA prohibits payments to any provider except where the provider furnished the information to determine the amount(s) due to the provider. The DME provider must supply the appropriate modifier to indicate that the appropriate documentation is on file. The OIG may request this documentation at anytime.

CMS's DME regional carriers reviewed claims and found that suppliers did not have appropriate documentation to support their claims and indicates that the claims submitted may be invalid and possibly should not have received payment. The OIG will determine if these payments were consistent with Medicare requirements.

The Code of Federal Regulations (CFR), 42 CFR § 405.371, authorizes the suspension of payments to the provider and suppliers if information indicates overpayment, fraud, willful misrepresentation, or aberrant billing practices. The OIG will assess CMS's safeguards to prevent payments to providers and suppliers that are suspended or excluded.

Medicare Part B Payments for Home Blood-Glucose-Testing Supplies

As stated in section 1862(a)(1)(A) of the Social Security Act, Medicare will not pay for items or services that are "not reasonable and necessary for the diagnosis and treatment of illness or injury or to improve the functioning of a malformed body member." The OIG reviews Medicare Part B payments made for home blood glucose test strips and lancet supplies. The review is based on information found in the local coverage determinations issued by the DME MACs. These policies identify certain elements that must be present in the physician's order for each glucose-testing supply billed to Medicare. In addition, the LCDs require that suppliers add a modifier to identify when the patient is insulin treated or non-insulin treated. The amount of supplies allowed differs depending on which modifier is used. The OIG determines if the payments to the DME supplier for home blood-glucose-testing equipment and supplies were appropriate and medically necessary.

Duplicate Payments to DME Suppliers with Multiple NPI Numbers

The OIG will continue its review of Part B payments for DME suppliers who have multiple national provider identifier (NPI) numbers. The NPI is described as the standard health identifier for health care providers. The Code of Federal Regulations (CFR), 45 CFR section 162.408, states that the National Provider System (NPS) assigns the NPI to health care providers. If certain conditions are met, a provider can obtain NPIs from the NPS for themselves or for any of their subparts. The OIG will determine if and to what extent a DME supplier has submitted duplicate Medicare claims using multiple NPIs.

DME Competitive Bidding Program

The OIG will review the process CMS used to conduct competitive bidding and subsequent pricing determinations for certain DMEPOS items and services in selected competitive bidding areas under rounds 1 and 2 of the competitive bidding program. MIPPA requires the OIG to conduct postaward audits to assess the process used by CMS for competitive bidding and subsequent pricing determinations under rounds 1 and 2.

As a separate review, the OIG will examine the extent to which participating suppliers in the competitive bidding program are soliciting physicians to prescribe certain brands or modes of delivery of covered items that are more profitable to suppliers. The OIG will also analyze billing patterns to identify changes resulting from competitive bidding.

Medicare Pricing for Parenteral Nutrition

The OIG plans to compare the Medicare's fee schedule for parenteral nutrition to fees paid by other sources of reimbursement. In 2009, Medicare paid more than $137 million for parenteral nutrition supplies. Previous OIG work found that Medicare allowances for major parenteral nutrition codes averaged 45 percent higher than Medicaid prices, 78 percent higher than prices available to Medicare risk contract health maintenance organizations, and 11 times higher than some manufacturers' contract prices.

Medicare Qualifications of Orthotists and Prosthetists

Medicare claims for orthotics and prosthetics will be examined to determine those that may have been paid to unqualified practitioners in 2009. The OIG will also assess whether CMS provided guidance to state licensing boards and the industry on the definition of a "qualified practitioner" of orthotics and prosthetics. No payment is supposed to be made for special and custom fabricated items unless provided by a qualified practitioner as defined in the statute. Previous OIG work found that $33 million in inappropriate Medicare payments were made in 1998 because the device did not meet the specifications billed, the device was not custom-fabricated, or the part billed was already included in the base code for a larger device. OIG concluded that the qualifications of orthotic suppliers varied, with noncertified suppliers most likely to provide inappropriate devices and services.

Medicare Enrollment and Monitoring for Suppliers of Durable Medical Equipment, Prosthetics, Orthotics, and Supplies

The OIG will review contractors' processes for enrolling and monitoring suppliers of DMEPOS. Medicare contractors must conduct prescreening, verification, validation, and final processing of Medicare provider enrollment applications. A recent OIG study found that suppliers omitted or provided inaccurate information on enrollment applications, which resulted in improper enrollment. The OIG will assess Medicare contractors' use of enrollment screening mechanisms and postenrollment monitoring to identify suppliers that pose fraud risks to Medicare.

Medicare Part B Payments for Lower-Limb Prostheses in 2009

The OIG will review Medicare payments for lower limb prostheses in 2009. In 2009, Medicare paid about $655 million for lower limb prostheses, which represented 82 percent of Medicare Part B payments for all prostheses. Over the last five years, payments for lower limb protheses increased by 27 percent. They will also assess the policies and practices that Medicare contractors have in place for lower limb prosthetic claims to prevent fraud, waste, and abuse.

Medicare Part B Payments for Drugs

The OIG plans to examine a number of drug issues related to Medicare Part B during the coming year. The OIG is required to compare average sales price (ASP) to available market price (AMP) and to notify the Secretary if the ASP for a selected drug exceeds the AMP by a threshold of 5 percent. In another review, widely available market prices (WAMP) for selected Part B prescription drugs are compared to ASPs for those drugs. The OIG is also required to compare ASPs to WAMPs for Part B covered drugs. If the OIG finds that the ASP of a drug exceeds the WAMP by 5 percent, CMS is required to base payment for the drug on the lesser of the WAMP or 103 percent of the AMP. This study will estimate the WAMPs of prescription drugs that have been identified in earlier OIG reports and compare the WAMPs to the drugs' ASPs.

In a review of trends and variations, the OIG will examine quarterly ASPs from the 2005 implementation of the payment methodology to the present. The OIG will determine the degree of fluctuation in ASPs from quarter to quarter and examine the potential monetary impact on Part B drug payments.

The *Medicare Benefits Policy Manual*, Pub. No. 100-02, chapter 15, section 50, states that Medicare Part B provides limited benefits for outpatient drugs that are covered when furnished "incident to" a physician's service. The covered drugs should not be usually self-administered by the patient. (The term "usually" here means more than 50 percent of the time for all Medicare beneficiaries who use the drug.) The OIG will determine whether Medicare payments for the Part B drugs, when associated with a physician service, were in accordance with Medicare requirements.

Part B immunosuppressive drug claims will be reviewed to determine whether they were prescribed and billed according to their Food and Drug Administration (FDA)-approved labels. Several FDA-approved labels for immunosuppressive drugs state that the drugs should not be used in combination with other immunosuppressive drugs. The review will also determine if Medicare paid for immunosuppressive drugs that should not have been used in combination with other immunosuppressive drugs.

The OIG will review Medicare payments for drugs and biologicals used on an off-label basis in cancer chemotherapeutic regimens. Medicare covers FDA-approved drugs used for off-label indications in anticancer chemotherapeutic regimens when such uses are supported in specified authoritative compendia. In 2007, Medicare payments for anticancer drugs totaled about $2.7 billion. This review will determine whether patients with particular indications were prescribed anticancer drugs approved by FDA for such indications before the use of off-label anticancer drugs. The agency will also examine whether there were improvements in the patients' medical conditions before the use of off-label drugs and how much Medicare could have saved had anticancer drugs continued to be used only within labeled uses.

Wet age-related macular degeneration (AMD) is the leading cause of blindness in the elderly. Medicare Part B pays for two drugs used to treat AMD. Lucentis is a drug specifically approved by FDA to treat wet AMD, and Avastin is approved to treat cancer with an off-label use as a treatment for wet AMD. CMS recently enacted and then reversed a decision to pay a lower amount for Avastin when used to treat wet AMD as the physicians claimed that the new payments were too low and would require them to prescribe the higher-priced Lucentis. The OIG will review physicians' acquisition costs and any additional compounding cost for Avastin when it is used to treat wet AMD. Further, the OIG will review national claims history data to identify nationwide usage patterns and payments for these two drugs. MACs have issued local coverage decisions allowing for reimbursement for Avastin off-label use to treat wet AMD. Initial results of the Comparison of Age-Related Macular Degeneration Treatments Trials (CATT) study that compares the safety and efficacy of the two drugs from the National Eye Institute of the National Institutes of Health (NIH) are expected in late 2010 or early 2011. The OIG plans to determine whether a significant savings can be recognized if Avastin or Lucentis is used more by ophthalmologists.

General Billing, Claims, and Coverage Issues

ASC X12N 837 (Version 4010) Professional Claim Format

Physicians and suppliers must submit all electronic Medicare Claims data to Medicare using the ASC X12N 837 claim format. The current version of the standards is 4010/4010A1 for health care transactions and the National Council for Prescription Drug Programs [NCPDP] version 5.1 for pharmacy transactions.

Modifications to the HIPAA Administrative Simplification rules were made on January 16, 2009. The current versions of the standards are to be replaced with version 5010 and version D.0, respectively. This Final Rule also adopted a new standard for Medicaid subrogation for pharmacy claims known as NCPDP 3.0.

Internal level I testing was to begin January 1, 2010. On January 1, 2011, level II testing with trading partners is to begin with payer acceptance of both versions 5010 and 4010A1. Full compliance with version 5010, D.O, and NCPDP 3.0 is required by January 1, 2012, except for small health plans, which must be compliant by January 1, 2013.

Note that errata for these versions replace the base versions for HIPAA compliance and must be fully implemented by January 1, 2012. For professional claims, this is version 005010X222A1; for institutional claims, version 005010X223A2; and for NCPDP claims, version D.0 April 2009.

Providers can keep up to date with the version 5010 schedule by accessing the CMS website links at http://www.cms.gov/ICD10/11a_Version_5010.asp#TopOfPage or http://www.cms.gov/ElectronicBilling EDITrans/18_5010D0.asp#TopOfPage.

Provider Taxonomy Codes

Provider taxonomy codes are 10-character, alphanumeric codes that identify the specialty of the provider. HIPAA regulations require the use of these taxonomy codes. Every time a provider or supplier is identified in the 837 claim, whether institutional or professional, the taxonomy code must be used to identify the provider or supplier's specialty.

The current list of provider taxonomy codes is available from http://www.wpc-edi.com. Regional DME MAC may be able to provide a current list.

Medical Necessity and DMEPOS

For DMEPOS items or services to be billed to a Medicare contractor, the physician or provider must have documentation demonstrating the medical necessity of the item. This information must be a part of the patient's medical record. For suppliers of DMEPOS items, an official order signed and dated by the ordering provider must be obtained. The order must detail the following:

- The patient's identifying information
- A description of the DMEPOS item
- The reason for the DMEPOS prescription, which can take the form of the ICD-9-CM code and/or diagnosis narrative information
- The start date of the order must be clearly specified
- If the order is for supplies that will be provided on a periodic basis, the order should include information on the quantity used, frequency of change, and duration of need (e.g., an order for surgical dressings might specify one 4x4 hydrocolloid dressing that is changed one to two times per week for one month or until the ulcer heals)
- The order must be sufficiently detailed, including all options or additional features that will be separately billed or that will require an upgraded code. The description can be a narrative description (e.g., lightweight wheelchair base) or a brand name/model number
- If the order is for a rented item or if the coverage criteria in a policy specify length of need, the order must include the length of need

- If the supply is a drug, the order must specify the name of the drug, concentration (if applicable), dosage, frequency of administration, and duration of infusion (if applicable)

The provider's signature must be an original signature. A faxed copy of the original order temporarily satisfies the requirement for most Medicare contractors, and allows the supplier to begin to fulfill the DMEPOS order so the patient can begin using the DMEPOS item as soon as possible. At some point, however, the supplier must obtain the original document from the provider. The supplier must then keep the original DMEPOS order on file. A copy of the order must be sent to the Medicare contractor when requested. If the item requires a Certificate of Medical Necessity (CMN), a separate provider written order is not necessary; the CMN acts as the original provider order. A copy of the CMN faxed to the supplier is considered sufficient documentation by federal auditors as long as the supplier retains the faxed copy and the provider retains the original.

The following are certain DMEPOS items for which the supplier must obtain the signed original detailed order before fulfilling the order:

- Seat-lift mechanisms
- Transcutaneous electrical nerve stimulator (TENS) units (purchase only)
- Power-operated vehicles
- Pressure reducing pads
- Mattress overlays, mattresses, and beds
- Other items as denoted by contractor local or regional coverage decisions

The first item requires only a written physician order; the remainder of the items requires CMNs to be completed by the provider and supplier.

Certificates of Medical Necessity

The Medicare program requires the completion of specific forms to establish the medical necessity of certain durable medical equipment, supplies, and services. Six of these particular forms, called Certificates of Medical Necessity (CMN), have been developed by the DME MAC. These forms have been given official form numbers by CMS and are generally referred to by these numbers. The form numbers are primarily used to identify each CMN submitted with electronic claims to the DME MAC.

Once a supplier receives a verbal or written order for a DMEPOS item that requires a CMN, the supplier generates a DMEPOS-specific CMN form and completes portions of the form. The supplier then sends it to the ordering provider for completion of patient-specific clinical information and final certification, which requires the provider to sign and date the order. The supplier must send the provider both sides of the CMN, as the reverse side of the form contains instructions for appropriate completion. The CMN forms cannot be modified in any way. Within the CMN forms there are specific sections for the DMEPOS supplier to fill out, and certain sections the provider must complete; in fact, the supplier is forbidden to assist the provider by completing these sections (see below).

The CMN forms generally follow a four-section format:

Section A	Patient and physician identifying information; HCPCS codes
	May be completed by the supplier
Section B	DMEPOS-specific information
	Completed by the physician, staff, or other clinician involved in the care of the patient; cannot be completed by the supplier
Section C	Narrative description of equipment and cost
	Completed by the supplier
Section D	Physician attestation, signature, and date
	Completed by the physician

CMNs are currently required for:

- Oxygen
- Pneumatic compression devices
- Osteogenesis stimulators
- Transcutaneous electrical nerve stimulators (TENS) (purchase only)
- Seat lift mechanisms

CMN Form Specifics

CMS issued guidance for certain aspects of the CMN. Previously faxed copies of the CMN from the provider were not considered valid documentation under CMS rules for the supplier to fulfill the DMEPOS order. In many cases, this resulted in both a delay of medical equipment being delivered to the patient and a delay in supplier reimbursement. As of CMS allowed the use of faxed copies of provider-completed CMNs to alleviate these situations. The faxed copy is all that is required to be kept on file by the supplier, as long as the ordering provider retains the original CMN. Note that if an audit were to be undertaken by Medicare contractors, the supplier would need to obtain the original CMN documents from the providers, or risk postpayment denial of the claims or assessment of overpayments, fines, or penalties.

DEPARTMENT OF HEALTH AND HUMAN SERVICES
CENTERS FOR MEDICARE & MEDICAID SERVICES

Form Approved
OMB No. 0938-0679

CERTIFICATE OF MEDICAL NECESSITY
CMS-848 — TRANSCUTANEOUS ELECTRICAL NERVE STIMULATOR (TENS)

DME 06.03B

SECTION A Certification Type/Date: INITIAL ___/___/___ REVISED ___/___/___ RECERTIFICATION ___/___/___

PATIENT NAME, ADDRESS, TELEPHONE and HIC NUMBER	SUPPLIER NAME, ADDRESS, TELEPHONE and NSC or applicable NPI NUMBER/LEGACY NUMBER
(_ _ _) _ _ _ - _ _ _ _ HICN _____	(_ _ _) _ _ _ - _ _ _ _ NSC or NPI # _____

PLACE OF SERVICE_____	HCPCS CODE	PT DOB __/__/__ Sex ___ (M/F) Ht. ___(in) Wt ___(lbs.)
NAME and ADDRESS of FACILITY *if applicable (see reverse)*		PHYSICIAN NAME, ADDRESS, TELEPHONE and applicable NPI NUMBER or UPIN
		(_ _ _) _ _ _ - _ _ _ _ UPIN or NPI # _____

SECTION B Information in this Section May Not Be Completed by the Supplier of the Items/Supplies.

EST. LENGTH OF NEED (# OF MONTHS): _____ 1-99 *(99=LIFETIME)* | DIAGNOSIS CODES (ICD-9): _____ _____ _____ _____

ANSWERS	ANSWER QUESTIONS 1-6 for purchase of TENS (Circle Y for Yes, N for No,)
Y N	1. Does the patient have chronic, intractable pain?
_____ Months	2. How long has the patient had intractable pain? (Enter number of months, 1 - 99.)
1 2 3 4 5	3. Is the TENS unit being prescribed for any of the following conditions? (Circle appropriate number) 1 - Headache 2 - Visceral abdominal pain 3 - Pelvic pain 4 - Temporomandibular joint (TMJ) pain 5 - None of the above
Y N	4. Is there documentation in the medical record of multiple medications and/or other therapies that have been tried and failed?
Y N	5. Has the patient received a TENS trial of at least 30 days?
___/___/___	6. What is the date that you reevaluated the patient at the end of the trial period?

NAME OF PERSON ANSWERING SECTION B QUESTIONS, IF OTHER THAN PHYSICIAN (Please Print):
NAME: _____ TITLE: _____ EMPLOYER: _____

SECTION C   Narrative Description of Equipment and Cost

(1) Narrative description of all items, accessories and options ordered; (2) Supplier's charge; and (3) Medicare Fee Schedule Allowance for each item, accessory, and option. (see instructions on back)

SECTION D   PHYSICIAN Attestation and Signature/Date

I certify that I am the treating physician identified in Section A of this form. I have received Sections A, B and C of the Certificate of Medical Necessity (including charges for items ordered). Any statement on my letterhead attached hereto, has been reviewed and signed by me. I certify that the medical necessity information in Section B is true, accurate and complete, to the best of my knowledge, and I understand that any falsification, omission, or concealment of material fact in that section may subject me to civil or criminal liability.

PHYSICIAN'S SIGNATURE_____ DATE ___/___/___

Form CMS-848 (09/05) EF 08/2006

For Section B of the CMN form, all information entered in support of the DMEPOS must be present in the patient's medical record; the CMN and the medical record documentation should match in essential information. A standing directive by CMS is that Section B of the CMN may not be completed by the supplier of the DMEPOS, even under the guidance or at the request of the ordering provider. The supplier can complete section C, Narrative Description of Equipment and Cost. If the supplier-entered information in Section C does not accurately reflect the information provided by the ordering provider, CMS will return the CMN unsigned to the supplier for correction.

Providers and suppliers should note that CMS, in its quest to halt fraud and abuse, has issued a directive related to correcting errors on the CMN forms. Similar to the long standing malpractice protocol involving the patient's medical record, CMS requires the incorrect information on the CMN to be struck through with a single line, the correct information entered just above the strike-through entry, and the provider's or supplier's initials annotated adjacent to the new entry. The correction must be dated as well. If the DMEPOS supplier feels that the corrected CMN may cause confusion, the supplier may request that a new CMN be completed with the accurate information.

Camera-ready copies of these forms are available on the websites of the DME MAC or at CMS website http://www.cms.hhs.gov/CMSForms/CMSForms/list.asp#TopOfPage. If more space is needed when completing Section C of these forms (Narrative Description of Equipment and Cost) then a special CMN—CMS Form 854, Section C Continuation Form—may be used to convey the remainder of the essential information. CMS Form 854 can only be used as an addendum to CMS forms 843 and 844, not with any other CMN form. If CMS Form 854 is used, it must be signed and dated (certified) by the ordering provider. The supplier must also keep it on file. For paper claim submitters, the form must accompany the primary form; for electronic submitters, the supplier need not transmit Form 854, but must retain it in case the form is requested by the DME MAC for review.

The CMN form for oxygen—CMS Form 484—includes the addition of Section C, the listing of the supplier's charge and Medicare fee schedule allowance for the equipment requested, as required by federal law. Section C also contains an area for a brief narrative description of the oxygen delivery system requested, whether it is compressed gas, liquid or concentrated, and stationary or portable. Other pertinent information should be listed in Section C (and confirmed by the ordering provider) such as the need for a cannula or mask, the prescribed oxygen flow rates, and so on.

Also contained within the CMS Form 484 is a revised question regarding the blood gas or oximetry test result that qualifies the oxygen for Medicare coverage. This question helps establish the medical necessity for the oxygen by asking if the test was performed "either with the patient in a chronic stable state as an outpatient, or within two days before discharge from an inpatient facility to [the patient's] home." If multiple tests have been performed, CMS views the most recent test as the qualifying results for home oxygen coverage. If the patient is one with a chronic cardiopulmonary condition requiring the use of oxygen, a test result reported for determining home oxygen coverage cannot be one that was obtained during an acute cardiopulmonary episode or acute exacerbation of the patient's disease process.

The physician currently responsible for the patient's pulmonary condition must complete the oxygen CMN. Suppliers must maintain their records so they can identify the new treating physicians and obtain new CMNs when necessary.

Providers and suppliers must be aware of a defined timeline when ordering and fulfilling orders for DMEPOS. If more than three months elapse from the time a CMN is completed by the ordering provider to the time the DMEPOS item is delivered, a new CMN must be completed. This directive ensures the continued medical necessity of the DMEPOS item, as a patient may no longer require the ordered item. The timeline is more prohibitive for an initial order for oxygen, which involves certain blood gases analysis. The order must be filled in 30 days for the supplier to be reimbursed. If this timeline is not met, a new CMN must be completed. The provider cannot complete the initial CMN for oxygen dispensation more than 30 days before the expected fulfillment of the order.

A copy of the initial CMN should accompany the following:

- All initial claims for the reported DMEPOS items or services
- Changes in the original
- Initial provision of nutrients and supplies

CMNs can be submitted both by electronic means and by paper submission. If the CMN is submitted in hard copy, the supplier need only include a copy of the front of the form. If the CMN is transmitted electronically in the NSF format, only information from Sections A, B, and D (not C) is required. The

HIPAA 837 professional claim format can accommodate all CMN fields.

CMN Cover Letters

A supplier must generate a cover letter for each CMN-required DMEPOS order to be sent to the provider for completion. These letters are seen as written confirmation of provider orders and are used as basic forums for communication between the ordering provider and the supplier. Traditionally the supplier has been limited in what to write in the letter in that it cannot influence the provider regarding the medical necessity of the DMEPOS item. However, CMS issued a statement about the use of cover letters for CMNs, in effect stating that it had no jurisprudence or regulatory control over CMN cover letters, and cannot restrict the information contained in them. It states that the burden of proof in terms of medical necessity for the DMEPOS remains with the ordering provider and the supplier.

The cover letters may include the following elements:

- An explanation of the section of the CMN to be completed by the ordering provider
- Instructions or guidance on where to send the completed CMN, and the expected time frame in which the CMN is to be returned to the supplier
- A request for a copy of any pertinent laboratory or other test results necessary for the order of the DMEPOS item
- Information related to CMS policy regarding coverage limitations or requirements for the DMEPOS being ordered of which the physician or provider should be aware

Modifier KX

Modifier KX is used on the CMS-1500 claim form to indicate that the DMEPOS supplier is maintaining medical necessity documentation in the supplier's files. This documentation only needs to be submitted to the DME MAC entity upon request. The DMEPOS supplier should create internal mechanisms to ensure the proper use of modifier KX. Improper use of the modifier may result in the submission of false claims. The OIG recommends that the DMEPOS supplier's written policies and procedures address the supplier's protocol for using this modifier.

Death of the Physician Who Completed the CMN

Suppliers are required to obtain new orders and new CMNs for customers whose originating physician has died. To avoid interruptions of payments for rentals, oxygen, or transfers of care, a grace period of 15 months from the date of death will be allowed for DME claims. At the end of the grace period, the supplier should have obtained new orders and CMNs. The supplier will then bill with the replacement physician's UPIN and CMN. This applies even to lifetime orders of oxygen.

Claims requiring CMNs that are signed by a deceased physician may be medical necessity denials. The supplier will have the opportunity to appeal any claims denied due to this reason. Claims denied due to the use of a deceased physician's UPIN would be denied using the message that the UPIN is invalid. These claims may also be appealed.

It is imperative that suppliers take note of this issue. Carriers' UPIN files have been updated and cross-matched against the AMA's deceased physician database and the Social Security Administration's database. Claims with a deceased physician's UPIN or CMN, whose date of service is after the physician's date of death, will be rejected.

Providers Prohibited from Charging for CMN Preparation

If a patient requires an item of DMEPOS, the completion of the CMN is considered a service to the patient rather than to the supplier. Providers cannot charge the patient or the supplier for the completion of the CMN. Section 4152 of the Omnibus Reconciliation Act of 1990 requires a provider to complete the CMN or DMEPOS order. The language in the statute does not authorize providers to separately charge the patient or the supplier for completing the CMN forms. Allegations of providers charging for completion of the CMN forms will be investigated as one or more of the following:

- Potential kickback situations under Section 1128B(b) of the Social Security Act
- A false representation with respect to the provider's actual charge for professional services furnished on or near the date of the DMEPOS order for the patient
- A potential assignment violation on claims for professional services on or near the date the provider orders the DMEPOS item for the patient
- A potential charge limit violation on unassigned claims for professional services on or near the date the provider ordered the DMEPOS item for the patient

The federal government has become aggressive in its efforts against fraud, waste, and abuse, and in doing so has actively included the patient in its campaigns.

DME Information Form

A DME Information Form (DIF) replaces the CMN for certain DME supplies. A DIF is completed and signed by the supplier. The DIF contains many of the same elements as the CMN, but does not require a narrative description of equipment and cost or a physician signature. DIFs are subject to the same requirements and restrictions as CMNs.

DIFs need to be completed to provide information for enteral and parenteral nutrition (PEN) and external infusion pumps.

Contractors may ask for supporting documentation beyond a CMN or DIF. Copies of CMNs and DIFs can be downloaded at http://www.cms.hhs.gov/CMSForms/CMSForms/list.asp#TopOfPage.

DMEPOS Prior Authorizations/ Advance Determination of Medicare Coverage

For reimbursement for some DMEPOS items, typically those requiring CMN forms, the items must have prior authorization or an advance determination of Medicare coverage (ADMC) from the DME MAC. For certain items of DMEPOS, an ADMC process must be undertaken before the delivery of the item to the patient (the DMERC entities will advise the providers and suppliers of these particular DMEPOS items). In these cases, the supplier must submit the CMN in advance of the claim for the purchase of the DMEPOS and specifically request an ADMC. The irony inherent in this process is that the prior authorization does not guarantee Medicare reimbursement for the item in question, and only indicates that the medical necessity criteria for the DMEPOS item have been met. A supplier or patient may request an ADMC before delivery of an item to determine whether payment for the item may be denied if:

- The item is a customized item
- The patient to whom the item is to be furnished, or the supplier, requests that such advance determination be made
- The item is not an inexpensive item

Customized DME is defined as items of DME that have been uniquely constructed or substantially modified for a specific patient according to the description and orders of the beneficiary's treating physician.

ADMCs are not initial determinations as no request for payment is being made and they cannot be appealed.

ADMCs must be made in writing. For submitters who usually transmit the CMN electronically with the claim, items subject to prior authorization require that both the CMN and the ADMC request be made by paper submission only. This documentation should be submitted to the DME MAC.

The Medicare contractor must render a written decision on an ADMC within 30 calendar days. An affirmative ADMC decision will provide the supplier and the patient assurance that, based on the information submitted with the request, Medicare medical necessity requirements have been met as established for the item.

An affirmative ADMC decision does not provide assurance that the patient meets Medicare eligibility requirements nor does it assure that any other Medicare requirements (MSP, etc.) have been met. Only upon submission of a complete claim can the Medicare contractor make a full and complete determination. An affirmative ADMC decision does not extend to the price that Medicare will pay for the item. An affirmative ADMC decision is valid for a period of six months from the date the decision is rendered. Medicare contractors reserve the right to review claims on a pre- or post-payment basis and may deny claims and take appropriate remedy if they determine that an affirmative ADMC decision was made based on incorrect information.

A negative ADMC decision communicates to the supplier and the patient that, based on the information submitted with the request, the patient does not meet the medical necessity requirements Medicare has established for the item. The negative ADMC decision should indicate why the request was denied. A patient or a supplier can resubmit an ADMC request if additional medical documentation is obtained that could affect the prior negative ADMC decision. However, requests may only be submitted once during a six-month period.

Local Coverage Determination (LCD)

Local coverage determinations (LCD) are contractor decisions developed to specify when clinical circumstances for a service are reasonable and necessary. They serve as an administrative and educational tool to assist providers in submitting claims correctly for payment. LCDs may apply to specific state regions, all submitters, or to a specific contractor. Each LCD lists the jurisdiction for which it applies. LCDs may be accessed at the contractor's website or through the CMS coverage database at http://www.cms.hhs.gov/mcd/search.asp.

Medicare Program Requirements

Provider/Supplier Identifiers

Federal laws mandate the use of specific codes to identify the provider or supplier of services on the claim. These national identifiers include:

- National Provider Number (NPI)
- Provider Identification Number (PIN) (Medicare)
- National Supplier Identification Number (NSIN)

The National Provider Identifier Number

The National Provider Identifier (NPI) number is part of the National Provider System developed by CMS and by various federal government and Medicaid state agencies. It was developed to standardize and simplify the provider and supplier enumeration process. Under this system, every provider and supplier is assigned an individual national identification number. This 10-digit number consists of a seven-digit base number, a one-digit mathematical algorithm, and a two-digit alphanumeric suffix to identify the provider setting or location. This number must be used on all claims filed to the DME MAC. Health care providers may apply for an NPI at http://nppes.cms.hhs.gov/NPPES/Welcome.do.

Keep NSC Files Updated

DMEPOS supplier standard number 2 requires that all suppliers notify the National Supplier Clearinghouse (NSC) with any change that is made to the Medicare enrollment application or Form CMS-855S within 30 days of the change. DMEPOS suppliers should use the March 2009 version of Form CMS-855S and should update the following information:

- List of products and services found in section 2.D
- Authorized official information in sections 6A and 15
- Correspondence address in section 2A2

This is important for suppliers who are involved in the Medicare DMEPOS Competitive Bidding Program. All suppliers must be sure that all information on their application form is current and up to date. For guidance on how to submit a change of information, please access the NSC website at http://www.palmettogba.com/nsc.

Accreditation

In November 2006, CMS approved 10 national accreditation organizations that accredit suppliers of durable medical equipment, prosthetics, orthotics, and supplies (DMEPOS) as meeting new quality standards under Medicare Part B. In order to enroll or maintain Medicare billing privileges, all DMEPOS suppliers must comply with the Medicare program's supplier standards (found at 42 CFR §424.57 (c)) and quality standards. The accreditation requirement applies to suppliers of durable medical equipment, medical supplies, home dialysis supplies and equipment, therapeutic shoes, parenteral/enteral nutrition, transfusion medicine and prosthetic devices, and prosthetics and orthotics. The Medicare Improvement for Patients and Providers Act of 2008 (MIPPA) specified professionals and other persons exempt from accreditation requirements. The Patient Protection and Affordable Care Act, Public Law 111-148, further exempted a pharmacy from accreditation if it meets all of the following criteria:

- Total billings by the pharmacy for DMEPOS are less than 5 percent of total pharmacy sales.
- The pharmacy has been enrolled as a supplier of durable medical equipment, prosthetics, orthotics, and supplies, and has been issued a provider number for at least five years.
- No final adverse action has been imposed on the pharmacy in the past five years.
- The pharmacy submits an attestation, as determined by CMS, that the pharmacy meets the first three criteria.
- The pharmacy agrees to submit materials, as requested, during the course of an audit conducted on a random sample of pharmacies selected annually.

Further information on the DMEPOS accreditation requirements, including a list of the accreditation organizations for DMEPOS suppliers, can be found at http://www.cms.gov/MedicareProviderSupEnroll/07_DMEPOSAccreditation.asp#TopOfPage.

Mandatory Provider and Supplier Claim Submission

The Omnibus Budget Reconciliation Act of 1989 (OBRA '89) mandates that the provider or supplier, within a one-year filing limit, must submit all patient claims for reimbursement when furnishing covered items on Medicare claims. This is true whether or not the provider is participating with the Medicare program. The provider or supplier is relieved of this obligation when furnishing noncovered items, unless the patient requests a Medicare payment determination (usually to receive a written denial from the Medicare program for secondary insurance purposes).

Claims to Medicare contractors are usually transmitted by CMS-1500 form, or by electronic means (called electronic data interchange [EDI] or electronic media claims [EMC]). Medicare carriers, DME MACs, and most major third-party payers do not accept practice superbills or encounter forms as appropriate formats for claim submissions.

In certain situations, a provider who has not entered into a private contract with the Medicare beneficiary (called an opt out agreement) does not have to submit a claim for a covered service for a Medicare patient. In these cases, typically the Medicare patient or the patient's legal representative decides not to authorize the provider to submit a claim, or the patient wishes not to divulge the confidential medical information that is on a claim to the Medicare program. A common example is when the patient does not want information about mental illness or a sexually transmitted disease (STD) to be disclosed to any person or entity. The Medicare patient has the latitude to change this order and later authorize the submission of the claim for the service. In this case, the provider is obligated to prepare and submit the claim.

Electronic DMEPOS Claims

Medicare requires providers to submit electronic media claims (EMC) using the professional 837 V4010 transmission format updated as appropriate with addendum information. An electronic claim is submitted via a central processing unit (CPU) to CPU transmission, tape, direct data entry, direct wire, or personal computer upload or download. A claim that is submitted via digital fax/OCR, diskette, or touch-tone telephone is not considered as an electronic claim.

A paper claim is submitted and received on paper, including fax print-outs. This also includes a claim that the contractor receives on paper and then reads electronically with OCR technology.

For the last 10 years, Medicare has been prohibited by regulation from paying clean electronic claims earlier than the 14th day after the receipt of the claim. This holding period is commonly referred to as the payment floor. The payment floor is 29 days effective January 1, 2006, for paper and non-HIPAA compliant electronic claims. Providers can avoid this added delay in payment by submitting HIPAA compliant clean electronic claims. CMS states that only claims using ANSI V004010 will be considered HIPAA-compliant (*Medicare Claims Processing Manual*, Pub. 100-04, chap. 1, sec. 80.2).

Clean claims do not require the MAC to investigate or develop them external to Medicare claims operations on a prepayment basis. These claims pass all edits, both contractor or MAC-specific and common working file (CWF), and are processed electronically.

For claims not considered clean, the Medicare contractor may need to do the following:

- Request additional information from the provider or supplier or other external source; this includes routine data not submitted with the claim, additional medical information, or information to resolve discrepancies detected within the claim and other documentation submitted for consideration

- Request information or assistance from another Medicare contractor; this includes development data obtained through the carrier-intermediary data exchange or requests for charge data from other contractors

- Develop or investigate Medicare Secondary Payer program information

- Request information from the provider or supplier necessary for a judicial coverage determination

- Perform sequential processing when an earlier claim is currently in development

- Perform outside claim development as a result of a common working file edit

The payment floor for paper claims is 29 calendar days. Clean electronic claims not paid by Medicare after 30 days will accrue interest, payable to the provider or supplier, beginning on the 31st day. The provider or supplier can also obtain automatic electronic funds transfer (EFT) and receive electronic remittance notices. In fact, a provider or supplier need not submit claims electronically to take advantage of EFT, as paper submitters can also receive EFT.

Funds deposited electronically are available in the provider's or supplier's bank account the day after the DME MAC transmits the EFT to the bank. Every EFT transaction has a tracking number in case a payment must be traced. Errors in EFT deposits usually occur when the provider or supplier has changed banks or closed the existing account currently being used for EFT by the DME MAC. All necessary information should be sent to the DME MAC as quickly as possible when the provider or supplier changes banks or bank accounts.

Many Medicare contractor supply the necessary EDI or EMC software programs free of charge; others charge a nominal fee or an inconsequential annual software maintenance fee. Certificates of Medical Necessity (CMNs) can be filed electronically as well, allowing the providers and suppliers of DMEPOS to forward all necessary documentation electronically. Physician orders, other than CMNs, currently do not have an electronic format for submission unless the note area within the electronic claim record is used for brief annotations.

Signature on File (SOF) Requirements

The patient's authorization for the release of confidential medical information is a necessary legal requirement to process medical claims. It is also a requirement by the Medicare program, state Medicaid programs, and all third-party payers, including managed care organizations. Providers and suppliers can retain in their files a blanket signature-on-file authorization form for each patient. In some cases, the patient's legal representative can complete the form. The signature-on-file authorization applies to any current and future services or items the provider or supplier may furnish to the patient. The signature-on-file form is valid for covered services only; it should not be confused with an advance beneficiary notice (ABN) for noncovered services or services deemed not medically necessary. It should be updated when the patient changes insurers, when benefits change, or when the patient's health status changes and a legal representative is assigned to care for the patient's legal matters. The signature-on-file document retained by the provider or supplier can be revoked by the patient or the patient's representative at any time.

Providers and suppliers using electronic claims processing with Medicare and other carriers must obtain the signature-on-file document. To implement this procedure, the supplier must incorporate the following language in addition to the patient's name and ID or policy number into the signature-on-file document to be acknowledged and signed by the patient or their legal representative:

> "I request that payment of authorized [Medicare or other carrier] benefits be made either to me or on my behalf for any services furnished me by [Name of provider/supplier], including physician services. I authorize any holder of medical or other information about me to release to the [Centers for Medicare and Medicaid Services or other insurance company] and its agents any information needed to determine these benefits or benefits for related services."

Many patient scenarios involve the use of a signature-on-file document, including the following:

- The patient signs the document
- The provider or supplier uses an SOF entry
- An illiterate or handicapped person acknowledges the signature-on-file authority given to the provider or supplier
- A legal representative for the patient provides the signature-on-file authorization

Beneficiary Right to Itemized Statements

Section 4311(b) of the Balanced Budget Act of 1997 provides Medicare patients the right to submit a written request to the provider or supplier for an itemized statement detailing the DMEPOS services or items furnished. Providers and suppliers must comply with the beneficiary's request within 30 days, or risk civil monetary penalties of $100 for each unfulfilled request. Once the patient receives the provider's or supplier's itemized statement, the patient can request the Medicare contractor to conduct a review for specific issues. These can be a range of issues including the following:

- The patient doesn't think these services or items were provided
- There are irregularities in the provider's or supplier's billing that seem suspicious to the patient
- The provider or supplier received overpayment

Medicare contractors routinely advise Medicare patients of their right to an itemized statement. The Explanation of Medicare Benefits (EOMB) and Medicare Summary Notice (MSN) contain the following statement:

> "You have a right to request an itemized statement that details each Medicare item or service you have received from your physician, hospital, or any other health supplier or health professional. Please contact them directly if you would like an itemized statement."

Providers and suppliers cannot charge for furnishing the Medicare patient the itemized statement. Itemization may mean providing the following information:

- Name of the patient
- Date of service
- Description of the service or item furnished
- Number of services or items furnished
- Provider or supplier charges

- Any internal tracking number used by the provider or supplier
- Amount paid by Medicare
- Patient's coinsurance liability
- Medicare claim number

The provider or supplier should also include the name and telephone number of the contact person at the provider/supplier's office if the patient has questions about the statement.

Private Contracting or Opting Out

The Balanced Budget Act of 1997, Section 4507, allows physicians and other practitioners to enter into private contracts with Medicare patients. This allows a Medicare patient and a provider to enter into an agreement in which neither party bills Medicare for services provided. The provider can bill the patient without dealing with Medicare coverage rules and billing requirements. This arrangement is known as an opt-out agreement.

The binding stipulation is that the provider is excluded from the Medicare program for all patients for two full years. CMS designed the two-year rule to prevent providers from committing fraud by billing both Medicare and the patient.

To enter into this arrangement the following conditions must be met:

- The provider cannot receive Medicare payment for any item or service, directly or on a capitated basis
- The provider cannot receive payment from an organization that receives Medicare payment for the item or service directly or on a capitated basis

Before any item or service is furnished on a private basis, the contract must be signed by the Medicare patient, and the provider must sign and file a written affidavit with the Department of Health and Human Services attesting that the provider will not submit any Medicare claim to the Medicare patient. Further, the affidavit must state that the provider will not receive any reimbursement for any item or service for a two-year period from the date the affidavit is signed.

By signing the opt out contract, the Medicare patient agrees to the following conditions:

- The patient will not submit a claim even though the services would be covered under Medicare
- The patient will be responsible to the provider for payments
- The patient understands that charge limits do not apply, meaning the provider can charge full fees
- The patient understands that Medigap plans do not make payments and that other supplemental plans may elect not to pay
- The patient understands that the patient has the right to have services from other physicians for whom Medicare payment would be made
- The patient understands that the private contract is not valid if entered into during an emergent or urgent health care situation, if the patient did not wish to enter into such a contract

If the provider has been excluded from the Medicare program (for whatever reasons), this information must be disclosed in the private contract. To reiterate an important fact, providers who opt out of the Medicare program in agreement with Medicare patients can charge any amount they wish for services.

Who Can Opt Out?

The opt-out or private contracting option is not available to all health care providers and suppliers who deal with the Medicare program. Providers authorized to opt out of the Medicare program and enter into private contracts with Medicare patients include the following:

- Doctors of medicine
- Doctors of osteopathy
- Physician assistants
- Nurse practitioners
- Clinical nurse specialists
- Certified registered nurse anesthetists
- Certified nurse midwives
- Clinical social workers
- Clinical psychologists

Health care providers not recognized under the law as having authorization to enter into private contract arrangements with Medicare patients include the following:

- Optometrists
- Chiropractors
- Podiatrists
- Dentists
- Oral surgeons
- Physical therapists in independent practice
- Occupational therapists in independent practice

General Billing, Claims, and Coverage Issues

Suppliers of DMEPOS

Suppliers are not approved at this time to enter into private contracts with Medicare patients. Providers who are suppliers of DMEPOS can opt out for services and items furnished, but cannot single out DMEPOS services and items for private contract arrangements while other services and items provided to Medicare patients remain within Medicare program parameters.

Suppliers may enter into private or other legal-type contracts with patients age 65 or older when those persons have chosen not to enroll in Medicare Part B. These patients are considered private-pay patients.

Opt Out Status and Medical Emergencies

CMS has made some revisions to the policy that allows providers or practitioners to opt out, and created a new modifier in relation to this policy. The modifier addresses emergent or urgent care situations. The revised policy states that during emergent or urgent care circumstances, a provider who has opted out of Medicare may treat a Medicare patient with whom the provider does not have a private contract, and may bill for the services. In this situation, the provider may not charge the patient more than what a nonparticipating provider would be permitted to charge, and must submit a claim to Medicare on the patient's behalf. Medicare will pay for covered services and items furnished in emergency or urgent situations when the patient has not signed a private contract with that provider.

CMS has created a HCPCS Level II modifier to alert Medicare carriers to this situation when reported by the provider:

GJ   Opt out physician or practitioner emergency or urgent service

This modifier must be used on claims for services rendered by an opt out provider for an emergency or urgent service.

For example, an opt out provider renders emergency care for a fractured limb to a Medicare patient with whom the provider does not have an individual opt out agreement. The provider bills Medicare for setting the fractured limb by reporting the appropriate CPT code with the emergency opt out modifier GJ and modifier 54, surgical care only. Then, to comply with the opt out rules, the provider has the patient sign a private contract to continue seeing the patient in follow up. If the patient does not agree to enter into this relationship with the treating provider, the patient must be referred to a Medicare-participating or nonparticipating provider (in either case, a provider not opted out of the Medicare program) who would be able to treat the patient and bill Medicare for the postoperative care using modifier 55, postoperative management only. In other words, once the patient no longer needs emergency or urgent care, the opt out provider cannot continue to treat the patient and bill Medicare for the follow up care if this is the patient's wish.

Termination of Opt Out Contracts

Buried within the federal regulations are rules allowing providers the option for early termination of the opt out status. To properly terminate the opt out arrangement with Medicare and the Medicare patients, a provider must:

- Have not previously opted out of Medicare
- Notify all Medicare contractors, with which the provider filed an affidavit, of the termination of the opt-out arrangement, no later than 90 days after the effective date of the opt out period
- Refund to each patient, with whom the provider has privately contracted, all payment collected in excess of the Medicare limiting charge (in the case of physicians) or in excess of the deductible and coinsurance (in the case of practitioners)
- Notify all patients, with whom the provider entered into private contracts, of the provider's decision to terminate the opt out arrangement, and of the patients rights to have claims filed on their behalf with Medicare for the services furnished during the opt out period

When the provider properly terminates the opt out arrangement in accordance with the above requirements, the provider will be reinstated in the Medicare program as if there had been no opt out status.

Medicare Secondary Payer Policies and DMEPOS

Under current federal regulations, it is possible for Medicare to make a secondary payment (e.g., act as the secondary insurer under the Medicare secondary payment (MSP) program), even if the primary insurer reimburses the provider or supplier more than the Medicare-allowed amount. In MSP cases, the patient has other insurance that is considered primary, and Medicare is considered the secondary insurer. A Medicare patient can expect to receive coverage through another primary insurer, such as the following:

- Employer group health plan coverage
- Automobile medical or no-fault insurance

© 2010 Ingenix

- Liability insurance
- Disability insurance
- Workers compensation
- Federal Black Lung program
- Veteran's Administration claims

When the Medicare contractor receives a claim as the secondary payer, the determination for amount of benefits will be the lower of two calculations:

- The amount Medicare would pay if there was no primary insurer
- The primary insurer's payment minus the higher of the Medicare allowance or primary insurer's allowance

Medicare's final MSP liability is the lower of the two calculations, which is then considered for payment at 100 percent.

For paper claims to be considered for Medicare secondary benefits, a copy of the primary insurer's explanation of benefits (EOB) or remittance notice must accompany the claim form for proper adjudication. If the primary insurance EOB is not submitted, Medicare will deny the claim.

Of particular interest to providers and suppliers of DMEPOS is that for all assigned claims, the secondary insurance claim must be prepared and submitted by the provider or supplier. This is true even in cases when the claim is unassigned (assignment was not accepted by the provider or supplier), but the patient furnishes a copy of the primary insurer's EOB and requests the provider or supplier to submit the claim to Medicare for secondary insurance determination.

Particular rules and regulations must be followed when submitting DMEPOS claims under the MSP for Medicare patients. Details of these rules and regulations fall outside of the scope of this publication; contact the Medicare contractor and the DME MAC for specific guidance.

The MSP can be confusing; the following checklist helps decipher the reason a claim has been denied by Medicare for secondary insurance payment:

- An EOB or denial from the primary insurer was not attached to the claim, or, for an electronic claim, the appropriate field was not completed
- The explanation of the denial code on the primary insurance EOB is missing. The reverse side of the EOB may have to be copied as it is common for this information to appear on the back of the EOB
- The date of service billed to Medicare does not match the date indicated on the primary insurer's EOB
- Charges submitted to Medicare do not match the charges submitted to the primary insurer as seen on the primary insurer's EOB
- Charges sent to Medicare on the secondary insurance claim are for the coinsurance amount only, instead of the full fees for the service
- The EOB attached to the Medicare claim is not from the primary insurance company on file with the Medicare contractor. A statement must be attached to the claim to alert the Medicare contractor in the event the primary insurance company has changed
- The CPT and HCPCS Level II codes on the claim do not match those submitted to the primary insurer

There is one designated contractor who will handle all coordination of benefit (COB) functions for the entire Medicare program. Group Health Incorporated (GHI) has been designated as the COB contractor. The payment safeguard functions have been assigned to one of 12 Program Safeguard Coordinators (PSCs). These PSCs have been assigned specific tasks and specific geographic areas. Your DME MAC should advise you of the PSC assigned to your area. In some cases, the PSC may be communicating directly with you on certain claims.

The DMEPOS Patient Waiver of Liability

Advance notice to a patient of the likelihood of denial means the patient was sufficiently apprised of the situation before having the item or service furnished. The patient must sign a waiver of liability that absolves the provider or supplier from liability for the item or service, and confirms the patient's financial obligation for the item or service should the payer, in fact, deny it. The waiver of liability should include the following:

- Date of service or date the item was furnished
- Identification of the service or DMEPOS item name; narrative description
- A summarized statement explaining that the payer is likely to deny payment due to its own medical necessity determination
- The patient's agreement to pay, signed and dated before the item is delivered

Obtaining the signed waiver of liability also ensures smoother claims processing and patient billing, as all aspects of the process are known. If the claim is submitted to the carrier for a noncovered or not medically necessary item or service, a denial will ensue. In this situation, patients who signed the liability waiver notice in advance are well aware of

General Billing, Claims, and Coverage Issues

their financial obligation and can be billed in person, either on the date-of-service or after the carrier's denial is received.

Providers and suppliers should explain to patients who sign a waiver of liability that it is the payer's own determination that has caused the patient to incur the financial liability for the DMEPOS service or item. In the view of the provider, the item is medically necessary. This medical necessity of the DMEPOS service or item may have to be explained to the patient in basic terms by a clinically trained staff member, if not the practitioner. Providers should always ensure the patient is fully aware of the financial liability before obtaining the patient's signature on the waiver form.

Medicare Coverage for Beneficiaries in State or Local Custody Under a Penal Authority

The OIG conducted a study in 2002 that determined that Medicare was incorrectly paying for services or items for beneficiaries that were in the custody of a state or local penal authority. Regulations in the Social Security Act prohibit Medicare payment for services that are paid directly or indirectly by any governmental entity. Medicare payment may be made only if the state or local law requires individuals to repay the cost of their medical services while in custody. The state or local government entity must also equally enforce these laws by billing all individuals, regardless of payer source, and must pursue the collection of this debt with the same vigor that it pursues other collection of debts.

CMS is attempting to enforce this regulation by adding fields to the CWF that contain the dates that a beneficiary is in state or local custody. All claims submitted will be checked against these date spans.

If a state or local government meets the requirements for payment as noted in the first paragraph, then the provider or supplier must append modifier QJ to claims. This is a line item modifier and it must be added to every service or item billed during the date span of the beneficiary's custody. Claims billed without a modifier for beneficiaries who are in custody will be denied.

If the state or local government does not require all individuals to repay the cost of their care and/or does not attempt to collect this payment from the individual, you will need to bill the appropriate governmental agency. State and local laws vary widely. If you are uncertain as to the details of your area, consult with an attorney or source at the government agency.

Medicaid is a federal program administered by each individual state. Medicaid may not follow the same regulations as Medicare does for this situation. Check with your state Medicaid agency for specific regulations pertaining to covered individuals who are in state or local custody.

Other payers including managed care organizations may or may not specifically address this situation. Coverage for individuals in state or local custody will most likely be addressed in the policy exclusion section of each insurance contract. If the policy does not specifically exclude coverage for this situation, you may bill the insurance carrier.

DMEPOS Claims Jurisdictions

In Section 911 of the Medicare Prescription Drug, Improvement, and Modernization Act (MMA), Congress mandated that the Secretary of Health and Human Services replace the current Medicare contracting system. The Centers for Medicare and Medicaid Services (CMS) must use competitive procedures to replace its current fiscal intermediaries (FI) and carriers with a uniform type of administrative entity, Medicare administrative contractors (MAC). These administrative contractors will process both institutional and professional claims in specified geographic jurisdictions of the country. MACs are to be phased in over the next few years with all jurisdictions to be operational by October 2011.

Home health and hospice will continue to have a specialty MAC separate from the other contractors.

As of August 2008, the SADMERC was replaced by the pricing, data analysis, and coding (PDAC) contractor. The PDAC is located in Fargo, North Dakota and is administered by Noridian Administrative Services, LLC (NAS): https://www.dmepdac.com/.

Palmetto GBA continues to provide the NSC services: http://palmettogba.com/palmetto/providers.nsf/DocsCatHome/National%20Supplier%20Clearinghouse.

For further information, please go to the CMS website at http://www.cms.hhs.gov/MedicareContractingReform/.

Each of the DME MACs processes a multitude of individual states' DMEPOS claims within established jurisdictions. DMEPOS claims must be filed to the local Medicare carrier or the DME MAC, depending on the services or DMEPOS furnished. Providers and suppliers must be sure to check with the

Medicare carrier bulletins and DME MAC bulletins for accurate claims point submissions, as there may be differences between carriers' guidelines.

The DME MACs adjudicate claims are based on the residence of the patient, not the place of service where the DMEPOS items were furnished (unless the claim in question is a foreign claim, in which case the site of service serves as the DME MAC jurisdiction marker). Suppliers must obtain the patient's permanent address, defined as the place of residence where the patient intends to spend more than six months of the calendar year. Using that information, the provider or supplier must submit the DMEPOS claim to the appropriate DME MAC entity.

DMEPOS Jurisdiction Tables

Each DME MAC entity issues a DMEPOS jurisdiction table on an annual basis (otherwise, this information is available from the DME MAC entity upon request). The tables indicate where the claims should be submitted and provide the HCPCS Level II codes (and code ranges) with general descriptions that must be reported for the DMEPOS items. (Items or services not listed can be referenced in the *Medicare Carriers Manual or the DME MAC Supplier Manual.*) The presence of a code in these tables does not guarantee that the Medicare contractor will accept the code, or that it represents a covered service.

Jurisdiction tables are generally issued in the spring. They are effective for July 1 of that year through June 30 of the following year. DMEPOS suppliers should review this table annually to note any changes and ensure that they are billing the correct contractor.

Medicare and DME MAC Claims Denials

Technical Denials

Coverage and exclusion determinations are defined in the Social Security Act, which are implemented through the following:

- Federal regulations and policies in the *Medicare Claims Processing Manual*
- Instructions from CMS
- Decisions made by the individual DME MAC entities that administer the Medicare program for specific items of DMEPOS

Many claim denials fall under the technical category of exclusions. The following are a few of these exclusions that preclude claim reimbursement:

- Disposable items and supplies used by patients at home, other than surgical dressings or supplies required for the effective use of covered DME, prosthetics, or orthotics
- Equipment that does not serve exclusive medical therapeutic functions
- Most oral or self-administered parenteral medications

Other services and items may be denied as not reasonable and necessary for the diagnosis and treatment of illness or injury or to improve the functioning of a malformed body member. These are generally national guidelines issued by CMS and are binding in all DME MAC jurisdictions. The DME MAC entities do have the authority to make medical necessity determinations on aspects of DMEPOS claims not defined by national CMS policy. There is a forced trend, however, for the national coalescence of CMS policy, which is expected to be in full effect in the next several years.

Experimental or investigational services, goods, and supplies are typically denied. Though the Medicare program has authorized coverage for several preventive medicine services and procedures, usually these services are excluded under the technical category as well.

Fragmented coding will lead to claims denials. This situation arises when an individual HCPCS code, one that includes several component items, is billed in addition to the codes for the component items. These are considered not separately payable items. Additionally, the National Correct Coding Initiative (CCI) edits contain many code combinations that, when reported together on a claim, will be denied due to one or more of the following reasons:

- Unbundling
- Using mutually exclusive codes
- Reporting sequential procedures/services
- Reporting separate procedures/services
- Reporting most extensive procedures
- Practicing certain standards of medical and surgical practice
- Including anesthesia in surgical procedures
- Reporting supplemental or add-on services

Truncated diagnosis coding is another coding error that frequently leads to claims denials. Codes having fourth or fifth digits but submitted with fewer digits are termed truncated. All ICD-9-CM diagnostic codes must be submitted at their highest level of specificity; codes should be expanded to the fourth or fifth digits, where applicable. Some codes only have three digits, however, and should not be appended with .0 or .00 to expand them to the fourth and fifth places.

The Advance Beneficiary Notice (ABN) of Noncoverage

The Medicare program puts forth great efforts to educate providers and suppliers. Updates, changes, and new policies are regularly published in bulletins, program memoranda, the Federal Register, and various program Internet web sites. Given this level of mass education, most physicians and health care professionals, including suppliers, are anticipating when a denial of reimbursement will occur for certain DMEPOS services or items.

For non-assigned claims, if Medicare adjudicates the claim as not medically necessary, the beneficiary is liable for payment to the provider or supplier. For assigned claims, the provider or supplier is usually held responsible for the item or service. The provider or supplier may not bill the patient for reimbursement. However, there are two major exceptions to this guideline:

- If the provider or supplier did not know or could not reasonably be expected to know that Medicare would not pay for the item, then payment would be made by Medicare to the provider or supplier. The provider or supplier would be expected to have knowledge of Medicare policy if:
  - a policy was published in Publication 100, Medicare bulletins, Medicare special reports, DME MAC Supplier Manual, or DME MAC;
  - the provider or supplier received notice of the policy from the DME MAC or Medicare carrier; or
  - there had been denials on similar claims in the past.
- If the supplier provided advance notice to the patient in writing before providing the item or service, and if the patient agreed to pay for the item or service if it was denied by Medicare, then the patient would be liable for payment to the provider or supplier.

Advance notice to the patient of the likelihood of denial by Medicare means the patient was sufficiently apprised of the situation before the item or service was furnished to them. Patients must sign an ABN, waiving the provider's responsibility and attesting to their ultimate financial obligation for the item or service should Medicare deny the item or service. The ABN must include the following:

- Date of delivery of the service or item
- Service or item name; narrative description
- A statement that Medicare is likely to deny payment
- An accurate reason why the provider or supplier believes that Medicare is likely to deny payment
- The patient's agreement to pay, signed and dated before the item is delivered

To communicate to the local Medicare contractor or the DME MAC entity that advance notice was furnished and is on file, the HCPCS code for the service or item furnished must be appended with modifier GA. This notifies Medicare that the appropriate guidelines were followed, and allows the patient to obtain a denial from Medicare. The claim in question can then be forwarded to the patient's secondary insurer for possible coverage of the service or item.

For services not covered by Medicare, modifier GZ should be used on claims to indicate that a service or item is expected to be denied, but must still be billed to Medicare to engage the patient's secondary insurance. This modifier is not reported for DMEPOS services or items expected to be denied due to medical necessity issues. Modifier GA must be reported instead.

Equipment and Service Upgrades

The upgrading of equipment and services usually refers to features or enhanced DMEPOS equipment or services that are over and above the covered DMEPOS item. For example: a service may be performed daily when it is covered only as a three times a week service; or a wheelchair may be provided with enhanced or additional equipment that is more than would be medically necessary. An upgrade is an item with features that go beyond what the physician ordered. The extent of, number of, duration of, or expense for an item, feature, or service may be more extensive and/or more expensive than the item or service that is considered reasonable and necessary under the payer's coverage requirements.

Upgraded equipment or services are usually offered in place of the covered equipment or service for one of three reasons:

- The patient may request features or enhancements beyond the usual
- The physician may order a specific item with the enhancements
- The supplier may offer the enhanced equipment or service at no charge.

The last reason may occur when a supplier prefers to carry only higher-level equipment in order to reduce inventory and repair costs. Many payers have specific guidelines for each scenario.

Most payers will generally pay only for the DMEPOS that is necessary for the patient's medical conditions. Specific restrictions and coverage is available from the payer. Many payers may treat upgrades in the same manner as Medicare, which has the most restrictive criteria.

Medicare Requirements for Upgrades

CMS has released several notices about the upgrades of equipment and services for Medicare beneficiaries. This service or equipment is normally not medically necessary. CMS states that guidelines for equipment upgrades apply to both assigned and unassigned claims.

If a supplier provides upgraded equipment at no charge, a modifier is required. Use the HCPCS code for the non-upgraded item and modifier GL. Modifier GL is defined as a medically unnecessary upgrade provided instead of standard item at no charge with no ABN issued. Additionally, the claim should contain only the charge for the non-upgraded item. Item 19 of the claim (or the attachment) must contain the make and model of the upgraded equipment. The supplier further needs to explain why this model is an upgrade. Payment is based on Medicare's payment for the non-upgraded equipment.

CMS will include a message on the Medicare Summary Notice (MSN) and on the remittance that tells the beneficiary that he/she is not liable for any additional charge as the result of receiving an upgraded item or service.

If a beneficiary requests an upgrade, the supplier should have the beneficiary sign an ABN. The ABN should be signed for both assigned and unassigned claims. The ABN should be used when the supplier expects Medicare to reduce the payment and issue a medical necessity partial denial of coverage for the expenses attributable to the upgrade. If an ABN is not signed, the supplier cannot collect from the beneficiary regardless of whether or not the claim was assigned.

The upgrade must be billed as two line items on the same claim. The first line of the claim would contain the HCPCS code for the upgraded DMEPOS item or service with modifier GA or modifier GZ appended. Use modifier GA if an ABN was signed or modifier GZ if no ABN was signed. The second line on the claim must include the appropriate HCPCS code for the DMEPOS that was ordered by the physician. Suppliers must append modifier GK to this line.

Modifier GK has the definition of "Actual item or service ordered by physician." Modifier GK cannot be billed alone. It must be used in conjunction with modifier GA or modifier GZ.

The charges submitted on the claim should be the supplier's full charge for the upgraded item or service and the full charge for the physician ordered item or service. Do not bill the expected Medicare allowable as the charge. Both of the DMEPOS items or services must appear in sequential order on the same claim. If the upgrade is within the same HCPCS code, suppliers must submit the two line items on the claim. The first line item for the upgraded DMEPOS should reflect the higher price.

The MSN and remittance will reflect the message that applies to ABNs. If an ABN was signed, the message will state that the beneficiary is liable for payment of the full charge or a portion of the full charge. If an ABN was not signed, the message will tell the beneficiary that they should not pay the supplier and that they are not liable for any charge.

If the physician orders an upgrade, the supplier should bill the HCPCS code for the upgraded item or service. There is no change from prior billing instructions on this issue. The carrier will review the claim and use its discretion to determine if the item or service will be covered. If the supplier believes that the ordered upgrade will not be covered, an ABN should be obtained. The ABN should explain that the physician ordered this upgrade, but Medicare may decide that it is not medically necessary.

In summary:

- An upgrade may be from one item to another within a single HCPCS code description. This would apply if one description is appropriate to either the non-upgraded item or service and the more expensive, enhanced item or service. An upgrade may also be a change from one HCPCS code to another similar HCPCS code

- An upgrade must be within the range of items or services ordered by the attending physician. The item or service must be medically appropriate for the beneficiary's medical condition. ABNs should not be used for substitutions of a different item or service that is not medically appropriate for the beneficiary's medical condition when the original item ordered was medically appropriate

- Having an ABN signed by the beneficiary does not release the supplier from any payment restrictions, coverage provisions, rules, or instructions that apply to the non-upgraded item or service. These issues still apply as if the

General Billing, Claims, and Coverage Issues

standard item or service were being provided rather than the upgrade
- If the standard item or service is covered on a rental basis, the upgraded item or service must be provided on a rental basis
- If a supplier has an ABN signed, the claim must indicate the upgraded item or service on the claim. The item or service must be billed with modifier GA when an ABN is signed or with modifier GZ if an ABN was not signed. The upgraded item or service must be listed in Item 19 or as an attachment to the claim whether it is billed on a CMS-1500 form or as an electronic claim
- Any denials should be medical necessity denials

Other Payers

For payers other than Medicare, the supplier should check coverage criteria for upgrades. Medicaid and managed care companies may require prior approval for an upgrade. Some payers may not make any provision for upgrades and may bar the supplier from billing the customer or insured. A supplier should issue a notice of non-coverage, similar to an ABN, if the payer will not cover more than the standard fee schedule amount.

Duplicate Claim Denials

Medicare Duplicate Claims Edits

A duplicate claim is defined as a claim for the same beneficiary, from the same provider or supplier, for the same date of service, for the same HCPCS code. In most circumstances this edit is a valid one.

There are, however, instances where the claim is legitimate and not a duplicate. For example, per CMS, if a pharmacy dispenses several drugs on one date of service, the pharmacy is entitled to a dispensing fee for each drug. Medicare will allow patients to have more than one disposable nebulizer, mastectomy bra, platform for walkers, and similar DME items as identified in the regulations and manuals. For these cases, the DME MAC can override the duplicate claim rejection and pay for all items.

If a duplicate claim rejection is received for a legitimate item, contact your DME MAC and request that they review the denial. If the item can legitimately be dispensed in quantities greater than one per day (or in the case of pharmacy dispensing fees, charged more than once per day), all items may be reimbursed.

Billing Medicare for Non-Covered Items or Services

There may be circumstances when a provider or supplier will submit a bill for a non-covered item or service to Medicare. These circumstances may include claim submission at the beneficiary's insistence or submission to obtain a denial for secondary-payer coverage.

Providers and suppliers may submit the claim with the appropriate modifier attached to the corresponding HCPCS code. Modifiers GA, GY, and GZ apply. If there is no specific HCPCS code to describe the item or supply, use A9270 Non-covered item or service. Code A9270 should be used when the item is statutorily non-covered and does not meet the definition of a Medicare benefit.

If you are billing A9270, describe the item or supply on the claim form or as a claim attachment.

The Purchase and Rental of DMEPOS Items

In many instances, Medicare patients have the option of purchasing or renting (leasing) certain items of DME. Expenses incurred for this are reimbursable if the following requirements are met:

1. The equipment meets the definition of DME under Medicare guidelines.
2. The equipment is necessary and reasonable for the treatment of the patient's illness or injury, or to improve the functioning of the patient's malformed body member.

Although an item may be classified as DME, it may not be covered for every patient presentation. The previous considerations will bar payment for equipment that cannot reasonably be expected to perform a therapeutic function, or will permit only partial payment when the type of equipment furnished substantially exceeds that required for the treatment of the illness or injury. Sufficient evidence of medical necessity is of particular importance in Medicare coverage determinations for items of DME.

DME is considered medically necessary (eligible for coverage) under the Medicare program when it can be expected to make a meaningful contribution to the treatment of the patient's illness or injury or to the improvement of the patient's malformed body member. In most cases, the provider's prescription for the equipment and other medical information available will be sufficient to establish that the equipment fully serves this purpose and meets this requirement for coverage.

© 2010 Ingenix

Even though an item of DME may serve a useful medical purpose, the Medicare carrier or DME MAC entity must also consider to what extent, if any, it would be reasonable for the Medicare program to pay for the item prescribed. The following considerations should be made:

- Is the expense of the DME item clearly disproportionate to the therapeutic benefits ordinarily derived from use of the equipment?
- Is the DME item substantially more costly than a medically appropriate and realistically feasible alternative pattern or regimen of care?
- Does the DME item essentially serve the same purpose as other equipment already available to the patient?

Claims for payment of equipment found to be not reasonable will be denied except in cases where it is determined that there exists a medically appropriate and realistically feasible alternative pattern or regimen of care for which payment could be made. In these exceptional cases, Medicare payment will be based on the reasonable charge for this alternative.

3. The equipment is used in the patient's home.

For purposes of purchase or rental of DME, a patient's home may be the patient's own dwelling, an apartment, a relative's home, a home for the aged, or some other type of institution. However, an institution may not be considered a patient's home under the following circumstances:

- It meets at least the basic requirement in the definition of a hospital (i.e., it is primarily engaged in providing diagnostic and therapeutic services or rehabilitation services to patients)
- It meets at least the basic requirement in the definition of a skilled nursing facility (i.e., it is primarily engaged in providing skilled nursing care and related services to inpatients, or rehabilitation services for injured, disabled, or sick persons)

If a patient is in an institution or distinct part of an institution that provides the services described above, then the patient is not entitled to have payment made for the purchase or rental of DME since such an institution may not be considered the patient's home.

Renting or Buying DME

The Medicare program provides the option of renting (leasing) certain items of DME, specifically costly items, rather than burdening the beneficiary with the need to purchase the item, alleviating the beneficiary's 20 percent coinsurance amount. The decision to rent or to purchase an item of DME resides strictly with the patient or the patient's legal representative. A rule of thumb in making the decision is to compare the rental charges for the anticipated number of months the DME will be medically necessary to the total purchase price of the item. Note that strict regulations exist under the Medicare program, as well as state agency Medicaid programs, for the renting of DME such as oxygen, walkers, hospital beds, TENS units, wheelchairs, and other items.

Renting DME and Capped Rental Parameters

A capped rental DME item is one in which the Medicare program will only reimburse the supplier for the rental of the item for a specified period of time. Suppliers must offer patients the option of converting capped rental DME to a purchased status during the DME's 10th continuous rental month (including power-driven wheelchairs not purchased when initially furnished). Patients have one month from the date the supplier makes the offer to accept the purchase option. If the patient does not accept the purchase option, payment continues on a rental basis not to exceed a period of continuous use of longer than 13 months.

After 13 months of rental payments made by Medicare, the supplier must continue to provide the item without charge—other than a charge for maintenance and servicing fees—until medical necessity ends or Medicare coverage ceases. If the patient accepts the purchase option, payment continues on a rental basis not to exceed a period of continuous use of longer than 13 months. On the first day after 13 continuous rental months during which Medicare payment is made, the supplier must transfer the title of the equipment to the patient.

Medicare payment is made on a monthly rental basis not to exceed a period of continuous use of the DME for 13 months or on a purchase option basis, or on a purchase basis for electric wheelchairs. For the first three rental months, the rental fee schedule is calculated to limit the monthly rental to 10 percent of the average allowed purchase price for new equipment during a base period, updated as necessary to account for inflation. For each of the remaining months, the monthly rental is limited to 7.5 percent of the average allowed purchase price.

All claims submitted to the DME MAC entity for consideration for reimbursement must show if the DME is rented or purchased. For a purchased DME, the claim must show whether the equipment is new or used. If the supplier does not indicate whether the equipment is new or used, the carrier will assume that the DME is used. Suppliers must also indicate on claims the amount of the rental or purchase charge. If this information is missing, or the purchase price appears to be out-of-line with charges of other suppliers for the same item, the carrier will make the buy or rent decision based on the prevailing charge for the item.

If interest or carrying charges are imposed on the patient because the supplier has made arrangements for the patient to pay deductible or coinsurance amounts in installments, these charges should be shown on the submitted documentation as well. DME suppliers must notify all patients of the purchase vs. rental options at the time the DME is obtained.

Special Parameters

When DME is available only for purchase, such as when the DME item must be custom made, then the claim is processed by the DME MAC as a DME purchase. When DME is available only as rented DME, then it will be reimbursed as a rented DME item. However, if a similar item of DME is available for purchase in the locality, the supplier must inform the patient that a similar item is available and that the DME MAC will make a rental vs. purchase determination for reimbursement. A similar item is a DME that meets the provider's prescription for the DME. DME is considered available for purchase in a locality if it is available by catalogue purchase in that locality.

There are also special parameters of DME purchase and rental when the DME is $120 or less (in which the DME MAC will generally not authorize a rental option and will cover the equipment outright, provided all other requirements are met or exceeded), and when the Medicare patient alleges financial hardship.

Oxygen Equipment

The Medicare Improvements for Patients and Providers Act of 2008 (MIPPA) repeals the transfer of ownership to the beneficiary for oxygen equipment after 36 months of rental. The supplier will retain ownership of the equipment and be required to provide necessary service to the equipment at no cost to the beneficiary.

DMEPOS Repairs and Maintenance

Payment for DME repairs and maintenance can be made under the Medicare program to both suppliers of DME and patients who have purchased (or are in the process of purchasing) the DME. This extends to payment for expendable and non-reusable items that are essential to the effective use of the DME.

Suppliers or renters of DME equipment usually recover the expenses incurred in maintaining the DME from the rental charges. Because of this, separately itemized charges billed to the Medicare program for repair, maintenance, and replacement of rented equipment are not covered, with a special exception for dialysis equipment. Payment is also not generally made for repair, maintenance, and replacement of patient-purchased equipment requiring frequent and substantial servicing, as well as capped rental equipment and oxygen equipment.

DME Repairs

The Medicare program covers repairs to DME that a patient has purchased or is in the process of purchasing when necessary to make the DME serviceable. If the expense for repairs exceeds the estimated expense of purchasing or renting another item of equipment for the remaining period of medical need, no payment will be made for the amount in excess.

DME Maintenance

The Medicare program does not cover the routine or periodic servicing of DME, such as testing, cleaning, regulating, and checking of the patient's equipment. The owner of the DME rather than by a retailer or some other person who may charge the patient generally performs routine maintenance. Normally, purchasers of DME are given operating manuals that describe the type of servicing an owner may perform to properly maintain the equipment. Thus, hiring a third-party contractor to do such work is viewed by the Medicare program as something done for the convenience of the supplier or patient, and is not covered. However, based on the manufacturer's recommendations, the Medicare program covers a more extensive maintenance or repair of the DME that must be performed by authorized technicians. This repair might include, for example, breaking down sealed components or performing tests that require specialized testing equipment not available to the supplier or patient.

Medicare covers the replacement of patient-owned DME in cases of loss or irreparable damage or wear, and in cases when replacement is required due to a change in the patient's condition. Expenses for replacement due to loss or irreparable damage may be reimbursed without a provider's order when Medicare determines the DME still meets the patient's medical needs. However, claims involving replacement equipment necessitated because of wear or a change in the patient's condition must be supported by a new provider's order.

Cases suggesting malicious damage, culpable neglect, or wrongful disposition of equipment will be investigated and denied if the Medicare carrier or

DME MAC determines that it is unreasonable to make program payment under the circumstances.

Reasonable charges for delivery of DME, whether rented or purchased, are covered if the supplier customarily makes separate charges for delivery and it is a common practice among other local suppliers.

Special DME Rental Scenario: Renal Dialysis Equipment

Generally, when renal dialysis equipment is leased by the supplier directly from the manufacturer, the rental charge tends to be closely related to the manufacturer's cost of the equipment. This means it does not include a margin for recovering the cost of repairs by the supplier beyond the initial warranty period. In view of physical distance and other factors that may make it impractical for the manufacturer to perform repairs, it is not feasible to make the manufacturer responsible for all repairs and include a margin for the additional costs. Reimbursement may be made for the repair and maintenance of home dialysis equipment leased directly from the manufacturer if the rental charge does not include a margin to recover these costs. Another stipulation for coverage of this equipment under the DME rental benefit is that the patient must be free to secure repairs locally in the most economical manner.

Whether the home renal dialysis equipment is being purchased by the patient, is owned outright, or is being leased, Medicare payment is to be made only after the initial warranty period for the equipment has expired. Generally, reimbursement for repairs, maintenance, and replacement parts for medically necessary home dialysis equipment is made in a lump sum payment. Where extensive repairs are required and the charge for repairing the item represents a substantial proportion of the purchase price of a replacement system, the Medicare program might make graduated payments instead of a lump-sum payment.

As in the case of the maintenance of purchased DME, the routine or periodic servicing of leased dialysis equipment, including most testing and cleaning, is not covered. While reimbursement will be made for more extensive maintenance and necessary repairs of leased dialysis equipment, the patient or family member is expected to perform those services for which the training for home or self-dialysis would have qualified them, such as the replacement of a light bulb.

Reasonable charges for travel expenses related to the repair of leased dialysis equipment are covered if the repair person customarily charges for travel, and this is a common practice among other repair persons in the patient's area. When a repair charge includes an element for travel, however, the location of other suitably qualified repair persons will be considered in determining the allowance for travel.

DMAC Billing Guidelines

The *Medicare Claims Processing Manual*, Pub. 100-4, chapter 20 details the billing rules for providers and suppliers who bill for DMEPOS. Several items are highlighted in the following list:

Once-a-Month Billing is the Maximum. DMEPOS claims should not be submitted to the DME MAC more than once a month. CMS advises the DME MAC entities to initiate review processes for claims to determine whether or not providers and suppliers are billing too frequently.

Submit DMEPOS Claims in Sequence. Claims must be submitted in sequence for each Medicare patient for continuous periods of service. For example, if certain capped rental equipment is being furnished to a patient from May through August, the supplier should submit the claim for May before submitting the claim for June, and so on.

DMEPOS is by Order Only. CMS warns that suppliers and manufacturers are not permitted to provide DMEPOS to patients unless the patient (or patient's legal representative) or the patient's provider has requested the DMEPOS. CMS says this "is to ensure that the DMEPOS are actually needed." This directive extends to prescription refills for medications and similar supplies as well. The patient "must specifically request refills of repetitive services or supplies before they are dispensed."

"A supplier may not initiate a refill of an order. The supplier must not automatically dispense a quantity of supplies on a predetermined basis." This is consistent with the DME MAC Supplier Manual, which states, "The description of the item (on an order) may be completed by someone other than the physician (usually the supplier). However, the physician must review the order and sign and date it to indicate agreement." But the supplier is prohibited from automatically mailing or delivering DMEPOS to a patient until it is requested.

Requests for Prescriptions. Considering the preceding official instructions to suppliers and manufacturers, CMS states that a request for a refill is different than a request for a renewal of a prescription. "The beneficiary or his/her representative will rarely keep track of when a prescription will run out. The physician is very unlikely to keep track of this either. The supplier is the one who will need to have the order on file and will know when the prescription will run out and a new order is needed." In these cases, the supplier is expected to take an active role in continuing the patient's prescription by contacting the physician to ask if the order should be renewed.

Appeals, Grievances, and Sanctions

Medicare Appeals

Providers and suppliers of DMEPOS have the right to request an adjustment or review of a claim felt to be inaccurately or unfairly adjudicated by the Medicare or DME Medicare administrative contractor (DME MAC) entity. In most cases, it behooves the provider or supplier to have specific internal protocol established for these claim re-evaluation options. There are important steps to follow when pursuing a re-evaluation of a claim determination.

If a supplier requests a review or other type of appeal on a nonassigned claim, the request must be made in writing and a patient authorization must accompany the request. Without the appropriate patient authorization, the request will be denied. Acceptable review requests must also include the following pieces of information:

- Beneficiary name
- Beneficiary date of birth
- Medicare health insurance claim (HIC) number
- Name and address of provider/supplier of item/ervice
- Date of initial determination
- Date of service for which the initial determination was issued (dates must be reported in a manner that comports with the Medicare claims filing instructions; ranges of dates are acceptable only if a range of dates is properly reportable on the Medicare claim form)
- Item and/or service, if any, at issue in the appeal

If the Medicare contractor or DME MAC entity return an initial claim for DMEPOS services or items to the supplier or provider, calling it unprocessable, then there are no immediate appeal rights. The claim must be refiled as a new claim.

CMS has determined that appeal rights should be granted only to the initial claim determination. Some providers and suppliers had been submitting another claim to extend the appeal time frame. Additional claims that duplicate the originally denied claim will be rejected as duplicates. DME MAC remittance remarks and beneficiary notices will be changed to state that the claim was a duplicate of a previously processed claim and that there are no appeal rights for a duplicate claim.

DMEPOS Claims Adjustments

When a claim is processed incorrectly due to an error made by the DME MAC, the provider or supplier can request an adjustment to the claim. In most cases this can be done over the telephone with a DME MAC representative. Examples of DME MAC errors necessitating claims adjustments include the following:

- Incorrect date of death
- Incorrect number of DMEPOS units or services
- Incorrect date of service

DMEPOS Claims Reviews

If a patient, provider, or supplier is dissatisfied with a claim determination for DMEPOS, the dissatisfied party has the right to request an appeal of the claim adjudication. A request for a claims appeal is now more commonly called a request for a review. DMEPOS claims denied due to medical necessity may only be appealed through the review process; claim adjustments cannot be made to these claims.

Parties who hold the right to request a review of a claim include the following:

- The patient
- The patient's choice of a representative
- A provider or supplier who has accepted assignment
- A supplier responsible for indemnification
- Medicaid state agency or the party authorized to act on behalf of the Medicaid state agency

Medicare has a five-level appeals process and each level must be completed before an appeal can proceed to the next level. The five levels are (1) redetermination, (2) reconsideration, (3) administrative law judge, (4) Departmental Appeals Board (DAB) review Appeals Council and (5) federal court review. The first two levels of appeal are the quickest and least costly for both the contractor and

© 2010 Ingenix

the provider. The majority of claims are resolved at one of these two levels.

Level One—Redeterminations

An initial review can be requested up to 120 days following the initial date of the claim determination, as indicated on the EOMB or electronic remittance notice. In most cases the review is considered an "independent, critical re-examination of the entire claim, by staff that did not participate in the initial decision, along with all medical necessity documentation submitted with the request." Reviews generally include the existing claim information—as originally submitted—along with any pertinent additional documentation, claim modifications, or other material evidence.

To help ensure that a request for a claim review is processed as swiftly and accurately as possible by the DME MAC entity, the following steps should be taken whenever appropriate:

- Be specific in the request, citing exactly what is to be reviewed by the DME MAC and why it is felt the review of the claim is necessary
- Clearly identify the patient and the claim in question by providing:
    - health insurance claim (HIC) number;
    - date of service;
    - internal control number assigned to the claim;
    - provider's or supplier's NSC number; and
    - provider's UPIN.
- Provide any other specific information that further identifies the claim, including:
    - surgery date;
    - equipment pick up or delivery date;
    - DMEPOS-specific model number, make of the DMEPOS; and
    - purpose or use of the DMEPOS.
- When requesting a review of a claim that involves the review of the CMN as well, be sure all required fields (questions) are completed; be certain the CMN has been certified (signed and dated by the physician or provider)
- Provide additional information that may support the need for the DMEPOS
- Highlight appropriate areas of EOMBs that are included with the request for review
- Ensure handwritten requests for review are completely legible

Requests for reviews do not have to be submitted on the CMS-20027 form, but can be made in writing, and must specifically cite the reason for the request for review. A telephone review can be requested if the claim correction will result in additional payment to the provider or supplier, and the review does not require a formal medical review of the case (many telephone reviews are considered claim adjustments and not true reviews). A request for review may be written on the EOMB if space allows, with any additional information annotated neatly on the EOMB or attached to it.

However, if writing directly on the EOMB will cause the information to appear messy and possibly confuse or mislead the DME MAC officials, it is probably best not to use the EOMB as the format to request the review.

Decisions in answer to the requests for reviews are typically provided within 45 days and must be completed within 60 days of receipt of the request.

If a provider or supplier is still dissatisfied with the outcome once a decision has been rendered by the DME MAC, the provider or supplier has a right to pursue the matter further. This is done by requesting a reconsideration.

The Qualified Independent Contractors (QIC) may be handling medical review appeals for your DME MAC.

Level Two—DMEPOS Reconsiderations

A reconsideration is defined as the second level of appeal following the review process. The reconsideration process essentially gives dissatisfied providers or beneficiaries the opportunity to present the reasons for their dissatisfaction with the way their claims were processed. A QIC adjudicator or clinical health panel conducts a new impartial review and an independent decision is rendered based on the information contained in the hearing file and medical documentation. The provider or beneficiary may request a hearing, in writing, within 180 days after the date of the first formal review determination.

The request for a reconsideration must include:

- The beneficiary's name
- The beneficiary's Medicare health insurance claim number
- The specific service and item for which the reconsideration is requested, and the specific date of service
- The name and signature of the party or representative of the party
- The name of the contractor that made the redetermination

As soon as practical, but no later than 30 days after the review, the QIC will issue a decision based on the record developed at the review.

Claimants still dissatisfied with the decision generated by the QIC can request an administrative law judge (ALJ) hearing, so long as the amount in question is $130.00 (singly or in aggregate). The request for an ALJ must be made within 60 days of the QIC review.

Signatures can be mailed, faxed, or submitted via a CMS approved portal application. A signature stamp or indication that a signature is on file is not acceptable by hard copy or fax.

Level Three—Administrative Law Judge Hearings
Although less than 1 percent of all claims processed ever go beyond the contractor (fiscal intermediary or carrier) level, there are three remaining appeal levels. It would be prudent to request a copy of the appeals file at this time. It will contain all of the information used thus far in the process.

A written request must be filed with the contractor or Health and Human Services Office of Medicare Hearing and Appeals (OMHA) field office within 60 days of the date of the QIC's decision. This is requesting an in-person hearing before a federal administrative law (ALJ) from the Office of Hearings and Appeals of the Social Security Administration. Following a QIC Review, and pending a requested ALJ hearing, the provider may submit additional information that might affect the appeal outcome.

Level Four—Departmental Appeals Board Review
If dissatisfied with the ALJ decision, the provider may request an Departmental Appeals Board (DAB) review Appeals Council. This appeal must also be in writing. The request must be received within 60 days of the ALJ decision. It may be submitted to the DAB or ALJ hearing office.

The DAB may review an ALJ's decision/dismissal if:

- There was an error of law
- The ALJ's decision/dismissal was not supported by substantial evidence
- The ALJ abused their discretion
- There is a broad policy or procedural issue that may affect the general public

The ALJs are required to follow all national coverage decisions published in a CMS manual or the *Federal Register*.

Level Five—Federal Court Review
If dissatisfied with the appeals council review, and if the amount in controversy exceeds $1,260.00, the provider may request a hearing before the federal court. This is an extremely expensive proposition and it rarely occurs. Considering the staggering legal fees it would cost to undertake this type of review, it is not often attempted. This final appeal requires the provider to have an attorney file the court papers and have legal representation.

LCD (Local Coverage Determination) Appeals (Reconsiderations)

The LCD reconsideration process is a mechanism by which interested parties can request a revision to an LCD. The whole LCD or any part of the LCD may be reconsidered. Reconsiderations are only accepted for LCDs published in final form. Requests are not accepted for other documents including:

- National Coverage Determinations (NCD)
- Coverage provisions in interpretive manuals
- Draft LCDs
- Template LCDs, unless or until they are adopted by the contractor
- Retired LCDs
- Individual claim determinations
- Bulletins, articles, training materials
- Any instance in which no LCD exists (i.e., requests for development of an LMRP)

LCD Reconsideration Requests

Requests should be submitted in writing. The request must identify the specific language the provider wants changed or deleted. The provider must also submit justification and published evidence to support the request. The level of evidence is the same as that needed to validate the need for a new LCD.

The contractor will determine whether the request is valid or invalid within 30 days. If the request is invalid, the contractor will respond, in writing, to the requestor explaining why the request was invalid.

If the request is determined valid, the contractor will make a final LCD reconsideration decision and notify the requestor of the decision with a rationale within 90 days.

If the contractor decides to not make any changes or to retire the LCD, the provider is notified within 90 days of the day of the request of the decision.

Third-Party Payer Appeals

Most private third-party payers grant the privilege to rebut or appeal a claim determination that is thought by the provider or supplier to have been inaccurately or unfairly adjudicated by the payer.

With the automated provider response systems in use by most major payers, some of the claims that require a reconsideration of benefits can be handled directly over the telephone. These cases frequently involve inaccurate coding and the omission of essential information. In these situations, all of the necessary information for correction or modification of the initial claim submission should be at hand during the telephone appeal. Not all requests for claim reconsideration can be handled in such a convenient fashion. Often a formal or written request for a claim appeal must be submitted to the payer.

A formal request for reconsideration of a claim determination must be made in writing and should be addressed to the payer's provider services unit or department. Many times the payer will provide special forms (such as a Provider Inquiry Form) that must be completed in lieu of a written request by letter. In cases where provider or supplier appeal correspondence to these units has resulted in procrastinated responses or have even been ignored by the payer (e.g., "We haven't received it. Can you send it again?" is a typical response reported by many practices), the payer's area representative can be a good resource in tracking down an appeal and in getting the matter expedited for a second determination. Generally, third-party payers have area representatives who are specifically assigned to geographical areas within the payer's purview.

The written request for an appeal must disclose the reasons the initial claim determination is felt to be inaccurate or unfair. Additional information and other supporting documentation for the service or item should be sent to the payer with the appeal request, including a copy of the original EOB form. The request for the appeal should always outline the reasons for the DMEPOS service or item in relation to the patient's clinical condition, and should detail the medical benefits the provider or supplier expects the patient to derive from the service or item. If a claim for a specialized item of DMEPOS is in question, the unique characteristics of the item, as well as the medical benefits anticipated from its use, should always be clearly discussed in the appeal request.

A claim that has been denied by the payer (not adjudicated or processed) does not usually require an appeal for reprocessing. A claim, once denied, is typically not recorded in the claim processing system, and does not need to undergo appeal procedures, but should simply be amended (in whatever way necessary to have it properly adjudicated) and resent to the payer.

The appeal process can vary among payers. Providers and suppliers should always ascertain the preferred appeal process for each payer. Much of this information can be gathered from the provider's or supplier's participating manual, or from the area payer representative. Some payers provide for an expedited appeal process in cases where delays in a claim reconsideration may be detrimental to the patient's health or long-term recovery potential. The time limit for filing an appeal should be noted and disclosed to all billing staff involved in appeals processes.

Additional Claims Determinations and Grievances

When the provider or supplier remains dissatisfied with the outcome of a claim appeal, most payers provide for yet another claim reconsideration request. These requests are almost uniformly required in writing, and like the written appeal request, they must outline why the physician, provider, or supplier feels the initial and appealed claim determinations were unsatisfactory.

Sometimes these secondary appeal requests are termed a medical director's review, as the plan medical director, or his/her staff will assess the situation and formulate a new claim determination. For some third-party payers, this step is considered the filing of a provider or supplier grievance and is handled by an independent grievance committee. The committee is usually composed of claims adjudication officials, clinical personnel, and the payer's medical director.

Often the outcome of an additional claim appeal, or a grievance filed in connection with a claim determination, is considered final. Participating providers and suppliers cannot bill the patient for the amount in dispute; however, another resource is available that might be of invaluable assistance: the state insurance commissioner.

Insurance Commissioner

Another avenue for providers and suppliers who feel a claim adjudication process has been unfairly undertaken by the third-party payer is to alert the state's insurance commissioner. While the state insurance commissioner's office does not enter into general payment amount disputes, since this is seen as a function of the participating contract that the provider or supplier enters into with the payer, it can assist in the following:

- Unfair reimbursement decisions
- General reimbursement determinations
- A payer's protracted reimbursement time
- A payer's denial to pay a claim for a DMEPOS service or item timely and correctly filed

The billing manager of the provider or supplier should become acquainted with the state's insurance commissioner's role in third-party payer disputes. The insurance commissioner's office can also supply the provider or supplier with essential information, such as:

- State requirements in force for payment floors for claim reimbursement
- A payer's rights when claim data submitted by the health care professional is incorrect or not specific
- Provider or supplier appeal rights, grievance rights, and rights to rebut sanctions established by the state

Any correspondence to the insurance commissioner's office should detail all of the necessary information to address the matter with the payer. Send a copy of the letter to the payer and the patient. The letter should also include copies of EOBs, appeal denial notices, or other third-party payer correspondence related to the claim in question. Copies of pertinent clauses of the provider's or supplier's participating contract should also be included.

Third-Party Payer Sanctions

The imposition of provider and supplier sanctions is a right reserved by the third-party payer, as specified in the participating contract. Sanctions can take the form of a written warning, or can be quite severe, resulting in termination from the plan and notification of the action by the payer to the National Practitioner Data Bank. Termination from the plan can result in isolation of the provider or supplier within the professional community, as this information must be disclosed upon application for privileges to hospitals and participation with other third-party payers and MCOs. severe sanction or termination from the plan occurs when the provider or supplier has rendered substandard care to a plan member. Substandard care, in most cases, means the care has resulted or can result in imminent harm to the patient, whether acute or long-term. Sanctions can also occur when the provider or supplier has breached the participating contract and has ignored fair warnings of such breach.

If a decision is made to terminate the provider or supplier from the plan due to perceived medical negligence, the payer will report the matter to the National Practitioner Data Bank. Termination from a participating contract with a third-party payer, for whatever reason, is generally performed in the following manner:

- The provider* is notified in writing of the termination
- The facts or basis of the termination are fully disclosed to the provider
- The provider's rights to appeal the termination are also fully disclosed
- The provider is apprised of the process to file an appeal of the payer's termination decision

*Provider = physician, other health care provider, or supplier.

The steps for notifying and educating the physician, provider, or supplier about sanctions to be imposed (other than termination from the plan) usually follow the same course as described above.

When the provider or supplier is terminated from the plan, the provider or supplier is typically held to the termination decision until the appeal has been filed and processed. If a reversal is concluded, then the provider or supplier will be reinstated to the plan and all records of the incident will be kept confidential within the plan's files. No record of the proceeding is sent to the National Practitioner Data Bank.

Fraud, Abuse, and Compliance

Introduction

The DMEPOS industry is under intense scrutiny by the federal government. Suppliers of DME, including providers who dispense DME and providers who certify the DME as medically necessary, have repeatedly surfaced as prominent targets for the Office of the Inspector General's (OIG's) annual work plan. This work plan focuses on almost every segment of the health care industry to expose areas of fraud, waste, and abuse. Physician practices, physician billing companies, DMEPOS suppliers, home health agencies, skilled nursing facilities, laboratories, and hospitals are all currently under the OIG's microscope. Given the fact that the OIG and other federal government agencies claim they have recouped inappropriate payments, overpayments, penalties, and fines of up to several billion dollars, it is unlikely that current aggressive fraud and abuse identification activities will subside.

The best and most powerful method of preventing or defending the provider and supplier's operations against fraud and abuse accusations is to prepare for such events. Preparation includes the following:

- Being fully aware of what composes fraud, abuse, and compliance
- Having a compliance plan that is reasonable and able to be practiced on a daily basis
- Performing internal self-audits

Questions that must be asked with each and every encounter or recertification include those that could incur an audit liability, such as:

- Is a copy of the original Certificate of Medical Necessity (CMN) on file for Medicare patients?
- Is the copy of the provider's order on file (that specifies the patient's exact clinical condition) in support of both the type of hospital bed ordered as well as hospital bed accessories?
- Is the need for the item and for specific accessories, including diagnosis, documented in the patient's clinical notes?

Definitions of Fraud and Abuse

CMS states that fraud occurs when a provider or supplier knowingly and willfully deceives the Medicare program, or misrepresents information, to obtain the benefit of monetary value, resulting in unauthorized Medicare payment to themselves or to another party.

The violator may act individually or in agreement with others, and may include a participating or nonparticipating provider, a supplier of DMEPOS, a Medicare patient, or even an individual or business entity unrelated to a patient.

Defrauding the Medicare program of federal monies includes but is not limited to the following practices:

- Billing for services or supplies that were not provided. This includes billing the Medicare program for no-show patients or DMEPOS clients
- Altering claim forms to obtain higher payment amounts
- Deliberately submitting claims for duplicate payment
- Soliciting, offering, or receiving a kickback, bribe, or rebate. Common examples of these practices are (1) paying an individual or business entity for the referral of a patient and (2) routinely waiving a patient's deductible or coinsurance
- Providing falsified CMN forms for patients not professionally known by the provider or supplier, or a supplier completing a CMN for the provider (in effect, ordering DMEPOS not originating from the provider's orders)
- Falsely representing the nature, level, or number of services rendered or the identity of the patient, dates of service, and so forth. This includes billing a telephone call as if it was an actual patient visit
- Being involved in collusion, whether between a provider and a patient or a provider and a supplier, resulting in higher costs or unnecessary charges to the Medicare program
- Using another person's Medicare card to authorize services for a different patient or non-Medicare patient
- Altering claims history records to generate fraudulent payment

- Repeatedly violating the assignment agreement or limiting charge amounts
- Falsely representing provider ownership in a clinical laboratory
- Using the Medicare program's name or logo without authorization. A person or entity may use neither the Medicare program's name nor logo in marketing or other efforts, and cannot use the Social Security emblem in advertising for items or services as Medicare approved

Most state Medicaid programs and many third-party payers follow the same basic outline for the definition of abuse.

CMS defines abuse of the federal Medicare program as "incidents or practices of providers, physicians, or suppliers of services and equipment which are inconsistent with accepted sound practices." Although often these incidents or practices cannot be considered flagrantly fraudulent, in some cases they may directly or indirectly result in unnecessary costs to the federal Medicare program. One of the most prevalent kinds of abuse is overutilization of medical and health care services.

Abuse of federal monies supporting the Medicare program includes but is not limited to the following practices:

- Excessive charges for services, procedures, or supplies
- Claims for services not medically necessary, or for services not medically necessary to the extent rendered. For instance, a panel of tests is ordered when, based upon the patient's working diagnosis, only a few of the tests within the panel were actually necessary
- Breaches of assignment agreements resulting in patients being billed for disallowed amounts
- Improper billing practices, such as when the provider exceeds the Medicare imposed limiting charge (115 percent of the Medicare—allowed amount for nonparticipating providers and for all providers of certain other services)
- The submission of claims to Medicare when another third-party payer, managed care organization (MCO), or workers compensation carrier is the primary payer
- Higher fee charges for Medicare patients than for non-Medicare patients

Again, many state Medicaid programs and third-party payers follow a similar definition when identifying abusive provider and supplier activities. Under the auspices of HIPAA, private payers have also been empowered to conduct fraud and abuse detection and prevention activities.

Definition of Compliance

Compliance is a broad term that has been applied to certain administrative aspects of health care in recent times. Compliance specifically encompasses the appropriate coding, billing (reporting), and documentation of medical services. In particular, being in compliance suggests the correct reporting of health care services to federal programs such as Medicare or the Children's Health Insurance Program (CHIP). This also applies to other federally funded programs, such as state Medicaid or medical assistance. Likewise, being in compliance is often germane to correctly documenting and billing health care services under participating contracts with third-party payers, such as Blue Cross/Blue Shield and Aetna/U.S. Healthcare. Compliance edicts may also be imposed by other payers, such as many of the common private or commercial third-party payers; MCOs, including preferred provider organizations (PPOs) and health maintenance organizations (HMOs); workers compensation carriers; and self-funded plans.

Noncompliance can lead to expulsion from private payers, hefty penalties, and possible criminal charges. Expulsion from a major health care plan such as Blue Cross/Blue Shield can permanently harm a provider's or supplier's DMEPOS business. Numerous payers consistently publish the names of sanctioned providers and suppliers. This can potentially lead to an irreparably damaged professional reputation for the exposed provider or supplier.

Criminal and Civil Statutes

Fraud and abuse against the Medicare program may be prosecuted under a variety of provisions of the United States code. A number of criminal and civil statutes are used to prosecute fraud and abuse cases involving the Medicare and Medicaid programs.

The laws used most commonly to prosecute for Medicare fraud and abuse include the Medicare-Medicaid Anti-Fraud and Abuse Amendments to the Social Security Act, the federal False Claims Act, Civil Monetary Penalties, and Assessments and Exclusion from Program Participation. It is a felony to steal from the Medicare program under these laws and depending on the validity of the case, penalties may result in criminal prosecution, civil proceedings, or administrative sanctions that may result in restitution, fines, imprisonment, and exclusion from the Medicare program.

In cases of suspected Medicare fraud and abuse, the United States attorney's office decides whether to file a civil suit or settle a case. Convicted individuals are required to pay back what was stolen plus additional

Fraud, Abuse, and Compliance

fines, and they are barred from doing business with Medicare in the future. The amount stolen plus additional money is paid to the government in the form of penalties and fines as further defined below. Administrative sanctions include taking action to exclude the provider from the Medicare program, referral to state licensing boards of medical or professional societies, or withdrawal of favorable waiver presumption.

CMS and the OIG have the authority to suspend, exclude, or terminate payment to providers, practitioners, and suppliers of Medicare services. The laws used to support this authority are described below.

Fraud Alerts

To keep providers and payers informed of fraud and abuse issues, OIG and CMS periodically issue national fraud alerts. The alerts are usually issued when there is a need to advise Medicare carriers, fiscal intermediaries (FIs), the quality improvement organizations (QIOs), providers, and beneficiaries about an activity that involves false claims. Not all of the alerts pertain to all providers, however, it is important for providers to keep abreast of the issues currently under investigation.

The alerts are for educational and informational purposes so that providers and suppliers can become more aware of fraudulent situations. Claims that are denied based on these fraud alerts will be denied based on facts obtained independent of the alerts.

OIG Fraud Alerts

The OIG issues special fraud alerts to address problems it is identifying in the health care industry. The alerts put the health care industry on notice that the OIG is pursuing certain abusive practices. They are the initial tools used to get providers to review their practices and comply with Medicare regulations. The OIG distributes the alerts directly to Medicare providers and publishes new fraud alerts in the Federal Register.

CMS National Fraud Alerts

CMS fraud alerts represent examples of fraudulent and abusive billing practices that are currently being investigated and hope to be prevented in the future. CMS issues national alerts when the fraud or abuse is perceived or has the potential to be widespread (i.e., crossing contractor [fiscal intermediary or carrier] jurisdictions).

Federal Fraud and Abuse Investigative Programs

The federal government's war on fraud and abuse has been aggressive over the past several years, and only continues to intensify. Spearheaded by the OIG of the Department of Health and Human Services (DHHS), the FBI, the Department of Justice (DOJ), and CMS, the federal government has been successful in consistently uncovering what it deems "fraudulent activities aimed at the Medicare and Medicaid programs." Whether or not the providers or suppliers actually intended to commit fraud is another matter; these successful efforts have fueled and increased the intensity and number of federal (and state) investigations, and there have been more indictments and convictions as a result.

A number of disparate programs and initiatives have evolved out of the DHHS. They include the following:

Annual OIG Workplan. In conjunction with CMS, the Public Health Service (PHS), and the Administrations for Children, Families, and Aging (all DHHS entities), the OIG Annual Workplan mission statement reads, in part, "We improve HHS programs and operations, and protect them against fraud, waste and abuse. By conducting independent and objective audits, evaluations and investigations, we provide timely, useful and reliable information and advice to Department officials, the Administration, the Congress, and the public." The OIG Workplan assists the DHHS in pursuing criminal convictions by recovering maximum dollar amounts through judicial and administrative methods, and recycling recouped program monies back into the federal programs.

Operation Restore Trust (ORT). This program was originally launched in five states to test several innovations in fighting Medicare and Medicaid fraud and abuse. It is now being expanded nationwide. ORT has been particularly adept at discovering Medicare overpayments to providers and hospitals.

Fraud and Abuse Hotline. HHS has expanded the 1-800-HHS-TIPS hotline for reporting fraud in the Medicare and Medicaid programs. Since 1995, more than 32,000 tips and complaints called into the program have warranted specific follow-up action.

Medicare Integrity Program

The Health Insurance Portability and Accountability Act (HIPAA) includes a provision formally establishing the Medicare Integrity Program (MIP). CMS has had a MIP in place for several years. This provision gives CMS the authority to enter into contracts with entities to promote the integrity of the Medicare program. MIP was established, in part, to strengthen CMS's ability to deter fraud and abuse in the Medicare program. There are basically two overall areas of concern. One area deals with the Coordination of Benefits (COB) functions that ensure that Medicare is appropriately paying for services when any other type of insurance covers the beneficiary.

The second area of concern is the safeguard or monitoring and integrity of the data and payment of Medicare services.

CMS has issued a pamphlet aimed at physicians, providers, and suppliers to provide information on the MIP. The information explains how the program works, answers questions, and promotes the goal of program integrity to pay it right the first time and to pay the right amount to the right provider, for the right service, to the right beneficiary.

Medicare has two prepayment review programs intended to assist in the identification of billing and reporting errors. These are the National Correct Coding Initiative (NCCI) Edits and the Medically Unlikely Edits (MUE).

CMS developed the NCCI to promote national correct coding methodologies and to control improper coding that leads to inappropriate payment in Medicare Part B claims. NCCI policies are based on coding conventions defined in the American Medical Association's (AMA's) Current Procedural Terminology (CPT) Manual, Healthcare Common Procedure Coding System (HCPCS) Manual, national and local Medicare policies and edits, coding guidelines developed by national societies, standard medical and surgical practice, or current coding practice. NCCI edits are updated quarterly. NCCI edits are available to the public on the NCCI website: http://www.cms.hhs.gov/NationalCorrectCodInitEd/.

CMS established units of service edits for Medicare Part B benefit claims, referred to as MUEs. An MUE for a CPT or HCPCS Level II code is the maximum units of service under most circumstances that a provider would report for a code for a single patient on a single date of service. Not all codes have an MUE, and not all MUEs are published.

MUEs are based on anatomic considerations, code descriptions, CPT coding instructions, established CMS policies, the nature of service or procedure, the nature of equipment, and clinical judgment. There are quarterly updates to MUEs on the same schedule as the quarterly updates to NCCI. CMS continues to add MUEs for additional HCPCS/CPT codes in these updates.

Providers and suppliers reporting DMEPOS items most likely will not be affected by the NCCI edits, but may find claims returned due to MUEs. Claim lines that pass the MUE edits continue to be processed. On facility claims, the claim is returned to the provider for correction when a line item fails the MUE. When a line item fails the MUE on physician and supplier claims, the line item is denied. Claim line denials can be appealed.

Program Safeguard Coordinators (PSCs)/ Zone Program Integrity Contractor (ZPIC)

- CMS has awarded Indefinite Delivery, Indefinite Quantity (IDIQ) contracts to PSCs or ZPICs to perform program integrity and data analysis activities as defined in specific task orders. A PSC or ZPIC can perform one, some, all, or any sub-set of the work associated with the following payment safeguard functions:
- Medical review
- Cost report audit
- Data analysis
- Provider education
- Fraud detection and prevention
- Medical utilization and fraud review including the review of claims, medical records, and medical necessity documentation and the analysis of utilization patterns for inappropriate use of services
- Identification of MSP situations

Among other activities, the PSCs or ZPICs will review claims on both a post- and prepayment basis. They will be able to deny claims for several reasons including services that are not covered, services that are not reasonable and necessary, and services that are not billed in compliance with local and national billing requirements. PSCs or ZPICs will do targeted claims reviews of services that are at high risk of being noncovered, misrepresented, or fraudulent. They will also do random reviews of all types of claims as well as task orders issued by CMS.

These organizations may be responsible also for conducting Coordinated Comprehensive Provider Reviews when they suspect fraud or abuse or that an overpayment has occurred. These reviews will involve a thorough analysis of a provider's processed claims and claims data, including medical records, beneficiary payment history, and other documentation.

Many companies submitted proposals to perform any or all of these functions. Contracts were awarded to one or more companies depending on the scope of each task order.

Program Integrity

The Medicare Program Integrity Manual (PIM), CMS Pub 100-8, is one of the completely online manuals, available on the Internet at http://www.cms.hhs.gov/Manuals/IOM/list.asp. The PIM details benefit integrity action taking place all across CMS and its contractors. The chapters in this manual are as follows:

Chapter 1	Overview of Medical Review (MR) and Benefit Integrity (BI) and Medicare Integrity Programs
Chapter 2	Data Analysis
Chapter 3	Verifying Potential Errors and Taking Corrective Actions
Chapter 4	Benefit Integrity
Chapter 5	Items and Services Having Special DME Review Considerations
Chapter 6	Intermediary MR Guidelines for Specific Services
Chapter 7	MR Reports
Chapter 8	Reserved for Future Use
Chapter 9	Reserved for Future Use
Chapter 10	Medicare Provider/Supplier Enrollment
Chapter 11	Fiscal Administration
Chapter 12	Comprehensive Error Rate Testing Program
Chapter 13	Local Coverage Determinations
Chapter 14	National Provider Identifier
Chapter 15	Medicare Enrollment Exhibits

This manual details the actions taken by medical review departments, gives information about the progressive corrective action program, discusses particular risk areas, and talks to contractors about dealing with the new program safeguard contractors.

Physician Order Fraud

The OIG's office published a special fraud alert in the Federal Register concerning physician liability for certifications in the provision of DMEPOS. The OIG's special fraud alerts typically address national trends in health care fraud, including potential violations of the Medicare anti-kickback statute. The special fraud alert related to DMEPOS specifically highlighted providers' responsibilities in making certifications for DMEPOS and the legal significance of these certifications.

The fraud alert addressed the following aspects of a provider's involvement in the DMEPOS certification process:

- The importance of physician and provider certification for Medicare patients
- How improper physician and provider certifications can foster fraud
- The potential consequences for knowingly signing a false or misleading certification, or signing such certification with reckless disregard for the truth

While the OIG believes that the actual incidence of providers who intentionally submit false or misleading CMN forms for durable medical equipment is relatively infrequent, provider laxity in reviewing and completing these certifications contributes to fraudulent and abusive practices by unscrupulous DMEPOS suppliers and home health agencies.

All providers should be aware that they are subject to criminal, civil, and/or administrative penalties if they sign a CMN form or physician order for DMEPOS knowing that the information relating to medical necessity is false, or if they sign a certification with reckless disregard for the truth of the information being submitted. While a provider can mistakenly sign a false or misleading certification (by simple, unintended negligence or by inadvertently agreeing to or omitting critical details), the provider may unwittingly facilitate the perpetration of supplier fraud. It is important that all providers and their coding or billing staff be aware of this information.

The OIG has found numerous examples of providers who have ordered DMEPOS—or more commonly have signed CMN forms—without reviewing the medical necessity for the item, or who have signed the CMN without even knowing the patient.

Certificate of Medical Necessity and DME MAC Information Form

Medicare requires claims for certain kinds of DME to be accompanied by a CMN form, signed and dated by the treating provider (unless the DME is prescribed as part of a plan of care for home health services). When a CMN is required, the provider or supplier must keep on file the CMN. The Medicare contractor may request these documents at any time.

A DME MAC Information Form (DIF) is completed and signed by the supplier. Narrative descriptions of the equipment, cost, and physician signatures are not required on a DIF. The supplier must keep a copy of the DIF.

Forms can be found at http://www.cms.gov/CMSForms/CMSForms/list.asp#TopOfPage.

Generally, a CMN form has four sections that must be completed:

- Section A contains general information on the patient, supplier, and provider. The supplier may complete section A.
- Section B contains the medical necessity justification for the DME. The supplier cannot complete this area. The provider, a nonphysician clinician involved in the care of the patient, or a physician employee must complete section B. If the provider did not personally complete Section B, the name of the person who did complete Section B and the person's title and employer must be specified.
- Section C contains a description of the equipment and its cost. The supplier completes section C.
- Section D is the treating provider's attestation and signature, which certifies that the provider has reviewed sections A, B, and C of the CMN, and that the information in Section B is true, accurate, and complete. Signature stamps and date stamps are acceptable.

By signing the CMN, the ordering provider attests to the following:

- He/she is the patient's treating provider and the information regarding the provider's address and unique physician identification number (UPIN) or National Provider Identifier (NPI) is correct
- The entire CMN, including the sections filled out by the supplier, was completed before the provider's signature
- The information in Section B relating to medical necessity is true, accurate, and complete to the best of the ordering provider's knowledge

Improper or Unauthorized CMN Forms

Unscrupulous suppliers and providers may steer other providers into signing or authorizing improper CMN forms. In some instances, the certification forms or statements are completed by DMEPOS suppliers and presented to the provider, who then signs the forms without verifying the actual need for the items or services. In many cases, the provider may obtain no personal benefit when signing these unverified orders, and is only accommodating the supplier or other provider. When the provider knows the information is false or acts with reckless disregard for the truth of the statement, the provider risks incurring criminal, civil, or administrative penalties.

Providers may receive compensation in exchange for their signatures. Compensation can take the form of cash payments, free goods, free or reduced rent, patient referrals, supplies, equipment, or free labor.

Even if the provider does not receive any financial or other benefits, they can be held liable for making false or misleading certifications. Such cases may trigger additional criminal and civil penalties under the anti-kickback statute.

The following are examples of inappropriate certifications uncovered by the OIG in the provision of DMEPOS items:

- At the prompting of a DMEPOS supplier, a provider signs a stack of blank CMN forms for transcutaneous electrical nerve stimulator (TENS) units. The CMNs are later completed with false information in support of fraudulent claims for the equipment. The false information purports to show that the provider ordered and certified the medical necessity for the TENS units for which the supplier has submitted claims.
- A provider accepts fees from a DMEPOS supplier for each prescription the provider signs for oxygen concentrators and nebulizers.
- A provider submits a claim with a UPIN/NPI that is different than the UPIN/NPI of the physician who signed the CMN. CMS recently reported that a study of DME claims revealed that a high volume were ordered or referred using UPINs/NPIs of deceased physicians. In these instances the physician who signed the CMN was alive, but the UPIN/NPI of a different deceased physician was submitted.

Fraud Related to CMN Forms and DMEPOS Orders

A provider is generally not personally liable for erroneous claims due to mistakes, inadvertence, or simple negligence. However, knowingly signing a false or misleading CMN form or DMEPOS order, or signing these documents with reckless disregard for the truth, can lead to serious criminal, civil, and administrative penalties, including the following:

- Criminal prosecution
- Fines as high as $10,000 per false claim, plus triple damages
- Administrative sanctions, including exclusion from participation in federal health care programs, withholding or recovery of payments, and disciplinary actions by state regulatory agencies or loss of license

Realigning Internal Operations

The internal operations of the provider's practice or supplier's medical equipment company should always be geared to securing patient understanding and acknowledgment of services rendered. This is a simple but effective tactic in avoiding frivolous malpractice accusations or suspicions of fraud and abuse under Medicare and state Medicaid programs. Most malpractice carriers would agree that the number of malpractice claims drops when there is effective communication between patients and providers. Patients must understand all of the billing processes and requirements related to securing their own medical care benefits for DMEPOS, so they do not misinterpret information and report it as possible fraud. Given that many Medicare patients are elderly, the likelihood of confusion about DMEPOS items and services is probably greater than if most were younger patients. If a legal guardian handles the patient's business affairs, the guardian should be aware of medical services provided to the patient.

This educational approach takes a combined effort by all staff members and may require a realignment of internal operations. Providers and clinical staff should always explain specific services before they are rendered, and why these services are needed. For medical providers, checkout staff should review the superbill or encounter form with each patient as the patient is departing, and explain the coinsurance and deductible rules. The supplier's technical and billing staff should review the needed DMEPOS item with the patient. Provider and supplier billing personnel should further reinforce this sometimes fragile bridge of understanding between the patient and the provider or supplier by (1) being clinically informed so they are able to answer questions about clinical services, and (2) being able to answer all billing questions with confidence.

The OIG's Compliance Program Guidance for the DMEPOS Industry

Released by the OIG in June 1999, the Compliance Program Guidance for the DMEPOS Industry is designed to assist in the elimination of fraud, waste, and abuse. The compliance program guidance is completely voluntary, and follows the basic outlines used in the OIG's program guidance for other areas of the health care community (hospitals, laboratories, home health agencies, etc.). It contains the seven major elements the OIG has determined as fundamental to an effective compliance program:

- Implementing written policies, procedures, and standards of conduct
- Designating a compliance officer and/or a compliance committee
- Conducting effective training and education programs for pertinent employees
- Developing effective lines of communication
- Enforcing standards through well-publicized disciplinary guidelines
- Conducting internal monitoring and auditing
- Responding promptly to detected offenses and developing corrective actions

Recognizing the size differentials of the organizations that make up the DMEPOS industry, the OIG crafted the compliance program guidance to be applicable in numerous DMEPOS settings regardless of company size, number of locations, type of DMEPOS items or services provided, or corporate structure. The actual applicability of the recommendations and guidelines provided in the compliance program depends on the circumstances of each individual DMEPOS provider or supplier.

The Federal Register dated October 5, 2000, contained an important notification for providers, particularly for the solo practitioner and for small group providers. Entitled "OIG Compliance Program for Individual and Small Group Physician Practices," this notice attempts to assist physician practices in the development of a useful compliance plan. It also forewarns providers about the importance of internal detection, prevention, and continual monitoring of health care fraud and abuse. The seven major elements listed above remain the same. The official appendices to this notification address reasonable and necessary services (including advice about the completion and certification of CMNs), physician relationships with hospitals, physician billing services, and other risk areas including kickbacks and unlawful advertising.

Lines of Communication

The OIG suggests that the DMEPOS supplier establish protocols to increase the communication among treating providers, the patients, and the DMEPOS supplier. It recommends that such protocols be included in the DMEPOS supplier's written policies and procedures. These protocols may include:

- The DMEPOS supplier periodically calling the patient to ensure the equipment is still being used and is operating properly
- The DMEPOS supplier periodically calling the treating provider to ensure the provided items continue to be medically necessary for a patient

In addition, it is recommended the DMEPOS supplier create mechanisms to ensure communication between different departments within its own company (such as sales and billing) to prevent the filing of incorrect claims.

Anti-Kickback and Self-Referral Concerns

The DMEPOS supplier must have established policies and procedures for compliance with federal and state laws, including the anti-kickback statute and the Stark physician self-referral law. These policies and procedures should address the following issues:

- The DMEPOS supplier's contracts and arrangements with actual or potential referral sources (such as providers) are reviewed by counsel (if appropriate) and comply with all applicable statutes and regulations, including the anti-kickback statute and the Stark physician self-referral law.

- The DMEPOS supplier will not submit or cause to be submitted to health care programs claims for patients who were referred to the DMEPOS supplier pursuant to contracts or financial arrangements that were designed to induce such referrals in violation of the anti-kickback statute or similar federal/state statute or regulation, or that otherwise violate the Stark physician self-referral law.

- The DMEPOS supplier does not offer a provider or other referral source more than fair market value for space rented to store items or supplies (e.g., consignment closet).

- The DMEPOS supplier does not offer or provide gifts, free services, or other incentives or things of value to patients, relatives of patients, physicians, home health agencies, nursing homes, hospitals, contractors, assisted living facilities, or other potential referral sources for the purpose of inducing referrals that violate any anti-kickback statute or federal or state statute or regulation.

Further, the OIG recommends that the written policies and procedures should specifically reference and take into account the OIG's safe harbor regulations, which describe those payment practices that are immune from criminal and administrative prosecution under the anti-kickback statute.

Auditing and Monitoring

Auditing and monitoring—two of the most important elements of a compliance program—must work in harmony toward a common goal.

Audits, according to the OIG's compliance program guidance, determine whether a provider is complying with laws governing medical coding and billing, marketing, and other high-risk areas. Audits can be done internally or externally.

Monitoring is the job of the compliance officer or a regulatory affairs or legal department worker. Monitoring includes identifying variations from an established baseline and then measuring improvement. Establish baselines when providing a new service or compliance program. Auditors can provide a basic listing of operations to use as the baseline to manage potential areas of vulnerability. Determine the root cause of any significant adverse variation from the baseline. Then, correct the problem and monitor it for a reasonable period to make sure the issue does not resurface.

Use on-site visits, interviews, questionnaires, forms and written materials reviews, and trend analyses to monitor compliance. Consider the following tips when monitoring:

- Stay independent of line management
- Maintain access to all personnel and documentation
- Present written evaluation reports to governing bodies
- Identify areas where corrective actions are needed

An ongoing internal evaluation or auditing process is critical to a successful compliance program. The extent and frequency of the evaluation or audit may vary depending on:

- The size of the provider's practice or the DMEPOS supplier's company
- The resources available
- The provider or supplier's prior history of noncompliance
- The risk factors that might be inherent in a particular DMEPOS supplier
- Although many monitoring techniques are available, one effective tool to promote and ensure compliance is the performance of regular, periodic compliance audits by internal or external auditors who have expertise in federal and state health care statutes, regulations, and other requirements. The audits should focus on the different aspects or departments of the provider or supplier, including external relationships with third-party contractors. At a minimum, these audits should address the DMEPOS provider and supplier's compliance with laws governing:

- Anti-kickback arrangements
- The physician self-referral prohibition
- Pricing
- Contracts
- Claim development and submission

- Reimbursement
- Sales (if appropriate)
- Marketing (if appropriate)

Whistleblowers

The OIG has stated that whistleblowers should be protected against employer and other retaliation, a concept embodied in the provisions of the False Claims Act. (See 31 U.S.C. ¤ 3730(h).) In many cases, employees become whistleblowers and report, incriminate, or sue their employers under the False Claims Act's "qui tam" provisions. They usually do this out of frustration because of the provider's or supplier's failure to take action when a questionable, fraudulent, or abusive situation is brought to the attention of the practice or company principal.

Billing Companies: OIG Guidelines

In 1998, the OIG released the Compliance Program Guidance for Third-Party Medical Billing Companies. In doing so, the OIG issued a statement that said, "This guidance, designed to assist companies that process bills for the nation's health care providers in preventing fraud, waste and abuse, affects virtually every segment of the health care industry."

According to the OIG, billing companies are becoming a vital segment of the national health care industry. Increasingly, health care providers and suppliers are relying on billing companies to assist them in processing claims in accordance with applicable statutes and regulations. Some health care providers are also consulting with billing companies to provide timely and accurate advice regarding reimbursement matters.

Billing companies are in a unique position to discover various types of fraud, waste, abuse, and billing errors on the part of the provider or supplier for whom they work. This unique access to information may place the billing company in a precarious position. On the one hand, the billing company's allegiance is to its client, the provider or supplier. On the other hand, the billing company should maintain a commitment to comply with the applicable federal and state laws, and the program requirements of federal, state, and private health care plans.

The OIG recognizes the importance of maintaining a positive and interactive communication between billing companies and the providers or suppliers they service. It is with this understanding that the OIG has addressed certain obligations for third-party medical billing companies with regard to provider and supplier misconduct. If the billing company finds evidence of misconduct on the part of the provider or supplier, it should refrain from the submission of questionable claims and notify the provider or supplier in writing within 30 days of such a determination. This notification should include all claim-specific information and the rationale for such a determination.

If the billing company discovers credible evidence of the provider's or supplier's continued misconduct, or flagrant fraudulent or abusive conduct, the company should (1) refrain from submitting any false or inappropriate claims, (2) terminate the contract, or (3) report the misconduct to the appropriate federal and state authorities within a reasonable time frame (i.e., no more than 60 days after determining that there is credible evidence of a violation).

When reporting misconduct to federal or state government officials, a billing company should provide all evidence relevant to the alleged violation of applicable federal or state law and the potential cost impact. Providers and suppliers should be aware that the compliance officer of the billing company, with guidance from governmental authorities, could be requested to continue to investigate the reported violation. Once the investigation is completed, the compliance officer may be required to notify the appropriate governmental authority of the outcome of the investigation, including a description of the impact of the alleged violation on the operation of the applicable health care programs or their patients. If the investigation ultimately reveals that criminal, civil, or administrative violations have occurred, the appropriate federal and state officials must be notified immediately.

Risk Assessment

The OIG has identified the following areas of risk as being particularly problematic for billing companies (but providers and suppliers who perform their own billing operations should also take note of this information):

- Billing for items or services not actually documented
- Unbundling of procedure codes
- Upcoding of procedure codes
- Failing to properly use modifiers
- Doing inappropriate balance billing
- Inadequately resolving overpayments
- Using computer software programs that encourage billing personnel to enter data in fields indicating services were rendered,

although they were not actually performed or documented
- Failing to maintain the confidentiality of information or records
- Willfully misusing provider or supplier identification numbers, which may result in improper billing
- Rendering outpatient services in connection with inpatient stays
- Doing duplicate billing in an attempt to gain duplicate payments
- Billing for discharge in lieu of transfer
- Providing billing company incentives that violate the anti-kickback statute or other similar federal or state statutes or regulations
- Participating in joint ventures
- Routinely waving copayments and billing third-party insurance only
- Providing discounts and professional courtesies

Billing Companies and DMEPOS Coding Services

Any billing company used by providers and suppliers of DMEPOS should have written policies and procedures concerning proper coding, and should reflect the current reimbursement principles set forth in applicable federal, state, or private-payer health care program requirements. The company's written policies and procedures should ensure that coding and billing are based on medical record documentation. Particular attention should be paid to issues of appropriate diagnosis codes, individual Medicare Part B claims (including documentation guidelines for evaluation and management services) and the use of patient discharge codes. The billing company should also institute a policy to require the coder or the coding department to review all rejected claims that pertain to diagnosis and procedure codes. Among the risk areas that billing companies should address while providing coding services are the following:

- Internal coding practices
- Assumption coding
- Alteration of the documentation
- Coding without proper documentation of all physician and other professional services
- Billing for services provided by unqualified or unlicensed clinical personnel
- Availability of all necessary documentation at the time of coding
- Employment of sanctioned individuals

Billing companies that provide coding services should maintain an up-to-date, user-friendly index for coding policies and procedures to ensure that specific information can be readily located. The billing company should ensure that essential coding materials, including quarterly updates, are readily accessible to all coding staff. These recommendations also apply to providers and suppliers who perform their own coding.

Billing companies that do not code bills for their clients should notify the provider or supplier to follow compliance safeguards with respect to the documentation of services rendered. The OIG recommends that billing companies that do not code for their clients incorporate in their contracts an agreement from each provider or supplier to address all coding compliance concerns.

Credit Balances

Credit balances occur when payments, allowances, or charge reversals posted to an account exceed the charges to the account. The matter of overpayments is of prime concern by the OIG and other federal officials. Providers and suppliers must establish or be aware of the billing company's policies and procedures for timely identification and resolution of these overpayments.

A billing company's information system should produce copies of individual patient accounts that reflect a credit balance, which simplifies tracking of these balances. Likewise, a credit balance report should be generated, typically on a monthly basis, for the timely reconciliation of these accounts. The billing company should always maintain a complete audit trail of all credit balances, and document the steps taken to reconcile the accounts.

Failure to notify authorities about an overpayment within a reasonable period of time could be interpreted as an attempt to conceal the overpayment from the government. That, in turn, could establish a basis for a criminal violation with respect to the billing company, as well as any individual who may be involved. For this reason, billing company compliance programs should ensure that overpayments are identified quickly, and encourage their provider and supplier clients to promptly return overpayments obtained from Medicare or other federal health care programs.

Fraud and Abuse by Medicare Patients

CMS maintains an incentive award program that enables patients who alert the Medicare program of possible acts of fraud and abuse to be eligible for rewards, if the reported information leads directly to the recovery of Medicare money. Under this program rewards of up to $1,000 can be paid to the reporting patients.

To receive a reward, the information reported on fraud and abuse must directly contribute to the recovery of Medicare funds for fraudulent activity not already under investigation by law enforcement agencies, the DHHS, state agencies, or Medicare's contractors. Rewards can be for 10 percent of the recovered Medicare overpayment, or a $1,000 maximum, and will be financed from the collected overpayments after all other fines and penalties have been recovered.

Medicare patients are being instructed to watch for and report the following activities related to provider and supplier services:

- Duplicate billing of services
- Charges for services not performed or items not dispensed
- Inappropriate or unnecessary services
- Charges billed for a more expensive procedure than the one received
- Low-cost new or used medical equipment, which is charged to the Medicare program as higher-cost or new equipment
- Services provided free to the patient but billed to Medicare
- CMN forms completed by the supplier or medial equipment vendor instead of the provider

Medicare patients or their legal representatives are being cautioned to carefully monitor all provider statements and Medicare Summary Notice (MSN). If a patient finds something suspicious, the patient is instructed to call the provider or supplier to discuss the matter. If the patient cannot obtain a satisfactory answer, or if the provider or supplier cannot be contacted, the patient is instructed to telephone the DHHS fraud and abuse hotline at (800) HHS-TIPS [(800) 447-8477]. Hotline operators are available to speak in English or Spanish. AARP information further advises patients who don't feel comfortable talking with their provider or supplier to call the hotline and report the matter in question.

The Health Insurance Portability and Accountability Act (HIPAA) of 1996

The HIPAA that has taken shape in Washington evolved from a straightforward effort to guarantee employees the right to transfer the security of their group health insurance coverage from one job to another—the "portability" of HIPAA's name. However, the biggest effect of HIPAA on those that provide health care services comes from the Administrative Simplification provisions of HIPAA.

HIPAA Administrative Simplification

The Administrative Simplification provisions of the HIPAA, Title II require the Department of Health and Human Services (HHS) to establish national standards for electronic health care transactions and national identifiers for providers, health plans, and employers. It also addresses the security and privacy of health data. HHS believes that by adopting these standards, the efficiency and effectiveness of the nation's health care system will increase by encouraging the widespread use of electronic data interchange in health care. This includes the transmission and processing of claims containing health care data. Any and all parties that submit or process health care claims are subject to regulations in HIPAA. DMEPOS suppliers must comply with HIPAA requirements.

Essentially, Administrative Simplification is several sets of regulations that deal with protecting the confidentiality of certain medical information and that contain standards for the safe and accurate exchange of that information

Privacy Standards

On December 28, 2000, the initial publication of the Standards for Privacy of Individually Identifiable Health Information Final Rule, was published. The purpose of these privacy requirements is five fold:

1. To limit the use and release of identifiable health information.

2. To give patients new rights to access their medical records and to know who else has accessed them.

3. To restrict most disclosures of personal health information to the minimum amount necessary to complete a given task.

4. To establish comprehensive federal criminal and civil sanctions for improper use and disclosure.

5. To establish new requirements for access of personal health information (PHI) by researchers and others.

Although these goals seem fairly simple and straightforward, HIPAA has established a complex set of requirements to meet them. Prior to beginning the steps for implementation of these complex requirements, determine if your organization is considered a "covered entity" under the HIPAA privacy regulations. Covered entities include all health plans, health care clearinghouses, and health care providers that transmit health information in electronic transactions covered under another part of the Administrative Simplification, the Standards for Electronic Transactions. Health care providers are defined as "any person or organization that furnishes, bills, or is paid for health care in the normal course of doing business." Most any provider of health care services that does billing in an electronic fashion will be a covered entity under HIPAA.

Transaction Standards and Code Sets

Modifications to Electronic Transactions and Code Sets proposal could modify the electronic transactions and code sets mandated by HIPAA; the notice of public rule making is expected at the first part of 2007. CMS announced the end of contingency planning in 2005, stating that claims not submitted in HIPAA compliant formats would be rejected for payment. Since this is a Medicare contractor issue, we suggest you contact your contractor's office for more information in relation to the acceptance of noncompliant claims forms.

Transaction Standards

HIPAA required that the secretary of HHS adopt standards for the electronic transfer of medical, billing, and administrative information within the health care systems. In addition, standardized code sets are vital under HIPAA for accurate and efficient electronic data interchange for diagnoses, procedures, and drugs. Overall, these standards are expected to reduce the administrative burdens on health care plans and providers by eliminating the estimated 400 different claim formats currently in use, and ultimately save the country's health care system $30 billion over the next 10 years.

The final rule concerning transaction standards and code sets was implemented in October 2000. Compliance was required by October 2002, although small health care plans had until October 2003 to comply. However, passage of H.R. 3323, Public Law 107-105 (also known as the Administrative Simplification Compliance Act) on January 3, 2002, delayed the implementation date for a year. Entities were able to receive the one-year extension, but only if they submitted a plan that showed how they would achieve compliance within the year.

On March 29, 2002, CMS released a model compliance plan to meet the extension requirements; a covered entity was able to submit its extension plan electronically through the CMS web site, and CMS provided an electronic confirmation of their receipt of the plan. Covered entities also had the option of submitting their own version of an extension plan on paper, but the downside to that approach is that they would receive no confirmation back from CMS that they had received it. Covered entities that did not submit a compliance plan (except for small health plans) needed to be compliant by the original date of October 16, 2002.

To discourage the return to the use of paper claims, entities are required to submit electronic, HIPAA-compliant claims to Medicare. The law does contain a provision to exempt providers with no electronic claims submission capability and small providers with less than 25 full-time employees for facilities and 10 for physician practices from this requirement.

Medicare and Medicaid claims need to be filed electronically by the October 2003 transactions set deadline with the exception of those claims that must be dropped to paper due to the use of unspecified codes. No specific information has been provided to deal with this situation. This latter situation becomes more problematic in light of the fact that the $1.50 per paper claim surcharge appears to be back in the picture.

These standards must be adopted by all government health care plans, including Medicare, Medicaid, the Military Health System for active duty and civilian personnel, and the health information programs of the Indian Health Service and the Veterans Administration. In addition, all private sector health plans (except certain small, self-administered plans) must use these standards, including managed care organization and ERISA plans, health care clearinghouses, and all health care providers who elect to submit or receive electronic transactions. The standards apply to electronic data interchange (EDI) only. They are not applicable to data that is stored, which can be in any format as long as it can be translated into the standard transaction format when necessary.

Although health care clearinghouses are required to comply with the standards, they may accept transactions that are not standardized in order to translate them into standard transactions for customers to send, or they may receive standard transactions and translate them into nonstandard formats for customers.

Use of these standards does not mean that a health plan has to change its payment policies. Although health plans have to accept and process bills submitted in the standard format, they do not have to provide benefits for any service or item that would not be paid prior to implementation of the standards, such as noncovered cosmetic procedures.

These standards are applicable to the following types of transactions:

- Health care claims and equivalent encounter information
- Enrollment and disenrollment in a health care plan
- Health insurance plan eligibility
- Health care payment and remittance advice
- Health insurance plan premium payments
- Health care claim status
- Certification and authorization of referrals
- Coordination of benefits

Although HIPAA also requires electronic submission standards for the first report of injury, these will be adopted at a future date. In addition, a standard for the electronic transmission of health care claims attachments will also be adopted.

The Health Insurance Portability and Accountability Act (HIPAA) of 1996

All of the transaction standards were created by standards development organizations in the private sector. With the exception of the retail pharmacy standards, all are from the Accredited Standards Committee. For purposes of electronic transactions, version 4010 of ANSI ASC X12N was selected.

The standards for retail pharmacy transactions are from the National Council for Prescription Drug Programs (NCPDP) since these standards are currently in widespread use. A February 20, 2003 final rule authorized the National Council for Prescription Drug Program's Telecommunication Standard Implementation Guide, version 5, release 1 (version 5.1), September 1999, and equivalent NCPDP Batch Standard Batch Implementation Guide, version 1, release 1 (version 1.1), January 2000, as the standards for transactions for the retail pharmacy sector.

Code Sets

The standard medical code sets, which are already in use by most health plans, health care clearinghouses, and health care providers, include:

- **ICD-9-CM, Volumes 1 and 2** (including the official ICD-9-CM guidelines for coding and reporting): required for diseases, injuries, impairments, other health problems and manifestations, and causes of injuries, diseases, impairments, and other health problems

- **ICD-9-CM, Volume 3** (including the official ICD-9-CM guidelines for coding and reporting): required for reporting diagnostic, preventive, therapeutic, or management procedures or actions taken by hospitals on inpatients

- **CPT**: required for reporting physician and other health care services

- **HCPCS Level II**: required for reporting physician and other health care services, equipment, supplies, substances, and other items used for health care services

- **CDT-4 (Current Dental Terminology)**: required for reporting dental services

- **National Drug Codes (NDC)**: required for reporting drugs and biologics by retail pharmacies

Reimbursement Guidelines

Many providers attempt to furnish items of DMEPOS as a convenience to their patients. Providers also furnish DMEPOS items to ensure that the proper application or fit of those items is achieved for maximum medical benefit to their patients. Very few providers actually proceed into DMEPOS dispensing with the idea that this activity will result in big profits. In this environment of stiff provider competition, however, the practice with an expansive service base will likely attract a larger and steadier patient base than a similar practice with a more limited scope of service. The one-stop shopping approach for medical services is a powerful tool in creating high patient volume and maintaining the fiscal health of the practice. This business principle is also true of DMEPOS supplier facilities.

DMEPOS Utilization and Authorization

Utilization, one of the most significant factors in the cost of medical care, is the primary focus of managed care and DMEPOS industry interface. To help control member utilization, the typical managed care policy requires the MCO member to obtain a provider order for any DMEPOS item. Under some MCO stipulations, this order can be generated by the treating specialist, who in turn must notify the MCO and receive authorization to either (1) dispense the item directly to the patient, or (2) allow the patient to obtain the item from a supplier. Under other MCO rules, the order for the DMEPOS must be routed from the specialist to the provider for approval, and then the MCO must be notified by the provider for final approval.

Prior authorizations, preauthorizations, and precertifications are mandatory (and many times burdensome) communications with the MCO generally required for performing special services (such as surgical procedures), making referrals, treating a patient in the emergency department (ED) admitting a patient to a skilled nursing facility, and ordering DMEPOS. This policy mandate affects all participating provider offices and involved suppliers as well.

Once approval is obtained from the MCO for the DMEPOS item, an authorization number or form is given to the provider. Providers should insist on receiving the MCO's permission in writing to obtain the DMEPOS item. The provider, whether a PCP or a specialist, must then contact the approved supplier and furnish the information necessary for DMEPOS dispensation. The supplier will need the patient's personal data (name, date of birth, address, etc.) and insurance information. In many cases, the supplier may also need information such as the following:

- Type of DMEPOS item with specific characteristics, if appropriate
- Patient's diagnosis
- Patient's prognosis
- Length of time the DMEPOS is needed (for items such as oxygen)
- Written physician order, personally signed and dated

These special reimbursement provisions clarify three basic facts:

- Which services and items are covered when pre-authorization is obtained from the plan
- Which services and items are specifically excluded
- Who is responsible for payment for excluded or noncovered items or services, and for covered items or services denied as not medically necessary when the patient has been given advance written notice of the probable denial

By signing the advance notice (similar to the Medicare program's ABN), the patient waives the provider's or supplier's liability and acknowledges financial responsibility for the item or service furnished. Obtaining the signed advance notice form ahead of time also ensures smoother claims processing and patient billing, as all facets of the process are known. If the claim is submitted to the carrier for a noncovered or not medically necessary item or service, a denial will ensue. Patients who signed the liability waiver notice in advance are aware of their financial obligation and can be billed on the date of service (for noncovered items) or after the carrier's denial is received (for items deemed not medically necessary).

PPS and Consolidated Billing

In an effort to contain costs, CMS has been instituting prospective payment systems (PPS) for each of its covered types of services. Acute care hospitals stays are reimbursed by diagnosis-related groups (DRGs). The payment is based on the patient's diagnoses, age, and procedures performed. The majority of the services provided to the hospital inpatient are covered in that one payment to the hospital.

CMS has expanded its cost containment efforts. A prospective payment system based on resource utilization was put into place for Skilled Nursing Facilities (SNFs) in 1999. A prospective payment system based on resource utilization for Home Health Agencies (HHAs) was instituted in 2000. Other PPS reimbursement plans have been instituted for hospital outpatients, long term acute care hospitals, and rehabilitation hospitals.

Customized prosthetic devices are excluded from these requirements for all PPS payments. A number of other items and services that are considered DMEPOS are included. Among the included items are ostomy supplies, surgical dressings, drugs, and some equipment.

Suppliers need to know the mechanics of the programs if they are going to enter into agreements with the SNF or HHA to provide DMEPOS. They also need to know what to do if their routine customer is now receiving SNF level services or HHA services.

Skilled Nursing Facilities

The consolidated billing requirement confers on the SNF the billing responsibility for the entire package of care that residents receive during a covered Part A SNF stay and physical, occupational, and speech therapy services received during a non-covered stay.

Exception: there are a limited number of services specifically excluded from consolidated billing and therefore separately payable.

For Medicare beneficiaries in a covered Part A stay, these separately payable services are:

- Physician's professional services
- Certain dialysis-related services, including covered ambulance transportation to obtain the dialysis services
- All ambulance services except when a medically necessary transport from one SNF to another SNF occurs, when the beneficiary is discharged from the first SNF and admitted to the second, and covered ambulance transportation to obtain dialysis
- Erythropoietin for certain dialysis patients
- Chemotherapy
- Chemotherapy administration services
- Radioisotope services
- Customized prosthetic devices
- Hospital's "facility charge" in connection with clinic services of a physician
- Certain cardiac catheterizations
- Certain computerized axial tomography (CT) scans
- Certain magnetic resonance imaging (MRIs)
- Certain radiation therapies
- Certain angiographies and lymphatic and venous procedures
- Emergency services
- Certain ambulatory surgeries involving the use of a hospital operating room
- Hospice care related to a beneficiary's terminal illness
- Screening services

A Part A covered stay means that the resident or patient meets Medicare coverage guidelines that deem they are receiving a skilled level of care. The patient's medical condition, potential for improvement, the intensity of the services provided, and their ability to perform daily functions are among the issues that are taken into account when determining if a patient is receiving skilled levels of care. Many long-term residents in SNFs or nursing homes are not receiving Medicare skilled levels of care. However even a long-term resident may have a status change that can change their level of care. A resident may have a cerebral vascular accident or may fall and break a bone. The resident would most likely be transferred to an acute care hospital. Upon the resident's return, they would probably qualify for skilled levels of care.

The SNF receives an all-inclusive payment for Part A covered stays. This payment depends on the resource utilization group (RUGs) to which their situation falls. The payment is intended to cover all services except those listed above. The payment does not change based upon the cost of the items or services.

Many DMEPOS supplies and some devices or equipment may not be billed separately by the SNF or by any other provider or supplier. These certain DMEPOS items are considered a part of the nursing home's PPS reimbursement. The supplier should bill the nursing home for these items and should have a formal agreement with the home for payment of these items.

If a patient in a nursing home is not receiving a skilled level of care and is not being reimbursed under Part A, then the supplier has a choice. Billing may be submitted directly by the supplier or may be submitted by the nursing home. Suppliers should have an agreement with the nursing home specifying which party will bill in these situations. Such an agreement will eliminate duplicate billing and concerns related to fraud and abuse. Only one party should submit the bill for the service. Do not bill the nursing home and then bill the DME MAC if the nursing home is taking too long to pay.

Home Health Agencies

CMS has a PPS program in place for Home Health Agencies (HHAs). Resource utilization groups take into account the patient's medical condition and the intensity of the services performed among other things to group HHA patients. If the patient is under a plan of care, many of the DMEPOS items should be billed to the Home Health Agency (HHA). The supplies are considered a part of the HHA's PPS reimbursement. The supplier should bill the HHA for these items and should have a formal agreement with the home for payment of these items.

The HHA must have its own physician order for the DMEPOS item. This is true even if the supplier has a long-standing order to supply an item, such as ostomy supplies to a patient or customer. Many DMEPOS items must be provided under an arrangement. If the supplier was unaware of the HHA services and there is no agreement with the HHA about the provision of the ostomy supplies, the supplies will not be reimbursed by any party. The patient has a freedom of choice that allows them to accept the HHA services. At that point, the HHA becomes responsible for all related care including the provision of many DMEPOS items.

If the patient is not on a plan of care or is not receiving Part A reimbursable services, the supplier may still be required to bill the HHA. Many DMEPOS items are subject to consolidated billing regulations. This means that the HHA must submit all charges for these services. The HHA will receive additional payment for these items. The supplier should bill the HHA for these items and should probably have an agreement with the home for payment of these items.

Applicable Consolidated Billing

The types of services, supplies, and equipment subject to consolidated billing regulations vary for SNFs and for HHAs. SNF regulations also vary depending upon whether the patient is receiving a skilled level of care and is covered under PPS. These items are usually listed by HCPCS code.

A provider or supplier may not be aware of changes in the customer's medical condition or types of care unless the supplier actively tracks all of their patients or customers. Even then, it may be difficult to make a determination. The supplier may only become aware of the issue upon receipt of a denial from the DME MAC. If the supplier routinely supplies nursing home or SNF patients, the supplier should work out an agreement with the SNF that would alert them prior to billing when billing should be sent to the SNF instead of the DMERC.

Financial Management Guidelines

This section of the Coders' Desk Reference for HCPCS reviews important areas of DMEPOS dispensing that every provider's practice and supplier's office should be intimately familiar with. Applying these formulas, tips, and guidelines will help to monitor profit and loss, and ultimately help the DMEPOS provider and supplier remain profitable.

DMEPOS dispensers should have knowledge of or develop the following:

- Financial formulas related to medical care used to regularly monitor the charges and reimbursements for DMEPOS items and services furnished

- Business formulas to monitor overhead and associated expenses

- Tips on how to perform a cost study and a reimbursement analysis

- Guidelines for doing a managed-care viability analysis to determine a managed-care plan's contribution or detriment to the business's bottom line; this should be done for both regular capitation or fee-for-service scenarios and for managed-care contracts that include DMEPOS as a carve-out service

- A checklist of simple office controls for tighter financial management

Financial Formulas

Financial management for DMEPOS providers and suppliers has become quite complicated over the past several years. A great deal of financial management concern has been placed on the numerous managed-care plans with which the DMEPOS provider and supplier must participate.

The DMEPOS provider and supplier must regularly monitor the financial trends of each health insurance plan they contract with by conducting a basic financial analysis of collections and accounts receivable (A/R). The fundamental structure of collections and A/R analysis begins with three key financial elements:

- Charges
- Adjustments
- Payments

Every provider and supplier's office should generate monthly financial information in these areas, either by a computerized billing system or by manual bookkeeping reports. These key elements, when used in the basic formulas provided in this section, will provide a snapshot of the provider and supplier's financial strength or weakness in terms of collections and A/R status.

Conducting Cost and Reimbursement Analyses

Becoming or remaining profitable when furnishing patients with DMEPOS items involves monitoring all aspects of the financial investment made to furnish those items. Patient charges, mandatory health insurance adjustments, and other types of adjustments and insurance and patient payments (reimbursements) must be meticulously followed and studied. Becoming or remaining profitable also involves tracking all associated costs for dispensing DMEPOS items. These costs are easy to track, and include a range of considerations from the actual purchase price of the DMEPOS item to the costs of any supplies used in furnishing the item. The payer must track reimbursement for the DMEPOS items because the profit margin for a single item of DMEPOS can vary greatly between one payer and another.

A cost and reimbursement analysis should be performed at least every six months, and no less than once every year.

DMEPOS Cost Study

The costs of furnishing DMEPOS items must be closely monitored, as many times escalating costs can out-rise reimbursement for those items, thereby nullifying any potential profits. If all of the costs are not tracked alongside the reimbursements, a deceptively healthy financial picture surrounding DMEPOS dispensing activities can emerge, fooling providers and suppliers into thinking the DMEPOS profit center is fiscally sound.

Typical costs associated with furnishing DMEPOS to patients, for both providers and suppliers, include the following:

- Actual item purchase price
- Shipping and freight charges
- Taxes
- Physician or provider time involved in the dispensation process
- Staff time involved in the dispensation process
- Office or medical supplies expended when ordering, receiving, and furnishing the items

Most of the information needed to perform the cost study is taken directly from the invoices for the DMEPOS items. Using a computerized spreadsheet gives the provider or supplier the ability to assign formulas to each cell for automatic calculations, resulting in a re-calculation of each DMEPOS item. This makes it convenient to keep all information current and to perform the study on a semi-annual basis. Many DMEPOS suppliers have software programs that can pull specific data fields, collate the data into a requested format, and dump the information into a report. In these cases, cost reports should be done more frequently than semi-annually simply because the convenience of obtaining this information makes it easier to monitor the cost data.

The final cost information for each DMEPOS item furnished, when considered in aggregate (the total number of each item dispensed on an annual basis), is the cost data that should be used in the final profit or loss determinations. Manufacturer and vendor discounts, such as that given for paying the amount due earlier than specified or those given when purchasing DMEPOS items in bulk, become important when considered on an annual basis. For example, a $2 early-pay discount received for each of 10 items paid early in one month (a total of $20 in savings) can add up to a considerable amount of savings over the space of a year.

The final calculated cost of each DMEPOS item should be organized by CPT or HCPCS Level II code and associated code description (instead of patient name, account number, etc.) for easy interface with reimbursement data. This will facilitate the next step in the financial analysis process—conducting a reimbursement analysis.

DMEPOS Reimbursement Analysis

The reimbursement analysis is the final portion of the financial management analysis needed to determine a particular DMEPOS item's profit or loss margin. Simply stated, the cost data are compared against the reimbursement information and a determination is made.

Reimbursement data for DMEPOS can come from a variety of sources, including the following:

- Health insurance payments (third-party payers, Medicare, Medicaid, managed-care plans, workers compensation carriers, private or self-funded plans)
- Patient copayments
- Patient coinsurance amounts (secondary insurance payments)
- Other patient payments (in the cases of insurance denials, noncovered items, self-pay patients, etc.)

The reimbursement analysis must also contain pertinent adjustment information, such as mandatory participating provider or supplier adjustments, courtesy and professional adjustments, and bad debt and charity write-offs.

Reimbursement information is obtained from the health insurance explanations of benefit forms (EOBs) or the explanations of Medicare benefit forms (EOMBs) that accompany each payment. These forms can vary widely in the type of payment information provided, but most will supply the following:

- The patient's name
- Plan identification number
- Provider's or supplier's name
- Provider's or supplier's plan identification number
- Date of service
- CPT or HCPCS Level II code for the DMEPOS item
- Modifier, if reported
- Diagnosis code linked to the CPT or HCPCS Level II code
- The provider's or supplier's charge
- The amount to be adjusted
- Patient copayment/coinsurance amounts
- Amount reimbursed

Some EOBs may only contain the patient and provider's or supplier's names, date of service, a description of the DMEPOS item and the amounts charged, adjusted, and reimbursed. In addition, most EOBs/EOMBs will note any amount applicable to the patient's annual deductible.

Reimbursement data is also obtained from the patient accounts for copayment and coinsurance amounts paid, deductibles collected, and retrieval of self-pay patient information. Self-pay patient information also includes patients with health insurance who, because the insurance did not cover the DMEPOS item, have paid for the item out of pocket when appropriate.

Like the cost study, the reimbursement analysis is set up in a spreadsheet format. The easiest method of setting up the spreadsheet is to arrange the CPT or HCPCS Level II codes and item descriptions horizontally (in the spreadsheet bars), from left to right, with the payer, charge, adjustment, and reimbursement information running vertically in the columns. Reimbursement for the items, whether received from the patient or from insurance carriers, must be tracked (entered onto the spreadsheet) by payer and CPT or HCPCS Level II code to dovetail with the previously collected cost data. DMEPOS volume data must be entered onto the spreadsheet as well to account for the number of specific items purchased and dispensed during the time period being studied.

Additional spreadsheets can be added when space does not allow for all of the information to be entered onto one spreadsheet.

Costs and Reimbursements

All of the information is to be considered individually and in aggregate when assessing the value of dispensing items of DMEPOS. In making the final determination, providers and suppliers should weigh the necessity of dispensing items against not dispensing items, especially if the items carry a significant margin of loss. This financial data must be assessed for each item of DMEPOS against such factors as:

- The item's necessity to other related DMEPOS items that carry a significant profit margin (supplies needed when using a certain DME apparatus)
- The possible loss of business because the patient prefers to obtain the related DME elsewhere, where all of the necessary DMEPOS items are available
- The impact of striking various unprofitable DMEPOS items from the service menu, thereby restricting provider options, forcing them to refer their patients to other suppliers

Glossary

An increasingly complex reimbursement climate means new terminology develops every year. The following glossary includes terms not only used when coding, it includes terms used by major insurers and the federal government.

AAPA. American Academy of Physician Assistants.

AAPC. American Academy of Professional Coders. National organization for coders and billers offering certification (CPC, CPC-H, and CPC-P) based upon physician-, outpatient facility-, or payer-specific guidelines.

AAPCC. Adjusted average per capita cost. Estimated average cost of Medicare benefits for an individual, based upon criteria including age, sex, institutional status, Medicaid, disability, and end-stage renal failure.

AAPPO. American Association of Preferred Provider Organizations.

abduction. Pulling away from a central reference line, such as moving away from the midline of the body.

abduction pillow. Device that immobilizes the hips and legs of hip surgery patients postoperatively.

ABN. Advance beneficiary notice.

abstractor. Person who selects and extracts specific data from the medical record and enters the information into computer files.

accrual. Amount of money set aside to cover a health care benefit plan's expenses based upon estimates using a combination of data, including the claims system and the plan's prior history.

ACLS. Advanced cardiac life support. Certification for health care professionals who have achieved proficiency in providing emergent care of cardiac and respiratory systems and medication management.

ACR. 1) American College of Radiology. 2) Adjusted community rate, calculation of what premium the plan charges to provide Medicare-covered benefits for greater frequency of use by participants.

ACR. 1) American College of Radiology. 2) Adjusted community rate, calculation of what premium the plan charges to provide Medicare-covered benefits for greater frequency of use by participants.

activities of daily living. Self-care activities often used to determine a patient's level of function such as bathing, dressing, using a toilet, transferring in and out of bed or a chair, continence, eating, and walking.

actuarial assumptions. Characteristics used in calculating the risks and costs of a plan, including age, sex, and occupation of enrollees; location; utilization rates; and service costs.

adduction. Pulling toward a central reference line, such as toward the midline of the body.

adjudication. Processing and review of a submitted claim resulting in payment, partial payment, or denial. In relationship to judicial hearings, it is the process of hearing and settling a case through an objective, judicial procedure.

admission. Formal acceptance of a patient by a health care facility.

ADS. Alternative delivery system. Any health care delivery system other than traditional fee-for-service.

advance beneficiary notice. Written communication with a Medicare beneficiary given before Part B services are rendered, informing the patient that the provider (including independent laboratories, physicians, practitioners, and suppliers) believes Medicare will not pay for some or all of the services to be rendered. Form CMS-R-131 form may be used for all situations where Medicare payment is expected to be denied. This revised form has been effective since March 1, 2009 and replaces the ABN-G (Form CMS-R-131G), ABN-L (Form CMS-R-131L), and NEMB (Form CMS-20007). (Note: Skilled nursing facilities (SNF) must use the revised ABN for items/services expected to be denied under Medicare Part B only.)

adverse selection. In health care contracting, the risk of enrolling members who are sicker than assumed and who will utilize expensive services more frequently.

age restriction. In health care contracting, limitation of benefits when a patient reaches a certain age.

age/sex rating. In health care contracting, structuring capitation payments based on members' ages and genders.

aggregate amount. Contracted maximum for which a member is insured for any single event in a health plan.

AHA. American Hospital Association. Health care industry association that represents the concerns of institutional providers. The AHA hosts the National Uniform Billing Committee (NUBC), which has a formal consultative role under HIPAA. The AHA also publishes <i>Coding Clinic for ICD-9-CM.</i>

AHIMA. American Health Information Management Association. Association of health information management professionals that offers professional and educational services, providing these certifications: RHIA, RHIT, CCS, CCS-P, CCA, CHDA, and CHPS.

Al-Anon, Alateen. Alcoholic support groups.

ALOS. Average length of stay. Utilization benchmark average compiled from the actual number of inpatient days calculated using factors such as geographical location and diagnosis.

AMA. American Medical Association. Professional organization for physicians. The AMA is the secretariat of the National Uniform Claim Committee (NUCC), which has a formal consultative role under HIPAA. The AMA also maintains the Current Procedural Terminology (CPT) coding system.

ambulatory surgery. Surgical procedure in which the patient is admitted, treated, and released on the same day.

AMCRA. American Managed Care Review Association.

AMLOS. Arithmetic mean length of stay. Average number of days patients within a given DRG stay in the hospital. The AMLOS is used to determine payment for outlier cases and to predict occupancy rates.

ANA. American Nursing Association.

AOA. American Osteopathic Association.

AP-DRG. All patient diagnosis-related group. 3M HIS made revisions and adjustments to the DRG system, now referred to as the All Patient DRGs. Early features of AP-DRGs included MDC 24, specifically devoted to HIV, and restructuring of the major diagnostic categories governing newborns.

APA. American Psychiatric Association.

APG. Ambulatory patient group. Reimbursement methodology developed for the Centers for Medicare and Medicaid Services.

apnea. Absence of breathing or breath.

apnea monitor. Device used to monitor breathing during sleep that sounds an alarm if breathing stops for more than the specified amount of time.

appeal. Specific request made to a payer for reconsideration of a denial or adverse coverage or payment decision and potential restriction of benefit reimbursement.

appropriateness of care. Proper setting of medical care that best meets the patient's care or diagnosis, as defined by a health care plan or other legal entity.

APR. Average payment rate. Amount of money CMS could pay an HMO for services provided to Medicare recipients under a risk contract.

ART. Accredited record technician. Former AHIMA certification describing medical records practitioners; now known as a registered health information technician (RHIT).

AS. Associate of Science.

ASN. Associate of Science, Nursing.

ASO. Administrative services only. Contractual agreement between a self-funded plan and an insurance company in which the insurance company assumes no risk and provides administrative services only.

assignment. In medical reimbursement, the arrangement in which the provider submits the claim on behalf of the patient and is reimbursed directly by the patient's plan. By doing so, the provider agrees to accept what the plan pays.

assignment of benefits. Authorization from the patient allowing the third-party payer to pay the provider directly for medical services. Under Medicare, an assignment is an agreement by the hospital or physician to accept Medicare's payment as the full payment and not to bill the patient for any amounts over the allowance amount, except for deductible and/or coinsurance amounts or noncovered services.

at risk. In medical reimbursement, a type of contract between Medicare and a payer or a payer and a provider in which the payer (in the case of Medicare) and the provider (in the case of the payer contracts) gets paid a set amount for care of a patient base. If costs exceed the amount the payer or provider were paid, the patients still receive care during the term of the contract.

attained age. In medical reimbursement, the age of the member as of the last birthday.

auditor. Professional who evaluates a provider's utilization, quality of care, or level of reimbursement.

AWP. *1)* Average wholesale price. Pharmaceutical price based on common data that is included in a pharmacy provider contract. *2)* Any willing provider. Describing statutes requiring a provider network to accept any provider who meets the network's usual selection criteria.

backlog. In medical reimbursement, the queue of claims that have not been adjudicated.

balance billing. Arrangement prohibited in Medicare regulations and some payer contracts whereby a provider bills the patient for charges not reimbursed by the payer.

basic coverage. Insurance providing coverage for hospital care.

basic health services. Defined set of benefits all federally qualified HMOs must offer enrollees.

BCBS. Blue Cross Blue Shield.

binder. Broad bandage that supports a body part.

board certification. Certification in a particular specialty based on the physician's demonstration of expertise and experience.

boarder. Individual who receives lodging, such as a parent, caregiver, or other family member, who is not a patient but may wish or need to be near the patient.

boarder baby. *1)* Newborn that remains in the nursery following discharge because the mother is still hospitalized. *2)* Premature infant who no longer needs intensive care but who remains for observation or to reach developmental milestones.

book of business. Payer's list of clients and contracts.

brace. Orthotic device that supports, in correct position, any moveable body part, and allows for limited movement. Medicare has a strict definition of a brace that includes only rigid or semirigid devices.

BSN. Bachelor of Science, Nursing.

Buck traction. Type of skin traction of the extremities maintained by using an apparatus such as a special splint, applied by dressings to the affected body part. Buck traction may be used on burn patients to hold the arm in a suspended upward position to prevent swelling, reduce skin shrinkage, and allow for greater range of motion with healing.

bundled. *1)* Gathering of several types of health insurance policies under a single payer. *2)* Inclusive grouping of codes related to a procedure when submitting a claim.

business coalition. Employers who form a cooperative to purchase health care less expensively.

cafeteria plan. Employer's offer of various services of many payers as separate elements in a health care plan.

Cap. *1)* Capitation. *2)* Contract maximum.

capitation. Contractual agreement whereby the provider is paid a fixed amount for treating enrolled patients regardless of utilization.

care unit. Specific department or facility within a hospital or long-term care facility designed and staffed for treating a particular type of patient.

carve-out. Medical benefits for a specific type of care considered covered by separate guidelines or not covered by the payer.

case management. Ongoing review of cases by professionals to assure the most appropriate utilization of services

case manager. Medical professional (usually a nurse or social worker) who reviews cases every few days to determine necessity of care and to advise providers on payers' utilization restrictions. Certifies ongoing care.

case mix index. Sum of all DRG relative weights for cases over a given period of time, divided by the number of Medicare cases.

casting. Material used for encasing a body part to immobilize it for injury repair; usually made from plaster or fiberglass.

casting tape. Material used for molding casts, usually made from fiberglass, but can be composed of plaster strips.

catastrophic case management. Method of reviewing ongoing cases in which the patient sustains catastrophic or extremely costly medical problems.

catchment area. Geographical area from which a health care organization draws its members.

CC. Complication or comorbid condition.

CCU. Coronary care unit. Facility dedicated to patients suffering from heart attack, stroke, or other serious cardiopulmonary problems.

CDC. Centers for Disease Control and Prevention.

census. In medical reimbursement, number and demographics of patients or members

Certificate of Medical Necessity. Form required by Medicare to establish the medical necessity of certain DMEPOS. It is completed by both the physician and the supplier, detailing the medical diagnosis and other information specific to the device ordered.

certification. Approval by a payer's case manager to continue care for a given number of days or visits.

CFR. Code of Federal Regulations.

cherry picking. In medical reimbursement, the practice of enrolling only healthy individuals and excluding those with existing problems.

chief complaint. In medical documentation, the presenting problem bringing the patient to the health encounter.

churning. 1) Performance-based reimbursement system emphasizing provider productivity. 2) When a provider sees a patient more than medically necessary with the intent of generating more revenue.

Civilian Health and Medical Program of the Uniformed Services. Federal program that covered the health benefits for families of all uniformed service employees. The program has been replaced by TRICARE.

CLA. Certified laboratory assistant.

claim. Statement of services rendered requesting payment from an insurance company or a government entity.

claim lag. Time incurred between the date of a claim and its submission for payment. *c. manual* Administrative guidelines used by claims processors to adjudicate claims according to company policy and procedure.

claim manual. Administrative guidelines used by claims processors to adjudicate claims according to company policy and procedure.

claims manager. Payer's manager who oversees the employee who processes routine claims.

claims reviewer. Payer employee who reviews claims like an auditor, looking at coding, prior authority, contract violations, etc.

CLIA. Clinical Laboratory Improvement Amendments. Requirements set in 1988, CLIA imposes varying levels of federal regulations on clinical procedures. Few laboratories, including those in physician offices, are exempt. Adopted by Medicare and Medicaid, CLIA regulations redefine laboratory testing in regard to laboratory certification and accreditation, proficiency testing, quality assurance, personnel standards, and program administration.

closed claim. Claim for which all apparent benefits have been paid.

closed panel. Arrangement in which a managed care organization contracts providers on an exclusive basis, restricting the providers from seeing patients enrolled in other payers' plans.

closed treatment. Realignment of a fracture or dislocation without surgically opening the skin to reach the site. Treatment methods employed include with or without manipulation, and with or without traction.

CMA. Certified medical assistant.

CMI. Case mix index. Sum of all DRG relative weights, divided by the number of Medicare cases. A low CMI may denote DRG assignments that do not adequately reflect the resources used to treat Medicare patients.

CMN. Certificate of medical necessity.

CMP. Competitive medical plan. Federal designation allowing plans to obtain eligibility to receive a Medicare risk contract without having to qualify as an HMO.

CMS. Centers for Medicare and Medicaid Services. Federal agency that administers the public health programs.

CMS-1500. Universal form used to file professional claims.

CMT. Certified medical transcriptionist.

COA. Certificate of authority. State license to operate as an HMO.

COB. Coordination of benefits. In health care contracting, method of integrating benefits payable when there is more than one group insurance plan so that the insured's benefits and the payment of insurance benefits from all sources do not exceed 100 percent of the allowed medical expenses.

COBRA. Consolidated Omnibus Reconciliation Act. Federal law that allows and requires past employees to be covered under company health insurance plans for a set premium, allowing individuals to remain insured when their current plan or position has been terminated.

coder. Professional who translates documented, written diagnoses and procedures into numeric and alphanumeric codes.

coding conventions. Each space, typeface, indentation, and punctuation mark determining how ICD-9-CM codes are interpreted. These conventions were developed to help match correct codes to the diagnoses documented.

coinsurance. Percentage of the allowed charges paid by a beneficiary toward the cost of care.

collagen. Protein based substance of strength and flexibility that is the major component of connective tissue, found in cartilage, bone, tendons, and skin.

collar. Device that encircles the neck to immobilize it, provide support, and/or severely limit its mobility.

commercial carriers. For-profit insurance companies issuing health coverage.

common working file. System of local databases containing total beneficiary histories developed by CMS to improve Medicare claims processing. Medicare fiscal intermediaries, and/or carriers, interact with these databases to obtain data on eligibility, utilization, Medicare secondary payer (MSP), and other detailed claims information.

community rating. Methodology of state and federal governments that require qualified HMOs to request the same amount of money for each member in a plan.

comorbidity. Preexisting condition that causes an increase in length of stay by at least one day in approximately 75 percent of cases. Used in DRG reimbursement.

comparative performance report. Report that provides an annual comparison of a physician's services and procedures with those of another physician in the same specialty and geographic area.

complex repair. Surgical closure of a wound requiring more than layered closure of the deeper subcutaneous tissue and fascia (i.e., debridement, scar excision, placement of stents or retention sutures, and sometimes site preparation or undermining that creates the defect requiring complex closure).

complication. Condition arising after the beginning of observation and treatment that modifies the course of the patient's illness or the medical care required, or an undesired result or misadventure in medical care.

component code. In CCI, the code following the comprehensive code that cannot be charged to Medicare when the comprehensive code is charged.

component coding. Coding a service that represents only a portion of the entire service provided, meant to standardize the reporting of interventional radiology services. Component coding allows a physician, regardless of specialty, to specifically identify and report those aspects of the service he or she provided, whether the procedural component, the radiological component, or both.

comprehensive codes. Code behind which component codes fall.

consultation. Advice or opinion regarding diagnosis and treatment or determination to accept transfer of care of a patient rendered by a medical professional at the request of the primary care provider.

continuity of coverage. In health care contracting, transfer of benefits from one plan to another without a lapse in coverage.

continuous positive airway pressure device. Pressurized device used to maintain the patient's airway for spontaneous or mechanically aided breathing. Often used for patients with mild to moderate sleep apnea.

contractor. Entity who enters into a contractual agreement with CMS to service a component of the Medicare program administration, for example, fiscal intermediaries, carriers, program safeguard coordinators.

conversion. In health care contracting, shifting a member under a group contract to an individual contract in accordance with contract terms and occurring with a change in employer benefits or when the covered person leaves the group.

conversion factor. *1)* Dollar value for each relative value unit. When this dollar amount is multiplied by the total relative value units, it yields the reimbursement rate for the service. *2)* National multiplier that converts the geographically adjusted relative value units into Medicare fee schedule dollar amounts that applies to all services paid under the MFS.

coordinated care. In health care contracting, system of health care delivery that influences utilization, quality of care, and cost of services. Managed care integrates financing and management with an employed or contracted organized provider network that delivers services to an enrolled population.

copayment. Cost-sharing arrangement in which a covered person pays a specified portion of allowed charges. In relation to Medicare, the copayment designates the specific dollar amount that the patient must pay and coinsurance designates the percentage of allowed charges.

correct coding initiative. Official list of codes from the Centers for Medicare and Medicaid Services' (CMS) National Correct Coding Policy Manual for Part B Medicare Carriers that identifies services considered an integral part of a comprehensive code or mutually exclusive of it.

corridor deductible. Fixed out-of-pocket amount the member must pay before benefits are available.

COT. Certified ophthalmic technician.

COTA. Certified occupational therapy assistant.

counseling. Discussion with a patient and/or family concerning one or more of the following areas: diagnostic results, impressions, and/or recommended diagnostic studies; prognosis; risks and benefits of management (treatment) options; instructions for management (treatment) and/or follow-up; importance of compliance with chosen management (treatment) options; risk factor reduction; and patient and family education.

Coverage Issues Manual. Revised and renamed the National Coverage Determination Manual in the CMS manual system, it contained national coverage decisions and specific medical items, services, treatment procedures, or technologies paid for under the Medicare program. This manual has been converted to the Medicare National Coverage Determinations Manual (NCD manual), Pub. 100-03.

covered charges. Charges for medical care and supplies that are medically necessary and met coverage and program guidelines.

covered person. Any person entitled to benefits under the policy, whether a member or dependent.

CPR. Computerized patient record. Computer application that allows all or most elements of a patient's medical record to be stored in a computerized database.

CPT. Current Procedural Terminology. Definitive procedural coding system developed by the American Medical Association that lists descriptive terms and identifying codes to provide a uniform language that describes medical, surgical, and diagnostic services for nationwide communication among physicians, patients, and third parties, used in outpatient reporting of services.

CPT codes. Codes maintained and copyrighted by the AMA and selected for use under HIPAA for noninstitutional and nondental professional transactions.

CPT modifier. Two-character code used to indicate that a service was altered in some way from the stated CPT or HCPCS Level II description, but not enough to change the basic definition of the service.

credentialing. 1) Reviewing the medical degrees, licensure, malpractice, and any disciplinary record of medical providers for panel and quality assurance purposes and to grant hospital privileges. 2) Coding certification.

critical care. Treatment of critically ill patients in a variety of medical emergencies that requires the constant attendance of the physician (e.g., cardiac arrest, shock, bleeding, respiratory failure, postoperative complications, critically ill neonate).

CRNA. Certified registered nurse anesthetist. Nurse trained and specializing in the administration of anesthesia. Anesthesia services rendered by a CRNA must be reported with HCPCS Level II modifier QX, QY, or QZ.

crosswalk. Cross-referencing of CPT codes with ICD-9-CM, anesthesia, dental, or HCPCS Level II codes.

CRT. Certified respiratory therapist.

CSO. Clinical service organization. Health care organization developed by academic medical centers to integrate medical school, faculty practice plan, and hospital.

CST. Certified surgical technologist.

CTLSO. Cervical-thoracic-lumbar-sacral orthosis.

custom fitted. Premanufactured orthotics that can be adjusted to fit the patient by bending, trimming, or other minimal efforts.

cutback. Reduction of the amount or type of insurance for a member who attains a specified age or condition (e.g., age 65, retirement).

daily benefit. Specified maximum benefit payable for room and board charges at a hospital.

database. Electronic store of utilization information used by payers to pay claims, negotiate contracts, and track utilization and cost of services.

DAW. Dispense as written. Notation from a physician to a pharmacist requesting that the brand name medication be given in lieu of a generic medication.

days per thousand. Standard unit of measurement of utilization determined by calculating the number of hospital days used in a year for each 1,000 covered lives.

DC. 1) Doctor of chiropractic medicine. 2) Discontinue. 3) Direct current.

decapitation. Inadequate capitation.

decubitus ulcer. Progressively eroding skin lesion produced by inflamed necrotic tissue as it sloughs off caused by continual pressure to a localized area, especially over bony areas, where blood circulation is cut off when a patient lies still for too long without changing position.

deductible. Predetermined dollar amount of covered billed charges that the patient must pay toward the cost of care.

diagnosis. Determination or confirmation of a condition, disease, or syndrome and its implications.

diagnostic. Examination or procedure to which the patient is subjected, or which is performed on materials derived from a hospital outpatient, to obtain information to aid in the assessment of a medical condition or the identification of a disease. Among these examinations and tests are diagnostic laboratory services such as hematology and chemistry, diagnostic x-rays, isotope studies, EKGs, pulmonary function studies, thyroid function tests, psychological tests, and other tests given to determine the nature and severity of an ailment or injury.

direct claim payment. Method where members deal directly with the payer rather than submitting claims through the employer.

direct contract model. Plan that contracts directly with individual private practice physicians rather than through an intermediary.

disarticulation. Removal of a limb through a joint.

discharge plan. Treatment plan by the provider for continued patient care after discharge that may include home care, the services of case managers or other health care providers, or transfer to another facility.

discharge status. Disposition of the patient at discharge (e.g., left against medical advice, discharged home, transferred to an acute care hospital, expired).

discharge transfer. Discharge of a patient from one facility to another.

disposition of patient. Description of the patient's status and destination at discharge (e.g., discharged to home) used for data and quality assurance purposes.

DME. Durable medical equipment. Medical equipment that can withstand repeated use, is not disposable, is used to serve a medical purpose, is generally not useful to a person in the absence of a sickness or injury, and is appropriate for use in the home. Examples of durable medical equipment include hospital beds, wheelchairs, and oxygen equipment.

DME MAC. Durable medical equipment Medicare administrative contractor. Entity where claims for specific DMEPOS must be submitted for processing and reimbursement (instead of the Medicare contractor).

DMEPOS. Durable medical equipment, prosthetics, orthotics, and supplies.

DO. Doctor of osteopathy.

DOS. Date of service. In health care contracting, day the encounter or procedure is performed or the day a supply is issued.

DPM. Doctor of podiatric medicine.

DRG. Diagnosis related group. Method CMS uses to pay hospitals for Medicare recipients based on a statistical system of classifying any inpatient stay into one of several hundred groups. It is a classification scheme whose patient types are defined by patients' diagnoses or procedures and, in some cases, by the patient's age or discharge status. Each DRG is intended to be medically meaningful and would ordinarily require approximately equal resource consumption as measured by length of stay and cost.

drug formulary. List of prescription medications preferred for use by a health plan and dispensed through participating pharmacies to covered persons.

DSM-IV. Diagnostic and Statistical Manual of Mental Disorders, Fourth Edition. Manual used by mental health workers as the diagnostic coding system for substance abuse and mental health patients

dual option. Offering of an HMO and traditional plan by one carrier.

dual-lead device. Implantable cardiac device (pacemaker or implantable cardioverter-defibrillator [ICD]) in which pacing and sensing components are placed in only two chambers of the heart.

DUR. Drug utilization review. Review to assure prescribed medications are medically necessary and appropriate.

DVM. Doctor of Veterinary Medicine.

dynamic flexion device. Highly specialized orthotic brace that allows for a controlled range of motion of a joint or joints during postoperative or post-traumatic convalescence.

E code. ICD-9-CM diagnosis code that describes the circumstance that caused an injury, not the nature of the injury. E codes are used to classify external causes of injury, poisoning, or other adverse effects. An E code should not be used as a principal diagnosis because the intermediary will reject the claim.

e.g.. For example.

E/M. Evaluation and management services. Assessment, counseling, and other services provided to a patient and reported through CPT codes.

E/M service components. Key components in determining the correct level of E/M codes are history, examination, and medical decision-making.

EAP. Employee assistance program. Services designed to help employees, their family members, and employers find solutions for workplace and personal problems that affect morale, productivity, or financial issues such as workplace stress, family/marital concerns, legal or financial problems, elder care, child care, substance abuse, emotional/stress issues, and other daily living concerns.

ecchymosis. Bruise.

EdD. Doctor of education.

EDI. Electronic data interchange. Transference of claims, certifications, quality assurance reviews, and utilization data via computer in X12 format. May refer to any electronic exchange of formatted data.

EHO. Emerging healthcare organizations. Hospitals and other providers that are emerging or affiliating.

elective admission. Admission made at the discretion of the patient and facility based on available resources.

electronic media claim. Automated claims processing method that uses a data storage tool to transfer claims data to the payer. EMC has been replaced by electronic data interchange (EDI).

ELOS. Estimated length of stay. Average number of days of hospitalization required for a given illness or procedure, based on prior histories of patients who have been hospitalized for the same illness or procedure.

emergency admission. Admission in which the patient requires immediate medical or psychiatric attention because of life-threatening, severe, and potentially disabling conditions.

emergency department. Organized hospital-based facility for the provision of unscheduled episodic services to patients who present for immediate medical attention. The facility must be available 24 hours a day.

emergency outpatient. Patient admitted for diagnosis and treatment of a condition requiring immediate attention but who will not stay at that facility or be transferred to another.

EMT. Emergency medical technician.

EMT-P. Paramedic.

encoder. Computer application that assists in the assignment of a diagnosis or procedure code and may also assign reimbursement categories and values.

encounter. Direct personal contact between a registered hospital outpatient (in a medical clinic or emergency department, for example) and a physician (or other person authorized by state law and hospital bylaws to order or furnish services) for the diagnosis and treatment of an illness or injury. Visits with more than one health professional that take place during the same session and at a single location within the hospital are considered a single visit.

enrollee. In medical reimbursement, person who subscribes to a specific health plan.

enrollment. Number of lives covered by the plan.

enteral nutrition. Feeding of a nutrient mixture directly into or just proximal to the upper end of the small bowel via a tube or through an existing stoma. Patients are usually able to absorb the nutrients.

EOB. Explanation of benefits. Statement mailed to the member and provider explaining claim adjudication and payment.

EOMB. Explanation of Medicare benefits. Explanation of Medicaid benefits. Explanation of member benefits. Typically sent to the provider and the patient, an explanation of how Medicare, Medicaid, or member benefits were paid, that is, the allowable amount paid, the coinsurance due to the provider or payable by the patient, or the reason why a claim may have been rejected or paid less or more than the original amount charged.

episode of care. One or more health care services received during a period of relatively continuous care by a hospital or health care provider.

EPO. 1) Epoetin alpha. 2) Exclusive provider organization. In health care contracting, an organization similar to an HMO, but the member must remain within the provider network to receive benefits. EPOs are regulated under insurance statutes rather than HMO legislation.

EPO. Exclusive provider organization. In health care contracting, an organization similar to an HMO, but the member must remain within the provider network to receive benefits. EPOs are regulated under insurance statutes rather than HMO legislation.

ERISA. Employee Retirement Income Security Act of 1974, Public Law 93-406. Mandates reporting, disclosure of grievance and appeals requirements, and fiduciary standards for private group life and health plans, and preempts state benefit mandates and premium tax laws for self-funded group health plans.

ESRD. End stage renal disease. Progression of chronic renal failure to lasting and irreparable kidney damage that requires dialysis or renal transplant for survival.

established patient. 1) Patient who has received professional services in a face-to-face setting within the last three years from the same physician or another physician of the same specialty who belongs to the same group practice. 2) For OPPS hospitals, patient who has been registered as an inpatient or outpatient in a hospital's provider-based clinic or emergency department within the past three years.

exclusions. Services excluded from a plan's coverage by the employer or payer because of risk or cost.

experience rating. In medical reimbursement, designation of a group's previous claims history to help determine premium rates.

explanation of benefits. Statement mailed to the member and provider explaining claim adjudication and payment.

explanation of Medicare benefits. Medicare statement mailed to the member and provider explaining claim adjudication and payment.

extramural birth. Infant born outside of a sterile environment.

extrication collar. Cervical collar with opening at the throat for patients who have a tracheotomy or tracheostomy.

fab fragment. Immunoglobulin molecule fragment that is antigen binding with a light and heavy chain.

facility. Place of patient care, including inpatient and outpatient, acute or long term.

facility of payment. Contractual relationship that permits the payer to pay someone other than the member or provider.

fact-oriented V codes. Codes that do not describe a problem or a service; they simply state a fact. These generally do not serve as an outpatient primary or inpatient principal diagnosis.

FAR. Federal acquisition regulations. Regulations of the federal government's acquisition of services.

FDA. Food and Drug Administration. Federal agency responsible for protecting public health by substantiating the safety, efficacy, and security of human and veterinary drugs, biological products, medical devices, national food supply, cosmetics, and items that give off radiation.

Federal Register. Government publication listing changes in regulations and federally mandated standards, including coding standards such as HCPCS Level II and ICD-9-CM.

federally qualified HMO. HMO that meets CMS guidelines for Medicare reimbursement.

fee schedule. List of codes and related services with pre-established billing amounts by a provider, or payment amounts by a payer that could be percentages of billed charges, flat rates, or maximum allowable amounts established by third-party payers. Medicare fee schedules apply to clinical laboratory, radiology, and durable medical equipment services.

FEHB. Federal Employee Health Benefits Program. Provides health plans to federal workers.

FEHBAR. Federal Employee Health Benefits Acquisition Regulations. Federal regulations for acquisition of health services used by government agencies and subcontractors.

FFS. Fee for service. 1) Payment for services, usually physician services, on a service-by-service basis rather than an alternative payment system like capitation. Fee-for-service arrangements may be discounted or undiscounted rates. 2) Situation in which the payer pays full charges for medical services.

FO. Finger orthosis.

formulary. List of prescription medications preferred for use by the health plan and dispensed through participating pharmacies to covered persons.

FPP. Faculty practice plan. Group practice developed around a teaching program or medical school.

fraternal insurance. Cooperative plan provided to members of an association or fraternal group.

FTE. Full time employee. Accounting equivalent of one full time employee that includes wages, benefits, and other costs.

gatekeeper. Primary care physician in a health care system in which a member's care must be provided by a primary care physician unless the physician refers the member to a specialist or approves the care provided by a specialist.

GHAA. Group Health Association of America. HMO trade organization.

global surgery package. Services included in a surgical procedure that include all of the elements needed to perform the procedure and routine follow-up care.

gm. Gram.

GMLOS. Geometric mean length of stay. Statistically adjusted value for all cases for a given diagnosis-related group, allowing for the outliers, transfer cases, and negative outlier cases that would normally skew the data. The GMLOS is used to determine payment only for transfer cases (i.e., the per diem rate).

government mandates. Services mandated by state or federal law, such as the correct use of ICD-9-CM codes.

grace period. Set number of days past the due date of a premium payment during which medical coverage may not be canceled and the premium payment may be made, or after employment termination. It varies by health plan contract and state law but is generally 30 to 60 days.

group model. HMO that contracts with a group of providers.

group practice. Group of providers that shares facilities, resources, and staff, and who may represent a single unit in a managed care network.

grouper. Computer application that assigns diagnosis-related groups (DRGs).

guidelines. Information appearing at the beginning of each of the six major sections of the CPT book. They also may appear at the beginning of subsections and code ranges. The information contained in the guidelines provides definitions, explanations of terms, and factors relevant to the section.

HCl. Hydrochloric acid.

HCPCS. Healthcare Common Procedure Coding System. *HCPCS Level I:* Healthcare Common Procedure Coding System Level I. Numeric coding system used by physicians, facility outpatient departments, and ambulatory surgery centers (ASC) to code ambulatory, laboratory, radiology, and other diagnostic services for Medicare billing. This coding system contains only the American Medical Association's Physicians' Current Procedural Terminology (CPT) codes. The AMA updates codes annually. *HCPCS Level II:* Healthcare Common Procedure Coding System Level II. National coding system, developed by CMS, contains alphanumeric codes for physician and nonphysician services not included in the CPT coding system. HCPCS Level II covers such things as ambulance services, durable medical equipment, and orthotic and prosthetic devices. *HCPCS modifiers:* Two-character code (AA-ZZ) that identifies circumstances that alter or enhance the description of a service or supply. They are recognized by carriers nationally and are updated annually by CMS.

Hct. Hematocrit.

heel cup. Plastic or rubber cup that fits into the back portion of the patient's shoe to provide protection, support, and stabilization.

HFO. Hand-finger orthosis.

HHA. Home health agency. Health care provider, licensed under state or local law, that provides skilled nursing and other therapeutic services. HHAs include visiting nurse associations and hospital-based home care programs. To participate in Medicare, an HHA must meet health and safety standards established by the U.S. Department of Health and Human Services (HHS). Home health services usually are provided in the patient's home, although some outpatient services performed in a hospital, SNF or rehabilitation center may be covered under home health if the equipment is required and cannot be used in the patient's home.

HHS. Health and Human Services. Cabinet department that oversees the operating divisions of the federal government responsible for health and welfare. HHS oversees the Centers for Medicare and Medicaid Services, Food and Drug Administration, Public Health Service, and other such entities.

HIAA. Health Insurance Association of America. Trade organization for payers.

hierarchy. Ranking or ordering of information or people.

HKAFO. Hip-knee-ankle foot orthosis.

HMO. Health maintenance organization. Medical health insurance coverage that pays claims based on a provider cost, per diem, or charge basis. Hospitals contract with an HMO to provide care at a contractually reduced price. HMO members pay a set monthly amount for coverage and are treated without additional cost, except for a copayment or deductible amount, payable by the patient. Like all managed care organizations, HMOs use a variety of mechanisms to control costs, including utilization management, discounted provider fee schedules, and financial incentives. HMOs use primary care physicians as gatekeepers and tend to emphasize preventive care.

hold harmless. Contractual clause stating that if either party is held liable for malpractice, the other party is absolved.

home health. Palliative and therapeutic care and assistance in the activities of daily life to home bound Medicare and private plan members.

horseshoe. U-shaped device that stabilizes or immobilizes the patella when used with a knee orthosis.

hospice. Organization that furnishes inpatient, outpatient, and home health care for the terminally ill. Hospices emphasize support and counseling services for terminally ill people and their families, pain relief, and symptom management. When the Medicare beneficiary chooses hospice benefits, all other Medicare benefits are discontinued, except physician services and treatment of conditions not related to the terminal illness.

hospital admission plan. Used to facilitate admission to the hospital and to assure prompt payment to the hospital.

hypopnea. Abnormal respiratory event lasting at least 10 seconds, with at least a 30 percent reduction in thoracoabdominal movement or airflow as compared to a baseline, and with at least a 4 percent oxygen desaturation.

IA. Intra-arterial.

IBNR. Incurred but not reported. Amount of money the payer's plan accrues to forestall unknown medical expenses.

ICD-10. International Classification of Diseases, Tenth Revision. Classification of diseases by alphanumeric code, used by the World Health Organization.

ICD-10-CM. International Classification of Diseases, Tenth Edition, Clinical Modification. Diagnostic coding system developed to replace ICD-9-CM in the United States. It is a clinical modification of the World Health Organization's ICD-10, already in use in much of the world, and used for mortality reporting in the United States. The implementation date for ICD-10-CM is October 1, 2013.

ICD-9-CM. International Classification of Diseases, Ninth Edition, Clinical Modification. Clinical modification of the international statistical coding system used to report, compile, and compare health care data, using numeric and alphanumeric (E codes and V codes) codes to help plan, deliver, reimburse, and quantify medical care in the United States.

ICF. Intermediate care facility. Health care facility that furnishes services to patients who do not require the degree of care provided by a hospital or skilled nursing facility or a step-down facility for patients who are leaving the hospital but who cannot be discharged to home because of continuing medical needs.

ID card. Wallet card carried by a plan member providing name, member and group numbers, effective dates, deductibles, and other information.

immediate maternity. Coverage provided for pregnancies that began prior to the date the member became insured.

immobilizer. Device used to restrain a part of the body, keeping the body part from moving.

implant. Material or device inserted or placed within the body for therapeutic, reconstructive, or diagnostic purposes.

in plan. Services chosen from a network provider.

incontestable clause. Provision in a policy that prohibits the plan from disputing coverage for certain conditions after a specified period of time.

INF. 1) Inferior. 2) Infusion.

infusion pump. Device that delivers a measured amount of drug or intravenous solution through injection over a period of time.

inpatient hospitalization. Period in which a patient is housed in a single hospital usually without interruption.

inpatient reimbursement. Payment to hospital for the costs incurred to treat a patient.

insoles. Rubber or plastic orthotics that fit inside the shoes to correct a deformity or help aid in the healing of an injury.

insurance carrier. Insurer or health plan that may underwrite, administer, or sell a range of health benefit programs.

intermediate repair. *1)* Surgical closure of a wound requiring closure of one or more of the deeper subcutaneous tissue and non-muscle fascia layers in addition to suturing the skin. *2)* Contaminated wounds with single layer closure that need extensive cleaning or foreign body removal.

internal skeletal fixation. Repair involving wires, pins, screws, and/or plates placed through or within the fractured area to stabilize and immobilize the injury.

IOL. Intraocular lens.

IPA. Individual practice association. Organization made up of providers who, along with the rest of a group, contract with payers at a discounted fee-for-service or capitated rate.

IPO. Individual practice organization. Organization made up of providers who, along with the rest of a group, contract with payers at a discounted fee-for-service or capitated rate.

IS. Information services. Administrators of the computer systems used by payers and providers.

IV. Intravenous.

JCAHO. Joint Commission on Accreditation of Healthcare Organizations. Organization that accredits health care organizations. In the future, the JCAHO may play a role in certifying these organizations' compliance with the HIPAA A/S requirements. Previously known as the Joint Commission for the Accreditation of Hospitals.

JD. Doctor of jurisprudence.

KAFO. Knee-ankle-foot orthosis. External apparatus utilized to improve motor control, gait stabilization, and reduce pain. The device is attached to the leg in order to help correct flexible deformities and to halt the progression of fixed deformities.

key components. Three components of history, examination, and medical decision making are considered the keys to selecting the correct level of E/M codes. In most cases, all three components must be addressed in the documentation. However, in established, subsequent, and follow-up categories, only two of the three must be met or exceeded for a given code.

KOH. Potassium hydroxide.

lag study. Report used by plan managers to determine how long claims are pending and how much is paid out each month.

lapse. Terminated policy.

late effect. Abnormality, dysfunction, or other residual condition produced after the acute phase of an illness, injury, or disease is over. There is no time limit on when late effects can appear.

LCD. Local coverage determination. Published decision by a fiscal intermediary or carrier regarding whether to cover a particular service or under what circumstances to cover it. The decision is valid only in the carrier's jurisdiction. LCDs replaced local medical review policies for CMS by year's end 2005.

LCSW. Licensed clinical social worker.

limiting charge. Maximum amount a nonparticipating physician or provider can charge for services rendered to a Medicare patient.

limits. In medical reimbursement, the ceiling for benefits payable under a plan.

line of business. Different health plans offered by a larger insurer or insurance broker as a product line.

lives. Unit of measurement used by plans to determine the number of people covered. Calculated by multiplying the number of members by 2.5.

local coverage determination. Statement of coverage and related usage specific to a Medicare contractor or designated geographic area.

long-term care facility. Nursing home or, more specifically, a facility offering extended, nonacute care to a resident patient whose illness does not require acute care.

loss ratio. Ratio between the cost to deliver medical care and the amount of money taken in by the plan.

LPN. Licensed practical nurse.

LSO. Lumbar sacral orthosis.

LVN. *1)* Licensed visiting nurse. *2)* Licensed vocational nurse.

MA. 1) Master of arts degree. 2) Medical assistant. 3) Mental age.

MAC. Maximum allowable charge. Amount set by the insurer as the highest amount that can be charged for a particular medical service or by a pharmacy vendor.

MAC. Medicare administrative contractor. One of 15 jurisdictional organizations that contract with CMS to adjudicate professional claims under Part A and Part B, responsible for daily claims processing, utilization review, record maintenance, dissemination of information based on CMS regulations, and whether services are covered and payments are appropriate. Four of the jurisdictions also include home health services. There are four separate MAC jurisdictions for DME services.

malingering. Feigning of illness, as the result of intentional deceit or as the result of mental illness.

managed health care. 1) Managing active cases to ensure care is the most appropriate, efficient, and effective. 2) System of health care meant to manage overall cost. 3) Method of health care whereby contracted physicians participate in managing health care costs.

mandated benefits. Services mandated by state or federal law such as child abuse or rape, not necessarily covered by insurers.

maximum allowable charge. Amount set by the insurer as the highest amount that can be charged for a particular medical service or by a pharmacy vendor.

MCE. Medical care evaluation.

mcg. Microgram.

MCO. Managed care organization. Generic term for various health benefit plans that provide coverage for health care services in conjunction with management and review of services provided to ensure that services are medically necessary and appropriate.

MD. Medical doctor.

MDC. Major diagnostic category. Dividing all possible principal diagnoses into mutually exclusive categories. These broad classifications of ICD-9-CM diagnoses are typically grouped by organ system.

ME. Medical examiner.

MEd. Master of education.

Medicaid. Joint federal and state program that covers medical expenses for people with low incomes and limited resources who meet the criteria. The benefits for recipients vary from state to state.

medical consultation. Advice or an opinion rendered by a physician at the request of the primary care provider.

medical loss ratio. Ratio between the cost to deliver medical care and the amount of money taken in by the plan.

medical meaningfulness. Patients in the same DRG can be expected to evoke a set of clinical responses that result in a similar pattern of resource use.

medical necessity. Medically appropriate and necessary to meet basic health needs; consistent with the diagnosis or condition and rendered in a cost-effective manner; and consistent with national medical practice guidelines regarding type, frequency, and duration of treatment.

Medicare. Federally funded program authorized as part of the Social Security Act that provides for health care services for people age 65 or older, people with disabilities, and people with end-stage renal disease (ESRD).

Medicare administrative contractor. Uniform type of Medicare administrative entity that will process both institutional and professional claims in specified geographic jurisdictions of the country. There will be 15 A/B MACs, four DME MACs, and four home health/hospice MACs. MACs will be phased in over the next few years with all jurisdictions operational by October 2011.

Medicare Fee Schedule. Fee schedule based upon physician work, expense, and malpractice designed to slow the rise in cost for services and standardize payment to physicians regardless of specialty or location of service with geographic adjustments.

Medicare Part A. Hospital insurance coverage that includes hospital, nursing home, hospice, home health, and other inpatient care. Claims are submitted to intermediaries for reimbursement.

Medicare Part B. Supplemental medical insurance that includes outpatient hospital care and physician and other qualified professional care. Claims from providers or suppliers other than a hospital are submitted to carriers for reimbursement. Hospital outpatient claims are submitted to their FI/MAC.

Medicare secondary payer. Specified circumstance when other third-party payers have the primary responsibility for payment of services and Medicare is the secondary payer. Medicare is secondary to workers' compensation, automobile, medical no-fault and liability insurance, EGHPs, LGHPs, and certain employer health plans covering aged and disabled beneficiaries. The MSP program prohibits Medicare payment for items or services if payment has been made or can reasonably be expected to be made by another payer, as described above.

Medicare supplement. Private insurance coverage that pays the Medicare deductible and copayments and may also pay the costs of services not covered by Medicare.

Medigap. Individual health insurance offered by a private entity to those persons entitled to Medicare benefits and is specifically designed to supplement Medicare benefits. It fills in some of the gaps in Medicare coverage by providing payment for some of the charges, deductibles, coinsurance amounts, or other limitations imposed by Medicare.

Medigap policy. Health insurance or other health benefit plan offered by a private company to those entitled to Medicare benefits. The policy covers charges not payable by Medicare because of deductibles, coinsurance amounts, or other Medicare-imposed limitations.

member. In medical reimbursement, subscriber of a health plan.

member months. In medical reimbursement, total of months each member was covered.

member services. In health care contracting, the payer department that works as a patient advocate to solve problems and may take claims appeals to a final committee after all other processes have been exhausted.

mental health substance abuse. Payer term for services rendered to members for emotional problems or chemical dependency.

mental or nervous. Payer term for services rendered to members for emotional problems or chemical dependency.

mEq. Milliequivalent.

MeSH. Medical staff-hospital organization.

MET. Multiple employer trust. Group of employers that join together to purchase health insurance using a self-funded approach to lower costs by the broadening membership pool to prevent an adverse selection.

MEWA. Multiple employer welfare association. Group of employers that join together to purchase health insurance using a self-funded approach to lower costs by the broadening membership pool to prevent an adverse selection.

mg. Milligram.

MHA. Master of health administration.

minor procedure. Self-limited procedure, usually with an assignment of 0 or 10 follow-up days by payers. A minor procedure may be considered by many payers to be part of the global package for a primary surgical service and cannot be billed separately from the primary procedure.

MIS. Management information system. Hardware and software facilitating claims management.

mixed model. HMO that includes both an open panel and closed panel option.

ml. Milliliter.

MLP. Midlevel practitioners. Professionals such as nurse practitioners, nurse midwives, physical therapists, physician assistants, and others who provide medical care but do so with physician input.

MLT. Medical laboratory technician.

modality. *1)* Form of imaging. These include x-ray, fluoroscopy, ultrasound, nuclear medicine, duplex Doppler, CT, and MRI. *2)* Any physical agent applied to produce therapeutic changes to biologic tissue; includes but is not limited to thermal, acoustic, light, mechanical, or electric energy.

modifier. Two-character code attached to a HCPCS code as a suffix to identify circumstances that alter or enhance the description of a service or supply.

morbidity rate. In health care contracting, an actuarial term describing predicted medical expense rate.

MP. Metacarpal phalangeal.

MPH. Master of public health. Advanced degree.

MSA. Medical savings account.

MSN. Master of science in nursing.

MSW. Master's in social work.

MT. Medical technologist.

multiple birth. Two or more infants delivered at the same time.

multiple employer group. Group of employers who contract together to subscribe to a plan, broadening the risk pool and saving money. Different from a multiple employer trust.

multiple-lead device. Implantable cardiac device (pacemaker or implantable cardioverter-defibrillator

[ICD]) in which pacing and sensing components are placed in at least three chambers of the heart.

NA. Nurse assistant.

NAHMOR. National Association of HMO Regulators.

NAIC. National Association of Insurance Commissioners. Organization of state insurance regulators.

national coverage determination. National policy statement granting, eliminating, or excluding Medicare coverage for a service, item, or test. NCDs state CMS policy regarding the circumstances under which the service, item, or test is considered reasonable and necessary or otherwise not covered for Medicare purposes. These polices apply nationwide.

National Supplier Clearinghouse. Entity that approves providers and medical equipment vendors as "suppliers" under the Medicare program, issuing an identification number to approved applicants.

national supplier identification number. Number with which providers or other health care professionals who disperse DMEPOS submit their claims. This number is obtained through an application to the National Supplier Clearinghouse, a centralized agency for DMEPOS suppliers.

NBICU. Newborn intensive care unit. Special care unit for premature and seriously ill infants.

NCD. National coverage determinations. National policy statements granting, eliminating, or excluding Medicare coverage for a service, item, or test. NCDs state CMS policy regarding the circumstances under which the service, item, or test is considered reasonable and necessary or otherwise not covered for Medicare purposes. These polices apply nationwide.

NCHS. National Center for Health Statistics. Division of the Centers for Disease Control and Prevention that compiles statistical information used to guide actions and policies to improve the public health of U.S. citizens. The NCHS maintains the ICD-9-CM coding system.

NCQA. National Committee for Quality Assurance. Organization that accredits managed care plans, or HMOs. In the future, the NCQA may play a role in certifying these organizations' compliance with the HIPAA A/S requirements.

ND. Doctor of naturopathy.

nebulization device. Device used to vaporize liquid medication for the airborne delivery of the medication to the patient. The medication is absorbed into the body via the respiratory tract. Medications can also be administered with a nebulizer to fragment and mobilize thick, excess mucous in the respiratory tract; these medications are broadly termed mucolytics.

NEC. Not elsewhere classifiable. Condition or diagnosis that is not provided with its own specified code in ICD-9-CM, but included in a more broadly defined code for other specified conditions.

neonatal period. Period of an infant's life from birth to the age of 27 days, 23 hours, and 59 minutes.

network model. Plan that contracts with multiple groups of providers, or networks, to provide care.

new patient. Patient who is receiving face-to-face care from a provider or another physician of the same specialty who belongs to the same group practice for the first time in three years. For OPPS hospitals, a patient who has not been registered as an inpatient or outpatient, including off-campus provider based clinic or emergency department, within the past three years.

newborn admission. Infant born in the facility.

normal delivery. Baby delivered without complication.

NOS. Not otherwise specified. Condition or diagnosis remains ill defined and is unspecified without the necessary information for selecting a more specific code.

NP. 1) Nurse practitioner. 2) Neuropsychiatry.

NPI. National provider identifier. Standard eight-digit alphanumeric provider identifier implemented under the Health Insurance Portability and Accountability Act of 1996 (HIPAA) requirements. The first seven digits identify the provider and the eighth position is a check digit. Providers are required to report their NPI number for electronic and paper billing.

O2. Oxygen.

OB. Obstetrician.

observation patient. Patient who needs to be monitored and assessed for inpatient admission or referral to another site for care

occupational therapy. Training, education, and assistance intended to assist a person who is recovering from a serious illness or injury perform the activities of daily life.

OIG. Office of Inspector General. Agency within the Department of Health and Human Services that is ultimately responsible for investigating instances of fraud and abuse in the Medicare and Medicaid and other government health care programs. OIG work plan Annual plan released by the Office of Inspector General (OIG) that details the areas of focus for fraud and abuse investigations.

OL. Outlier threshold. Component that figures in the reimbursement calculation for a DRG.

open enrollment period. Time period during which subscribers in a health benefit program have the opportunity to re-enroll or select an alternative health plan being offered to them, usually without evidence of insurability or waiting periods.

open panel. Arrangement in which a managed care organization that contracts with providers on an exclusive basis is still seeking providers.

OPL. Other party liability. In coordination of benefits, the decision that the other plan is the primary plan.

orthosis. Derived from a Greek word meaning "to make straight," it is an artificial appliance that supports, aligns, or corrects an anatomical deformity or improves the use of a moveable body part. Unlike a prosthesis, an orthotic device is always functional in nature.

orthotic. Use of a mechanical orthopedic device that compensates for, supports, corrects, or prevents deformities.

osteogenesis stimulator. Device used to stimulate the growth of bone by electrical impulses or ultrasound.

ostomy. Artificial (surgical) opening in the body used for drainage or for delivery of medications or nutrients.

OTR. Occupational therapist registered.

out of plan. In health care contracting, services of a provider who is not a member of the preferred provider network.

out of service area. In health care contracting, medical care received out of the geographic area that may or may not be covered, depending on the plan.

outlier. Case classified to a specific DRG but with exceptionally high costs compared with other cases classified to the same DRG. The fiscal intermediary or MAC makes a payment in addition to the original DRG amount for these situations. A cost outlier is paid an amount in excess of the cut-off threshold for a given DRG. The day outlier no longer applies.

outpatient. Patient who receives care without being admitted for inpatient or residential care.

outpatient visit. Encounter in a recognized outpatient facility.

overutilization. Services rendered by providers more frequently than usual.

PA. 1) Physician assistant. Medical professional who receives additional training and can assess, treat, and prescribe medications under a physician's review. 2) Posteroanterior. 3) Pulmonary artery. 4) HCPCS Level II modifier used to denote a surgical or other invasive procedure that was performed on the wrong body part.

paneled. In health care contracting, provider contracted with an HMO.

par provider. Provider who is participating in a health plan or Medicare program.

parenteral nutrition. Nutrients provided subcutaneously, intravenously, intramuscularly, or intradermally for patients during the postoperative period and in other conditions, such as shock, coma, and renal failure.

partial disability. Congenital or acquired inability to perform part of one's job.

partial hospitalization. Situation in which the patient only stays part of each day over a long period. Cardiac, rehabilitation, and chronic pain patients, for example, could use this service.

partial payment. Payment to a provider or member with the expectation that other payments will be forthcoming before the claim is closed.

PAS norms. Based on a professional activity study performed regularly by the Commission on Professional and Hospital Activities and broken out by average length of stay (ALOS) by region.

PATOS. Payment (received) at the time of service.

PBM. Prescription benefit managers. HMO staff who monitor amount and use of drugs prescribed.

PCP. Primary care physician. Physician who makes an initial diagnosis and referral and retains control over the patient and utilization of services both in and outside of the plan.

pediatric patient. Patient usually younger than 14 years of age.

peer review. Evaluation of the quality of the total health care provided by medical staff with equivalent training, such as a physician-to-physician or nurse-to-nurse evaluation.

PEPM. Per employee per month.

PEPP. Payment error prevention program. Program to help reduce Medicare PPS inpatient hospital payment errors.

per diem reimbursement. In health care contracting, reimbursement to an institution based on a set rate per day rather than on a charge-by-charge basis.

percutaneous skeletal fixation. Treatment that is neither open nor closed. In this procedure, the injury site is not directly visualized. Instead, fixation devices (pins, screws) are placed to stabilize the dislocation using x-ray guidance.

perinatal death. Stillborn births and neonatal deaths.

pessary. Device placed in the vagina to support and reposition a prolapsing or retropositioned uterus, rectum, or vagina.

PharmD. Doctor of pharmacy.

PhD. Doctor of philosophy.

PHO. Physician-hospital organization.

physician assistant. Medical professional who receives additional training and can assess, treat, and prescribe medications under a physician's review.

PIN. Physician identification number.

plan manager. Payer employee managing all of the contracts and contract negotiations for one or more specific plans.

PMPM. Per member per month.

PMPY. Per member per year.

pneumatic splint. Splint filled with air or gas to provide circumferential protection and support.

pooling. Health payers' practice of combining risk.

POS. Point of service. Health benefit plan allowing the covered person to choose to receive a service from a participating or nonparticipating provider, with different benefit levels associated with the use of participating providers.

posting date. Date a charge is posted to a patient account by the provider, frequently not the same as the actual date of service, but usually within five days of the actual date of service.

PPA. Preferred provider arrangement. Similar to a PPO.

PPO. Preferred provider organization. Program that establishes contracts with providers of medical care. Usually the benefit contract provides significantly better benefits and lower member cost for services received from preferred providers, encouraging covered persons to use these providers, who may be reimbursed on a discounted basis.

PPS. Prospective payment system. Reimbursement methodology that uses predetermined rates for each type of discharge, procedure, service, or item based on a standard type of case. For hospital inpatients, the Medicare PPS system of DRGs was implemented in 1983 to hold down the rising cost of health care. For hospital outpatients, OPPS has been based on ambulatory payment classifications effective August 1, 2000. For skilled nursing facilities, it is based on the RUG-IV system, and for home health it is based on the HHRGs.

precertification. Preadmission certification. Approval in advance of a procedure or hospital stay by a payer employee, who considers the diagnosis, the planned treatment, and expected length of stay.

preexisting condition. Symptom that causes a person to seek diagnosis, care, or treatment for which medical advice or treatment was recommended or received by a physician within a certain time period before the effective date of medical insurance coverage. The preexisting condition waiting period is the time the beneficiary must wait after buying health insurance before coverage begins for a condition that existed before coverage was obtained.

premature delivery. Infant delivered with time of gestation less than 37 weeks.

presenting problem. Disease, condition, illness, injury, symptom, sign, finding, complaint, or other reason for the patient encounter

primary care. Basic or general health care, traditionally provided by family practice, pediatrics, and internal medicine practitioners.

primary diagnosis. Current, most significant reason for the services or procedures provided.

principal diagnosis. Condition established after study to be chiefly responsible for occasioning the admission of the patient to the hospital for care.

principal procedure. Procedure performed for definitive treatment rather than for diagnostic or exploratory purposes, or that was necessary to treat a complication. Usually related to the principal diagnosis.

PRO. Peer review organization. Organization that contracts with CMS to conduct preadmission, preprocedure, and postdischarge medical reviews and determine medical necessity, appropriateness, and quality of certain inpatient and outpatient surgical procedures for which payment may be made in whole or in part under the Medicare program.

problem-oriented V codes. ICD-9-CM codes that identify circumstances that could affect the patient in the future but are neither a current illness nor an injury. Use these codes to describe an existing circumstance or problem that may influence future medical care.

prodrug. Inactive drug that goes through a metabolic process when given resulting in a chemical conversion that changes the drug into an active pharmacological agent.

professional association plans. Plan provided by a professional association that affords self-employed professionals (e.g., physicians, CPAs, lawyers) less expensive coverage.

program safeguard coordinator. Contractor charged with maintaining the integrity of the Medicare program. Duties include data analysis, audit, review, and monitoring related to beneficiary information (such as COB data), medical review, cost reports, provider education, and fraud detection and prevention.

prosthetic. Device that replaces all or part of an internal body organ or body part, or that replaces part of the function of a permanently inoperable or malfunctioning internal body organ or body part.

provider. All-inclusive, generic term for people or institutions that provide health care. The provider may be a physician, hospital, pharmacy, other facility, or other health care provider.

PSC. Program safeguard coordinators.

PT. Physical therapy.

PTA. Physical therapy assistant.

PTMPY. Per thousand members per year.

QA. Quality assurance. Monitoring and maintenance of established standards of quality for patient care.

QM. Quality management. Monitoring and maintenance of established standards of quality.

RBRVS. Resource-based relative value scale. Fee schedule introduced by CMS to reimburse physician Medicare fees based on the amount of time and resources expended in treating patients with adjustments for overhead costs and geographical differences.

reasonable and customary. Fees charged for medical services that are considered normal, common, and in line with the prevailing fees in the provider's geographical area.

referral. Approval from the primary care physician to see a specialist or receive certain services. May be required for coverage purposes before a patient receives care from anyone except the primary physician.

regional medical center. Hospital that provides comprehensive services to a large regional area but that may not be a tertiary care facility. Largely used in the west where facilities may serve hundreds of square miles.

rehabilitation. Restoration of physical and mental functions to allow the usual daily activities of life.

reimbursement. Payment of actual charges or allowable incurred as a result of accident or illness.

reinsurance. Insurance purchased by an HMO, insurance company, or self-funded employer from another insurance company to protect itself against all or part of the losses that may be incurred in the process of honoring the claims of its participating providers, policy holders, or employees and covered dependents.

relative weight. Assigned weight that is intended to reflect the relative resource consumption associated with each DRG. The higher the relative weight, the greater the payment to the hospital. The relative weights are calculated by CMS and published in the final prospective payment system rule.

review committee. Multidisciplinary committee that considers denied cases being appealed, catastrophic cases, or fee-for-service cases.

RHIA. Registered health information administrator. Accreditation for medical record administrators, previously known as a registered records administrator (RRA), through AHIMA.

RHIT. Registered health information technician. Accreditation for medical records practitioners, previously known as accredited records technician (ART), through AHIMA.

Glossary

rib belt. Device that encircles the abdomen and provides support for injured ribs while they heal.

risk contract. Contract between Medicare and a payer or a payer and a provider in which the payer (in the case of Medicare) and the provider (in the case of the payer contracts) receive a set amount for care of a patient base. If costs exceed the amount the payer or provider was paid, the patients still receive care during the term of the contract.

risk factor reduction. Reduction of risk in the pool of health plan members.

risk manager. Person charged with keeping financial risk low, including malpractice cases.

risk pool. Pool of people who will be in the insured group, their medical and mental histories, other factors such as age, and their predicted health.

RN. Registered nurse.

RPh. Registered pharmacist.

RPT. Registered physical therapist.

RRA. Registered records administrator.

RRT. Registered respiratory therapist.

rush charge. Charge for expeditious test results.

RVS. Relative value study. Guide that shows the relationship between the time, resources, competency, experience, severity, and other factors necessary to perform procedures that is multiplied by a dollar conversion factor to determine a monetary value for the procedure.

RVU. Relative value unit. Value assigned a procedure based on difficulty and time consumed. Used for computing reimbursement under a relative value study.

SACH. Solid ankle, cushion heel.

sanction. Imposition of penalties or exclusion of a provider for fraud or infractions such as an inappropriate use of services, providing procedures that may harm the patient, or applying inferior techniques.

schedule. Listing of amounts payable for specific procedures.

second opinion. Medical opinion obtained from another health care professional, relevant to clinical evaluation, before the performance of a medical service or surgical procedure. Includes patient education regarding treatment alternatives and/or to determine medical necessity.

secondary insurer. In a COB arrangement, the insurer that reimburses for benefits pending after payment by the primary insurer.

self-funded plan. Plan where the risk is assumed by the employer rather than the insurer. The employer generally pays claims directly from a general fund account that may be managed by a third party.

self-insured. Individual or organization that assumes the financial risk of paying for health care.

self-pay patients. Patients who pay for medical care out-of-pocket.

SEO. Shoulder-elbow orthosis.

separate procedures. Services commonly carried out as a fundamental part of a total service, and as such usually do not warrant a separate identification. They are noted in the CPT book with the parenthetical phrase (separate procedure) at the end of the description, and are payable only when they are performed alone.

service date. Date a charge is incurred for a service.

service plan. *1)* Plan that has contracts with providers but is not a managed care plan. *2)* Another name for Blue Cross/Blue Shield plans.

service-oriented V codes. ICD-9-CM codes that identify or define examinations, aftercare, ancillary services, or therapy. Use these V codes to describe the patient who is not currently ill but seeks medical services for some specific purpose such as follow-up visits. You can also use this type of V code as a primary diagnosis for outpatient services when the patient has no symptoms that can be coded and screening services are provided.

shadow pricing. Setting rates just below a competitor's rates. Maximizes profits but raises medical costs.

short-stay patients. In medical reimbursement, inpatients admitted for 48 hours or less, or outpatients who stay 24 hours or less.

sick baby. Infant with medical complications not resulting from premature birth.

simple repair. Surgical closure of a superficial wound, requiring single layer suturing of the skin (epidermis, dermis, or subcutaneous tissue).

skeletal traction. Applying a pulling force directly on the long axis of bones by inserted wires or pins and using weights and pulleys to keep the bone in proper alignment.

skin traction. Application of a pulling force to a limb accomplished by a device fixed to felt dressings or strappings on the body surface.

small subscriber group aggregate. Aggregate of professional associations, small business, or other entities formed to be considered a single, large subscriber group.

SNF. Skilled nursing facility. Institution or a distinct part of an institution that is primarily engaged in providing skilled nursing care and related services for residents who require medical or nursing care; or rehabilitation services for the rehabilitation of injured, disabled, or sick persons.

SO. 1) Shoulder orthosis. 2) Sacroiliac orthosis.

SOF. Signature on file.

softgoods or soft goods. DMEPOS industry term for medical devices such as braces, splints, joint supports and protectors, cervical pillows, and other similar orthopaedic-oriented items.

specimen. Tissue cells or sample of fluid taken for analysis, pathologic examination, and diagnosis.

splint. Brace or support for an anatomical structure after surgery or injury.

split inventory technique. Keeping highly-utilized DMEPOS easily accessible to staff, while keeping surplus in a central storage area.

SSA. Social Security Act.

SSN. Social security number.

staff model. HMO that employs its own providers.

standard anesthesia formula. Reimbursement formula that consists of base units plus time units plus modifying units (e.g., physical status and qualifying circumstances) plus other allowed unit/charges that is multiplied by a conversion factor.

stat charge. Charge for expeditious test results.

state insurance commission. State group that approves insurance certificates for each state and regulates the industry based on statutes.

steering. Providing financial incentives to plan members to use the managed care provider panel.

stockinet. Material used to wrap an injured body part before applying a cast; usually of breathable material to wick moisture away from skin.

stop loss. In health care contracting, a form of reinsurance that protects health insurance above a certain limit and minimizes risks for providers.

subrogation. Recovery of monies or benefits from a third party who is liable for the payment.

subsidiary codes. Services that are not included as part of the primary procedure but that are not performed alone and may be identified as each additional, or list-in-addition-to services. Phrases that help identify subsidiary codes include, but are not limited to: each additional, list in addition to, and done at time of other major procedure

substantial comorbidity. Preexisting condition that will, because of its presence with a specific principal diagnosis, cause an increase in the length of stay by at least one day in approximately 75 percent of the cases.

substantial complication. Condition that arises during the hospital stay that prolongs the length of stay by at least one day in approximately 75 percent of the cases.

subtraction. Removal of an overlying structure to better visualize the structure in question by imposing one x-ray on top of another.

superbill. Multipurpose sheet used for all patient encounters that typically contains a check-off list of ICD-9-CM diagnosis codes, evaluation and management codes, and procedure and HCPCS Level II codes in the outpatient setting.

supplemental health services. Optional services that a health plan may cover or provide.

support. Article that provides stabilization, but not immobilization, to an injured or disabled body part.

surgical package. Normal, uncomplicated performance of specific surgical services, with the assumption that, on average, all surgical procedures of a given type are similar with respect to skill level, duration, and length of normal follow-up care.

swing bed. Bed used for acute or long-term care, depending on the patient's need and the hospital's level of occupancy. Swing beds typically are available in small and rural hospitals. A swing-bed patient may be admitted and discharged from acute care and readmitted to a swing bed to receive skilled or intermediate levels of care. At times, the patient may remain in the same bed while changes occur in his or her care, charges, and payment.

TCC. Transitional care center. Facility used in lieu of an extended care facility or before discharge to an extended care facility.

technical component. Portion of a health care service that identifies the provision of the equipment, supplies, technical personnel, and costs attendant to the performance of the procedure other than the professional services.

TEFRA. Tax Equity and Fiscal Responsibility Act. Protects the rights of full-time employees to remain on the company's health plan to age 69.

tertiary care facility. Hospital providing specialty care to patients referred from other hospitals because of the severity of their injuries or illnesses.

therapeutic. Act meant to alleviate a medical or mental condition.

therapeutic procedure. Treatment of a pathological or traumatic condition through the use of activities performed to treat or heal the cause or to effect change through the application of clinical skills or services that attempt to improve function.

therapeutic services. Services performed for treatment of a specific diagnosis. These services include performance of the procedure, various incidental elements, and normal, related follow-up care.

thermoplastic. Item that can be softened by heat, but hardens upon cooling.

third-party administrator. Firm that performs administrative functions for a self-funded plan but assumes no risk.

third-party payer. Public or private organization that pays for or underwrites coverage for health care expenses for another entity, usually an employer (e.g., Blue Cross Blue Shield, Medicare, Medicaid, commercial insurers).

THKAO. Thoracic-hip-knee-ankle orthosis.

three-digit diagnostic codes. Codes used only when no fourth or fifth digit is available. There are only about 100 codes at the highest level of specificity in the three-digit form. Most payers, including Medicare, do not accept three-digit codes when higher levels of specificity exist.

time limit. In health care contracting, a set number of days in which a claim can be filed according to the payer or state insurance commission.

TPA. Third-party administrator. Firm that performs administrative functions for a self-funded plan but assumes no risk.

TPL. Third party liability. Payer liable for the cost of an illness or injury, such as auto or homeowner insurer.

TQM. Total quality management. Concept that quality is an organic part of a plan's service and a provider's care and can be quantified and constantly improved.

traction. Drawing out or holding tension on an area by applying a direct therapeutic pulling force.

transcutaneous electrical nerve stimulator. Device that delivers a controlled amount of electricity to an area of the body to stimulate healing and/or to mitigate post-surgical or post-traumatic pain.

transfer. Transfer between hospitals occurs when a patient is admitted to a hospital, discharged, and subsequently admitted to another hospital for additional treatment once the patient's condition has stabilized or a diagnosis has been established.

treatment plan. Plan of care established by the provider outlining specific deficits and planned treatment that may be submitted to the case manager when seeking certification for a plan member.

triage. Medical screening of patients to determine priority of treatment based on severity of illness or injury and resources at hand.

triple option. Offering of an HMO, indemnity plan, and preferred provider organization by one insurance firm.

uCi. Microcurie.

UCR. Usual, customary, and reasonable. Fees charged for medical services that are considered normal, common, and in line with the prevailing fees in a given geographical area.

unbundling. Separately packaging costs or services that might otherwise be billed together including billing separately for health care services that should be combined according to the industry standards or commonly accepted coding practices.

underwriting. Evaluating and determining the financial risk a member or member group has on an insurer.

unlisted procedure. Procedural descriptions used when the overall procedure and outcome of the procedure are not adequately described by an existing procedure code. Such codes are used as a last resort and only when there is not a more appropriate procedure code.

unspecified. Term in ICD-9-CM that indicates more information is necessary to code the term to further specificity. In these cases, the fourth digit of the code is always 9.

upcoding. Practice of billing a code that represents a higher reimbursement than the code for the procedure actually performed.

UPIN. Unique physician identification number. Number unique to each physician, assigned by CMS, to identify physicians and suppliers who provide medical services or supplies to Medicare beneficiaries. It is a six-character, alphanumeric identification number designed to track payment and utilization information for individual physicians. The attending physician and operating physician identification numbers are required when billing for Medicare services.

URAC. Utilization Review Accreditation Commission. Accrediting body of case management.

urgent admission. Admission in which the patient requires immediate attention for treatment of a physical or psychiatric problem.

USP. United States pharmacopoeia.

USPHS. United States Public Health Service.

utilization review. Formal assessment of the medical necessity, efficiency, and/or appropriateness of health care services and treatment plans on a prospective, concurrent, or retrospective basis.

utilization review nurse. Nurse who evaluates cases for appropriateness of care and length of service and can plan discharge and services needed after discharge.

V code. Part of ICD-9-CM codes, V codes describe circumstances that influence a patient's health status and identify reasons for medical encounters resulting from circumstances other than a disease or injury already classified in the main part of ICD-9-CM.

volume. *1)* Number of services performed. *2)* Number of patients. *3)* Number of patients in a DRG during a specific time.

weighting. Assigning more worth to a fee based on the number of times it is charged, weighting the resource-based relative value fees for an area.

well-baby care. Medical services, immunizations, and regular provider visits considered routine for an infant.

withhold. Percentage of payment to providers held by an HMO until the cost of referral or services has been determined. If the provider goes over the amount determined appropriate, the HMO keeps that amount.

workers' compensation. State-governed system designated to administer and regulate the provision and cost of medical treatment and wage losses arising from a worker's job-related injury or disease, regardless of who is at fault. In exchange, the employer is protected from being sued.

wraparound plan. Insurance or health plan coverage for copays and deductibles not covered under a member's base plan.

ZPIC. Zone Program Integrity Contractor. CMS newly created entity currently being transitioned to replace the existing Program Safeguard Contractors (PSC). These contractors will be responsible for ensuring the integrity of all Medicare-related claims under Parts A and B (hospital, skilled nursing, home health, provider, and durable medical equipment claims), Part C (Medicare Advantage health plans), Part D (prescription drug plans), and coordination of Medicare-Medicaid data matches (Medi-Medi).

Medicare Guidelines for Selected Topics

Diabetic Supplies and Services

CMS generally defines diabetes mellitus as a condition of abnormal glucose metabolism diagnosed using the following criteria: a fasting blood sugar greater than or equal to 126 mg/dL on two different occasions; a two-hour post-glucose challenge greater than or equal to 200 mg/dL on two different occasions; or a random glucose test greater than 200 mg/dL for a person with symptoms of uncontrolled diabetes.

Medicare

Insulin and Syringes

When insulin is furnished to inpatients in a covered hospital stay it is covered and payment is included in the reimbursement for the inpatient stay. For outpatient services, insulin is a self-administrable drug that is not covered unless administered in an emergency situation, such as to a patient in a diabetic coma.

Insulin syringes are covered only when they are furnished incident to a physician's professional services. To be covered under this provision an insulin syringe must have been used by the physician or under his or her direct personal supervision, and the insulin injection must have been given in an emergency situation (e.g., diabetic coma). Home use of an insulin syringe by a diabetic is not covered.

Blood Glucose Monitors and Related Supplies

Blood glucose monitors are meter devices that read color changes produced on specially treated reagent strips by glucose concentrations in the patient's blood. There are several different types of blood glucose monitors. Medicare coverage of these devices varies depending on both the type of device and the medical condition of the patient for whom the device is prescribed.

Reflectance colorimeter devices used for measuring blood glucose levels in clinical settings are not covered as durable medical equipment for use in the home because the need for frequent professional re-calibration makes them unsuitable for home use.

Some types of blood glucose monitors that use a reflectance meter specifically designed for home use by diabetic patients may be covered as durable medical equipment, subject to the conditions and limitations described below.

Lancets, reagent strips, and other supplies necessary for the proper functioning of the device are also covered for patients for whom the device is indicated. Coverage of home blood glucose monitors and related supplies is limited to patients meeting the following conditions:

- The patient has diabetes (ICD-9-CM codes 250.00–250.93) that is being treated by a physician.

- The patient's physician states that the patient is capable of being trained to use the particular device prescribed in an appropriate manner. In some cases, the patient may not be able to perform this function, but a responsible individual can be trained to use the equipment and monitor the patient to assure that the intended effect is achieved. This is permissible if the patient's physician properly documents it in the medical record.

- The glucose monitor and related accessories and supplies have been ordered by the physician who is treating the patient's diabetes and the treating physician maintains records reflecting the care provided including, but not limited to, evidence of medical necessity for the prescribed frequency of testing.

- The device is designed for home use rather than clinical.

There is a blood glucose monitoring system designed especially for use by those with visual impairments. The monitors used in such systems are identical in terms of reliability and sensitivity to the standard blood glucose monitors described above. They differ by having such features as voice synthesizers, automatic timers, and specially designed arrangements of supplies and materials to enable the visually impaired to use the equipment without assistance. These blood glucose monitoring systems are covered under Medicare if the following conditions are met:

- The patient and device meet the conditions listed above for coverage of standard home blood glucose monitors.
- The patient's physician certifies that a visual impairment is severe enough to require use of this special monitoring system.

The additional features and equipment for use with these monitors justifies a higher reimbursement amount than allowed for standard blood glucose monitors.

Supplies used in home glucose monitoring are covered when the monitor is covered. The supplier must have an order that is signed and dated by the treating physician. The order for home blood glucose monitors and/or diabetic testing supplies must include all of the following elements:

- Item to be dispensed
- Quantity of items to be dispensed
- Specific frequency of testing
- Whether the patient has insulin-treated or non-insulin-treated diabetes
- Treating physician's signature
- Date of the treating physician's signature
- Start date of the order (only required if the start date is different from the signature date)

An order that states "as needed" will result in those items being denied as not medically necessary. The supplier is required to have a renewal order from the treating physician every 12 months. This renewal order must also contain the information specified above.

An order for supplies must also meet the following criteria:

- The patient has nearly exhausted the supply of test strips and lancets or useful life of one lens shield cartridge previously dispensed.
- When the treating physician has ordered a frequency of testing that exceeds utilization guidelines, there must be documentation in the patient's medical record stating the specific reason.
- The treating physician has seen the patient and has evaluated his or her diabetes control within six months prior to ordering strips and lancets or lens shield cartridges that exceed utilization guidelines.
- If refills of supplies that exceed utilization guidelines are dispensed, there must be documentation in the physician's records (e.g., a specific narrative statement that adequately documents the frequency at which the patient is actually testing or a copy of the beneficiary's log) or in the supplier's records (e.g., a copy of the beneficiary's log) stating the patient is testing at a frequency that corroborates the quantity of supplies that have been dispensed. If the patient is regularly using quantities of supplies that exceed utilization guidelines, new documentation must be present at least every six months.

The quantity of test strips, lancets, and replacement lens shield cartridges that are covered depends on the usual medical needs of the diabetic patient.

Suppliers must not dispense a quantity of supplies exceeding a beneficiary's expected utilization. Suppliers should stay attuned to atypical utilization patterns on behalf of their clients and verify with the ordering physician that the atypical utilization is, in fact, warranted. Regardless of utilization, a supplier must not dispense more than a three-month quantity of glucose testing supplies at a time.

Suppliers may contact the treating physician to renew an order; however, the request for renewal may only be made with the patient's continued monthly use of testing supplies and only with the patient's request to the supplier for order renewal.

Laser skin piercing devices are not medically necessary. If a laser skin piercing device is ordered for use with a covered home blood glucose monitor, payment will be based on the allowance for the least costly medically appropriate alternative. Since the laser skin-piercing device is not medically necessary, replacement lens shield cartridges are also not medically necessary. If replacement lens shields are ordered, payment will be based on the allowance for the least costly medically appropriate alternative (A4259).

Alcohol or peroxide and Betadine or pHisoHex are not covered since these items are not required for the proper functioning of the device.

Urine test reagent strips or tablets are not covered since they are not used with a glucose monitor.

The ICD-9-CM diagnosis code describing the condition that necessitates glucose testing must be included on each claim for the monitor, accessories, and supplies.

If the patient is being treated with insulin injections, modifier KX must be appended to the code for the monitor and each related supply on every claim submitted. Modifier KX must not be used for a patient who is not receiving insulin injections. If the patient is not being treated with insulin injections, modifier KS must be appended to the code for the monitor and each related supply on every claim submitted.

Hospital Use of Glucometers

Glucometers are simple devices that determine blood glucose. Most are FDA-approved for home use by the patient. All home use of these devices automatically qualifies under the CLIA waiver. Some of these devices are also reimbursable when used by health care professionals in a facility under the CLIA waiver. Professional use of these devices is reviewed on a case-by-case basis.

Diabetes Self-Management Training

Medicare covers outpatient diabetes self-management training (DSMT) services when furnished by a certified provider who meets certain quality standards. DSMT is intended to educate beneficiaries in the successful self-management of diabetes. The program includes instructions in self-monitoring of blood glucose, education about diet and exercise, an insulin treatment plan developed specifically for the patient who is insulin-dependent, and motivation for patients to use the skills for self-management.

Medicare covers the initial training for a patient who has one or more of the following medical conditions present prior to the physician's or nonphysician practitioner's order:

- New onset diabetes or a patient with diabetes who is newly eligible for Medicare
- Inadequate glycemic control as evidenced by a glycosylated hemoglobin (HbA1C) level of 8.5 percent or more on two consecutive HbA1C determinations three or more months apart in the year before the patient begins receiving training
- Change in treatment regimen from diet control to oral diabetes medication, or from oral diabetes medication to insulin
- High risk for complications based on inadequate glycemic control (documented acute episodes of severe hyperglycemia occurring in the past year during which the beneficiary needed emergency room visits or hospitalization)
- High risk based on at least one of the following documented complications:
  - Lack of feeling in the foot or other foot complications such as foot ulcers, deformities, or amputation
  - Pre-proliferative or proliferative retinopathy or prior laser treatment of the eye
  - Kidney complications related to diabetes, when manifested by albuminuria, without other cause, or elevated creatinine

The physician or qualified nonphysician practitioner treating the condition must order the training. The order must include a statement signed by the physician indicating the service is needed, the number of initial or follow-up hours ordered, the topics to be covered in training, and a determination as to whether individual or group training is appropriate.

The condition requiring training must be documented in the medical record maintained by the referring physician or qualified nonphysician practitioner. Patients are eligible to receive follow-up training each calendar year following the year in which they have been certified as requiring initial training. When training under the order is changed, the physician or qualified nonphysician practitioner treating the patient must sign the training order or referral. A copy must be maintained in the patient's file in the DSMT program's records.

Providers billing these codes must provide a copy of the American Diabetes Association's or the Indian Health Service's Education Recognition Program certificate prior to submitting the first claim.

CMS will not reimburse services rendered to a patient in the hospital or SNF, hospice care, nursing home, or in an RHC/FQHC.

Initial DSMT cannot exceed 10 hours. It must be furnished within a continuous 12-month period. Except for one hour, training must be furnished in a group setting, unless there are no group sessions available within two months of when the training is ordered, the beneficiary has documented special needs, or the physician orders additional insulin training.

Follow-up training can consist of no more than two hours of individual or group training per year. Group training consists of two to 20 individuals. Follow-up training must follow the year during which initial training occurred. The physician must document the specific medical condition the training must address.

Medical Nutrition Therapy Services

Medicare covers medical nutrition therapy (MNT) services when furnished by a registered dietitian or nutrition professional meeting certain requirements. The benefit is available for beneficiaries with diabetes or renal disease when a physician makes the referral.

Medicare will cover an initial three-hour visit for an assessment, follow-up visits for interventions not to exceed two hours, and reassessments as necessary during the 12-month period beginning with the initial assessment ("episode of care") to assure compliance with the dietary plan.

For Medicare purposes, MNT is a separate benefit from DSMT. A patient may receive the full amount of both benefits in the same period, which is 10 hours of initial DSMT and three hours of MNT. However, providers are not allowed to bill DSMT and MNT on the same date of service for the same patient.

Medicare will cover MNT if the following conditions are met:

- The treating physician makes a referral and indicates a diagnosis of diabetes or renal disease.
- The number of hours covered in an episode of care are not exceeded unless a second referral is received from the treating physician.

MNT services may be provided on an individual or group basis without restrictions. MNT services are not covered for beneficiaries receiving maintenance dialysis.

The referring physician must maintain documentation in the patient's medical record. Referrals must be made for each episode of care and reassessments prescribed as a result of a change in medical condition or diagnosis.

Additional hours of MNT services may be covered when the treating physician determines there is a change of diagnosis or medical condition that necessitates diet modification.

A qualified registered dietitian or nutrition professional must provide MNT services. In order to file Medicare claims for MNT, a registered dietitian/nutrition professional must be enrolled as a provider in the Medicare program and meet the qualification requirements. Registered dietitians and nutrition professionals must accept assignment. These services can be billed to the FI when performed in a hospital outpatient setting if the nutritionist or registered dietitian reassigns the patient's benefits to the hospital. There is no facility fee payment for these services.

MNT may be billed with CPT codes 97802, 97803, or 97804. HCPCS Level II codes G0270 and G0271 are reported for reassessment and subsequent intervention following a second referral in the same year for a change in diagnosis, medical condition, or treatment regimen.

Dressings

Medicare

Coverage of surgical dressings are limited to primary and secondary dressings required for the treatment of a wound caused by or treated by a surgical procedure that has been performed by a physician or other health care professional. Surgical dressings required after debridement of a wound are also covered, irrespective of the type of debridement, as long as the debridement was reasonable and necessary and was performed by a health care professional acting within the scope of his or her legal authority when performing this function. Surgical dressings are covered for as long as they are medically necessary.

Primary dressings are therapeutic or protective coverings applied directly to wounds or lesions on the skin or caused by an opening to the skin. Secondary dressing materials that serve a therapeutic or protective function and that are needed to secure a primary dressing are also covered. Items such as adhesive tape, roll gauze, bandages, and disposable compression material are examples of secondary dressings. Some items, such as transparent film, may be used as a primary or secondary dressing.

Elastic stockings, support hose, foot coverings, leotards, knee supports, surgical leggings, gauntlets, and pressure garments for the arms and hands are examples of items that are not ordinarily covered as surgical dressings.

Porcine skin dressings are covered if reasonable and necessary for the individual patient as a dressing for burns, donor sites of a homograft, and decubiti and other ulcers. Gradient pressure dressings are Jobst elasticized heavy-duty dressings and are covered when used to reduce hypertrophic scarring and joint contractures following burn injury.

Surgical dressings furnished to an inpatient in a hospital or skilled nursing facility are considered therapeutic items covered under the inpatient stay. Supplies including surgical dressings furnished to an inpatient for use only outside the hospital are not usually covered as inpatient hospital services. However, a temporary supply that is medically necessary to permit or facilitate the patient's discharge from the hospital and is required until the patient can obtain a continuing supply is covered as an inpatient hospital service.

Surgical dressings applied on an outpatient basis in a hospital or skilled nursing facility are covered when provided in connection with a clinic visit or a practitioner's treatment of the outpatient.

If a physician or non-physician practitioner applies surgical dressings as part of a professional service that is billed to Medicare, the surgical dressings are considered incident to the professional services of the health care practitioner.

Surgical dressings used by a home health agency in its visits are generally considered routine supplies that are included in the cost per visit of home health care services. Routine supplies would not include those supplies that are specifically ordered by the physician or are essential to HHA personnel in order to effectuate the plan of care.

When surgical dressings are not covered incident to the services of a health care practitioner and are obtained by the patient from a supplier (e.g., drugstore, physician, or other health care practitioner that qualifies as a supplier) on an order from a physician or other health care professional, the surgical dressings are covered separately under Part B. These dressings would be billed by the supplier to the DME MAC.

Consolidated Billing

All surgical dressings and related supplies dispensed to a nursing home patient/resident or home health services recipient are included in the consolidated billing requirements and each provider's prospective payment system (PPS).

For home health services recipients, all billing related to these items must be performed by the home health agency. For nursing home patients/residents receiving skilled care reimbursed under Part A, these items are considered to be a component of the inpatient stay. If a source other than the skilled nursing facility dispenses these items, the source must look to the nursing home for payment and cannot bill Medicare directly for these items. If the nursing home patient/resident is not receiving a skilled level of care and is not being reimbursed under Part A, then suppliers have a choice. The first option is for the supplier to bill these items directly to the DME MAC. The second option is for the supplier to bill the nursing home directly and the home would bill Medicare.

Drugs, Biologicals, and Radiopharmaceuticals

Medicare

Drugs, biologicals, and radiopharmaceuticals for use in a hospital or skilled nursing facility that are ordinarily furnished by the hospital for the care and treatment of inpatients are covered. Payment is included in the reimbursement for the inpatient Part A covered stay.

Drugs and biologicals furnished by a hospital to an inpatient for use outside the hospital are, in general, not covered as inpatient hospital services. When a drug or biological is deemed medically necessary to permit or facilitate the patient's departure from the hospital, and a limited supply is required until the patient can obtain a continuing supply, the limited supply is covered as an inpatient hospital service.

Medicare Part B provides limited benefits for outpatient drugs. The program covers drugs that are furnished "incident to" a physician's service provided that the drugs are not usually self-administered by the patients who take them.

When reporting concurrent administration for drugs and biologicals that are mixed together, hospitals should report the HCPCS code and quantity of each product. If the hospital is compounding drugs that have no assigned HCPCS code, the hospital should report the unlisted HCPCS Level II drug code J9999 or J3490.

Generally, drugs, biologicals, and radiopharmaceuticals are covered only if all of the following requirements are met:

- They meet the definition of drugs or biologicals
- They are of the type that is not usually self-administered
- They meet all the general requirements for coverage of items as incident to a physician's services
- They are reasonable and necessary for the diagnosis or treatment of the illness or injury for which they are administered according to accepted standards of medical practice
- They are not excluded as noncovered immunizations
- They have not been determined by the Food and Drug Administration (FDA) to be less than effective

The drug must be approved for marketing by the FDA and must be used for indications specified on the labeling.

In order to meet all the general requirements for coverage under the incident-to provision, an FDA approved drug or biological must:

- Be of a form that is not usually self-administered
- Must be furnished by a physician
- Must be administered by the physician or by auxiliary personnel employed by the physician and under the physician's personal supervision

The charge, if any, for the drug, biological, or radiopharmaceutical must be included in the physician's bill, and the cost must represent an expense to the physician. Drugs, biologicals, and radiopharmaceuticals furnished by other health care professionals must also meet these requirements.

Self-administrable Drugs

Medicare Part B does generally not cover drugs that can be self-administered, such as those in pill form or those self-injected. Certain self-administered drugs are covered. Examples of self-administered drugs that are covered include blood-clotting factors, drugs used in immunosuppressive therapy, erythropoietin for dialysis patients, osteoporosis drugs for certain homebound patients, certain oral cancer drugs, and drugs that are necessary for the effective use of Durable Medical Equipment (DME) or prosthetic devices. It is up to the Medicare contractor to determine is a self-administrable drug is covered. Contractors have proscribed instructions to follow when determining if a self-administrable drug is covered. Generally if the drug and route of administration is medically reasonable and necessary the drug will be covered. If a drug is available in both oral and injectable forms, the injectable form of the drug must be medically reasonable and necessary as compared to using the oral form. Self-administrable drugs that are integral to a procedure (e.g., eye drops used prior to or in cataract surgery) are covered.

Antineoplastic Drugs

Antineoplastic drugs, biologicals, or radiopharmaceuticals are covered on an inpatient or outpatient basis for FDA-approved uses. Coverage of off-label uses of antineoplastic drugs, biologicals, or radiopharmaceuticals is dependent upon the Medicare contractor. Check local coverage determinations that may be specific to the contractor.

CMS will cover off-label use of oxaliplatin, irinotecan, cetuximab, or bevacizumab when used in one of nine clinical trials identified by CMS and sponsored by the National Cancer Institute. A list of clinical trials is available at http://cms.hhs.gov/coverage/download/id90b.pdf. When billing for oxaliplatin, irinotecan, cetuximab, or bevacizumab used in one of the nine clinical trials identified by CMS and sponsored by the National Cancer Institute, modifier QR must be appended to the HCPCS Level II code. ICD-9-CM diagnosis code V70.7 must be reported as a secondary diagnosis.

Oral Antineoplastic Drugs

Oral antineoplastic drugs are covered if it has the same active ingredient as the injectable drug. It may have a different chemical composition than the injectable drug but body metabolizing of the drug must result in the same chemical composition in the body. A cancer diagnosis code must be reported when billing for these HCPCS Level II codes. If there is no cancer diagnosis the claim will be denied.

Oral Antiemetic Drugs

Medicare covers oral antiemetic drugs when used as full therapeutic replacement for intravenous dosage forms as part of a cancer chemotherapeutic regimen when the drug is administered or prescribed by a physician for use immediately before, at, or within 48 hours after the time of administration of the chemotherapeutic agent. A cancer diagnosis code must be reported when billing for these HCPCS codes.

The allowable period of covered therapy includes day one, the date of service of the chemotherapy drug (beginning of the time of treatment), plus a period not to exceed two additional calendar days, or a maximum period up to 48 hours. Some drugs are limited to 24 hours; some to 48 hours. The hour limit is included in the narrative description of the HCPCS Level II code.

The oral antiemetic drug should be prescribed only on a per chemotherapy treatment basis. For example, only enough of the oral antiemetic for one 24- or 48-hour dosage regimen (depending upon the drug) should be prescribed/supplied for each incidence of chemotherapy treatment. These drugs may be supplied by the physician in the office, by an inpatient or outpatient provider (e.g., hospital, CAH, SNF, etc.), or through a supplier (e.g., a pharmacy).

The physician must indicate on the prescription that the beneficiary is receiving the oral antiemetic drug as full therapeutic replacement for an intravenous antiemetic drug as part of a cancer chemotherapeutic regimen. When the drug is provided by a facility, the patient's medical record maintained by the facility must be documented to reflect that the patient is receiving the oral antiemetic drug as full therapeutic replacement for an intravenous antiemetic drug as part of a cancer chemotherapeutic regimen.

Take-home Supplies of Oral Antiemetic and Antineoplastic Drugs

Hospitals, including CAHs, cannot bill the contractor for take-home supplies of oral anti-cancer drugs, oral antiemetic drugs, or inhalation drugs, in addition to the previous prohibition on immunosuppressive drugs. Hospitals can bill the contractor and be paid for only a single day's dose administered or dispensed during a defined encounter in a hospital outpatient department. Medicare has specifically defined this encounter as "an encounter with a physician or mid-level professional (e.g., a physician assistant or nurse practitioner) during which one or more specimens are collected for laboratory work, treatment is monitored (including anticancer drugs, either oral or infused), and a drug is administered."

A problem arises only when more than a single day's supply of a drug is dispensed to the patient for take-home use. The hospital has three choices:

1. The hospital may dispense the drugs and not charge for them. They cannot bill the patient for covered drugs and these drugs are covered under Part B in most circumstances.
2. The hospital may issue a prescription for the drugs.
3. The hospital can enroll as a pharmacy supplier with the DME MAC and bill the dispensed drugs and a dispensing fee to the DME MAC via the National Council for Prescription Drug Programs (NCPDP) electronic transaction.

Claims for SNF patients in a non-covered stay, or for hospital or SNF inpatients that have exhausted Part A benefits (TOB 12X or 22X) are not affected. TOBs 12X and 22X would be billed to the contractor as usual. Payment is dependent on the applicable reimbursement methodology for the type of hospital (e.g., OPPS for OPPS hospitals or reasonable cost for CAHs and non-OPPS hospitals).

Drugs Used in DME

Drugs and biologicals that are necessary for the effective use of durable medical equipment are covered if they are reasonable and necessary for treatment of the illness or injury or to improve the functioning of a malformed body member. These drugs and biologicals include those which must be put directly into the equipment in order to achieve the therapeutic benefit of the durable medical equipment or to assure the proper functioning of the equipment (e.g., tumor chemotherapy agents used with an infusion pump or heparin used with a home dialysis system).

Drugs and biologicals dispensed for use in DME must be billed to the DME MAC by a supplier who possesses a current license to dispense prescription drugs in the state in which the drug is dispensed. A supplier that is not the entity that dispenses the drugs or biologicals cannot purchase the item used in conjunction with DME for resale to the beneficiary.

Immunosuppressive Drugs

Immunosuppressive drugs are covered following discharge from a hospital for a Medicare covered organ transplant. Covered drugs include those immunosuppressive drugs that have been specifically labeled as such and approved for marketing by the FDA. (This is an exception to the standing drug policy that permits coverage of FDA-approved drugs for non-labeled uses, where such uses are found to be reasonable and necessary in an individual case.)

Covered drugs also include those prescription drugs, such as prednisone, that are used in conjunction with immunosuppressive drugs as part of a therapeutic regimen reflected in FDA-approved labeling for immunosuppressive drugs. Antibiotics, hypertensives, and other drugs that are not directly related to organ rejection are not covered

Prescriptions for immunosuppressive drugs generally should be non-refillable and limited to a 30-day supply. The 30-day guideline is necessary because dosage frequently diminishes over a period of time, and further, it is not uncommon for the physician to change the prescription from one drug to another. Unless there are special circumstances, contractors will not consider a supply of drugs in excess of 30 days to be reasonable and necessary and will deny payment. OPPS hospitals cannot dispense and bill for 30-day supplies of immunosuppressive drugs unless they are enrolled DME suppliers.

Hemophilia Clotting Factors

Medicare covers blood-clotting factors for hemophilia patients competent to use such factors to control bleeding without medical supervision, and items related to the administration of such factors. For purposes of Medicare Part B coverage, hemophilia encompasses the following conditions:

- Factor VIII deficiency (classic hemophilia)
- Factor IX deficiency (also termed plasma thromboplastin component (PTC) or Christmas factor deficiency)
- von Willebrand's disease

The amount of clotting factors determined to be necessary to have on hand and thus covered under this provision is based on the historical utilization pattern or profile developed by the contractor for each patient. It is expected that the treating source (e.g., a family physician or comprehensive hemophilia diagnostic and treatment center) have such information.

Unanticipated occurrences involving extraordinary events, such as automobile accidents or inpatient hospital stays, will change this base line data and should be appropriately considered. In addition, changes in a patient's medical needs over a period of time require adjustments in the profile.

Medicare will cover anti-inhibitor coagulant complex (AICC) for patients with hemophilia A and inhibitor antibodies to factor VIII who have major bleeding episodes and who fail to respond to other, less expensive therapies.

Reimbursement is based upon the least expensive medically necessary blood clotting factors. Blood clotting factors are available both in virally inactivated forms and a recombinant form. The FDA has determined that both varieties are safe and effective. Therefore, unless the prescription specifically calls for the recombinant form, payment is based on the less expensive, non-recombinant forms.

Consolidated Billing

For nursing home patients/residents receiving skilled care reimbursed under Part A, these items are considered to be a component of the inpatient stay. If a source other than the skilled nursing facility dispenses these items, the source must look to the nursing home for payment and cannot bill Medicare directly for these items. If the nursing home patient/resident is not receiving a skilled level of care and is not being reimbursed under Part A, then suppliers must bill these items directly to the DME MAC. Drugs and biologicals dispensed to home health services recipients must be billed directly by the supplier.

Medicare pays for drugs in one of three ways: some drugs are paid on a cost basis; some under its Prospective Payment System (PPS) plans; but for most drugs outside of a facility setting, Medicare pays the lower of billed charges or the payment limit based on the Average Sales Price (ASP).

The items paid for under this last method include but are not limited to drugs furnished incident to a physician's service, immunosuppressive drugs furnished by pharmacies, drugs furnished by pharmacies under the durable medical equipment benefit, covered oral anticancer drugs, and blood clotting factors. The table below indicates the payment methodology for drugs and biologicals by type and setting.

Enteral Nutrition

Medicare

These nutrient solutions, devices, and accessories are billed to the DME MAC and not to facility or professional contractors. In place of a CMN, a DME information form (DIF) needs to be completed to provide information for enteral and parenteral nutrition (PEN). For PEN, this form is CMS-10126. A DIF is completed and signed by the supplier. It does not require a narrative description of equipment and cost or a physician signature. DIFs are subject to the same requirements and restrictions as CMNs. This form must be submitted with the CMS-1500 claim form. Electronic filers can use the electronic CMN format.

Typical examples of conditions that would qualify for coverage are anatomic in nature, such as head and neck cancer with reconstructive surgery; and disorders impairing motility, such as a central nervous system disease leading to interference with the neuromuscular mechanisms of ingestion, of such severity that the patient cannot be maintained with oral feeding. However, claims for Part B coverage of enteral nutrition therapy for these and any other conditions must be approved on a case-by-case basis. Enteral therapy is not covered for clinical reasons like anorexia, nausea associated with mood disorders, or end stage renal disease.

The patient must have permanent impairment. However, this judgment does not preclude the possibility that the patient will improve. If, in the judgment of the provider, the condition is of long and/or indefinite duration (at least three months), then the test of permanence is considered to be met.

Baby food and other regular grocery products that can be blended and used with the enteral system will be denied as non-covered. Of special note: Ensure will only be covered if the criteria for parenteral and enteral nutrition (PEN) therapy are met; Medicare does not reimburse for Ensure if it is taken orally.

A total daily calorie intake of 20-35 cal/kg/day is considered sufficient to achieve or maintain appropriate body weight in most patients. The ordering provider must document the medical necessity for a caloric intake outside this range in an individual patient. This information must be available to the DME contractor on request.

Consolidated Billing

For nursing home patients/residents receiving skilled care reimbursed under Part A, these items are considered to be a component of the inpatient stay. If a source other than the skilled nursing facility dispenses these items, the source must look to the nursing home for payment and cannot bill Medicare directly for these items. If the nursing home patient/resident is not receiving a skilled level of care and is not being reimbursed under Part A, then suppliers must bill these items directly to the DME MAC. Enteral solutions, supplies, and accessories dispensed to home health services recipients should be billed directly by the supplier.

Documentation Standards

Additional documentation must be included with the first claim for enteral nutrition if the nutrient solutions are to be delivered via a pump, or if special nutrient solutions are needed. Refer to the DME MAC Supplier Manual for specific instructions.

Each claim must contain a physician's written order or prescription and sufficient medical documentation (e.g., hospital records, clinical findings from the attending physician, etc.) to permit an independent conclusion that the patient's condition meets the requirements of the prosthetic device benefit, and that enteral nutrition therapy is medically necessary. Allowed claims are to be reviewed at periodic intervals of no more than three months by the contractor's medical consultant or specially trained staff, and additional medical documentation considered necessary should be obtained as part of this review. (Note: DME MACs may have differing recertification requirements, e.g., every six months instead of every three months.)

An interval recertification for continued coverage of the PEN therapy, usually three to six months (depending on the DME contractor policy), must include a provider's statement describing the continued need for parenteral nutrition. Some recertifications must include specific test results; refer to the DME MAC Supplier Manual for these rules.

If there are changes in the patient's condition causing the reporting of different codes other than those initially certified with the original CMN, or if the patient has an interval of two or more months since the previous enteral nutrition administration, or if the method of administration changes from syringe or gravity to that of a pump, a new CMN and/or recertification must be filed.

The ordering physician is expected to see the patient within 30 days before the initial certification or required recertification (but not revised certifications). If the physician does not see the patient within this timeframe, he/she must document the reason why and describe what other monitoring methods were used to evaluate the patient's enteral nutrition needs.

Hospital Beds

Medicare

Hospital beds used in facilities are considered part of the routine equipment. Their cost should be included in the room and board charges. Specialty beds are generally considered to be included with the definition of routine equipment. Facilities are advised to check with their contractor if there are questions about the appropriateness of additional charges for rented specialty beds

A fixed height hospital bed for use in the patient's home is covered when:

- The patient's condition requires positioning of the body, for example, to alleviate pain, promote good body alignment, prevent contractures, and avoid respiratory infections, in ways not feasible in an ordinary bed. Elevation of the head/upper body less than 30 degrees does not usually require the use of a hospital bed. When the patient requires the head of the bed to be elevated more than 30 degrees due to congestive heart failure, chronic pulmonary disease, or problems with aspiration, pillows or wedges must have been considered and ruled out.

- The patient's condition requires special attachments, such as traction equipment, that cannot be fixed and used on an ordinary bed.

A physician's prescription and additional documentation must establish the medical necessity for a hospital bed for home use. The physician's prescription and supplementing documentation when required must accompany the initial claim. If the stated reason for the need for a hospital bed is the patient's condition requires positioning, the prescription or other documentation must describe the medical condition (e.g., cardiac disease, chronic obstructive pulmonary disease, quadriplegia or paraplegia) and also the severity and frequency of the symptoms of the condition. If the stated reason for requiring a hospital bed is the patient's condition requires special attachments, the prescription must describe the patient's condition and specify the attachments that require a hospital bed.

It is up to the Medicare contractor to determine if a variable height feature of a hospital bed is approved for coverage and is considered medically necessary for one of the following conditions:

- Severe arthritis and other injuries to lower extremities (e.g., fractured hip). The condition requires the variable height feature to assist the patient to ambulate by enabling the patient to place his or her feet on the floor while sitting on the edge of the bed

- Severe cardiac conditions where the patient is able to leave the bed, but must avoid the strain of "jumping" up or down

Coders' Desk Reference for HCPCS

- Spinal cord injuries, including quadriplegic and paraplegic patients, multiple limb amputee, and stroke patients. Those patients who are able to transfer from bed to a wheelchair, with or without help
- Other severely debilitating diseases and conditions, if the variable height feature is required to assist the patient to ambulate.

A heavy duty extra wide hospital bed is covered if the patient meets criteria for hospital bed and weighs more than 350 pounds, but less than 600 pounds. An extra heavy-duty hospital bed is covered if the patient meets criteria for a hospital bed and the patient's weight exceeds 600 pounds.

Electric powered adjustments to lower and raise head and foot may be covered when the provider's medical staff determines that the patient's condition requires frequent change in body position and/or there may be an immediate need for a change in body position (i.e., no delay can be tolerated) and the patient can operate the controls and cause the adjustments. Exceptions may be made in cases of spinal cord injury and brain damaged patients. A total electric hospital bed is not covered, as the height adjustment feature is a convenience feature.

An air-fluidized bed uses warm air under pressure to set small ceramic beads in motion that simulate the movement of fluid. The patient's body weight is evenly distributed over a large surface area, which creates a sensation of floating. Medicare payment for home use of the air-fluidized bed for treatment of pressure sores can be made if such use is reasonable and necessary for the individual patient.

An air-fluidized bed may be considered reasonable and necessary when:

- The patient has a stage three full thickness tissue loss or stage four deep tissue destruction pressure sore
- The patient is bedridden or chair bound as a result of severely limited mobility
- In the absence of an air-fluidized bed, the patient would require institutionalization
- The air-fluidized bed is ordered in writing by the patient's attending physician based upon a comprehensive assessment and evaluation of the patient after completion of a course of conservative treatment designed to optimize conditions that promote wound healing. This course of treatment must have been at least one month in duration without progression toward wound healing. This month of prerequisite conservative treatment may include some period in an institution as long as there is documentation available to verify that the necessary conservative treatment has been rendered
- Use of wet-to-dry dressings for wound debridement, begun during the period of conservative treatment and which continue beyond 30 days, will not preclude coverage of air-fluidized bed. Should additional debridement again become necessary, while a patient is using an air-fluidized bed (after the first 30-day course of conservative treatment), it will not cause the air-fluidized bed to become not covered. In all instances documentation verifying the continued need for the bed must be available.
- A trained adult caregiver is available to assist the patient with activities of daily living, fluid balance, dry skin care, repositioning, recognition and management of altered mental status, dietary needs, prescribed treatments, and management and support of the air-fluidized bed system and its problems such as leakage
- A physician directs the home treatment regimen and reevaluates and recertifies the need for the air-fluidized bed on a monthly basis
- All other alternative equipment has been considered and ruled out

Conservative treatment must include:

- Frequent repositioning of the patient with particular attention to relief of pressure over bony prominences, usually every two hours
- Use of a specialized support surface (Group II) designed to reduce pressure and shear forces on healing ulcers and to prevent new ulcer formation
- Necessary treatment to resolve any wound infection
- Optimization of nutrition status to promote wound healing
- Debridement by any means (including wet to dry dressings that do not require an occlusive covering) to remove devitalized tissue from the wound bed
- Maintenance of a clean, moist bed of granulation tissue with appropriate moist dressings protected by an occlusive covering, while the wound heals

Home use of the air-fluidized bed is not covered under any of the following circumstances:

- The patient has coexisting pulmonary disease (the lack of firm back support makes coughing ineffective and dry air inhalation thickens pulmonary secretions)

- The patient requires treatment with wet soaks or moist wound dressings that are not protected with an impervious covering such as plastic wrap or other occlusive material
- The caregiver is unwilling or unable to provide the type of care required by the patient on an air-fluidized bed
- Structural support is inadequate to support the weight of the air-fluidized bed system (it generally weighs 1,600 pounds or more)
- Electrical system is insufficient for the anticipated increase in energy consumption
- Other known contraindications exist

Coverage of an air-fluidized bed is limited to the equipment itself. Payment for this covered item may only be made if the written order from the attending physician is furnished to the supplier prior to the delivery of the equipment. Payment is not included for the caregiver or for architectural adjustments such as electrical or structural improvement.

For hospital beds used in the home, an order for each item billed must be signed and dated by the treating physician, kept on file by the supplier, and made available to the DME contractor upon request. Items billed to the DME contractor before a signed and dated order has been received by the supplier must be submitted with modifier EY added to each affected HCPCS Level II code.

If the patient does not meet any of the coverage criteria for any type of hospital bed it will be denied as not medically necessary. If documentation does not support the medical necessity of the type of bed billed, payment will be based on the allowance for the least costly medically appropriate alternative.

If the patient's condition requires bedside rails, they can be covered as an integral part of, or an accessory to, a hospital bed. Trapeze equipment is covered if the patient needs this device to sit up because of a respiratory condition, to change body position for other medical reasons, or to get in or out of bed. A bed cradle is covered when it is necessary to prevent contact with the bed coverings. If a patient's condition requires a replacement innerspring mattress or foam rubber mattress it will be covered for a patient owned hospital bed.

A bed board or an over bed table is not covered since it is not primarily medical in nature.

Infusion Pumps, External; Equipment and Supplies

Medicare

Injectable drugs administered in a physician's office, with or without a pump, must be billed to the local carrier and not the DME MAC.

Payment is made if all of the requirements for Medicare reimbursement are met and the applicable DME MAC entity's medical necessity policies for the external infusion pump have been followed.

An external infusion pump is covered for the indications as detailed below:

I. Administration of deferoxamine for the treatment of chronic iron overload

II. Administration of chemotherapy for the treatment of primary hepatocellular carcinoma or colorectal cancer when this disease manifestation cannot be resected or when the patient refuses surgical excision of the tumor

III. Administration of morphine when used in the treatment of intractable pain caused by cancer

IV. Administration of continuous subcutaneous insulin for the treatment of diabetes mellitus, type-I, which has been documented by a serum C-peptide level < 0.5 mcg/L, if either of the following criteria (a) or (b) are met:

a. The patient has completed a comprehensive diabetes education program; has been on a program of multiple daily injections of insulin (i.e., at least three injections per day), with frequent self-adjustments of insulin dose for at least six months prior to initiation of the insulin pump; and has documented frequency of glucose self-testing an average of at least four times per day during the two months prior to initiation of the insulin pump, and meets one or more of the following criteria (1-5) while on the multiple injection regimen:

1. Glycosylated hemoglobin level (HbA1C) less than 7 percent
2. History of recurring hypoglycemia
3. Wide fluctuations in blood glucose before mealtime
4. Dawn phenomenon with fasting blood sugars frequently exceeding 200 mg/dL
5. History of severe glycemic excursions

b. The patient with type-I diabetes has been on an external insulin infusion pump prior to enrollment in Medicare and has documented frequency of glucose self-testing an average of at least four times per day during the month prior to Medicare enrollment.

In addition to meeting Criterion A or B above, the following general requirements must be met:

The patient with diabetes must be insulinopenic per the updated fasting C-peptide testing requirement, or, as an alternative, must be beta cell autoantibody positive. The updated fasting C-peptide testing requirement is:

- Insulinopenia is defined as a fasting C-peptide level that is less than or equal to 110 percent of the lower limit of normal of the laboratory's measurement method.

- For patients with renal insufficiency and creatinine clearance (actual or calculated from age, gender, weight, and serum creatinine) 50 ml/minute, insulinopenia is defined as a fasting C-peptide level that is less than or equal to 200 percent of the lower limit of normal of the laboratory's measurement method.

- Fasting C-peptide levels will only be considered valid with a concurrently obtained fasting glucose 225 mg/dL.

- Levels only need to be documented once in the medical records.

For patients who have purchased an external insulin infusion pump prior to April 1, 2000, insulin and supplies used with the pump are covered during the period of covered use of the pump as long as the patient is a type-I diabetic as evidenced by a serum C-peptide level less than 0.5 mcg/L.

Continued coverage of an external insulin pump requires that the patient be seen and evaluated by the treating physician at least every three months. In addition, the external insulin infusion pump must be ordered and follow-up care rendered by a physician who manages multiple patients on continuous subcutaneous insulin infusion therapy, and who works closely with a team, including nurses, diabetic educators, and dietitians who are knowledgeable in the use of continuous subcutaneous insulin infusion therapy.

V. Administration of other drugs is covered if either of the following sets of criteria (1) or (2) is met:

Criteria set 1:

- Parenteral administration of the drug in the home is reasonable and necessary

- An infusion pump is necessary to safely administer the drug

- The drug is administered by a prolonged infusion of at least eight hours because of proven improved clinical efficacy

- The therapeutic regimen is proven or generally accepted to have significant advantages over intermittent bolus administration regimens or infusions lasting less than eight hours

Criteria set 2:

- Parenteral administration of the drug in the home is reasonable and necessary

- An infusion pump is necessary to safely administer the drug

- The drug is administered by intermittent infusion (each episode of infusion lasting less than eight hours), which does not require the patient to return to the physician's office prior to the beginning of each infusion

- Systemic toxicity or adverse effects of the drug is unavoidable without infusing it at a strictly controlled rate as indicated in the Physicians Desk Reference, American Medical Association's drug evaluations, or the U.S. pharmacopeia drug information

Coverage for the administration of other drugs, based on criteria set (1) or (2), using an external infusion pump, is limited to the following situations (a) to (e):

1. Administration of the anticancer chemotherapy drugs cladribine, fluorouracil, cytarabine, bleomycin, floxuridine, doxorubicin (non-liposomal), vincristine, or vinblastine by continuous infusion over at least eight hours when the regimen is proven or generally accepted to have significant advantages over intermittent administration regimens

2. Administration of narcotic analgesics (except meperidine) in place of morphine to a patient with intractable pain caused by cancer, who has not responded to an adequate oral/transdermal therapeutic

regimen and/or cannot tolerate oral/ transdermal narcotic analgesics

3. Administration of the following antifungal or antiviral drugs: acyclovir, foscarnet, amphotericin B, and ganciclovir. Liposomal amphotericin B is covered for patients who meet one of the following criteria:

    - The patient has suffered some significant toxicity that would preclude the use of standard amphotericin B and is unable to complete the course of therapy without the liposomal form
    - The patient has significantly impaired renal function
    - Payment for the liposomal form will be based on the allowance for the least-costly medically appropriate alternative, standard amphotericin B, unless accompanied by a statement from the provider substantiating the medical need for the liposomal form of amphotericin B for a particular patient

4. Administration of parenteral inotropic therapy, using the drugs dobutamine, milrinone, and/or dopamine, for patients with congestive heart failure and depressed cardiac function if a patient meets all of the following criteria:

    - Dyspnea at rest is present despite treatment with maximum or near maximum tolerated doses of digoxin, a loop diuretic, and an angiotensin converting enzyme inhibitor or another vasodilator (e.g., hydralazine or isosorbide dinitrate), used simultaneously (unless allergic or intolerant). Doses are within the following ranges (lower doses will be covered only if part of a weaning or tapering protocol from higher dose levels):
        - Dobutamine 2.5-10 mcg/kg/min
        - Milrinone 0.375-0.750 mcg/kg/min
        - Dopamine < 2 mcg/kg/min
    - Invasive hemodynamic studies performed within six months prior to the initiation of home inotropic therapy show (a) cardiac index (CI) is less than or equal to 2.2 liters/min/meter squared and/or pulmonary capillary wedge pressure (PCWP) is greater than or equal to 20 mm Hg before inotrope infusion on maximum medical management and (b) at least a 20 percent increase in CI and/or at least a 20 percent decrease in PCWP during inotrope infusion at the dose initially prescribed for home infusion

    - There has been an improvement in patient well being (less dyspnea, improved diuresis, improved renal function, and/or reduction in weight), with the absence of dyspnea at rest at the time of discharge and the capability of outpatient evaluation by the prescribing provider at least monthly

    - In the case of continuous infusion, there is documented deterioration in clinical status when the drug is tapered or discontinued under observation in the hospital, or, in the case of intermittent infusions, there is documentation of repeated hospitalizations for congestive heart failure despite maximum medical management

    - Any life threatening arrhythmia is controlled prior to hospital discharge and there is no need for routine electrocardiographic monitoring at home

    - The patient is maintained on the lowest practical dose, and efforts to decrease the dose of the drug or the frequency/duration of infusion are documented during the first three months of therapy

    - The patient's cardiac symptoms, vital signs, weight, lab values, and response to therapy are routinely assessed and documented in the patient's medical record

5. Administration of parenteral epoprostenol for patients with pulmonary hypertension if they meet the following disease criteria:

    - The pulmonary hypertension is not secondary to pulmonary venous hypertension (e.g., left-sided atrial or ventricular disease, left-sided valvular heart disease, etc.) or disorders of the respiratory system (e.g., chronic obstructive pulmonary disease, interstitial lung disease, obstructive sleep apnea or other sleep disordered breathing, alveolar hypoventilation disorders, etc.)

    - The patient has primary pulmonary hypertension or pulmonary hypertension that is secondary to one of the following conditions:
        - connective tissue disease

- thromboembolic disease of the pulmonary arteries
- human immunodeficiency virus (HIV) infection
- cirrhosis
- diet drugs
- congenital left-to-right shunts
• If these conditions are present, the following criteria must be met:
  - the pulmonary hypertension has progressed despite maximal medical and/or surgical treatment of the identified condition
  - the mean pulmonary artery pressure is greater than 25 mm Hg at rest or greater than 30 mm Hg with exertion
  - the patient has significant symptoms from the pulmonary hypertension (i.e., severe dyspnea on exertion, and either fatigability, angina, or syncope)
  - treatment with oral calcium channel blocking agents has been tried and failed, or has been considered and ruled out
6. Administration of gallium nitrate for the treatment of symptomatic cancer-related hypercalcemia (ICD-9-CM diagnosis code 275.42). Generally, patients should have serum calcium (corrected for albumin) equal to or greater than 12 mg/dl.

The recommended usage for gallium nitrate is daily for five consecutive days. Use for more than five days will be denied as not medically necessary. More than one course of treatment for the same episode of hypercalcemia will be denied as not medically necessary.

Other Supplies

External infusion pumps and related drugs and supplies will be denied as not medically necessary when the criteria described by the above indications are not met. When an infusion pump is covered, the drug necessitating the use of the pump and necessary supplies are also covered. When a pump has been purchased by the Medicare program, other insurer, or the patient, or the rental cap has been reached, the drug necessitating the use of the pump and supplies are covered as long as the coverage criteria for the pump are met.

An IV pole is covered only when a stationary infusion pump is covered. It is considered not medically necessary if it is billed with an ambulatory infusion pump.

Supplies used with an external infusion pump (excluding external insulin infusion pumps) are covered during the period of covered use of an infusion pump. Allowance is based on the number of cassettes or bags prepared. For intermittent infusions, no more than one cassette or bag is covered for each dose of drug. For continuous infusion, the concentration of the drug and the size of the cassette or bag should be maximized to result in the fewest cassettes or bags in keeping with good pharmacologic and medical practice. Drugs and supplies that are dispensed, but not used for unforeseen circumstances (e.g., emergency admission to hospital, drug toxicity, etc.) are covered. Suppliers are expected to anticipate changing needs for drugs (e.g., planned hospital admissions, drug level testing with possible dosage change, etc.) in their drug and supply preparation and delivery schedule.

Charges for drugs administered via a DME infusion pump may only be billed by the entity that actually dispenses the drug to the Medicare patient, and that entity must be permitted under all applicable federal, state, and local laws and regulations to dispense drugs. Drugs and related supplies and equipment billed by a supplier who does not meet these criteria will be denied as not medically necessary.

The DME MAC does not process claims for implantable infusion pumps or drugs and supplies used in conjunction with an implantable infusion pump. Hospitals submit claims for these items to their intermediary. Claims for implantable pumps, drugs, and supplies from other providers are billed to the local carrier.

Drugs used in a DME infusion pump should be coded using the appropriate HCPCS codes or NDC number. If the drug does not have a distinct code, then use the unclassified drug code J7799. Do not use J9999; this code is not valid for claims billed to the DME MAC.

Any entity billing drugs to a DME MAC must use the NDC number.

Medicare Noncovered Items/Services

External insulin infusion pumps for type-II diabetics, including insulin-treated type-II diabetics, will be denied as not medically necessary.

An external infusion pump and related drugs and supplies will be denied as not medically necessary in the home setting for the treatment of thromboembolic disease and/or pulmonary embolism by heparin infusion.

An infusion controller device has been considered by the Medicare program as not medically necessary.

Documentation Standards

For an item to be considered for coverage and payment by Medicare, the information submitted by the supplier must be corroborated by documentation in the physician's medical records that Medicare coverage criteria have been met. The patient's medical records include the provider's office records, hospital records, nursing home records, home health agency records, or records from other health care professionals. This documentation must be available to the DME MAC upon request.

An order for the item that has been signed and dated by the treating provider and a DIF (CMS form 10125) that has been filled out, signed, and dated by the treating provider must be kept on file by the supplier. For external infusion pumps, an ICD-9-CM diagnosis code (specific to the fifth digit) describing the condition that necessitates the pump must be included on each order and DIF for the pump, drug/insulin, and/or supplies.

If a patient begins using an infusion for one drug and subsequently the drug is changed or if another drug is added, a revised DIF must be submitted for use of the pump with the new or additional drug. In the case of an additional drug, all drugs for which the pump is used should be included on the revised DIF.

If an inotropic drug is ordered, the initial claim must include a copy of the order (prescription and documentation from the treating physician), which includes information relating to each of the criteria defined in the aforementioned guidelines. This must include the before and after inotropic drug infusion values.

Medical necessity related to specific clinical data may not be completed by the supplier or by anyone in a financial relationship with the supplier. If coverage criteria as stated in the Medicare policy are not met, the claim should be accompanied by a letter from the physician detailing the patient's history (e.g., dates of past hospitalization for heart failure, prior use of parenteral inotropics and the results, etc.). If invasive hemodynamic studies were not performed, a letter and any supporting documentation should accompany the claim explaining the rationale for not performing the tests.

Lens

Medicare

Refractive lenses are covered when they are medically necessary to restore the vision normally provided by the natural lens of the eye of an individual lacking the organic lens because of surgical removal or congenital absence. Covered diagnoses are limited to Pseudophakia (ICD-9-CM code V43.1), Aphakia (ICD-9-CM code 379.31), and congenital Aphakia (ICD-9-CM code 743.35). Lenses provided for other diagnoses will be denied as noncovered.

Aphakia is the absence of the lens of the eye. Pseudophakia is an eye in which the natural lens has been replaced with an artificial intraocular lens (IOL).

After each cataract surgery with insertion of an intraocular lens (ICD-9-CM code V43.1), coverage is limited to one pair of eyeglasses or contact lenses. Replacement glasses and lenses are noncovered. If a patient has a cataract extraction with IOL insertion in one eye, subsequently has a cataract extraction with IOL insertion in the other eye, and does not receive spectacles or cataract lenses between the two surgical procedures, Medicare covers only one pair of eyeglasses or contact lenses after the second surgery. If a patient has a pair of eyeglasses, has a cataract extraction with IOL insertion, and receives only new lenses, but not new frames after the surgery, the benefit would not cover new frames at a later date (unless it follows subsequent cataract extraction in the other eye).

Refractive lenses are covered even though the surgical removal of the natural lens occurred before Medicare entitlement.

For patients who are aphakic who do not have an IOL (ICD-9-CM codes 379.31 and 743.35), the following lenses or combinations of lenses are covered when determined to be medically necessary:

- Lenses in frames for far vision and lenses in frames for near vision
- Contact lenses for far vision (including for cases of binocular and monocular aphakia); payment will be made for the contact lenses, as well as lenses in frames for near vision to be worn at the same time as the contact lens, and lenses in frames to be worn when the contacts have been removed

When billing claims for a progressive lens, use the appropriate code for the standard bifocal (V2200-V2299) or trifocal (V2300-V2399) lens, and a second line item using V2781 for the difference between the charge for the progressive lens and the standard lens.

If aphakia is the result of the removal of a previously implanted lens, the date of the surgical removal of the lens must accompany the claim.

Medicare Noncovered Items/Services
Lenses used as sunglasses (pseudophakic patient) in addition to regular prosthetic lenses are not covered.

Ostomy Devices and Supplies

Medicare
Ostomy bags supplies and necessary accessories required for attachment are covered as prosthetic devices. This coverage also includes irrigation and flushing equipment and other items and supplies directly related to ostomy care, whether the attachment of a bag is required.

Ostomy supplies are exempt DME in a hospital setting under certain restrictions. When the ostomy supply is associated with the surgery that created the opening or a revision to the opening, it is an exempt DME item. In that situation, hospitals bill their intermediary. If the ostomy supply is used in other circumstances it does not qualify as an exempt DME. Freestanding ambulatory surgery centers are also allowed the same exemptions as hospitals.

They may bill the items listed as exempt DME to their carrier.

Ostomy supplies used in the home for routine care must be dispensed and billed by a DME supplier.

Consolidated Billing
All ostomy devices, supplies, and accessories dispensed to a nursing home patient/resident or home health services recipient are included in the consolidated billing requirements and each provider's prospective payment system (PPS).

For home health services recipients, all billing related to these items must be performed by the home health agency. For nursing home patients/residents receiving skilled care reimbursed under Part A, these items are considered to be a component of the inpatient stay. If a source other than the skilled nursing facility dispenses these items, the source must look to the nursing home for payment and cannot bill Medicare directly for these items. If the nursing home patient/resident is not receiving a skilled level of care and is not being reimbursed under Part A, then suppliers have a choice. The first option is for the supplier to bill these items directly to the DME MAC. The second option is for the supplier to bill the nursing home directly and the home would bill Medicare.

Oxygen (O_2) and O_2 Equipment

Medicare
Oxygen furnished to hospital inpatients is covered as a part of the inpatient stay as a supply. Oxygen furnished to hospital outpatients is covered as a part of the outpatient visit or surgery. Routine supplies furnished by the physician in the course of performing his or her services (e.g., gauze, ointments, bandages, and oxygen) are covered. Charges for such services and supplies must be included in the physician's bill.

Home oxygen and oxygen equipment is covered by Medicare as reasonable and necessary only for patients with significant hypoxemia who meet the medical documentation, laboratory evidence, and health conditions as specified below.

Coverage is available for patients with significant hypoxemia in the chronic stable state (e.g., not during a period of acute illness or an exacerbation of their underlying disease) when the patient has:

- A severe lung disease, such as chronic obstructive pulmonary disease, diffuse interstitial lung disease, cystic fibrosis, bronchiectasis, widespread pulmonary neoplasm

- Hypoxia-related symptoms or findings that might be expected to improve with oxygen therapy (e.g., pulmonary hypertension, recurring congestive heart failure due to chronic cor pulmonale, erythrocytosis, impairment of the cognitive process, nocturnal restlessness, and morning headache)

If the patient has one of these conditions the following further requirements apply:

- Group I—Patients with significant hypoxemia evidenced by any of the following:

  – An arterial PO_2 at or below 55 mm Hg or an arterial oxygen saturation at or below 88 percent, taken at rest, breathing room air

  – An arterial PO_2 at or below 55 mm Hg or an arterial oxygen saturation at or below 88 percent, taken during sleep for a patient who demonstrates an arterial PO_2 at or above 56 mm Hg or an arterial oxygen saturation at or above 89 percent, while awake; or a greater than normal fall in oxygen level during sleep (a decrease in arterial PO_2 more than 10 mm Hg or decrease in arterial oxygen saturation more than 5 percent) associated with symptoms or signs reasonably attributable to hypoxemia (e.g., impairment of cognitive processes and nocturnal restlessness or insomnia). In either of these cases, coverage is provided only for use of oxygen during sleep, and then only one type of unit will be covered. Portable oxygen would not be covered in this situation

- An arterial PO_2 at or below 55 mm Hg or an arterial oxygen saturation at or below 88 percent, taken during exercise for a patient who demonstrates an arterial PO_2 at or above 56 mm Hg, or an arterial oxygen saturation at or above 89 percent, during the day while at rest. In this case, supplemental oxygen is provided during exercise if there is evidence the use of oxygen improves the hypoxemia that was demonstrated during exercise when the patient was breathing room air

- Group II—Patients whose arterial PO_2 is 56 to 59 mm Hg or whose arterial blood oxygen saturation is 89 percent, if there is evidence of:
  - Dependent edema suggesting congestive heart failure
  - Pulmonary hypertension or cor pulmonale, determined by measurement of pulmonary artery pressure, gated blood pool scan, echocardiogram, or "P" pulmonale on EKG (P wave greater than 3 mm in standard leads II, III, or AVF)

- Erythrocythemia with a hematocrit greater than 56 percent

- Group III—The Medicare contractor's reviewing physician will review on a case-by-case basis instances where oxygen is ordered for patients arterial PO_2 levels at or above 60 mm Hg or arterial blood oxygen saturation at or above 90 percent.

Initial claims for oxygen services must include a completed CMN (CMS form 484) to establish whether coverage criteria are met and to ensure that the oxygen services provided are consistent with the physician's prescription or other medical documentation. The documentation must indicate the other forms of treatment that have been tried (e.g., medical and physical therapy directed at secretions, bronchospasm, and infection) and that these treatments have not been sufficiently successful.

The medical and prescription information in section B of the CMN can be completed only by the treating physician, the physician's employee, or another clinician (e.g., nurse, respiratory therapist, etc.) as long as that person is not the DME supplier.

Although hospital discharge coordinators and medical social workers may assist in arranging for physician-prescribed home oxygen, they do not have the authority to prescribe the services. Suppliers may not enter this information. While this section may be completed by a non-physician clinician or a physician employee, it must be reviewed and the CMN must be signed by the attending physician.

Claims for oxygen must also be supported by medical documentation in the patient's record. Separate documentation is used with electronic billing. This documentation may be in the form of a prescription written by the patient's attending physician who has recently examined the patient, usually within a month of the start of therapy, and must specify:

- A diagnosis of the disease requiring home use of oxygen
- The oxygen flow rate
- An estimate of the frequency, duration of use (e.g., 2 liters per minute, 10 minutes per hour, 12 hours per day), and duration of need (e.g., six months or lifetime) Note that a prescription for "Oxygen PRN" or "Oxygen as needed" does not meet this requirement

The attending physician should specify the type of oxygen delivery system to be used (e.g., gas, liquid, or concentrator).

New medical documentation written by the patient's attending physician must be submitted in support of revised oxygen requirements when there has been a change in the patient's condition and need for oxygen therapy. Repeat arterial blood gas studies are appropriate when evidence indicates that an oxygen recipient has undergone a major change in his or her condition relevant to home use of oxygen.

A physician's certification of medical necessity for oxygen equipment must include the results of specific testing before coverage can be determined. Initial claims for oxygen therapy must include the results of a blood gas study that has been ordered and evaluated by the attending physician. This is usually in the form of a measurement of the partial pressure of oxygen (PO_2) in arterial blood. A measurement of arterial oxygen saturation obtained by ear or pulse oximetry is also acceptable when ordered and evaluated by the attending and performed under his or her supervision or when performed by a qualified provider or supplier of laboratory services.

When the arterial blood gas and the oximetry studies are both used to document the need for home oxygen therapy and the results are conflicting, the arterial blood gas study is the preferred source of documenting medical need. Blood gas tests can be conducted by a hospital certified to do such tests. The conditions under which the laboratory tests are performed must be specified in writing and submitted with the initial claim (i.e., at rest, during exercise, or during sleep).

It is expected that virtually all patients who qualify for home oxygen coverage for the first time have recently been discharged from a hospital where they have had arterial blood gas tests; these hospital tests can be submitted in support of initial claims for home oxygen. If more than one arterial blood gas test is performed during the patient's hospital stay, the test result obtained closest to, but no earlier than two days prior to the hospital discharge date, is required as evidence of the need for home oxygen therapy. For those patients whose initial oxygen prescription did not originate during a hospital stay, blood gas studies should be done while the patient is in the chronic stable state (i.e., not during a period of an acute illness or an exacerbation of the underlying disease).

Medicare Noncovered Items/Services

Conditions for which oxygen therapy is not covered include:

- Angina pectoris in the absence of hypoxemia. This condition is generally not the result of a low oxygen level in the blood, and there are other preferred treatments.
- Breathlessness without cor pulmonale or evidence of hypoxemia. Although intermittent oxygen use is sometimes prescribed to relieve this condition, it is potentially harmful and psychologically addicting.
- Severe peripheral vascular disease that results in clinically evident desaturation in one or more extremities. There is no evidence that increased PO_2 improves the oxygenation of tissues with impaired circulation.
- Terminal illnesses that do not affect the lungs.

The Medicare program assumes any delivery charges for home O_2 equipment are included in the price charged for the equipment. Separate reimbursement for delivery is not typically paid and separate charges are prohibited from being charged.

Medicare does not reimburse for O_2 when the Medicare beneficiary is traveling on an airplane.

Oxygen equipment that is purchased is not eligible for Medicare coverage.

Claims for supplies and accessories, including drugs, will be denied if submitted in advance of claims for the base equipment. If the DME MAC cannot determine that the patient either owns or rents the O_2 base equipment, the supplies and accessories will be denied payment. A denial may also occur if the DME MAC cannot establish whether or not the patient meets the medical necessity requirements for the base O_2 equipment.

Consolidated Billing

If oxygen and related equipment are dispensed to a nursing home patient/resident receiving skilled care reimbursed under Part A, these items are considered to be a component of the inpatient stay. If a source other than the skilled nursing facility dispenses these items, the source must look to the nursing home for payment and cannot bill Medicare directly for these items. If the nursing home patient/resident is not receiving a skilled level of care and is not being reimbursed under Part A, then suppliers should bill these items directly to the DME MAC. For home health services recipients, suppliers should bill these items to the HHA as they are included in consolidated billing requirements.

Parenteral Nutrition

Medicare

For parenteral nutrition therapy to be covered under Part B, the claim must be accompanied by the physician's or provider's certified DIF, and there must be evidence of written medical documentation to permit an independent conclusion that the requirements of a prosthetic device benefit are met, and that parenteral nutrition therapy is medically necessary. An example of a condition that would typically qualify for coverage is a massive small bowel resection resulting in severe nutritional deficiency in spite of adequate oral intake. However, coverage of parenteral nutrition therapy for this and any other condition must be approved (certified) on a case-by-case basis initially and at periodic intervals of no more than three months by the carrier's medical consultant or specially trained staff, relying on medical and other documentation as the carrier may require.

Nutrient solutions for parenteral therapy are routinely covered. However, Medicare will not pay for more than one month's supply of nutrients at any one time. Claims submitted retroactively (vs. prospectively, for qualified providers) may include multiple months.

Reimbursement for nutrient solutions is based on the reasonable charge for the solution components (vs. a pre-mixed solution). However, if the patient's medical record establishes that the patient, due to physical or mental state, is unable to safely or

Medicare Guidelines for Selected Topics

effectively mix the solution, and there is no family member or other person who can assist the patient, payment can be made on the basis of the reasonable charge for the more expensive premixed solutions. The medical record must include a signed statement from the attending physician that attests that the premixed solutions are required.

The patient must have a (a) condition involving the small intestine and/or its exocrine glands that significantly impairs the absorption of nutrients or (b) disease of the stomach and/or intestine that is a motility disorder and impairs the ability of nutrients to be transported through the gastrointestinal (GI) system. There must be objective evidence supporting the clinical diagnosis.

Parenteral nutrition is noncovered for the patient with a functioning gastrointestinal tract whose need for parenteral nutrition is only due to the following:

- A swallowing disorder
- A temporary defect in gastric emptying, such as a metabolic or electrolyte disorder
- A psychological disorder impairing food intake, such as depression
- A metabolic disorder inducing anorexia, such as cancer
- A physical disorder impairing food intake, such as the dyspnea of severe pulmonary or cardiac disease
- A side effect of a medication
- Renal failure and/or dialysis

Parenteral nutrition is covered in any of the following situations:

A. The patient has undergone recent (within the past three months) massive small bowel resection leaving less than five feet of small bowel beyond the ligament of Treitz.

B. The patient has a short bowel syndrome that is severe enough that the patient has net gastrointestinal fluid and electrolyte malabsorption, such that on an oral intake of 2.5 to 3.0 liters/day, the enteral losses exceed 50 percent of the oral/enteral intake and the urine output is less than 1 liter/day.

C. The patient requires bowel rest for at least three months and is receiving intravenously 20-35 cal/kg/day for treatment of symptomatic pancreatitis with/without pancreatic pseudocyst, severe exacerbation of regional enteritis, or a proximal enterocutaneous fistula where tube feeding distal to the fistula is not possible.

D. The patient has complete mechanical small bowel obstruction where surgery is not an option.

E. The patient is significantly malnourished (10 percent weight loss over three months or less and serum albumin less than 3.4 gm/DL) and has severe fat malabsorption (fecal fat exceeds 50 percent of oral/enteral intake on a diet of at least 50 gm of fat/day as measured by a standard 72 hour fecal fat test).

F. The patient is significantly malnourished (10 percent weight loss over three months or less and serum albumin less than 3.4 gm/Dl) and has a severe motility disturbance of the small intestine and/or stomach that is unresponsive to prokinetic medication, and is demonstrated either (1) scintigraphically (solid meal gastric emptying study demonstrates that the isotope fails to reach the right colon by six hours following ingestion), or (2) radiographically (barium or radiopaque pellets fail to reach the right colon by six hours following administration). These studies must be performed when the patient is not acutely ill and is not on any medication that would decrease bowel motility. Unresponsiveness to prokinetic medication is defined as the presence of daily symptoms of nausea and vomiting while taking maximal doses.

For criteria A through F above, the conditions are deemed to be severe enough that the patient would not be able to maintain weight and strength on only oral intake or tube enteral nutrition. Patients who do not meet criteria A through F above must meet criteria 1 and 2, which is modification of diet and pharmacologic intervention, plus criteria G and H below:

G. The patient is malnourished (10 percent weight loss over three months or less and serum albumin less than 3.4 gm/Dl).

H. A disease or clinical condition has been documented as being present and it has not responded to altering the manner of delivery of appropriate nutrients (e.g., enteral therapy — slow infusion of nutrients through a tube with the tip located in the stomach or jejunum).

The following are some examples of moderate abnormalities that would require a failed trial of tube enteral nutrition before parenteral nutrition would be covered:

- Moderate fecal fat malabsorption that exceeds 25 percent of oral/enteral intake on a diet of at least 50 gm of fat/day as measured by a standard 72 hour fecal fat test

- Diagnosis of malabsorption with objective confirmation by methods other than 72-hour fecal fat test (e.g., Sudan stain of stool, d-xylose test, etc.)
- Gastroparesis that has been demonstrated (a) radiographically or scintigraphically as described in F above with the isotope or pellets failing to reach the jejunum in three to six hours, or (b) by manometric motility studies with results consistent with an abnormal gastric emptying, and which is unresponsive to prokinetic medication
- A small bowel motility disturbance that is unresponsive to prokinetic medication, demonstrated with a gastric to right colon transit time between three to six hours
- A small bowel resection leaving greater than five feet of small bowel beyond the ligament of Treitz
- A short bowel syndrome that is not severe (as defined in B)
- A mild to moderate exacerbation of regional enteritis, or an enterocutaneous fistula
- A partial mechanical small bowel obstruction where surgery is not an option as long as the following criteria are met: 1a) a permanent condition of the alimentary tract is present that has been deemed to require parenteral therapy because of its severity (criteria A-F); or 1b) a permanent condition of the alimentary tract is present that is unresponsive to standard medical management (criterion H); and 2) the person is unable to maintain weight and strength (criterion G)

If the coverage requirements for parenteral nutrition are met, medically necessary nutrients, administration supplies, and equipment are covered.

There are specific guidelines that contain stipulations for patients who require intradialytic parenteral nutrition (IDPN), as well as parameters of coverage for total caloric daily intake; nutrition solutions containing little or no amino acids and/or carbohydrates; solutions with proteins outside of the range of 0.8-1.5 gm/kg/day; dextrose concentration less than 10 percent, or lipid use; and guidelines for patients with the ability to obtain partial nutrition from oral intake or a combination of oral/enteral (or even oral/enteral/parenteral) intake.

Consolidated Billing

For nursing home patients/residents receiving skilled care reimbursed under Part A, these items are considered to be a component of the inpatient stay. If a source other than the skilled nursing facility dispenses these items, the source must look to the nursing home for payment and cannot bill Medicare directly for these items. If the nursing home patient/resident is not receiving a skilled level of care and is not being reimbursed under Part A, then suppliers must bill these items directly to the DME MAC. Parenteral solutions, supplies, and accessories dispensed to home health services recipients should be billed directly by the supplier.

Documentation Standards

Additional documentation must be included with the first claim for parenteral nutrition, depending on the type of solution that is medically necessary.

An interval recertification for continued coverage of the PEN therapy, usually three to six months (depending on the DME MAC policy), must include a physician's statement describing the continued need for parenteral nutrition. Some recertifications must include specific test results; refer to the DME MAC Supplier Manual for these rules.

The ordering physician is expected to see the patient within 30 days before the initial certification or required recertification (but not revised certifications). If the physician does not see the patient within this timeframe, the provider must document the reason why and describe what other monitoring methods were used to evaluate the patient's nutrition needs.

If there are changes in the patient's condition that cause the reporting of different codes other than those initially certified with the original DIF, a new DIF and/or recertification must be filed.

Pressure Reducing Support Surfaces: Groups I, II, and III

Medicare

General Coverage: Codes E0185 and E0197-E0199 identified as "pressure pad for mattress" describe nonpowered pressure reducing mattress overlays. These devices are designed to be placed on top of a standard hospital or home mattress. A gel/gel-like mattress overlay (E0185) is characterized by a gel or gel-like layer with a height of 2 inches or greater. An air mattress overlay (E0197) is characterized by interconnected air cells having a cell height of 3 inches or greater that are inflated with an air pump. A water mattress overlay (E0198) is characterized by a filled height of 3 inches or greater. A foam mattress overlay (E0199) is characterized by all of the following:

- Base thickness of 2 inches or greater and peak height of 3 inches or greater if it is a convoluted overlay (e.g., egg crate-type), or an overall

height of at least 3 inches if it is a non-convoluted overlay
- Foam with a density and other qualities that provide adequate pressure reduction
- Durable, waterproof cover

Codes E0186, E0187, and E0196 describe nonpowered pressure-reducing mattresses. A foam mattress (E0184) is characterized by all of the following:

- Foam height of 5 inches or greater
- Foam with a density and other qualities that provide adequate pressure reduction
- Durable, waterproof cover
- Can be placed directly on a hospital bed frame

An air, water, or gel mattress (E0186, E0187, E0196) is characterized by all of the following:

- Height of 5 inches or greater of the air, water, or gel layer (respectively)
- Durable, waterproof cover
- Can be placed directly on a hospital bed frame

Codes E0180, E0181, E0182, and A4640 describe powered pressure-reducing mattress overlay systems (alternating pressure or low air loss). They are characterized by all of the following:

- An air pump or blower that provides either sequential inflation and deflation of air cells or a low interface pressure throughout the overlay
- Inflated cell height of the air cells through which air is being circulated 2.5 inches or greater
- Height of the air chambers, proximity of the air chambers to one another, frequency of air cycling (for alternating pressure overlays), and air pressure provide adequate patient lift, reduce pressure, and prevent bottoming out

The staging (grading) of pressure ulcers used in Medicare's policy follows:

- Stage I—nonblanchable erythema of intact skin
- Stage II—partial thickness skin loss involving epidermis and/or dermis
- Stage III—full thickness skin loss involving damage or necrosis of subcutaneous tissue that may extend down to, but not through, underlying fascia
- Stage IV—full thickness skin loss with extensive destruction, tissue necrosis, or damage to muscle, bone, or supporting structures

"Bottoming out" is the finding that an outstretched hand, placed palm up between the undersurface of the overlay or mattress and the patient's bony prominence (coccyx or lateral trochanter), can readily palpate the bony prominence. This bottoming out criterion should be tested with the patient in the supine position with their head flat, in the supine position with their head slightly elevated (no more than 30 degrees), and in the side-lying position.

A group I mattress overlay or mattress (A4640, E0181-E0187, E0196-E0199) is covered if the patient meets criterion 1 or criteria 2 or 3 and at least one of criteria 4 through 7:

Criteria:

1. Completely immobile (i.e., patient cannot make changes in body position without assistance)
2. Limited mobility (i.e., patient cannot independently make changes in body position significant enough to alleviate pressure)
3. Any stage pressure ulcer on the trunk or pelvis
4. Impaired nutritional status
5. Fecal or urinary incontinence
6. Altered sensory perception
7. Compromised circulatory status

When the coverage criteria for a group I overlay or mattress are not met, a claim will be denied as not medically necessary unless there is clear documentation that justifies the medical necessity for the item in the individual case. A group I support surface billed without modifier KX (see later in this section) will usually be denied as not medically necessary.

A foam overlay or mattress that does not have a waterproof cover is not considered durable (i.e., DME) and will be denied as noncovered by the Medicare program.

The support surface provided for the patient should be one in which the patient does not bottom out.

Clinical information for Group I support surfaces: Patients needing pressure-reducing support surfaces should have a care plan that has been established by the patient's physician or home care nurse, which is documented in the patient's medical records, and which generally should include the following:

- Education of the patient and caregiver on the prevention and/or management of pressure ulcers

- Regular assessment by a nurse, physician, or other licensed health care practitioner
- Appropriate turning and positioning
- Appropriate wound care (for a stage II, III, or IV ulcer)
- Appropriate management of moisture/incontinence
- Nutritional assessment and intervention consistent with the overall plan of care

Note: Products containing multiple components are categorized according to the clinically predominant component (usually the topmost layer of a multi-layer product). For example, a product with 3 inch powered air cells on top of a 3 inch foam base would be coded as a powered overlay (E0181), not as a powered mattress (E0277).

Group II support surfaces: E0277 describes a powered pressure-reducing mattress (alternating pressure, low air loss, or powered flotation without low air loss) that is characterized by all of the following:

- An air pump or blower that provides either sequential inflation and deflation of the air cells or a low interface pressure throughout the mattress
- Inflated cell height of the air cells through which air is being circulated is 5 inches or greater
- Height of the air chambers, proximity of the air chambers to one another, frequency of air cycling (for alternating pressure mattresses), and air pressure provide adequate patient lift, reduce pressure, and prevent bottoming out
- A surface designed to reduce friction and shear
- Can be placed directly on a hospital bed frame

Code E0193 describes a semielectric or total electric hospital bed with a fully integrated powered pressure-reducing mattress that has all of the characteristics defined previously under code E0277 characteristics.

Code E0371 describes an advanced nonpowered pressure-reducing mattress overlay that is characterized by all of the following:

- Height and design of individual cells that provide significantly more pressure reduction than a group I overlay, and prevent bottoming out
- Total height of 3 inches or greater
- A surface designed to reduce friction and shear

Documented evidence to substantiate that the product is effective for the treatment of conditions described by the coverage criteria for group II support surfaces

Code E0372 describes a powered pressure reducing mattress overlay (low air loss, powered flotation without low air loss, or alternating pressure) that is characterized by all of the following:

- An air pump or blower that provides either sequential inflation and deflation of the air cells or a low interface pressure throughout the overlay
- Inflated cell height of the air cells through which air is being circulated is 3.5 inches or greater
- Height of the air chambers, proximity of the air chambers to one another, frequency of air cycling (for alternating pressure overlays), and air pressure to provide adequate patient lift, reduce pressure, and prevent bottoming out
- A surface designed to reduce friction and shear

Code E0373 describes an advanced nonpowered pressure-reducing mattress that is characterized by all of the following:

- Height and design of individual cells that provide significantly more pressure reduction than a group I mattress, and prevent bottoming out
- Total height of 5 inches or greater
- A surface designed to reduce friction and shear
- Can be placed directly on a hospital bed frame

The staging of pressure ulcers for group II support surfaces is the same as that for group I support surfaces.

A group II support surface is covered if the patient meets criterion 1, 2, and 3; criterion 4; or criterion 5 and 6.

Criteria:

1. Multiple stage II pressure ulcers located on the trunk or pelvis
2. Patient on a comprehensive ulcer treatment program for at least the past month, which includes the use of an appropriate group 1 support surface
3. The ulcers have worsened or remained the same over the past month
4. Large or multiple stage III or IV pressure ulcer on the trunk or pelvis

5. Recent myocutaneous flap or skin graft for a pressure ulcer on the trunk or pelvis (surgery within the past 60 days)
6. The patient on a group II or III support surface immediately prior to a recent discharge from a hospital or nursing facility (discharge within the past 30 days)

The comprehensive ulcer treatment described in criterion two above should generally include:

- Education of the patient and caregiver on the prevention and/or management of pressure ulcers
- Regular assessment by a nurse, physician, or other licensed health care practitioner (usually at least weekly for a patient with a stage III or IV ulcer)
- Appropriate turning and positioning
- Appropriate wound care (for a stage II, III, or IV ulcer)
- Appropriate management of moisture/incontinence
- Nutritional assessment and intervention consistent with the overall plan of care

If the patient is on a group II surface, a care plan should be established by the physician or home care nurse that includes the above elements. The support surface provided for the patient should be one in which the patient does not bottom out.

When a group II surface is covered following a myocutaneous flap or skin graft, coverage generally is limited to 60 days from the date of surgery.

When the stated coverage criteria for a group II mattress or bed are not met, a claim will be denied as not medically necessary unless there is clear documentation that justifies the medical necessity for the item in the individual case. A Group II support surface billed without modifier KX will usually be denied as not medically necessary.

Clinical Information for Group II Support Surfaces: Continued use of a group II support surface is covered until the ulcer is healed, or if healing does not continue, there is documentation in the medical record to show that: (1) other aspects of the care plan are being modified to promote healing, or (2) the use of the group II support surface is medically necessary for wound management.

Appropriate use of modifier KX is the responsibility of the supplier billing the DME MAC. The supplier should maintain adequate communication on an ongoing basis with the clinician providing the wound care, in order to accurately determine that use of modifier KX still reflects the clinical conditions that meet the criteria for coverage of a group II support surface, and that adequate documentation exists in the medical record reflecting these conditions. Such documentation should not be submitted with a claim, but should be available for review if requested by the DME MAC.

In cases where a group II product is inappropriate, a group I or III support surface could be covered if coverage criteria for that group are met.

Group III support surfaces: Code E0194 for an air-fluidized bed is a device employing the circulation of filtered air through silicone-coated ceramic beads creating the characteristics of fluid. The staging of pressure ulcers for group III support surfaces is the same as that for groups I and II.

An air-fluidized bed is covered only if all of the following criteria are met:

- The patient has a stage III (full thickness tissue loss) or stage IV (deep tissue destruction) pressure sore
- The patient is bedridden or chair bound as a result of severely limited mobility
- In the absence of an air-fluidized bed, the patient would require institutionalization
- The air-fluidized bed is ordered in writing by the patient's attending physician based upon a comprehensive assessment and evaluation of the patient after conservative treatment has been tried without success

Treatment should generally include the following:

- Education of the patient and caregiver on the prevention and/or management of pressure ulcers
- Assessment by a physician, nurse, or other licensed health care practitioner at least weekly
- Appropriate turning and positioning
- Use of a group II support surface, if appropriate
- Appropriate wound care
- Appropriate management of moisture/incontinence
- Nutritional assessment and intervention consistent with the overall plan of care

The patient must generally have been on the conservative treatment program for at least one-month prior to use of the air-fluidized bed, with worsening or no improvement of the ulcer. Generally, the evaluation must be performed within a week prior to initiation of therapy with the air-fluidized bed. An air-fluidized bed will be covered under the following circumstances:

- A trained adult caregiver is available to assist the patient with activities of daily living, fluid balance, dry skin care, repositioning, recognition and management of altered mental status, dietary needs, prescribed treatments, and management and support of the air-fluidized bed system and its problems, such as leakage
- A physician directs the home treatment regimen, and reevaluates and recertifies the need for the air-fluidized bed on a monthly basis
- All other alternative equipment has been considered and ruled out

An air-fluidized bed will be denied as not medically necessary under any of the following circumstances:

- The patient has coexisting pulmonary disease (the lack of firm back support makes coughing ineffective and dry air inhalation thickens pulmonary secretions)
- The patient requires treatment with wet soaks or moist wound dressings that are not protected with an impervious covering, such as plastic wrap or other occlusive material
- The caregiver is unwilling or unable to provide the type of care required by the patient on an air-fluidized bed
- Structural support is inadequate to support the weight of the air-fluidized bed system (it generally weighs 1,600 pounds or more)
- The electrical system is insufficient for the anticipated increase in energy consumption
- Other known contraindications exist

Payment is not included for the caregiver or for architectural adjustments, such as electrical or structural improvement.

If the stated coverage criteria for an air-fluidized bed are not met, the claim will be denied as not medically necessary unless there is clear documentation that justifies the medical necessity for the item in the individual case.

Clinical Information for Group III Support Surfaces: The continued medical necessity of an air-fluidized bed must be documented by the treating physician every month. Continued use of an air-fluidized bed is covered until the ulcer is healed, or, if healing does not continue, there is documentation to show the following:

- Other aspects of the care plan are being modified to promote healing
- The use of the bed is medically necessary for wound management

Documentation Standards

Group I Support Surfaces

An order for the overlay or mattress, which is signed and dated by the treating physician, must be kept on file by the supplier. The written order must be obtained prior to the delivery of the item.

For Medicare beneficiaries, the supplier should obtain all necessary information prior to dispensing the pressure-reducing support surface. A DME MAC data collecting form, Statement of Ordering Physician Group I Support Surfaces, should be provided to the treating physician for completion. Questions pertaining to medical necessity on any form used to collect this information may not be completed by the supplier or anyone in a financial relationship with the supplier. This statement must be supported by information in the patient's medical record, which would be available to the DME MAC on request. Do not send this form to the DME MAC unless specifically requested.

Group II Support Surfaces

An order for the mattress or bed, which is signed and dated by the treating provider, must be kept on file by the supplier. The written order must be obtained prior to the delivery of the item.

For Medicare beneficiaries, the supplier should obtain all necessary information prior to dispensing the pressure-reducing support surface. A DME MAC data collecting form, Statement of Ordering Physician Group II Support Surfaces, should be provided to the treating physician for completion. Questions pertaining to medical necessity on any form used to collect this information may not be completed by the supplier or anyone in a financial relationship with the supplier. This statement must be supported by information in the patient's medical record, which would be available to the DMERC on request. Do not send this form to the DMERC unless specifically requested.

Group III Support Surfaces

An order for the bed, which has been signed and dated by the attending physician who is caring for the patient's wounds, must be kept on file by the supplier. The written order must be obtained prior to the delivery of the air-fluidized bed.

Prosthetic and Orthotic Devices

Medicare

Prosthetic devices (other than dental) are covered under Part B when the device replaces all or part of an internal body organ or replaces all or part of the function of a permanently inoperative or malfunctioning internal body organ. Orthotics, which include leg, arm, back, and neck braces; trusses; and artificial limbs and eyes are covered under Part B when furnished incident to physician services or on a physician's order.

A brace includes rigid and semi-rigid devices that are used for the purpose of supporting a weak or deformed body member or restricting or eliminating motion in a diseased or injured part of the body. Back braces include, but are not limited to, special corsets (e.g., sacroiliac, sacrolumbar, dorsolumbar corsets) and belts. A terminal device (e.g., hand or hook) is covered under this provision whether the patient requires an artificial limb. Stump stockings and harnesses (including replacements) are also covered when these appliances are essential to the effective use of the artificial limb. Elastic stockings, garter belts, and similar devices do not come within the scope of the definition of a brace.

Replacements or repairs of such devices are covered when furnished incident to physician services or on a physician's orders. Adjustments to an artificial limb or other appliance required by wear or by a change in the patient's condition are covered when ordered by a physician. Adjustments, repairs, and replacements are covered even when the item has been in use before the user enrolled in Part B of the program so long as the device continues to be medically required.

Prefabricated prosthetics and orthotics, other than ostomy supplies, are exempt DME that may be billed by the nursing home or hospital to the FI. When furnished to inpatients in a Part A covered stay, the prefabricated prosthetics and orthotics is included in the inpatient reimbursement. When the patient is not in a covered Part A inpatient stay or is an outpatient, separate payment will be made under the DMEPOS fee schedule. Customized prosthetics and orthotics should be billed directly by the supplier to the DME MAC.

Please note that there are nine states that currently require an orthotist or prosthetist furnish orthotics and prosthetics. As of October 2005, the nine states include Alabama, Florida, Illinois, New Jersey, Ohio, Oklahoma, Rhode Island, Texas, and Washington. When a supplier from one of these states bills customized fabricated orthotics and prosthetics to the DME MAC, the supplier must have a specialty code that includes orthotists or prosthetists or Medicare will deny the claim.

Consolidated Billing

For nursing home patients/residents receiving skilled care reimbursed under Part A, non-customized prosthetics and orthotics are considered to be a component of the inpatient stay. If a source other than the skilled nursing facility dispenses these items, the source must look to the nursing home for payment and cannot bill Medicare directly for these items. If the nursing home patient/resident is not receiving a skilled level of care and is not being reimbursed under Part A, then suppliers may bill these items to the facility or directly to the DME MAC. Prosthetics and orthotics dispensed to home health services recipients are exempt from consolidated billing requirements and may be billed directly by the supplier.

Ankle-Foot Orthosis (AFO) and Knee-Ankle-Foot Orthosis (KAFO); Related Additions and Replacements; Repairs

Medicare

For an item to be considered for Medicare coverage under the orthotic benefit category, it must be a rigid or semirigid device used for the purpose of supporting a weak or deformed body member or restricting or eliminating motion in a diseased or injured part of the body.

A nonambulatory AFO may be either an ankle contracture splint or a foot drop splint.

AFOs and KAFOs that are molded-to-patient-model (custom fabricated) are covered for ambulatory patients when the basic coverage criteria listed previously are met and one of the following criteria are met:

- The patient could not be fit with a prefabricated AFO
- The condition necessitating the orthosis is expected to be permanent or of longstanding duration (more than six months)
- There is a need to control the knee, ankle, or foot in more than one plane
- The patient has a documented neurological, circulatory, or orthopedic status that requires custom fabricating over a patient model to prevent tissue injury
- The patient has a healing fracture that lacks normal anatomical integrity or anthropometric proportions

If the specific criteria for a molded-to-patient-model orthosis are not met, but the criteria for a prefabricated, custom fitted orthosis are met, payment will be based on the allowance for the least costly medically appropriate alternative.

The allowance for the labor involved in replacing an orthotic component that is coded with the miscellaneous code L4210 is separately payable in addition to the allowance for that component.

Claims for prefabricated or custom fabricated devices that contain a concentric adjustable torsion style mechanism in the knee or ankle joint and that are being used to treat a joint contracture should be coded as E1810 Dynamic adjustable knee extension/flexion device or E1815 Dynamic adjustable ankle extension/flexion device for the device itself and the interface material (represented by code E1820). If a concentric adjustable torsion style mechanism in the knee or ankle joint is used in a custom-fabricated orthosis to provide and assist function to joint motion during ambulation, it should be coded as L2999.

Medicare Noncovered Items/Services

Evaluation of the patient, measurement and/or casting, and fitting of the orthosis are included in the allowance for the orthosis. There is no separate payment for these services.

If the expense for repairs exceeds the estimated expense of providing another entire orthosis, no payment will be made for the amount in excess.

The allowance for the labor involved in replacing an orthotic component is included in the allowance for that component.

Modifiers

If an AFO or KAFO is used solely for the treatment of edema and/or for the prevention or treatment of a heel pressure ulcer, modifier GY should be added to the base code and any related addition code. A short narrative statement should be documented in the medical record explaining why modifier GY is reported, such as "Used to prevent pressure ulcer," "Used to treat pressure ulcer," or "Used to treat edema." This statement should be entered in the HAO record of an electronic claim or attached to a hard copy claim.

Facial Prosthesis

Medicare

Modifications may be billed to Medicare when they occur more than 90 days after delivery of the prosthesis and they are required because of a change in the patient's condition.

Repairs are covered when there has been accidental damage or extensive wear to the prosthesis that can be repaired. The expense for the repairs cannot exceed the estimated expense for a replacement prosthesis.

Replacement of a facial prosthesis is covered in cases of loss or irreparable damage or wear or when required because of a change in the patient's condition that cannot be accommodated by modification of the existing prosthesis. When replacement involves a new impression/moulage rather than use of a previous master model, the reason for the new impression/moulage must be clearly documented in the supplier's records and be available to the DME MAC on request.

Claims for facial prostheses from non-physicians provided in an office or nursing home setting are submitted to the DME MAC. Claims for facial prostheses from physicians in these settings are submitted to the local carrier. Claims for facial prostheses provided in an outpatient hospital setting are submitted to the local intermediary. Facial prostheses provided in an inpatient hospital setting are included in the payment made to the hospital and should not be submitted to the DME MAC. Implanted prosthesis anchoring components should not be billed to the DME MAC.

If an ocular prosthesis is dispensed to the patient as an integral part of a facial prosthesis, the supplier of the facial prosthesis must bill the ocular prosthesis component.

When a new ocular prosthesis component is provided as an integral part of an orbital, upper facial, or hemi-facial prosthesis, it should be billed using code V2623 or V2629 on a separate claim line. When a replacement facial prosthesis utilizes an ocular component from the prior prosthesis, the ocular prosthesis code should not be billed.

If a facial prosthesis has a component that is used to attach it to a bone-anchored implant or to an internal prosthesis (e.g., maxillary obturator), that component should be billed separately using code L8048. This code should not be used for implanted prosthesis anchoring components.

When a prosthesis is needed for adjacent facial regions, a single code must be used to bill for the item whenever possible. For example, if a defect involves the nose and orbit, this should be billed using the hemi-facial prosthesis code and not separate codes for the orbit and nose. This would apply even if the prosthesis is fabricated in two separate parts.

Medicare Noncovered Items/Services
Follow-up visits that occur more than 90 days after delivery and that do not involve modification or repair of the prosthesis are not covered.

Modifiers
When a replacement prosthesis is fabricated from a new impression/moulage, modifier KM should be added to the code. When a replacement prosthesis is fabricated using a previous master model, modifier KN should be added to the code.

The right (RT) and left (LT) modifiers should be used with facial prosthesis codes when applicable. If bilateral prostheses using the same code are billed on the same date of service, the code should be entered on a single claims line using modifiers LT and RT and billed with 2 units of service.

Lower Limb Prostheses; Related Additions and Replacements; Miscellaneous Prostheses and Services

Medicare
Prostheses are covered when furnished incident to physician's services or on a physician's order.

Accessories (e.g., stump stockings for the residual limb, harness [including replacements]) are covered when these appliances aid in or are essential to the effective use of the artificial limb. A lower limb prosthesis is covered when the patient:

- Will reach or maintain a defined functional state within a reasonable period of time
- Is motivated to ambulate

This information must be documented in the medical record.

A functional status level is a determination of the medical necessity for certain components/additions to the prosthesis. Potential functional ability is based on the reasonable expectations of the prosthetist and ordering physician, considering factors including, but not limited to:

- The patient's past history (including prior prosthetic use if applicable)
- The patient's current condition, including the status of the residual limb and the nature of other medical problems
- The patient's desire to ambulate

Clinical assessments of patient rehabilitation potential should be based on the following classification levels:

- Level 0: The patient does not have the ability or potential to ambulate or transfer safely with or without assistance and a prosthesis does not enhance their quality of life or mobility.
- Level 1: The patient has the ability or potential to use a prosthesis for transfers or ambulation on level surfaces at fixed cadence. This is typical of the limited and unlimited household ambulator.
- Level 2: The patient has the ability or potential for ambulation with the ability to traverse low-level environmental barriers such as curbs, stairs, or uneven surfaces. This is typical of the limited community ambulator.
- Level 3: The patient has the ability or potential for ambulation with variable cadence. This is typical of the community ambulator who has the ability to traverse most environmental barriers, and may have vocational, therapeutic, or exercise activity that demands prosthetic utilization beyond simple locomotion.
- Level 4: The patient has the ability or potential for prosthetic ambulation that exceeds basic ambulation skills, exhibiting high impact, stress, or energy levels. This is typical of the prosthetic demands of the child, active adult, or athlete.

Basic lower extremity prostheses include a single axis, constant friction knee. Coverage is extended only if there is sufficient clinical documentation of functional need for the technologic design feature of a given type of knee prosthesis. This information must be retained in the physician or prosthetist's files.

Any prosthesis or prosthetic component provided in an inpatient hospital setting should not be submitted to the DME MAC.

The submitted charge for replacements reflects both the cost of the component and the labor associated with the removal, replacement, and finishing of that component. Labor associated with replacement should not be reported using L7520.

Adjustments to a prosthesis due to wear or by change in the patient's condition are covered under the initial provider's order for the prosthesis for the life of the prosthesis.

Repairs to a prosthesis are covered when necessary to make the prosthesis functional.

If the expense for repairs exceeds the estimated expense of purchasing another entire prosthesis, no payments can be made for the amount of the excess. Maintenance, which may be necessitated by manufacturer's recommendations or the construction of the prosthesis (and must be performed by the prosthetist), is covered as a repair.

Replacement of a prosthesis or prosthetic component is covered in cases of loss or irreparable damage or wear, or when required because of a change in the patient's condition. Expenses for replacement of a prosthesis or prosthetic components required because of loss or irreparable damage may be reimbursed without a provider's order when it is determined that the prosthesis, as originally ordered, still fulfills the patient's medical needs. However, claims involving replacement of a prosthesis or major component (foot, ankle, knee, socket) necessitated by wear or a change in the patient's condition must be supported by a new provider's order. When the DMERC determines that malicious damage, culpable neglect, or wrongful disposition of the prosthesis has occurred, an investigation will be undertaken to determine whether it is unreasonable to make program payment under the circumstances.

Medicare Non-Covered Items/Services

A prosthesis will be denied as not medically necessary if the patient's potential functional level is 0. The above functional levels are reflected in modifiers K0 through K4.

The following items are included in the reimbursement for a prosthesis and are not separately billable to Medicare:

- Evaluation of the residual limb and gait
- Fitting of the prosthesis
- Cost of base component parts and labor contained in HCPCS base codes
- Repairs due to normal wear or tear within 90 days of delivery
- Adjustments of the prosthesis or the prosthetic component made when fitting the prosthesis or component, and for 90 days from the date of delivery when the adjustments are not necessitated by changes in the residual limb or the patient's functional abilities
- Routine periodic servicing, such as testing, cleaning, and checking of the prosthesis, is noncovered

Speech Generating Devices and Speech Aids

Medicare

Electronic speech aids are covered as prosthetic devices when the patient has had a laryngectomy or his or her larynx is permanently inoperative. There are two types of speech aids. One operates by placing a vibrating head against the throat and the other amplifies sound waves through a tube that is inserted into the user's mouth.

A tracheostomy-speaking valve is covered as an element of the trachea tube, which makes the tube more effective. The trachea tube and valve are covered prosthetic devices.

Augmentative and alternative communication devices or communicators, which are generally referred to as speech generating devices, are covered prosthetic devices if the contractor's medical staff determines that the patient suffers from a severe speech impairment and that the medical condition warrants the use of a device.

Speech generating devices are defined as speech aids that provide an individual who has severe speech impairment with the ability to meet his or her functional speaking needs. Speech generating devices include the following characteristics:

- Dedicated speech device, used solely by the individual who has a severe speech impairment
- Digitized speech output, using prerecorded messages, less than or equal to eight minutes recording time
- Digitized speech output, using prerecorded messages, greater than eight minutes recording time
- Synthesized speech output that requires message formulation by spelling and device access by physical contact with the device-direct selection techniques
- Synthesized speech output that permits multiple methods of message formulation and multiple methods of device access
- Software that allows a laptop computer, desktop computer, or personal digital assistant (PDA) to function as a speech generating device

Devices that would not meet the definition of speech generating devices and are not covered are characterized by:

- Devices that are not dedicated speech devices, but are devices that are capable of running software for purposes other than for speech generation (e.g., devices that can also run a

word processing package, an accounting program, or perform other than non-medical function).
- Laptop computers, desktop computers, or PDAs that may be programmed to perform the same function as a speech generating device, are not covered since they are not primarily medical in nature and do not meet the definition of DME. For this reason, they cannot be considered speech-generating devices for Medicare coverage purposes.
- A device that is useful to someone without severe speech impairment is not considered a speech-generating device for Medicare coverage purposes.

A tracheostomy-speaking valve and electronic speech aids are devices that may be billed by any facility just as any other exempt prosthetic and orthotic. Speech generating devices must be supplied and billed by an enrolled DME supplier.

Transcutaneous Electrical Nerve Stimulation

Medicare

Transcutaneous electrical nerve stimulation (TENS) is an accepted modality as a rehabilitation therapy. TENS may be used for the relief of acute postoperative pain and its use is covered under Medicare. TENS may be covered whether used as an adjunct to the use of drugs or as an alternative to drugs in the treatment of acute pain resulting from surgery. TENS, when used for acute postoperative pain, is expected to be necessary for relatively short periods of time, usually 30 days or less. TENS devices, whether durable or disposable, may be used in furnishing this service. TENS devices are considered supplies when used for the purpose of treating acute postoperative pain. As such they may be hospital supplies furnished to inpatients covered under Part A, or supplies incident to a physician's service when furnished in connection with surgery done on an outpatient basis, and covered under Part B.

When TENS is used for chronic pain, the TENS device may be covered as DME. An assessment of the effectiveness of the TENS to treat chronic pain should be made before the device is prescribed. This assessment usually involves attachment of a transcutaneous nerve stimulator to the surface of the skin over the peripheral nerve to be stimulated. The patient uses it on a trial basis and its effectiveness in modulating pain is monitored by the physician or physical therapist.

When used for the treatment of chronic, intractable pain, the TENS unit must be used by the patient on a trial basis for a minimum of one month (30 days), but not to exceed two months. Document the medical necessity for such services that are furnished beyond the first month. The trial period must be monitored by the physician to determine the effectiveness of the TENS unit in modulating the pain. For coverage of a purchase, the physician must determine whether the patient is likely to derive a significant therapeutic benefit from continuous use of a TENS. The medical records must document a reevaluation of the patient at the end of the trial period, must indicate how often the patient used the TENS unit, the typical duration of use each time, and the results.

If TENS significantly alleviates pain, it may be considered as primary treatment. If it produces no relief or greater discomfort than the original pain, then the TENS therapy cannot be covered.

The physician or physical therapist providing the services usually furnishes the equipment necessary for assessment. Where the physician or physical therapist advises the patient to rent the TENS from a supplier during the trial period rather than supplying it himself or herself, Medicare payment may be made for rental of the TENS, as well as for the services of the physician or physical therapist who is evaluating its use.

A four lead TENS unit may be used with two leads or four leads, depending on the characteristics of the patient's pain. If it is ordered for use with four leads, the medical record must document why two leads are insufficient to meet the patient's needs.

During the rental of a TENS unit from a DME supplier, supplies for the unit are included in the rental allowance. There is no additional allowance for electrodes, lead wires, batteries, etc. If a TENS unit (E0720 or E0730) is purchased, the allowance includes lead wires and one month's supply of electrodes, conductive paste or gel (if needed), and batteries.

When supplied by a DME supplier, separate payment may be made for DME replacement supplies when they are medically necessary and are used with a TENS unit that has been purchased. If two TENS leads are medically necessary, then a maximum of one unit of HCPCS Level II code A4595 would be allowed per month. If four leads were necessary, a maximum of two units per month would be allowed. If the use of the TENS unit is less than daily, the frequency of billing for the TENS supply code should be reduced proportionally.

There should be no billing and there will be no separate allowance for replacement electrodes, conductive paste or gel, replacement batteries, or a battery charger used with a TENS unit.

When supplied by a DME supplier, replacement of lead wires will be covered when they are inoperative due to damage and the TENS unit is still medically necessary. Replacement more often than every 12 months would rarely be medically necessary. Other supplies, including but not limited to the following, will not be separately allowed: adapters (e.g., snap, banana, alligator, tab, button, clip), belt clips, adhesive remover, additional connecting cable for lead wires, carrying pouches, or covers.

TENS can ordinarily be delivered to patients through the use of conventional electrodes, adhesive tapes, and lead wires. There may be times where it might be medically necessary for certain patients receiving TENS treatment to use, as an alternative to conventional electrodes, adhesive tapes and lead wires, a form-fitting conductive garment (i.e., a garment with conductive fibers that are separated from the patient's skin by layers of fabric).

A form-fitting conductive garment (and medically necessary related supplies) may be covered under the program only when it has been approved by the FDA and it has been prescribed by a physician for use in delivering covered TENS treatment. Additionally one of the medical indications below must be met:

- The patient cannot manage without the conductive garment because there is such a large area or so many sites to be stimulated and the stimulation would have to be delivered so frequently that it is not feasible to use conventional electrodes, adhesive tapes, and lead wires.
- The patient cannot manage without the conductive garment for the treatment of chronic intractable pain because the areas or sites to be stimulated are inaccessible with the use of conventional electrodes, adhesive tapes, and lead wires.
- The patient has a documented medical condition such as skin problems that preclude the application of conventional electrodes, adhesive tapes, and lead wires.
- The patient requires electrical stimulation beneath a cast to treat disuse atrophy, where the nerve supply to the muscle is intact, or to treat chronic intractable pain.
- The patient has a medical need for rehabilitation strengthening (pursuant to a written plan of rehabilitation) following an injury where the nerve supply to the muscle is intact.

TENS treatments performed in a facility or professional office are billed as a rehabilitation therapy modality. TENS devices when used by the patient in the home for covered therapy would be billed by the DME supplier to the DME MAC.

When the TENS is rented or purchased from a DME supplier, an order for each item billed must be signed and dated by the treating physician, kept on file by the supplier, and made available to the DME MAC upon request. Items delivered before the supplier has received a signed written order must be submitted with modifier EY added to each affected HCPCS Level II code.

When the TENS purchased from a DME supplier, a CMN (CMS form 848) must be completed, signed, and dated by the treating physician. The CMN must be kept on file by the supplier and made available to the DME MAC on request. The CMN may act as a substitute for a written order if it contains all the required elements of an order. The initial claim must include a copy of the CMN. A TENS CMN is not necessary for rentals.

Urological Supplies

Medicare

Permanent urinary retention is defined as retention that is not expected to be medically or surgically corrected in that patient within three months.

Most use in hospitals is on a temporary basis, which means that these items do not meet the definition of DME. When used on a temporary basis, these supplies should be billed without a HCPCS Level II code using revenue codes 0270, 0271, or 0272 as routine supplies. If the patient is permanently impaired and the supplies qualify as DME, then they should be reported with a HCPCS Level II code under revenue code 0274 as orthotics and prosthetics.

If the catheter or the external urinary collection device meets the coverage criteria, then the related supplies that are necessary for their effective use are also covered.

The patient must have a permanent impairment of urination. This does not require a determination that there is no possibility that the patient's condition may improve sometime in the future. If the medical record, including the judgment of the attending physician, indicates the condition is of long and indefinite duration (ordinarily at least three months), the test of permanence is considered met.

When urological supplies are furnished in a physician's office, they may be billed to the DME MAC only if the patient's condition meets the definition of permanence. The use of a urological supply for the treatment of chronic urinary tract infection or other bladder condition in the absence of permanent urinary incontinence or retention is not covered by Medicare. Since the patient's urinary system is functioning, the criteria for coverage under the prosthetic benefit provision are not met.

Nonroutine catheter changes are covered when documentation substantiates medical necessity, such as for the following indications:

- The catheter is accidentally removed (e.g., pulled out by the patient)
- A malfunction of catheter has occurred (e.g., the balloon does not stay inflated, a hole has developed in the catheter)
- The catheter is obstructed by encrustation, mucous plug, blood clot, etc.
- There is a history of recurrent obstruction or urinary tract infection for which it has been established that an acute event is prevented by a scheduled change at intervals of less than once per month

A urinary drainage collection system will be covered for routine changes of the urinary drainage collection system, as noted in the following table.

Additional charges will be allowed for medically necessary non-routine changes when the documentation substantiates the medical necessity (e.g., obstruction, clotting of blood, or chronic, recurrent urinary tract infection).

If there is a catheter change and an additional drainage bag change within a month, the combined utilization for the items should be considered when determining if additional documentation should be submitted with the claim for appropriate adjudication.

Intermittent irrigation of an indwelling catheter requires the use of certain supplies. These supplies are covered when they are used on an as-needed (nonroutine) basis in the presence of acute obstruction of the catheter. Supplies for the routine intermittent irrigation of a catheter will be denied as not medically necessary. Routine irrigation is defined as being performed at predetermined intervals. In some cases, the DMERC may request a copy of the order for irrigation and documentation in the patient's medical record of the presence of acute catheter obstruction when irrigation supplies are billed.

Covered supplies for medically necessary nonroutine irrigation of a catheter include either an irrigation tray or an irrigation syringe, and sterile saline or sterile water. When syringes, trays, sterile saline, or water are used for routine irrigation, they will be denied as not medically necessary. Irrigation solutions containing antibiotics and chemotherapeutic agents will be denied as noncovered. Irrigating solutions such as acetic acid or hydrogen peroxide used for the treatment or prevention of urinary obstruction will be denied as not medically necessary. Irrigation supplies that are used for care of the skin or perineum of incontinent patients are noncovered.

Supplies for the continuous irrigation of an indwelling catheter are covered if there is a history of obstruction of the catheter and the patency of the catheter cannot be maintained by intermittent irrigation in conjunction with medically necessary catheter changes. Continuous irrigation as a primary preventive measure (i.e., there is no history of catheter obstruction) will be denied as not medically necessary. Documentation must substantiate the medical necessity of catheter irrigation and, in particular, continuous irrigation as opposed to intermittent irrigation. The medical records must also indicate the rate of solution administration and the duration of need. This documentation may be requested by the DME MAC.

Covered supplies for medically necessary continuous bladder irrigation include a three-way Foley catheter, irrigation tubing set, and sterile saline or sterile water. Payment for irrigating solutions such as acetic acid or hydrogen peroxide will be based on the allowance for sterile water or sterile saline.

Continuous irrigation is a temporary measure. Continuous irrigation for more than two weeks is rarely medically necessary. The patient's medical records should indicate this medical necessity; these medical records may be requested by the DMERC entity.

For each episode of covered sterile catheterization, Medicare will cover the following:

- One catheter and an individual packet of lubricant
- An intermittent catheter kit

The kit code should be used for billing even if the components are packaged separately rather than together as a kit. If sterile catheterization is not medically necessary, sterile supplies will be denied as not medically necessary.

Male external catheters (condom type) or female external urinary collection devices are covered for patients who have permanent urinary incontinence when used as an alternative to an indwelling catheter. The utilization of male external catheters generally should not exceed 35 per month. Greater use of these devices must be accompanied by documentation that supports the medical necessity of the increased quantity.

Adhesive strips or tape used with a male external catheter are included in the allowance for the catheter and are not separately payable. If adhesive strips or tape are used with the male external catheter, payment will be denied as not medically necessary.

When billing for urological supplies furnished in a physician's office for a permanent impairment, use the place of service code (POS) corresponding to the patient's current place of residence (POS=12); do not use POS 11 for the physician's office.

Medicare Noncovered Items/Services

Other supplies used in the management of incontinence include, but are not limited to, the following items:

- Creams, salves, lotions, barriers (liquid, spray, wipes, powder, paste), or other skin care products
- Catheter care kits
- Adhesive remover (coverage remains for use with ostomy supplies)
- Catheter clamp or plug
- Disposable underpads, e.g., Chux pads
- Diapers, drip collectors, or incontinent garments, disposable or reusable
- Drainage bag holder or stand
- Urinary suspensory without leg bag
- Measuring container
- Urinary drainage tray
- Gauze pads and other dressings (coverage remains under other benefits, e.g., surgical dressings)
- Other incontinence products not directly related to the use of a covered urinary catheter or external urinary collection device

These items will be denied as noncovered because they are not prosthetic devices, nor are they required for the effective use of a prosthetic device.

Irrigation solutions containing antibiotics and chemotherapeutic agents should be coded A9270 Non-covered item or service. Irrigating solutions such as acetic acid or hydrogen peroxide that are used for the treatment or prevention of urinary obstruction should be coded A4321 Therapeutic agent for urinary catheter irrigation.

Catheter insertion trays will be denied as not medically necessary for clean, nonsterile intermittent catheterization.

Catheters and related supplies will be denied as noncovered if it is expected that the condition will be temporary.

If the patient's condition is expected to be temporary, urological supplies may not be billed to the DMERC. In this situation, they are considered supplies provided incident to a physician's service, and payment is included in the allowance for the physician's services, which are processed by the local carrier.

Urological supplies, that are not used with, or for which use is not related to covered catheters or external urinary collection devices (i.e., drainage and/or collection of urine from the bladder), will be denied as noncovered.

The use of leg bags for bedridden patients will be denied as not medically necessary.

Irrigation solutions containing antibiotics and chemotherapeutic agents will be denied as noncovered.

Consolidated Billing

All urological supplies dispensed to a nursing home resident or home health recipient are included in the consolidated billing requirements and the Prospective Payment System (PPS) reimbursement. This means that the supplier will need to know the patient status when the supplies are dispensed.

For patients in a nursing home: If the patient is receiving skilled nursing level care and is covered under Part A benefits, the supplies may not be billed separately by the SNF or by any other provider or supplier. This would be duplicate billing. The supplies are considered a part of the nursing home's PPS reimbursement. The DME supplier should bill the nursing home for these items and should probably have an agreement with the home for payment of these items.

If a patient in a nursing home is not receiving a skilled nursing level of care and is not being reimbursed under Part A, then the DME supplier has a choice: billing may be submitted directly by the supplier or may be submitted by the nursing home. DME suppliers should have an agreement with the nursing home specifying which party will bill in these situations. Such an agreement will eliminate duplicate billing and concerns related to fraud and abuse. Only one party should submit the bill for the service. Do not bill the nursing home and then bill the DME MAC if the nursing home is taking too long to pay.

For patients receiving home health services: If the patient is under a plan of care, urological supplies should be billed to the Home Health Agency (HHA). The supplies are considered a part of the HHA's PPS reimbursement. The DME supplier should bill the HHA for these items and should probably have an agreement with the home for payment of these items.

The HHA must have an order for the urological supplies and the supplies must be provided under an arrangement. If the supplier was unaware of the HHA services and there is no agreement with the HHA about the provision of the supplies, the supplies will not be reimbursed by any party. The patient has the freedom to accept the HHA services. At that point, the HHA becomes responsible for all related care, including the provision of urological supplies, but excluding any other DME.

If the patient is not on a plan of care or is not receiving Part A reimbursable services, the supplier must still bill the HHA. These urological supplies are subject to consolidated billing regulations. This means that the HHA must submit all charges for these services. The HHA will receive additional payment for these items. The supplier should bill the HHA for these items and should probably have an agreement with the home for payment of these items.

Documentation Standards

The order on file must include the type of supplies ordered and the approximate quantity to be used per unit of time. There must be a statement indicating whether the patient has permanent or temporary urinary incontinence or retention, or other indication for use of a catheter or urinary collection device. If the order indicates permanent urinary incontinence or urinary retention, and if the item is a catheter, an external urinary collection device, or a supply used with one of these items, modifier KX should be added to the code for each urological supply on each claim submitted.

When billing for quantities of supplies greater than those approved for coverage, the claim must include documentation supporting the medical necessity for the higher utilization.

The initial claim for catheters or kits used for sterile intermittent catheterization in the home must be accompanied by documentation supporting the medical necessity for sterile technique.

Wheelchairs and Power Mobility Devices

Physicians, physician assistants, nurse practitioners, or clinical nurse specialists may prescribe wheelchairs and power mobility devices (PMD). Wheelchairs and PMDs do not require a CMN. The treating practitioner must conduct a face-to-face examination of the beneficiary and write a written prescription for the PMD. The written prescription must be signed and dated by the treating practitioner who performed the face-to-face examination. The written prescription must include the beneficiary's name, the date of the face-to-face examination, the diagnoses and conditions that the PMD is expected to modify, a description of the item, and the length of need. This written prescription for the PMD must be received by the supplier within 45 days after the face-to-face examination. For those instances of a recently hospitalized beneficiary, the supplier must receive the written prescription within 45 days after the date of discharge from the hospital.

The face-to-face examination requirement does not apply when only accessories for PMDs are ordered, nor does it apply for the ordering of replacement PMDs. A replacement PMD would be the same device as previously ordered. For instance, if a beneficiary has a POV but would like to replace the POV with a power wheelchair, a face-to-face examination would need to be conducted.

Prior to dispensing a PMD, the DME supplier must obtain from the treating practitioner who performed the face-to-face examination the written prescription accompanied by supporting documentation of the beneficiary's need for the PMD in the home. Supporting documentation of the patient's need for the PMD in the home must accompany the prescription. This documentation must be specific to the patient's PMD evaluation and may include the history, physical examination, diagnostic tests, and summary of findings, diagnoses, and treatment plans. Submit only those parts of the medical record that clearly demonstrate medical necessity, including the history of events that led to the request for the PMD, the mobility deficits to be corrected by the PMD, documentation demonstrating that other treatments do not obviate the need for the PMD, documentation that the patient lives in an environment that supports the use of the PMD, and documentation that the patient or caregiver is capable of operating the PMD.

CMS will pay a separate add-on payment in addition to the office visit for the additional physician and treating practitioner work and resources required for submitting pertinent parts of the medical record. Report HCPCS Level II code G0372 Physician service required to establish and document the need for a power mobility device (use in addition to primary evaluation and management code), to obtain this add-on payment. Code G0372 must be reported on the same claim as the E/M code.

Medicare Noncovered Codes

The following is a list of Medicare noncovered HCPCS Level II codes (as indicated in the HCPCS code set master file):

A0021	A4566	A9300	E2230
A0080	A4570	B4100	E8000
A0090	A4575	E0172	E8001
A0100	A4580	E0203	E8002
A0110	A4590	E0231	G0122
A0120	A4627	E0232	G0219
A0130	A4670	E0240	G0235
A0140	A6000	E0241	G0252
A0160	A6413	E0242	G0255
A0170	A6530	E0243	G0282
A0180	A6533	E0244	G0295
A0190	A6534	E0245	G0428
A0200	A6535	E0270	G9013
A0210	A6536	E0273	G9014
A0225	A6537	E0274	G9016
A0380	A6538	E0315	G9050
A0390	A6539	E0446	G9051
A0888	A6540	E0481	G9052
A0998	A6541	E0625	G9053
A4210	A6544	E0638	G9054
A4232	A6549	E0641	G9055
A4250	A9152	E0642	G9056
A4252	A9153	E0936	G9057
A4261	A9180	E0970	G9058
A4264	A9270	E1085	G9059
A4266	A9273	E1086	G9060
A4267	A9274	E1089	G9061
A4268	A9275	E1090	G9062
A4269	A9276	E1130	G9147
A4466	A9277	E1140	H0001
A4490	A9278	E1250	H0002
A4495	A9279	E1260	H0003
A4500	A9280	E1285	H0004
A4510	A9281	E1290	H0005
A4520	A9282	E1300	H0006
A4554	A9283	E1358	H0007

H0008	H1003	J7307	S0093
H0009	H1004	J8499	S0104
H0010	H1005	J8515	S0106
H0011	H1010	J8565	S0108
H0012	H1011	K0740	S0109
H0013	H2000	L2861	S0117
H0014	H2001	L3215	S0122
H0015	H2010	L3216	S0126
H0016	H2011	L3217	S0128
H0017	H2012	L3219	S0132
H0018	H2013	L3221	S0136
H0019	H2014	L3222	S0137
H0020	H2015	L3891	S0138
H0021	H2016	L7600	S0139
H0022	H2017	L8692	S0140
H0023	H2018	M0075	S0142
H0024	H2019	M0076	S0145
H0025	H2020	M0100	S0148
H0026	H2021	M0300	S0155
H0027	H2022	M0301	S0156
H0028	H2023	P2031	S0157
H0029	H2024	P7001	S0160
H0030	H2025	Q0144	S0164
H0031	H2026	Q3026	S0166
H0032	H2027	S0012	S0169
H0033	H2028	S0014	S0170
H0034	H2029	S0017	S0171
H0035	H2030	S0020	S0172
H0036	H2031	S0021	S0174
H0037	H2032	S0023	S0175
H0038	H2033	S0028	S0176
H0039	H2034	S0030	S0177
H0040	H2035	S0032	S0178
H0041	H2036	S0034	S0179
H0042	H2037	S0039	S0181
H0043	J1055	S0040	S0182
H0044	J1825	S0073	S0183
H0045	J1826	S0074	S0187
H0046	J3520	S0077	S0189
H0047	J3535	S0078	S0190
H0048	J3570	S0080	S0191
H0049	J7300	S0081	S0194
H0050	J7302	S0088	S0195
H1000	J7303	S0090	S0197
H1001	J7304	S0091	S0199
H1002	J7306	S0092	S0201

Medicare Noncovered Codes

S0207	S0610	S2205	S3708
S0208	S0612	S2206	S3711
S0209	S0613	S2207	S3713
S0215	S0618	S2208	S3800
S0220	S0620	S2209	S3818
S0221	S0621	S2225	S3819
S0250	S0622	S2230	S3820
S0255	S0625	S2235	S3822
S0257	S0630	S2260	S3823
S0260	S0800	S2265	S3828
S0265	S0810	S2266	S3829
S0270	S0812	S2267	S3830
S0271	S1001	S2270	S3831
S0272	S1002	S2300	S3833
S0273	S1015	S2325	S3834
S0274	S1016	S2340	S3835
S0280	S1030	S2341	S3837
S0281	S1031	S2342	S3840
S0302	S1040	S2344	S3841
S0310	S2053	S2348	S3842
S0315	S2054	S2350	S3843
S0316	S2055	S2351	S3844
S0317	S2060	S2360	S3845
S0320	S2061	S2361	S3846
S0340	S2065	S2400	S3847
S0341	S2066	S2401	S3848
S0342	S2067	S2402	S3849
S0390	S2068	S2403	S3850
S0395	S2070	S2404	S3851
S0400	S2079	S2405	S3852
S0500	S2080	S2409	S3853
S0504	S2083	S2411	S3854
S0506	S2095	S2900	S3855
S0508	S2102	S3000	S3860
S0510	S2103	S3005	S3861
S0512	S2107	S3600	S3862
S0514	S2112	S3601	S3865
S0515	S2115	S3620	S3866
S0516	S2117	S3625	S3870
S0518	S2118	S3626	S3890
S0580	S2120	S3628	S3900
S0581	S2140	S3630	S3902
S0590	S2142	S3645	S3904
S0592	S2150	S3650	S3905
S0595	S2152	S3652	S4005
S0601	S2202	S3655	S4011

S4013	S5121	S8037	S9001
S4014	S5125	S8040	S9007
S4015	S5126	S8042	S9015
S4016	S5130	S8049	S9024
S4017	S5131	S8055	S9025
S4018	S5135	S8080	S9034
S4020	S5136	S8085	S9055
S4021	S5140	S8092	S9056
S4022	S5141	S8096	S9061
S4023	S5145	S8097	S9075
S4025	S5146	S8100	S9083
S4026	S5150	S8101	S9088
S4027	S5151	S8110	S9090
S4028	S5160	S8120	S9097
S4030	S5161	S8121	S9098
S4031	S5162	S8185	S9109
S4035	S5165	S8186	S9117
S4037	S5170	S8189	S9122
S4040	S5175	S8210	S9123
S4042	S5180	S8262	S9124
S4981	S5181	S8265	S9125
S4989	S5185	S8270	S9126
S4990	S5190	S8301	S9127
S4991	S5199	S8415	S9128
S4993	S5497	S8420	S9129
S4995	S5498	S8421	S9131
S5000	S5501	S8422	S9140
S5001	S5502	S8423	S9141
S5010	S5517	S8424	S9145
S5011	S5518	S8425	S9150
S5012	S5520	S8426	S9152
S5013	S5521	S8427	S9208
S5014	S5522	S8428	S9209
S5035	S5523	S8429	S9211
S5036	S5550	S8430	S9212
S5100	S5551	S8431	S9213
S5101	S5552	S8450	S9214
S5102	S5553	S8451	S9325
S5105	S5560	S8452	S9326
S5108	S5561	S8460	S9327
S5109	S5565	S8490	S9328
S5110	S5566	S8940	S9329
S5111	S5570	S8948	S9330
S5115	S5571	S8950	S9331
S5116	S8030	S8990	S9335
S5120	S8035	S8999	S9336

Medicare Noncovered Codes

S9338	S9446	S9988	T2005
S9339	S9447	S9989	T2007
S9340	S9449	S9990	T2010
S9341	S9451	S9991	T2011
S9342	S9452	S9992	T2012
S9343	S9453	S9994	T2013
S9345	S9454	S9996	T2014
S9346	S9455	S9999	T2015
S9347	S9460	T1000	T2016
S9348	S9465	T1001	T2017
S9349	S9470	T1002	T2018
S9351	S9472	T1003	T2019
S9353	S9473	T1004	T2020
S9355	S9474	T1005	T2021
S9357	S9475	T1006	T2022
S9359	S9476	T1007	T2023
S9361	S9480	T1009	T2024
S9363	S9482	T1010	T2025
S9364	S9484	T1012	T2026
S9365	S9485	T1013	T2027
S9366	S9490	T1014	T2028
S9367	S9494	T1015	T2029
S9368	S9497	T1016	T2030
S9370	S9500	T1017	T2031
S9372	S9501	T1018	T2032
S9373	S9502	T1019	T2033
S9374	S9503	T1020	T2034
S9375	S9504	T1021	T2035
S9376	S9529	T1022	T2036
S9377	S9537	T1023	T2037
S9379	S9538	T1024	T2038
S9381	S9542	T1025	T2039
S9401	S9558	T1026	T2040
S9430	S9559	T1027	T2041
S9433	S9560	T1028	T2042
S9434	S9562	T1029	T2043
S9435	S9590	T1030	T2044
S9436	S9810	T1031	T2045
S9437	S9900	T1502	T2046
S9438	S9970	T1503	T2048
S9439	S9975	T1505	T2049
S9441	S9976	T1999	T2101
S9442	S9977	T2001	T4521
S9443	S9981	T2002	T4522
S9444	S9982	T2003	T4523
S9445	S9986	T2004	T4524

T4525	V2788	V5200	V5260
T4526	V5008	V5210	V5261
T4527	V5010	V5220	V5262
T4528	V5011	V5230	V5263
T4529	V5014	V5240	V5264
T4530	V5020	V5241	V5265
T4531	V5030	V5242	V5266
T4532	V5040	V5243	V5267
T4533	V5050	V5244	V5268
T4534	V5060	V5245	V5269
T4535	V5070	V5246	V5270
T4536	V5080	V5247	V5271
T4537	V5090	V5248	V5272
T4538	V5095	V5249	V5273
T4539	V5100	V5250	V5274
T4540	V5110	V5251	V5275
T4541	V5120	V5252	V5298
T4542	V5130	V5253	V5336
T4543	V5140	V5254	V5362
T5001	V5150	V5255	V5363
T5999	V5160	V5256	V5364
V2025	V5170	V5257	
V2702	V5180	V5258	
V2787	V5190	V5259	

HCPCS Lay Descriptions

A0021

A0021 Ambulance service, outside state per mile, transport (Medicaid only)

Lay Description

This code represents a per mile charge for ambulance transportation outside of the state where the ambulance provider is based. This code is used only for Medicaid claims. Consult the local Medicaid office in the state that the provider is located for further definition and usage requirements.

A0080-A0210

A0080 Nonemergency transportation, per mile — vehicle provided by volunteer (individual or organization), with no vested interest
A0090 Nonemergency transportation, per mile — vehicle provided by individual (family member, self, neighbor) with vested interest
A0100 Nonemergency transportation; taxi
A0110 Nonemergency transportation and bus, intra- or interstate carrier
A0120 Nonemergency transportation: mini-bus, mountain area transports, or other transportation systems
A0130 Nonemergency transportation: wheelchair van
A0140 Nonemergency transportation and air travel (private or commercial) intra- or interstate
A0160 Nonemergency transportation: per mile — caseworker or social worker
A0170 Transportation ancillary: parking fees, tolls, other
A0180 Nonemergency transportation: ancillary: lodging, recipient
A0190 Nonemergency transportation: ancillary: meals, recipient
A0200 Nonemergency transportation: ancillary: lodging, escort
A0210 Nonemergency transportation: ancillary: meals, escort

Lay Description

These codes provide for reporting nonemergency transportation and related ancillary services. Different types of vehicles used and/or the areas traveled, as well as additional fees are specified in these codes. This range reports nonemergency transport services such as a vehicle provided by a volunteer or family member; wheelchair van, taxi, bus, or air transport (private or commercial); mountainous area transport, or transportation outside the state. Examples of ancillary services include parking fees and tolls, lodging or meals for the recipient or for the escort, and per mile transportation of a caseworker or social worker.

A0225

A0225 Ambulance service, neonatal transport, base rate, emergency transport, one way

Lay Description

Use this code for the emergency transport of a neonate by ambulance, one way only, at base rate.

A0380

A0380 BLS mileage (per mile)

Lay Description

A basic life support (BLS) ambulance is one that provides transportation plus the equipment and staff needed for such basic life support services as controlling bleeding, splinting fractures, treating shock, delivering babies, and performing cardio-pulmonary resuscitation (CPR). BLS transport is reported on a per mile basis.

Medicare Information

Report the actual charge for the ambulance mileage.

A0382

A0382 BLS routine disposable supplies

Lay Description

Basic life support (BLS) routine disposable supplies include such items as cervical collar, gauze, dressings, and ice packs. Report a unit of one for all routine disposable supplies that are used.

Medicare Information

Under the ambulance fee schedule, payment for supplies and ancillary services furnished incident to the ambulance transport are included in the ground base rates and in the two air base rates. Medicare will not make a separate, additional payment for supplies and services under the fee schedule. Such items and services include, but are not necessarily limited to, drugs, supplies, EKGs, waiting time, and extra attendants.

A0384

A0384 BLS specialized service disposable supplies; defibrillation (used by ALS ambulances and BLS ambulances in jurisdictions where defibrillation is permitted in BLS ambulances)

Lay Description

Specialized disposable basic life support (BLS) defibrillation supplies include such items as defibrillator electrodes (AED), pacing pads, combination pads, and gel pads. This code is used in jurisdictions where defibrillation is permitted in BLS ambulances.

A0390

A0390 ALS mileage (per mile)

Lay Description

Advanced life support (ALS) mileage is paid on a per mile basis based on the patient's condition. Some local governments may require an ALS response for all calls, but Medicare pays only for the level of service provided, and then only when the service is medically necessary. This applies to ground and air transports.

Medicare Information

Report the actual charge for the ambulance mileage.

A0392

A0392 ALS specialized service disposable supplies; defibrillation (to be used only in jurisdictions where defibrillation cannot be performed in BLS ambulances)

Lay Description

Specialized disposable advanced life support (ALS) defibrillation supplies include such items as defibrillator electrodes (AED), pacing pads, combination pads, and gel pads. Report A0392 only in jurisdictions where defibrillation cannot be performed in basic life support (BLS) ambulances.

A0394

A0394 ALS specialized service disposable supplies; IV drug therapy

Lay Description

Specialized disposable advanced life support (ALS) IV drug therapy supplies include items such as IV start kits, IV tubing, disposable armboard, catheter, pump sets, micro drip, and Y-site tubing. Report this code once for all IV drug therapy supplies used.

A0396

A0396 ALS specialized service disposable supplies; esophageal intubation

Lay Description

Specialized disposable advanced life support (ALS) esophageal intubation supplies, which are used for airway management, include such items as esophageal obturator, esophageal gastric tube, stylette, inflation syringe, endotracheal tube, laryngoscope blade, cricotracheotomy kits, and disposable bag valve mask.

A0398

A0398 ALS routine disposable supplies

Lay Description

Advanced life support (ALS) routine disposable supplies include such items as EKG electrodes, cervical collar, gauze, and dressings. Report a unit of one for all routine disposable supplies that are used.

Medicare Information

Under the ambulance fee schedule, payment for supplies and ancillary services furnished incident to the ambulance transport are included in the ground base rates and in the two air base rates. Medicare will not make a separate, additional payment for supplies and services under the fee schedule. Such items and services include, but are not necessarily limited to, drugs, supplies, EKGs, waiting time, and extra attendants.

A0420

A0420 Ambulance waiting time (ALS or BLS), one-half (1/2) hour increments

Lay Description

This code reports ambulance waiting time for both BLS and ALS services. Time is reported in one-half hour increments. Do not report waiting time of less than one-half hour. Report one unit for each half-hour increment or portion thereof for waiting times of one-half hour or more.

Medicare Information

Unless unusual, ambulance waiting time is considered be included within the total time spent picking up and transporting a patient. Separate payment is not allowed for ambulance waiting time unless that waiting time is extraordinarily long or there are unusual circumstances. Documentation to support charges for waiting time must accompany the claim. The Medicare contractor will determine whether waiting time is warranted and payable.

A0422

A0422　Ambulance (ALS or BLS) oxygen and oxygen supplies, life sustaining situation

Lay Description

This code reports the oxygen and oxygen supplies used in a life-sustaining situation during ambulance transportation (ALS or BLS). There are two levels of ambulance service, basic medical care or basic life support (BLS) and advanced emergency medical care or advanced life support (ALS). Basic ambulance service requires at least one member of the ambulance crew to be certified at the basic EMT level and trained in patient assessment, the recognition of signs and symptoms regarding illness and injury, and in the use of proper procedures when rendering basic emergency medical care. Advanced ambulance service requires at least one of the ambulance crew to be additionally certified to provide emergency procedures, which at a minimum include defibrillation and/or synchronized cardioversion, but may also include administration of intravenous solutions, intubation, and administration of emergency drugs.

A0424

A0424　Extra ambulance attendant, ground (ALS or BLS) or air (fixed or rotary winged); (requires medical review)

Lay Description

This code reports charges for an additional ambulance attendant for both ground (BLS and ALS) and air (fixed wing and rotary transports). The need for an additional ambulance attendant must be substantiated by report.

Medicare Information

Coverage and separate payment for extra ambulance attendants is allowed if medically necessary in unusual circumstances. Documentation to support charges for extra attendants must accompany the claim. The Medicare contractor will determine whether the extra attendant is warranted and payable.

A0425

A0425　Ground mileage, per statute mile

Lay Description

This code reports ground mileage. Mileage and reimbursement rates are generally defined by and under the jurisdiction of state statutes.

Medicare Information

For covered transports, mileage is a component of ambulance fee schedule reimbursement. For Medicare purposes, mileage refers to "loaded miles." CMS defines loaded miles as the number of miles that the patient is transported in the ambulance vehicle. There is a predetermined rate per statute mile that applies to all types of ground transport, except paramedic intercepts. There is a separate rate for air miles that applies to air transports. Providers and suppliers must report all medically necessary mileage in a single line item. An additional payment is made for points of patient pickup in a rural area.

A0426-A0427

A0426　Ambulance service, advanced life support, nonemergency transport, level 1 (ALS 1)
A0427　Ambulance service, advanced life support, emergency transport, level 1 (ALS 1 — emergency)

Lay Description

Advanced life support, non-emergency transport, level 1 (ALS 1) is the transportation by ground ambulance vehicle and the provision of medically necessary supplies and services. Report A0427 for advanced life support, emergency ambulance transport, level 1 (ALS 1-emergency), which includes the provision of an ALS assessment or at least one ALS intervention. Advanced life support intervention means a procedure that is in accordance with state and local laws, beyond the scope of authority of an emergency medical technician-basic (EMT-Basic).

Medicare Information

In A0426, report the "Service Units" for each ambulance trip provided during the billing period. In A0426, the service unit is always equal to one. The total charges should include the actual charge for the ambulance service including all supplies used for the ambulance trip but excluding the charge for mileage.

A0428-A0429

A0428　Ambulance service, basic life support, nonemergency transport, (BLS)
A0429　Ambulance service, basic life support, emergency transport (BLS, emergency)

Lay Description

Basic life support, non-emergency transport (BLS) is transportation by ground ambulance vehicle and the provision of medically necessary supplies and services, including BLS ambulance services as defined by state laws. The ambulance must be staffed by an individual who is qualified in accordance with state and local laws as an emergency medical technician-basic (EMT-Basic). These laws may vary from state to state or within a state. For example, only in some jurisdictions is an EMT-Basic permitted to operate limited equipment onboard the vehicle, assist more qualified personnel in performing assessments and interventions, and establish a peripheral intravenous (IV) line. Report A0429 when medically necessary BLS transport services are supplied in the context of an emergency response.

Medicare Information

In A0428, report the "Service Units" for each ambulance trip provided during the billing period. In A0428, the service unit is always equal to one. The total charges should include the actual charge for the ambulance service including all supplies used for the ambulance trip but excluding the charge for mileage.

A0430-A0431

A0430   Ambulance service, conventional air services, transport, one way (fixed wing)

A0431   Ambulance service, conventional air services, transport, one way (rotary wing)

Lay Description

Fixed wing (FW) ambulance (airplane) conventional air service (A0430) is the transportation by a fixed wing aircraft that is certified by the Federal Aviation Administration (FAA) as a fixed wing air ambulance along with the provision of medically necessary services and supplies. This code is reported for one-way transport service. Rotary wing (RW) ambulance (helicopter) conventional air service (A0431) is the transportation by helicopter that is certified by the Federal Aviation Administration (FAA) as a rotary wing ambulance, including the provision of medically necessary supplies and services. This code is reported for one-way transport service.

Medicare Information

Report the "Service Units" for each ambulance trip provided during the billing period. In A0430, the service unit is always equal to one. The total charges should include the actual charge for the ambulance service including all supplies used for the ambulance trip but excluding the charge for mileage.

A0432

A0432   Paramedic intercept (PI), rural area, transport furnished by a volunteer ambulance company which is prohibited by state law from billing third-party payers

Lay Description

Paramedic intercept (PI) services are advanced life support (ALS) services provided with the ambulance transport by a volunteer ambulance company that is prohibited from doing any third party billing by state laws. Use this code for PI services provided in a rural area.

Medicare Information

The entity providing the ALS paramedic intercept service must:

- Be certified as qualified to provide ALS services in accordance with CFR 410.41 of the regulations
- Bill all recipients of ALS paramedic services, whether or not they are Medicare beneficiaries

Payment is based on the actual charge or the ALS rate minus 40 percent of the BLS rate, whichever is lower.

A0433

A0433   Advanced life support, level 2 (ALS 2)

Lay Description

Advanced life support, level 2 (ALS 2) is the transportation by ground ambulance vehicle and the provision of medically necessary supplies and services including at least three separate administrations of one or more medications by intravenous push/bolus or by continuous infusion (excluding crystalloid fluids), or ground ambulance transport and the provision of at least one ALS 2 procedures, such as manual defibrillation/cardioversion, endotracheal intubation, central venous line, cardiac pacing, chest decompression, surgical airway, or intraosseous line.

Medicare Information

Report the "Service Units" for each ambulance trip provided during the billing period. In A0433, the service units is always equal to one. The total charges should include the actual charge for the ambulance service including all supplies used for the ambulance trip but excluding the charge for mileage.

A0434

A0434   Specialty care transport (SCT)

Lay Description

Specialty care transport (SCT) is hospital-to-hospital transportation of a critically injured or ill beneficiary by a ground ambulance vehicle, including the provision of medically necessary supplies and services, at a level of service beyond the scope of the EMT-Paramedic. SCT is necessary when a beneficiary's condition requires ongoing care that must be furnished by one or more health professionals in an appropriate specialty area (e.g., emergency or critical care nursing, emergency medicine, respiratory care, cardiovascular care, or a paramedic with additional training).

Medicare Information
Report the "Service Units" for each ambulance trip provided during the billing period. In A0434, the service units is always equal to one. The total charges should include the actual charge for the ambulance service including all supplies used for the ambulance trip but excluding the charge for mileage.

A0435-A0436
A0435 Fixed wing air mileage, per statute mile
A0436 Rotary wing air mileage, per statute mile

Lay Description
Report A0435 for each statute mile a patient is transported in a fixed wing airplane. Report A0436 for each statute mile a patient is transported in a rotary wing aircraft.

Medicare Information
For air ambulance services, the fee schedule payment is calculated using:

- A nationally uniform base rate for fixed wing and a nationally uniform base rate for rotary wing
- A geographic adjustment factor (GAF) for each ambulance fee schedule area (GPCI)
- A nationally uniform loaded mileage rate for each type of air service
- A rural adjustment to the base rate and loaded mileage for services furnished in a rural area

A0888
A0888 Noncovered ambulance mileage, per mile (e.g., for miles traveled beyond closest appropriate facility)

Lay Description
Mileage for an ambulance trip is covered only to the nearest, appropriate facility. However, there are instances when a beneficiary requests to be transported to a facility that is not the closest appropriate facility. In these situations, there is additional mileage that is not covered. Use A0888 to report these additional, noncovered miles. This policy applies to both ground and air ambulance services.

Medicare Information
Medicare has a long-standing policy that mileage for an ambulance trip is covered only to the nearest, appropriate facility. However, Medicare recognizes that there are instances when a beneficiary may request to be transported to a facility that is not the closest appropriate facility. In these situations, there would be additional mileage that is not covered by Medicare. This policy applies to both ground and air ambulance services. In addition to the base rate and mileage ambulance lines, providers must report a third line for non-covered ambulance miles.

A0998
A0998 Ambulance response and treatment, no transport

Lay Description
When an ambulance is dispatched and treatment is provided to the patient without the patient being transported to another site, the service is reported with A0998.

A0999
A0999 Unlisted ambulance service

Lay Description
This code is used for any ambulance service that is not described by other HCPCS Level II codes. It should be used as a last resort and only when there is not a more appropriate procedure code. When reporting an unlisted code, provide a detailed explanation of the services in remarks, billing notes, or as an attachment.

A4206-A4209
A4206 Syringe with needle, sterile, 1 cc or less, each
A4207 Syringe with needle, sterile 2 cc, each
A4208 Syringe with needle, sterile 3 cc, each
A4209 Syringe with needle, sterile 5 cc or greater, each

Lay Description
A sterile syringe with a needle is used for injecting or withdrawing liquids into or from any vessel or cavity. Each may vary in size and content capacity. Report A4206 for a 1 cc syringe, A4207 for a 2 cc syringe, A4208 for a 3 cc syringe, and A4209 for a 5 cc or greater size syringe.

A4210
A4210 Needle-free injection device, each

Lay Description
This code reports a needle free injection instrument. These could be injectors such as hypodermic jet pressure powered devices for insulin injections.

A4211
A4211 Supplies for self-administered injections

Lay Description
Patients may administer injectable medications, such as insulin or calcitonin, themselves. Supplies for self-administered injections are rarely covered unless an emergency situation exists.

Medicare Information

When a drug that is usually injected by the patient (e.g., insulin or calcitonin) is injected by the physician, it is excluded from coverage unless administered in an emergency situation (e.g., diabetic coma).

A4212

A4212   Noncoring needle or stylet with or without catheter

Lay Description

Noncoring needles or stylets are most often used to cleanly penetrate rubber self-sealing septums that are part of indwelling ports and pumps. The reservoirs on these surgically implanted devices can be refilled numerous times when noncoring needles are used.

A4213

A4213   Syringe, sterile, 20 cc or greater, each

Lay Description

This code reports supply of a sterile syringe with a capacity of 20 cc or greater. Syringes of this size may be used for injection of medications by intravenous or intraarterial push. These types of syringes may also be used for wound irrigation.

A4215

A4215   Needle, sterile, any size, each

Lay Description

This code reports any sterile size needle. This code is for a single needle and may be reported multiple times if more than one needle is used.

Medicare Information

Sterile needles used to administer or perform covered services are considered incidental supplies in a hospital, skilled nursing facility, or physician office. Separate payment is not made. Reimbursement is considered to be included in the payment for the procedure. Sterile needles used by a home health agency for covered home health visits are generally considered routine supplies that are included in the cost per visit for home health care services.

Under certain circumstances, such as supplies necessary for home dialysis, a separate payment for sterile needles may be allowed. In these instances, billing and coverage is determined by the specific circumstances (e.g., supplies for home dialysis patients covered under Method II that are billed by the DME supplier).

A4216-A4217

A4216   Sterile water, saline and/or dextrose, diluent/flush, 10 ml
A4217   Sterile water/saline, 500 ml

Lay Description

Sterile water, saline, or dextrose for injection or irrigation is reported with A4216-A4217. Report A4216 for 10 ml vial of sterile water, saline, and/or dextrose and A4217 for 500 ml of sterile water or saline.

Medicare Information

Sterile water used for irrigation or as an injection in conjunction with covered services are considered an incidental supply in a hospital, skilled nursing facility, or physician office. Separate payment is not made. Reimbursement is considered to be included in the payment for the procedure. Sterile water used by a home health agency for covered home health visits is generally considered a routine supply that is included in the cost per visit for home health care services.

Under certain circumstances, such as supplies necessary for home dialysis, a separate payment for sterile water may be allowed. In these specific instances, billing and coverage is determined by the specific circumstances (e.g., supplies for home dialysis patients covered under Method II that are billed by the DME supplier).

A4218

A4218   Sterile saline or water, metered dose dispenser, 10 ml

Lay Description

A metered dose dispenser of sterile saline or water may be used with a nebulizer or inhaler for dispensing inhalation medications. A metered dose dispenser delivers a precise amount of sterile saline or water for use in the device. This allows proper dilution of the medication. Report A4218 for a 10 ml metered dose dispenser of sterile saline or water.

Medicare Information

Sterile water used in conjunction with a covered service is considered an incidental supply in a hospital, skilled nursing facility, or physician office. Separate payment is not made. Reimbursement is considered to be included in the payment for the procedure. Sterile water used by a home health care agency is generally considered a routine supply that is included in the cost per visit. Certain circumstances, such as supplies necessary for DME use, may allow separate payment for sterile water. In those specific instances, billing and coverage is determined by the specific circumstances (e.g., supplies for a nebulizer or metered dose dispenser may be covered when the dispenser itself is covered).

A4220

A4220   Refill kit for implantable infusion pump

Lay Description

Implantable infusion pumps are typically small, biocompatible, stainless steel units that are surgically placed subcutaneously near the target drug delivery area. A refillable reservoir delivers a constant, prescribed rate of liquid drug to the target site. Drug delivery may be by spring or piston pressure against the reservoir. Routes of administration include intravenous, intra-arterial, intraperitoneal, and intraventricular. Code A4220 reports a refill kit for an implanted pump. The kit may contain appropriate noncoring needles, filters, connectors, and other items, but not the drug itself.

Medicare Information

Implantable infusion pumps are covered by Medicare for 5-FUdR therapy for unresected liver or colorectal cancer and for opioid drug therapy for intractable pain. Report drugs separately. Medicare covers incontinence appliances and care supplies when the medical record indicates incontinence is permanent or of long and indefinite duration. Medicare claims fall under the jurisdiction of the DME regional carrier for a permanent condition, and under the local carrier when provided in the physician's office for a temporary condition.

A4221

A4221   Supplies for maintenance of drug infusion catheter, per week (list drug separately)

Lay Description

Drug infusion catheters embrace a range of approaches, including peripheral intravenous lines, peripherally inserted central catheters (PICC), and centrally inserted intravenous lines. Maintenance supplies for such drug infusion catheters may include flush solutions, dressings, cannulas, and needles. This code is not drug specific.

Medicare Information

Supplies for the maintenance of a parenteral drug infusion catheter are covered during the period of covered use of an infusion pump. They are also covered for the weeks in between covered infusion pump use, not to exceed four weeks per episode. More than one unit of service per week is not separately allowed.

Supplies (including dressings) used in conjunction with a durable infusion pump (E0779, E0780, E0781, E0791, K0455), but excluding external insulin infusion pumps (E0784), are included in A4221 and A4222. Other codes should not be used for the separate billing of these supplies.

Code A4230 infusion set for external insulin pump, nonneedle cannula type and A4231 infusion set for external insulin pump, needle type are not valid for claim submission to the DME MAC because they are included in A4221.

Supplies used with an external insulin infusion pump are covered during the period of covered use of an infusion pump and are billed using A4221 and A4232. Catheter insertion devices for use with external insulin infusion pump infusion cannulas are included in the allowance for A4221 and are not separately payable.

Note: See chapter titled "Medicare Guidelines," under "Infusion Pumps, External; Equipment and Supplies," for additional Medicare billing and documentation information.

A4222-A4223

A4222   Infusion supplies for external drug infusion pump, per cassette or bag (list drugs separately)

A4223   Infusion supplies not used with external infusion pump, per cassette or bag (list drugs separately)

Lay Description

Code A4222 reports infusion supplies for external drug infusion pumps, which may be portable units worn on belts outside the body or larger stationary units. Use this code per cassette or bag, with drugs, such as diluting solutions, tubing, and other administration supplies, such as port caps listed separately. Code A4223 reports infusion supplies not used with an external infusion pump, per cassette or bag. These codes are not drug specific.

A4230-A4231

A4230   Infusion set for external insulin pump, nonneedle cannula type

A4231   Infusion set for external insulin pump, needle type

Lay Description

These codes report infusion supplies pertaining to external insulin pumps. These are portable, battery-operated devices worn by the patient on a belt or sling. The device connects to a drug reservoir and the system is designed to deliver continuous subcutaneous insulin therapy over an extended period of time. The device usually delivers insulin into subcutaneous fat in the abdominal region and the infusion set must be changed out every few days. Code A4230 reports an infusion set for a non-needle cannula style pump and may include a specialty insertion device. Code A4231 reports the more conventional needle insertion infusion. Cassettes or bags are included, as are diluting solutions, tubing, and other administration supplies, such as port caps. This code is drug specific to insulin.

Medicare Information

See the chapter titled "Medicare Guidelines," under "Infusion Pumps, External; Equipment and Supplies," for Medicare information.

A4232

A4232   Syringe with needle for external insulin pump, sterile, 3 cc

Lay Description

This code is designated for a syringe with needle for external insulin pump, sterile, 3 cc. Code A4232 describes the insulin reservoir for use with the external insulin infusion pump (E0784). The reservoir may be either glass or plastic and includes the needle for drawing up the insulin. This code does not include the insulin for use in the reservoir.

A4233-A4236

A4233   Replacement battery, alkaline (other than J cell), for use with medically necessary home blood glucose monitor owned by patient, each
A4234   Replacement battery, alkaline, J cell, for use with medically necessary home blood glucose monitor owned by patient, each
A4235   Replacement battery, lithium, for use with medically necessary home blood glucose monitor owned by patient, each
A4236   Replacement battery, silver oxide, for use with medically necessary home blood glucose monitor owned by patient, each

Lay Description

Glucometers with associated accessories and supplies are used for patients with all types of diabetes mellitus to monitor blood glucose, and are available in a variety of models. A replacement battery for a medically necessary, patient-owned home blood glucose monitor (glucometer) is reported based on the type of battery required. Report A4233 for an alkaline battery other than J cell; A4234 for an alkaline battery J cell; A4235 for a lithium battery; and A4236 for a silver oxide battery.

Medicare Information

Medicare National Coverage Determinations Manual, Pub. 100–3, chap. 1, part 4, sec. 40.3 details coverage criteria for home blood glucose monitors. When the blood glucose monitor is covered, the associated supplies such as batteries may be covered.

A4244-A4248

A4244   Alcohol or peroxide, per pint
A4245   Alcohol wipes, per box
A4246   Betadine or pHisoHex solution, per pint
A4247   Betadine or iodine swabs/wipes, per box
A4248   Chlorhexidine containing antiseptic, 1 ml

Lay Description

Glucometers and associated accessories and supplies are used for patients with all types of diabetes mellitus to monitor blood glucose levels. Supplies used in monitoring blood glucose levels include a variety of antiseptics and antimicrobials to cleanse the skin prior to piercing the skin to obtain a blood sample to perform the glucose test. Report A4244 for each pint of alcohol or peroxide. Alcohol wipes are reported per box with A4245. Betadine, pHisoHex, and iodine are other types of anti-infective solutions used on the skin and are available in both pints or individually wrapped swabs or wipes. Report A4246 per pint of Betadine or pHisoHex and A4247 per box of Betadine or iodine swabs or wipes. A chlorhexidine containing antiseptic such as Hibiclens may also be used to prevent skin infections. Chlorhexidine has antiseptic activity and an antimicrobial effect against a wide range of microorganisms. Report A4248 per 1 ml of chlorhexidine.

Medicare Information

Glucometers and associated accessories and supplies are used for patients with all types of diabetes mellitus to monitor blood glucose levels. Supplies used in monitoring blood glucose levels include a variety of antiseptics and antimicrobials to cleanse the skin prior to piercing the skin to obtain a blood sample to perform the glucose test. Report A4244 for each pint of alcohol or peroxide. Alcohol wipes are reported per box with A4245. Betadine, pHisoHex, and iodine are other types of anti-infective solutions used on the skin and are available in both pints or individually wrapped swabs or wipes. Report A4246 per pint of Betadine or pHisoHex and A4247 per box of Betadine or iodine swabs or wipes. A chlorhexidine containing antiseptic such as Hibiclens may also be used to prevent skin infections. Chlorhexidine has antiseptic activity and an antimicrobial effect against a wide range of microorganisms. Report A4248 per 1 ml of chlorhexidine.

A4250-A4259

A4250 Urine test or reagent strips or tablets (100 tablets or strips)
A4252 Blood ketone test or reagent strip, each
A4253 Blood glucose test or reagent strips for home blood glucose monitor, per 50 strips
A4255 Platforms for home blood glucose monitor, 50 per box
A4256 Normal, low, and high calibrator solution/chips
A4257 Replacement lens shield cartridge for use with laser skin piercing device, each
A4258 Spring-powered device for lancet, each
A4259 Lancets, per box of 100

Lay Description

Glucometers and associated accessories and supplies are used for patients with all types of diabetes mellitus to monitor blood glucose levels, and are available in a variety of models. Accessories and supplies for these devices range from alcohol prep pads to lancets for piercing the skin to obtain the required blood sample to perform the test. Many of these supplies must be used each time the test is performed and are not reusable. Many diabetics require frequent, if not daily, blood glucose monitoring, whether or not the patient is on insulin. For Type I diabetes mellitus patients who require insulin (the patient's body does not manufacture insulin and therefore it must come from an external source, such as injections), blood glucose monitoring is a life-sustaining requirement. The accessories and supplies are medically necessary to properly and accurately perform the blood glucose monitoring. Blood glucose test or reagent strips are used with home glucose monitoring devices and are usually covered for insulin-dependent diabetics whose monitor has been prescribed by the physician. Code A4250 represents 100 strips or tablets used to test urine, A4252 represents one blood ketone test or reagent strip, and A4253 reports 50 strips for a home glucose monitoring system. Platforms are used with lancing devices to prevent cross infection and to control depth of penetration of the lancing device. Report A4255 per box of 50 platforms. Calibrator solutions or chips are used with a home glucose monitoring device to check the integrity of the glucometer and the test strips. Calibrator solutions or chips are provided in normal, low, and high levels, and are reported with A4256. Lancing devices use lasers or springs. Use of a laser device requires a lens shield cartridge. A replacement lens shield cartridge used with a laser skin piercing device is reported with A4257. A spring piercing device for a lancet is reported with A4258. A lancet is a pointed surgical knife with two edges. Report A4259 for each box of 100 lancets used.

Medicare Information

See chapter titled "Medicare Guidelines," under "Diabetics Supplies and Services," for Medicare billing and documentation information.

A4261

A4261 Cervical cap for contraceptive use

Lay Description

A cervical cap is a thimble shaped latex device that covers the cervix and is used with a spermicide as a barrier method of contraception. Report A4261 for a cervical cap used as a contraceptive.

A4262-A4263

A4262 Temporary, absorbable lacrimal duct implant, each
A4263 Permanent, long-term, nondissolvable lacrimal duct implant, each

Lay Description

Report A4262 for use of a temporary, absorbable tear duct implant. Report A4263 when a permanent, long-term nondissolvable lacrimal duct implant is used.

Medicare Information

Always report A4262 and A4263 concurrent to the implant procedure.

Medicare will not allow separate payment for silicone punctal plugs (A4263) or temporary plugs (A4262), as these are included in the procedure.

A4264

A4264 Permanent implantable contraceptive intratubal occlusion device(s) and delivery system

Lay Description

An intratubal occlusion device is a permanent, implantable, contraceptive occlusive device and system used for nonincisional sterilization. This process is performed using a hysteroscopic approach. The system is comprised of a micro-insert implantable stainless steel inner coil with polyester fibers and a super-elastic nitinol outer anchoring coil. The micro-insert, when released, expands to conform and anchor in the fallopian tube.

A4265

A4265 Paraffin, per pound

Lay Description

Paraffin is a waxy, white, tasteless, odorless mixture of solid hydrocarbon made from petroleum. It is often used as the base for an ointment or wound dressing. Report A4265 for each pound used.

A4266

A4266 Diaphragm for contraceptive use

Lay Description

A diaphragm is a rubber or plastic cup that fits over the cervix uteri and is used for contraceptive purposes. Report A4266 when a diaphragm is supplied to the patient.

A4267-A4268

A4267 Contraceptive supply, condom, male, each
A4268 Contraceptive supply, condom, female, each

Lay Description

A condom is a thin, flexible sheath used by a man to prevent pregnancy and/or sexually transmitted diseases. Report A4267 for each male condom supplied. Report A4268 if the contraceptive supplied is a condom made for sheathing the internal anatomy of the female.

A4269

A4269 Contraceptive supply, spermicide (e.g., foam, gel), each

Lay Description

Spermicides are contraceptive agents used to kill spermatozoa. Report A4269 for each supply of spermicide.

A4270

A4270 Disposable endoscope sheath, each

Lay Description

This code reports the use of a disposable sheath that covers an endoscope, a device consisting of a tube and optical system for viewing the inside of a hollow organ or cavity.

A4280

A4280 Adhesive skin support attachment for use with external breast prosthesis, each

Lay Description

Report A4280 for the adhesive skin support attachment used with a breast prosthesis, a man-made substitute for a missing breast.

A4281-A4286

A4281 Tubing for breast pump, replacement
A4282 Adapter for breast pump, replacement
A4283 Cap for breast pump bottle, replacement
A4284 Breast shield and splash protector for use with breast pump, replacement
A4285 Polycarbonate bottle for use with breast pump, replacement
A4286 Locking ring for breast pump, replacement

Lay Description

A breast pump is used to extract the milk from a lactating mother. Report A4281 for replacement tubing for the breast pump; A4282 for a replacement adapter used with the breast pump; A4283 for a replacement cap for the breast pump bottle; A4284 for a breast shield and splash cover replacement for the breast pump; A4285 for a replacement polycarbonate bottle for use with the breast pump; and A4286 for the replacement of the locking ring on the breast pump.

A4290

A4290 Sacral nerve stimulation test lead, each

Lay Description

There are five pairs of spinal or sacral nerves. Report A4290 for each test lead used in a sacral nerve stimulation examination.

A4300

A4300 Implantable access catheter, (e.g., venous, arterial, epidural subarachnoid, or peritoneal, etc.) external access

Lay Description

A catheter is a tube inserted into the body to evacuate or inject fluids into body cavities. Report A4300 for an implantable external access catheter (e.g., venous, arterial, epidural subarachnoid, peritoneal, etc.).

A4301

A4301 Implantable access total catheter, port/reservoir (e.g., venous, arterial, epidural, subarachnoid, peritoneal, etc.)

Lay Description

This code reports the supply of an integrated vascular port/reservoir and catheter designed for subdermal implantation. The system is designed for patients requiring regular or continuous intravenous or intra-arterial infusion of drugs. The system may be used to deliver any of a variety of medicines, particularly those for oncology therapy. In some instances, the implanted port and catheter delivers drugs to the spinal cord (epidural), the brain (subarachnoid), or to the abdominal (peritoneal) cavity. Implantable infusion pumps are typically small biocompatible stainless steel units that are surgically placed subcutaneously near the site of optimal drug delivery. The port and reservoir can be smaller in diameter than a nickel coin. A refillable reservoir delivers a constant, prescribed rate of liquid drug to the target site. Typically, the reservoir features a rubber diaphragm that can be penetrated by a non-coring needle to refill the drug.

A4305-A4306

A4305 Disposable drug delivery system, flow rate of 50 ml or greater per hour
A4306 Disposable drug delivery system, flow rate of less than 50 ml per hour

Lay Description

These disposable drug delivery systems comprise devices that deliver liquid drugs by the elastic pressure of the reservoir container. The term elastomeric infusion pump may be used. Report A4305 for a flow rate of 50 ml or greater per hour and A4306 for a flow rate of less than 50 ml per hour. These codes are not drug specific.

A4310-A4316

A4310 Insertion tray without drainage bag and without catheter (accessories only)
A4311 Insertion tray without drainage bag with indwelling catheter, Foley type, 2-way latex with coating (Teflon, silicone, silicone elastomer or hydrophilic, etc.)
A4312 Insertion tray without drainage bag with indwelling catheter, Foley type, 2-way, all silicone
A4313 Insertion tray without drainage bag with indwelling catheter, Foley type, 3-way, for continuous irrigation
A4314 Insertion tray with drainage bag with indwelling catheter, Foley type, 2-way latex with coating (Teflon, silicone, silicone elastomer or hydrophilic, etc.)
A4315 Insertion tray with drainage bag with indwelling catheter, Foley type, 2-way, all silicone
A4316 Insertion tray with drainage bag with indwelling catheter, Foley type, 3-way, for continuous irrigation

Lay Description

Urinary catheters and external urinary collection devices are used to drain or collect urine from a patient who has permanent urinary incontinence or permanent urinary retention. Supplies or accessories are also used with the catheters and are part of the service provided.

Medicare Information

See chapter titled "Medicare Guidelines," under "Urological Supplies," for Medicare billing and documentation information.

A4320-A4322

A4320 Irrigation tray with bulb or piston syringe, any purpose
A4321 Therapeutic agent for urinary catheter irrigation
A4322 Irrigation syringe, bulb or piston, each

Lay Description

These codes are reported for cleaning and irrigation items for incontinence care. Report A4320 for an irrigation tray with bulb or piston syringe, used with sterile water; A4321 if a therapeutic agent is used for urinary catheter irrigation; A4322 for each irrigation syringe, bulb, or piston.

Medicare Information

See chapter titled "Medicare Guidelines," under "Urological Supplies," for Medicare billing and documentation information.

A4326

A4326 Male external catheter with integral collection chamber, any type, each

Lay Description

Male external catheters (condom-type) are used by patients who have permanent urinary incontinence as an alternative to an indwelling catheter. A male external catheter is used over the external genitalia as an incontinence guard. This code reports a male external catheter with integral collection chamber, any type, each.

Medicare Information

Specialty type male external catheters, such as those that inflate or include a faceplate, are covered only when documentation substantiates the medical necessity for such a catheter. Payment will be based on the least costly, but medically appropriate alternative if documentation does not substantiate medical necessity.

Note: See chapter titled "Medicare Guidelines," under "Urological Supplies," for additional Medicare billing and documentation information.

A4327-A4328

A4327 Female external urinary collection device; meatal cup, each
A4328 Female external urinary collection device; pouch, each

Lay Description
A female external urinary collection device is used to collect urine as it passes to the outside of the body. Report A4327 for each metal cup that is an external urinary collective device or A4328 for each pouch used.

Medicare Information
See chapter titled "Medicare Guidelines," under "Urological Supplies," for Medicare billing and documentation information.

A4330

A4330 Perianal fecal collection pouch with adhesive, each

Lay Description
Report A4330 for a perianal stool collection pouch that uses adhesive.

A4331

A4331 Extension drainage tubing, any type, any length, with connector/adaptor, for use with urinary leg bag or urostomy pouch, each

Lay Description
Extension drainage tubing is used with a urostomy pouch or latex urinary leg bag for patients who are ambulatory or are chair or wheelchair bound but not bedridden. Report this code for any type, any length of extension drainage tubing with the connector or adaptor.

Medicare Information
Extension tubing will be covered when used with a latex urinary leg bag, but is not separately covered for A4314, A4315, A4316, A4354, A4357, A4358, and A5105. The allowance for the tubing is included in the payment for these codes.

Note: See chapter titled "Medicare Guidelines," under "Urological Supplies," for additional Medicare billing and documentation information.

A4332-A4334

A4332 Lubricant, individual sterile packet, each
A4333 Urinary catheter anchoring device, adhesive skin attachment, each
A4334 Urinary catheter anchoring device, leg strap, each

Lay Description
Report A4332 for each individual sterile packet of lubricant and A4333 for each adhesive skin attachment used as a urinary catheter anchoring device. Report A4334 if the anchoring device is a leg strap.

Medicare Information
Adhesive catheter anchoring devices and catheter leg straps are covered items. More than three anchor devices per week or one leg strap per month will be denied as not medically necessary unless the claim is accompanied by documentation justifying a larger quantity.

Nonsterile lubricating gel would be covered for use with clean nonsterile catheterization technique. Eight units of service (8 oz.) can be covered per month. An individual packet of lubricant is not medically necessary for clean, non-sterile intermittent catheterization.

Note: See chapter titled "Medicare Guidelines," under "Urological Supplies," for additional Medicare billing and documentation information.

A4335

A4335 Incontinence supply; miscellaneous

Lay Description
Incontinence supplies are leak proof undergarments worn by the patient who cannot retain or control the release of urine, semen, or feces. This code reports miscellaneous incontinence supplies.

A4336

A4336 Incontinence supply, urethral insert, any type, each

Lay Description
Urethral inserts are designed for the female patient to manage and/or treat urinary incontinence. A self-inserted, single use, disposable intra-urethral device results in instant control of severe stress urinary incontinence (SUI). This insert is a small, latex free, narrow silicone tube that is totally encased in a soft, thin, mineral oil-filled sleeve. The sleeve forms a balloon at the internal tip and a soft, oval shaped external retainer at the opposite end. The device is inserted using a disposable applicator.

A4338-A4346

A4338 Indwelling catheter; Foley type, 2-way latex with coating (Teflon, silicone, silicone elastomer, or hydrophilic, etc.), each
A4340 Indwelling catheter; specialty type, (e.g., Coude, mushroom, wing, etc.), each
A4344 Indwelling catheter, Foley type, 2-way, all silicone, each
A4346 Indwelling catheter; Foley type, 3-way for continuous irrigation, each

Lay Description
Indwelling catheters remain in the body for a period of time. Report A4338 for each two-way, Foley type latex with coating catheter. Report A4340 for each specialty-type indwelling catheter (e.g., coude, mushroom, wing, etc.). Report A4344 for each Foley type, two-way indwelling catheter made of silicone. Report A4346 for each three-way catheter used for continuous irrigation.

Medicare Information
Indwelling catheters are covered at a quantity of no more than one catheter per month for routine catheter maintenance.

When a specialty indwelling catheter or an all-silicone catheter is used, there must be documentation in the patient's medical record of the medical necessity for the catheter rather than a straight Foley-type catheter with coating (such as recurrent encrustation, inability to pass a straight catheter, or sensitivity to latex). This documentation may be requested by the DME MAC. If documentation is requested and does not substantiate medical necessity, payment will be made based on the least costly, but medically appropriate alternative.

A three-way indwelling catheter, either alone or with other components, will be covered only if continuous catheter irrigation is medically necessary.

Note: See chapter titled "Medicare Guidelines," under "Urological Supplies," for additional Medicare billing and documentation information.

A4349

A4349 Male external catheter, with or without adhesive, disposable, each

Lay Description
Male external catheters (condom-type) are used by patients who have permanent urinary incontinence as an alternative to an indwelling catheter. A male external catheter is used over the external genitalia as an incontinence guard. Report A4349 for each disposable male external catheter with or without adhesive.

Medicare Information
See the chapter titled "Medicare Guidelines," under "Urological Supplies," for Medicare information.

A4351-A4353

A4351 Intermittent urinary catheter; straight tip, with or without coating (Teflon, silicone, silicone elastomer, or hydrophilic, etc.), each
A4352 Intermittent urinary catheter; Coude (curved) tip, with or without coating (Teflon, silicone, silicone elastomeric, or hydrophilic, etc.), each
A4353 Intermittent urinary catheter, with insertion supplies

Lay Description
Urinary catheterization involves insertion of a drainage tube up the urethra and into the bladder where it is often held in place by an inflated balloon. For these indwelling catheters, a reservoir is typically attached to contain the drained urine, which, for many patients, may be monitored for volume and tested for content. This code range, however, reports intermittent catheterization, a treatment approach for certain urinary disorders, and patient profiles. The catheter is inserted using antiseptic technique by the patient or a caregiver four times a day, or more often as needed. A topical anesthetic may be employed and the catheter is lubricated. The bladder is completely voided into a container and the catheter withdrawn after each procedure. The catheter may be disinfected and reused, or discarded.

A4354

A4354 Insertion tray with drainage bag but without catheter

Lay Description
This code reports the supply of a urinary catheterization insertion tray. This type of sterile tray typically includes a preloaded syringe, absorbent pads, drapery, gloves, and lubricants. A drainage bag or graduated container is included in the code description, but the catheter itself is specifically excluded. Report A4354 for supply of an insertion tray with drainage bag but without catheter.

A4355

A4355 Irrigation tubing set for continuous bladder irrigation through a 3-way indwelling Foley catheter, each

Lay Description
This code reports the supply of a specific continuous bladder irrigation set. Bladder catheterization is generally called for in patients unable to void urine naturally and following certain surgeries.

Continuous irrigation is usually temporary and may be required in certain circumstances involving obstructions. The bladder is a sterile environment and sterile hardware and technique is ordinarily required to catheterize it. A Foley catheter features a balloon tip that is inflated upon entry into the bladder to hold the device in place (indwelling). A three-way catheter features a lumen for urine drainage, one to inflate and deflate the Foley balloon, and one for irrigation fluids and medications.

A4356

A4356 **External urethral clamp or compression device (not to be used for catheter clamp), each**

Lay Description

This code reports the supply of external urethral clamps, also known as penile clamps, Cunningham clamps, or Knuttsen clamps. These reusable metal devices fit over the penis. Typically, soft foam that contours to the shape of the penis is compressed, closing off the urethra. Compression on the devices must be relieved every several hours.

A4357

A4357 **Bedside drainage bag, day or night, with or without antireflux device, with or without tube, each**

Lay Description

Patients with urinary ostomies may use a bedside drainage bag during the day or night. The bedside drainage bag is used for the collection of urinary output from a urinary pouch. It is sometimes necessary, especially at night, for the bag to be connected to the pouch to prevent urinary overflow and excessive weight in the pouch, which could cause urinary leakage and disruption of the pouch seal. The bag is made of a high grade PVC and can hold up to 2,000 cc. Report A4357 for a bedside drainage bag with or without tube and with or without an anti-reflux device, which prevents urinary back flow.

Medicare Information

See the chapter titled "Medicare Guidelines," under "Urological Supplies," for Medicare information.

A4358

A4358 **Urinary drainage bag, leg or abdomen, vinyl, with or without tube, with straps, each**

Lay Description

Leg or abdomen urinary drainage bags are indicated for patients who are ambulatory or are chair or wheelchair bound but not bedridden. The vinyl bag can be used with either a suprapubic or Foley catheter for the purpose of urine collection and typically holds up to 1000 cc. The bag is held in place next to the abdomen or around the leg by woven straps. This code describes a drainage bag, with or without tubing.

Medicare Information

Leg bags are covered for patients who are ambulatory or are chair- or wheelchair-bound.

Payment will be made for either a vinyl leg bag or a latex leg bag. The use of both bags is considered not medically necessary by Medicare. The medical necessity for drainage bags containing gel matrix or other material, intended to be disposed of on a daily basis, has not been established. Payment for these types of bags will be based on the allowance and usual frequency of change for the least costly, but medically appropriate alternative.

Note: See chapter titled "Medicare Guidelines," under "Urological Supplies," for additional Medicare billing and documentation information.

A4360

A4360 **Disposable external urethral clamp or compression device, with pad and/or pouch, each**

Lay Description

A disposable, external urethral clamp or compression device is designed for a male patient to manage and/or treat light to moderate urinary incontinence. It works by minimizing urinary incontinence by means of mechanical compression of the urethra, eliminating the leakage of urine and allowing the bladder to fill. If there is leakage that breaks through from the urethra, the moisture is restricted to the disposable pouch or pad.

A4361

A4361 **Ostomy faceplate, each**

Lay Description

An ostomy faceplate is a solid interface between the patient's skin and the pouch. It is usually made of plastic, rubber, or encased metal. It does not have an adhesive property and there is no pectin-based or karaya material that is an integral part of the faceplate. It can be taken off the skin and reattached repeatedly. It is held on by means of a separate adhesive and/or an elastic belt. Use this code to report each ostomy faceplate.

Medicare Information

Supplies related to ostomy care are a covered benefit, including catheters, catheter supplies, ostomy bags, and other supplies.

The quantity of ostomy supplies needed by a patient is determined by the type of ostomy, its location, its construction, and the condition of the skin surface surrounding the stoma. There will be variation according to individual patient need. The medical necessity for using a greater quantity of supplies than usually expected for the patient's condition must be well documented in the patient's medical record and may be requested by the DME MAC.

There is seldom medical necessity for closed colostomy or ileostomy pouches rather than drainable pouches. The medical necessity of a closed pouch must be well documented in the patient's medical record and may be requested by the

DME MAC.

If provided in the physician's office for a temporary condition, the item is incident to the physician's service and billed to the local carrier. If provided in the physician's office or other place of service for a permanent condition, the item is a prosthetic device and billed to the DME MAC.

A4362, A5121-A5122

A4362 Skin barrier; solid, 4 x 4 or equivalent; each
A5121 Skin barrier; solid, 6 x 6 or equivalent, each
A5122 Skin barrier; solid, 8 x 8 or equivalent, each

Lay Description

Skin barriers are an interface between the patient's skin and the pouching system. They are used to create an adhesive seal between the skin and the pouch. Barriers can be curved with a built in convexity creating a more adhesive bond to the patient's skin and better protrusion of the stoma. These codes represent solid ostomy skin barriers that are used independently, usually with a pouch that does not have its own integral skin barrier. Report A4362 for a 4X4 or equivalent skin barrier; see A5121 for a 6X6 or equivalent barrier; and A5122 for an 8X8 or equivalent solid ostomy skin barrier.

Medicare Information

See the chapter titled "Medicare Guidelines," under "Ostomy Devices and Supplies," for Medicare information.

A4363

A4363 Ostomy clamp, any type, replacement only, each

Lay Description

An ostomy clamp is a closure accessory used to prevent spillage from an open-ended (drainable) ostomy pouch. An ostomy clamp is provided with

the purchase of an ostomy bag and is not billed separately. Report A4363 only for replacement of the ostomy clamp.

Medicare Information

See chapter titled "Medicare Guidelines," under "Ostomy Devices and Supplies," for Medicare billing and documentation information.

A4364, A5126

A4364 Adhesive, liquid or equal, any type, per oz
A5126 Adhesive or nonadhesive; disk or foam pad

Lay Description

Adhesive liquids are applied directly to the skin or to a protective barrier, such as a disk or foam pad, providing increased bonding of ostomy devices. These adhesives are in liquid form or are equal to a liquid available in bottles or spray cans. They are rubber based or acrylic based and non-toxic. Proper application of adhesives is a thin, light coat on the desired area. Adhesives can be removed with petroleum-based solvents. Report A4364 for liquid adhesive or equal, per ounce and A5126 for an adhesive or non-adhesive disk or foam pad.

Medicare Information

See the chapter titled "Medicare Guidelines," under "Ostomy Devices and Supplies," for Medicare information.

A4366

A4366 Ostomy vent, any type, each

Lay Description

A separate ostomy vent can be added to the ostomy pouch to allow the release of gas and is reported with A4366. This code must not be used for pouches in which a vent with a filter is incorporated in the pouch by the manufacturer.

Medicare Information

See chapter titled "Medicare Guidelines," under "Ostomy Devices and Supplies," for Medicare billing and documentation information.

A4367

A4367 Ostomy belt, each

Lay Description

An ostomy belt is used to secure and conceal ostomy appliances. They are made of lightweight cotton and Lycra/elastic. Belts are designed to be used with one or two-piece systems for left, right, or center stomas and vary in width depending on the patient's need. Some belts provide a pocket for the appliance that has a Velcro closure that allows for easy emptying.

A4368

A4368   Ostomy filter, any type, each

Lay Description

An ostomy filter prevents the buildup of gas trapped in the pouch by allowing the gas to be effectively expelled through a vent. Filters may be incorporated into a pouch, inserted into a venting ring on the pouch, or attached to the pouch exterior. They may also include deodorizing materials such as charcoal for the vented gas. Code A4368 describes an ostomy filter, any type.

Medicare Information

Supplies related to ostomy care are a covered benefit, including catheters, catheter supplies, ostomy bags, and other supplies.

The quantity of ostomy supplies needed by a patient is determined by the type of ostomy, its location, its construction, and the condition of the skin surface surrounding the stoma. There will be variation according to individual patient need. The medical necessity for using a greater quantity of supplies than usually expected for the patient's condition must be well documented in the patient's medical record and may be requested by the DME MAC.

There is seldom medical necessity for closed colostomy or ileostomy pouches rather than drainable pouches. The medical necessity of a closed pouch must be well documented in the patient's medical record and may be requested by the DME MAC.

If provided in the physician's office for a temporary condition, the item is incident to the physician's service and billed to the local carrier. If provided in the physician's office or other place of service for a permanent condition, the item is a prosthetic device and billed to the DME MAC.

Medicare Information

See the chapter titled "Medicare Guidelines," under "Ostomy Devices and Supplies," for Medicare information.

A4369-A4373

A4369   Ostomy skin barrier, liquid (spray, brush, etc.), per oz
A4371   Ostomy skin barrier, powder, per oz
A4372   Ostomy skin barrier, solid 4 x 4 or equivalent, standard wear, with built-in convexity, each
A4373   Ostomy skin barrier, with flange (solid, flexible or accordian), with built-in convexity, any size, each

Lay Description

This range of codes reports skin care and conditioning supplies for patients fitting adhesive pouches over an ostomy, a surgically created opening through the skin to divert bowel contents into an external container or pouch. Peristomal skin can become difficult to care for over time due to the irritating nature of fecal material, enzymes, and the repeated application and removal of adhesives. Barriers are an interface between the patient's skin and the pouching system and have a variety of options such as built-in convexity, locking or non-locking flanges, and use with or without faceplates. Barriers offer a level of protection to the skin while providing a surface to adhere the ostomy faceplate.

A4375-A4378

A4375   Ostomy pouch, drainable, with faceplate attached, plastic, each
A4376   Ostomy pouch, drainable, with faceplate attached, rubber, each
A4377   Ostomy pouch, drainable, for use on faceplate, plastic, each
A4378   Ostomy pouch, drainable, for use on faceplate, rubber, each

Lay Description

These codes represent drainable ostomy pouches. Ostomy pouches are used by patients who have had a surgically created opening for diversion of the urine or feces. An ostomy faceplate is a solid interface between the patient's skin and the pouch. It is usually made of plastic, rubber, or encased metal. It can be taken off the skin and reattached repeatedly. It is held on by means of a separate adhesive and/or an elastic belt.

Medicare Information

Ostomy devices and supplies are covered prosthetics. Hospitals may be paid for these items only when they are dispensed at the time of the surgery that created the ostomy, or at the time of a surgical revision. Routine and replacement supplies are considered DMEPOS and must be billed by the supplier.

A4379-A4384

A4379 Ostomy pouch, urinary, with faceplate attached, plastic, each
A4380 Ostomy pouch, urinary, with faceplate attached, rubber, each
A4381 Ostomy pouch, urinary, for use on faceplate, plastic, each
A4382 Ostomy pouch, urinary, for use on faceplate, heavy plastic, each
A4383 Ostomy pouch, urinary, for use on faceplate, rubber, each
A4384 Ostomy faceplate equivalent, silicone ring, each

Lay Description

These codes represent urinary ostomy pouches for use on barrier, with flange. Urinary ostomy pouches are used by patients who have had a surgically created opening for diversion of the urine. An ostomy faceplate is a solid interface between the patient's skin and the pouch. It is usually made of plastic, heavy plastic, rubber, or silicone. It can be taken off the skin and reattached repeatedly. It is held on by means of a separate adhesive and/or an elastic belt. Report A4379 for a urinary pouch with plastic faceplate attached; A4380 for one with a rubber faceplate attached; and A4381 for a urinary ostomy pouch to be used on a plastic faceplate (not attached). Report A4382 for a urinary pouch for use on a heavy plastic faceplate; A4383 for one used on a rubber faceplate, and A4384 for an ostomy faceplate equivalent, silicone ring.

A4385

A4385 Ostomy skin barrier, solid 4 x 4 or equivalent, extended wear, without built-in convexity, each

Lay Description

An ostomy is a surgically created opening through the skin to divert bowel contents into an external container or pouch. Peristomal skin can become difficult to care for over time due to the irritating nature of fecal material, enzymes, and the repeated application and removal of adhesives. Barriers are an interface between the patient's skin and the pouching system and have a variety of options such as built-in convexity, locking or non-locking flanges, and use with or without faceplates. Barriers offer a level of protection to the skin while providing a surface to adhere the ostomy faceplate. Report A4385 for a solid skin barrier, 4-inch square patch style, with extended wear features. The unit will not feature built-in convexity.

A4387-A4390

A4387 Ostomy pouch, closed, with barrier attached, with built-in convexity (1 piece), each
A4388 Ostomy pouch, drainable, with extended wear barrier attached, (1 piece), each
A4389 Ostomy pouch, drainable, with barrier attached, with built-in convexity (1 piece), each
A4390 Ostomy pouch, drainable, with extended wear barrier attached, with built-in convexity (1 piece), each

Lay Description

An ostomy pouch is a device used for the collection of stomal or urinary output for patients who have undergone procedures causing either a temporary or permanent interference with normal excretion. The ostomy pouch with barrier attached, is a one-piece system in which a solid barrier serving to create an adhesive seal is part of the ostomy pouch. The barrier may be either pectin-based or karaya-based for normal wear, or pectin-based with special additives for extended wear. The pouch may contain an opening at the bottom through which the contents can be drained, or be sealed without an outlet.

Medicare Information

Ostomy devices and supplies are covered prosthetics. Hospitals may be paid for these items only when they are dispensed at the time of the surgery that created the ostomy, or at the time of a surgical revision. Routine and replacement supplies are considered DMEPOS and must be billed by the supplier.

A4391-A4393

A4391 Ostomy pouch, urinary, with extended wear barrier attached (1 piece), each
A4392 Ostomy pouch, urinary, with standard wear barrier attached, with built-in convexity (1 piece), each
A4393 Ostomy pouch, urinary, with extended wear barrier attached, with built-in convexity (1 piece), each

Lay Description

These codes represent urinary ostomy pouches. Urinary ostomy pouches are for use with patients who have had a surgically created opening for diversion of the urine. The ostomy pouch with barrier attached is a one-piece system in which a solid barrier serving to create an adhesive seal is part of the pouch. The barrier may be either pectin-based or karaya-based for normal wear, or pectin-based with special additives for extended wear. The use of convexity is commonly indicated when a pouch seal is unable to fasten properly for an acceptable length of time or when persistent skin irritation occurs even without leakage.

Medicare Information
Ostomy devices and supplies are covered prosthetics. Hospitals may be paid for these items only when they are dispensed at the time of the surgery that created the ostomy, or at the time of a surgical revision. Routine and replacement supplies are considered DMEPOS and must be billed by the supplier.

A4394-A4395

A4394   Ostomy deodorant, with or without lubricant, for use in ostomy pouch, per fl oz

A4395   Ostomy deodorant for use in ostomy pouch, solid, per tablet

Lay Description
These codes report deodorants for use with ostomy pouches, devices for collecting stomal or urinary output in patients who have undergone procedures causing either a temporary or permanent interference with normal excretion. Deodorants are available in liquid or solid form and eliminate urine and fecal odors. Report A4394 for liquid, with or without lubricant, per fluid ounce and A4395 for solid per tablet.

Medicare Information
See the chapter titled "Medicare Guidelines," under "Ostomy Devices and Supplies," for Medicare information.

A4396

A4396   Ostomy belt with peristomal hernia support

Lay Description
This code reports an ostomy belt with peristomal hernia support. Ostomy belts are used to secure and conceal ostomy appliances. They are made of lightweight cotton and Lycra/elastic. Belts are designed to be used with one or two-piece systems for left, right, or center stomas and vary in width depending on the patient's need. Some belts provide a pocket for the appliance that has a Velcro closure that allows for easy emptying. This ostomy belt utilizes a rigid hernia support plate in the pouch pocket of the belt to provide necessary support for a herniated stoma.

A4397-A4400

A4397   Irrigation supply; sleeve, each
A4398   Ostomy irrigation supply; bag, each
A4399   Ostomy irrigation supply; cone/catheter, with or without brush
A4400   Ostomy irrigation set

Lay Description
Irrigation sets are used in the cleaning and maintenance of sigmoid colostomies. Full kits include all supplies necessary for proper irrigation of colostomies, such as a waterbag regulator, cone, faceplate, belt, and sleeves. Report A4397 for an irrigation sleeve; A4398 for an irrigation bag used for holding the warm water necessary for flushing out the ostomy; A4399 for a cone/catheter including brush; and A4400 for a complete set. Replacement of an irrigation ostomy bag or cone/catheter, including brush, every three months would be appropriate.

Medicare Information
See the chapter titled "Medicare Guidelines," under "Ostomy Devices and Supplies," for Medicare information.

A4402

A4402   Lubricant, per oz

Lay Description
The lubricants used for ostomy supplies are water soluble, greaseless, odorless gels. These gels lubricate ostomy supplies such as catheters to reduce irritation. Report A4402 per ounce of a lubricating gel used with ostomy supplies.

Medicare Information
See the chapter titled "Medicare Guidelines," under "Ostomy Devices and Supplies," for Medicare information.

A4404

A4404   Ostomy ring, each

Lay Description
This code is used to report an ostomy ring. An "o" ring is a round rubber ring used as an additional security measure to hold a pouch clip closed. It can be found in any hardware store and looks like a thick, black ring.

Medicare Information
See the chapter titled "Medicare Guidelines," under "Ostomy Devices and Supplies," for Medicare information.

A4405-A4406

A4405 Ostomy skin barrier, nonpectin-based, paste, per oz
A4406 Ostomy skin barrier, pectin-based, paste, per oz

Lay Description

Pastes are applied directly to the skin to act as a protective sealant beneath ostomy appliances. They may have a synthetic or natural base. Report A4405 for each ounce of non-pectin based paste (e.g., karaya) required for skin sensitive to synthetic barriers. Report A4406 for each ounce of paste if it is pectin-based.

Medicare Information

Ostomy devices and supplies are covered prosthetics. Hospitals may be paid for these items only when they are dispensed at the time of the surgery that created the ostomy, or at the time of a surgical revision. Routine and replacement supplies are considered DMEPOS and must be billed by the supplier.

A4407-A4411

A4407 Ostomy skin barrier, with flange (solid, flexible, or accordion), extended wear, with built-in convexity, 4 x 4 in or smaller, each
A4408 Ostomy skin barrier, with flange (solid, flexible or accordion), extended wear, with built-in convexity, larger than 4 x 4 in, each
A4409 Ostomy skin barrier, with flange (solid, flexible or accordion), extended wear, without built-in convexity, 4 x 4 in or smaller, each
A4410 Ostomy skin barrier, with flange (solid, flexible or accordion), extended wear, without built-in convexity, larger than 4 x 4 in, each
A4411 Ostomy skin barrier, solid 4 x 4 or equivalent, extended wear, with built-in convexity, each

Lay Description

An ostomy skin barrier (wafer) with built-in convexity is one in which an outward curve is usually achieved with plastic embedded in the barrier, allowing better protrusion of the stoma and adherence to the skin. Skin barriers are an interface between the patient's skin and the pouching system. They are used to create an adhesive seal between the skin and the pouch.

Medicare Information

Ostomy devices and supplies are covered prosthetics. Hospitals may be paid for these items only when they are dispensed at the time of the surgery that created the ostomy, or at the time of a surgical revision. Routine and replacement supplies are considered DMEPOS and must be billed by the supplier.

A4412-A4413

A4412 Ostomy pouch, drainable, high output, for use on a barrier with flange (2 piece system), without filter, each
A4413 Ostomy pouch, drainable, high output, for use on a barrier with flange (2-piece system), with filter, each

Lay Description

These codes report the supply of a high-output, drainable ostomy pouch to be used with a two-piece barrier with flange system. These pouches have been specifically designed for high stomal output. A high-output ostomy pouch must have a capacity of greater than or equal to 0.75 liters, an anti-reflux valve, and a large bore solid spout with cap or plug. Report A4412 for each high-output ostomy pouch without filter and A4413 for each high-output ostomy pouch with filter.

Medicare Information

See chapter titled "Medicare Guidelines," under "Ostomy Devices and Supplies," for Medicare billing and documentation information.

A4414-A4415

A4414 Ostomy skin barrier, with flange (solid, flexible or accordion), without built-in convexity, 4 x 4 in or smaller, each
A4415 Ostomy skin barrier, with flange (solid, flexible or accordion), without built-in convexity, larger than 4 x 4 in, each

Lay Description

These codes represent ostomy skin barriers with a flange, solid, flexible, or accordion type, without built-in convexity, not specified as extended wear. Skin barriers are an interface between the patient's skin and the pouching system. They are used to create an adhesive seal between the skin and the pouch. Report A4414 for each barrier that is 4 sq inches or smaller and A4415 for each one larger than 4 sq inches.

Medicare Information

Ostomy devices and supplies are covered prosthetics. Hospitals may be paid for these items only when they are dispensed at the time of the surgery that created the ostomy, or at the time of a surgical revision. Routine and replacement supplies are considered DMEPOS and must be billed by the supplier.

A4416-A4420, A4423

A4416 Ostomy pouch, closed, with barrier attached, with filter (1 piece), each
A4417 Ostomy pouch, closed, with barrier attached, with built-in convexity, with filter (1 piece), each
A4418 Ostomy pouch, closed; without barrier attached, with filter (1 piece), each
A4419 Ostomy pouch, closed; for use on barrier with nonlocking flange, with filter (2 piece), each
A4420 Ostomy pouch, closed; for use on barrier with locking flange (2 piece), each
A4423 Ostomy pouch, closed; for use on barrier with locking flange, with filter (2 piece), each

Lay Description

These codes represent ostomy pouches that are for use with patients who have had a surgically created opening for diversion of stool. Ostomy pouches collect the stomal output, in this case feces, and can be drainable or closed. Drainable pouches have an opening at the bottom through which fecal contents can be emptied. Closed pouches have a sealed bottom with no outlet for feces. Ostomy pouches described by A4416-A4420 are closed pouches. There are also one-piece and two-piece systems. One-piece systems are supplied "with barrier attached" or "without barrier attached." Two-piece systems have a locking or non-locking flange that is coupled to a skin barrier with flange. Skin barriers are an interface between the patient's skin and the pouching system and have a variety of different options such as built-in convexity, filters, locking or non-locking flanges, and use with or without faceplates.

Medicare Information

See chapter titled "Medicare Guidelines," under "Ostomy Devices and Supplies," for Medicare billing and documentation information.

A4421

A4421 Ostomy supply; miscellaneous

Lay Description

Miscellaneous ostomy supplies for which a more specific code is not available are reported with A4421.

A4422

A4422 Ostomy absorbent material (sheet/pad/crystal packet) for use in ostomy pouch to thicken liquid stomal output, each

Lay Description

Absorbent material such as sheets, pads, or crystals is added to the ostomy pouch to thicken the liquid output from the stoma. These materials draw liquid away from the stoma to minimize irritation, reduce splashing when emptying the pouch, and facilitate in venting of gas. Report this code for absorbent material, any type.

A4423

A4423 Ostomy pouch, closed; for use on barrier with locking flange, with filter (2 piece), each

Lay Description

Please refer to codes A4416–A4420 for the description, coding, and billing information.

A4424-A4427

A4424 Ostomy pouch, drainable, with barrier attached, with filter (1 piece), each
A4425 Ostomy pouch, drainable; for use on barrier with nonlocking flange, with filter (2-piece system), each
A4426 Ostomy pouch, drainable; for use on barrier with locking flange (2-piece system), each
A4427 Ostomy pouch, drainable; for use on barrier with locking flange, with filter (2-piece system), each

Lay Description

These codes represent drainable ostomy pouches. Ostomy pouches are for use with patients who have had a surgically created opening for diversion of the urine. The ostomy pouch with barrier attached is a one-piece system in which a solid barrier serving to create an adhesive seal is part of the ostomy pouch. The barrier may be either pectin-based or karaya-based for normal wear, or pectin-based with special additives for extended wear. Filters prevent the buildup of gas trapped in the pouch by allowing the gas to be effectively expelled through a vent. A flange or plastic ring on both the pouch and skin barrier secures the barrier and the pouch. Report A4424 for a drainable pouch with barrier attached and filter, each; A4425 for one used on a barrier with nonlocking flange and filter (two piece system), each; A4426 for a pouch used on a barrier with locking flange (two piece system); and A4427 for a pouch used on a barrier with locking flange and filter (two piece system).

Medicare Information

Ostomy devices and supplies are covered prosthetics. Hospitals may be paid for these items only when they are dispensed at the time of the surgery that created the ostomy, or at the time of a surgical revision. Routine and replacement supplies are considered DMEPOS and must be billed by the supplier.

A4428-A4434

A4428 Ostomy pouch, urinary, with extended wear barrier attached, with faucet-type tap with valve (1 piece), each
A4429 Ostomy pouch, urinary, with barrier attached, with built-in convexity, with faucet-type tap with valve (1 piece), each
A4430 Ostomy pouch, urinary, with extended wear barrier attached, with built-in convexity, with faucet-type tap with valve (1 piece), each
A4431 Ostomy pouch, urinary; with barrier attached, with faucet-type tap with valve (1 piece), each
A4432 Ostomy pouch, urinary; for use on barrier with nonlocking flange, with faucet-type tap with valve (2 piece), each
A4433 Ostomy pouch, urinary; for use on barrier with locking flange (2 piece), each
A4434 Ostomy pouch, urinary; for use on barrier with locking flange, with faucet-type tap with valve (2 piece), each

Lay Description

These codes represent urinary ostomy pouches. Urinary ostomy pouches are for use with patients who have had a surgically created opening for diversion of the urine. The ostomy pouch with barrier attached, is a one-piece system in which a solid barrier serving to create an adhesive seal is part of the ostomy pouch. The barrier may be either pectin-based or karaya-based for normal wear, or pectin-based with special additives for extended wear. The use of convexity is commonly indicated when a pouch seal is unable to fasten properly for an acceptable length of time or when persistent skin irritation occurs even without leakage. A flange or plastic ring on both the pouch and skin barrier secures the barrier and the pouch.

Medicare Information

Ostomy devices and supplies are covered prosthetics. Hospitals may be paid for these items only when they are dispensed at the time of the surgery that created the ostomy, or at the time of a surgical revision. Routine and replacement supplies are considered DMEPOS and must be billed by the supplier.

A4450-A4452

A4450 Tape, nonwaterproof, per 18 sq in
A4452 Tape, waterproof, per 18 sq in

Lay Description

Tape is used to hold on a wound cover and can be an elastic roll gauze or non-elastic roll gauze. Additional tape is usually not required when a wound cover with an adhesive border is used. Tape change is determined by the frequency of wound cover change. Report A4450 once for each 18 sq inches of non-waterproof tape and A4452 once for each 18 sq inches of waterproof tape.

Medicare Information

When a wound cover with an adhesive border is being used, no other dressing would be used on top of it and additional tape is usually not required. Reasons for use of additional tape would have to be well documented. An adhesive border is usually more binding than that obtained with separate taping, and is therefore indicated for use with wounds requiring less-frequent dressing changes.

Usual use for wound covers measuring 16 square inches or less is up to two units per dressing change; wound covers measuring 16 to 48 square inches is up to three units per dressing change; wound covers measuring greater than 48 square inches is up to four units per dressing change.

A4455-A4456

A4455 Adhesive remover or solvent (for tape, cement or other adhesive), per oz
A4456 Adhesive remover, wipes, any type, each

Lay Description

Adhesives sometimes require adhesive remover or solvent for complete removal. They are usually petroleum based. Adhesive remover or solvent for removal of tape, cement, or other adhesive is reported per ounce with A4455. Report adhesive remover wipes with A4456.

Medicare Information

See chapter titled "Medicare Guidelines," under "Ostomy Devices and Supplies," for Medicare billing and documentation information.

A4458

A4458 Enema bag with tubing, reusable

Lay Description

This code reports the supply of a reusable enema bag and tubing. Traditionally, these are heavy gauge rubber bags that hold about two quarts of liquid. An enema bag is designed to hang about 18 inches above the patient in the SIMM's position (lying on the side). Tubing from the bag is inserted into the

A4461-A4463

A4461 Surgical dressing holder, nonreusable, each
A4463 Surgical dressing holder, reusable, each

Lay Description

An abdominal dressing holder is usually a slightly elastic garment that may be worn over surgical dressings where adhesives might pose problems or among patients with limited mobility. The device typically opens from side panels, allowing for easy access to the dressings. Report A4461 each nonreusable abdominal dressing holder. Report A4463 for each reusable abdominal dressing holder.

Medicare Information

See the chapter titled "Medicare Guidelines," under "Dressings," for Medicare information.

A4465

A4465 Nonelastic binder for extremity

Lay Description

A nonelastic extremity binder is used for the treatment of lymphedema. These binders apply a gentle, gradient pressure to the affected extremity by use of a sleeve in combination with adjustable straps that provide compression. The sleeve slides over the affected extremity and then the compression bands are adjusted. Some models have gauges that assess the pressure applied over any region of the extremity. These gauges ensure that compression applied to the patient's limb is consistently applied and in the proper range to provide optimal results.

A4466

A4466 Garment, belt, sleeve or other covering, elastic or similar stretchable material, any type, each

Lay Description

Garment, belt, sleeve or other covering made of elastic or a similar stretchable material, any type/each. This code may apply to devices, such as splints, that are not rigid or semi-rigid and/or support devices which are made up of elastic, neoprene, or a similar stretchable material. Elastic garments are considered to be elastic even if they have flexible plastic or metal stays. If a garment made with elastic material has a rigid plastic or metal component, it is considered a nonelastic orthosis for purposes of Medicare coverage and coding.

rectum. Fluid from the bag is allowed to drain into the colon. The fluid is retained for a short duration and the patient voids contents of the colon/rectum.

A4470

A4470 Gravlee jet washer

Lay Description

The Gravlee Jet Washer is a sterile, disposable, diagnostic device for detecting endometrial cancer by obtaining a tissue sample. The use of this device is indicated where the patient exhibits clinical symptoms or signs suggestive of endometrial disease, such as irregular or heavy vaginal bleeding. The tissue obtained is preserved by the addition of an equal amount of Papanicolaou fixative to the irrigation solution from which a cell block is prepared to give a histologic specimen. The use of the Gravlee jet washer should not be confused with a diagnostic curettage.

Medicare Information

The Gravlee jet washer is a disposable device used to detect endometrial cancer. It is covered only in patients exhibiting clinical symptoms or signs suggestive of endometrial disease.

A4480

A4480 VABRA aspirator

Lay Description

The VABRA aspirator is a vacuum operated device designed to collect endometrial samples for biopsy. The cervix may be first accessed by a sounding device to assist in dilation. A pipette tip from the VABRA device is inserted into the vaginal canal, through the cervical os, and into the endometrial lining of the uterus. Retraction of an outer sleeve of the cannula creates a gentle suction to collect the specimen. The specimen is stabilized in neutral fluid and prepared for analysis. Collection of the endometrial tissues may be timed to a particular phase of the menstrual cycle for optimal results. Report A4480 for supply of each disposable VABRA aspirator.

A4481

A4481 Tracheostoma filter, any type, any size, each

Lay Description

This code reports the supply of a filter designed to fit the opening of a tracheostomy. Typically, this device is a soft foam filter disk to cover the air entry of a tracheal stoma. The filter may be designed to interface with a silicon button fitted to the stoma.

A4483

A4483 Moisture exchanger, disposable, for use with invasive mechanical ventilation

Lay Description

Patients on mechanical ventilation lose the advantage of natural moisturizing effects of air flowing over the mucous membranes of the sinuses and nasopharynx. This code reports provision of a disposable moisture exchange device fitted to the mechanical ventilation system.

A4490-A4510

A4490 Surgical stockings above knee length, each
A4495 Surgical stockings thigh length, each
A4500 Surgical stockings below knee length, each
A4510 Surgical stockings full-length, each

Lay Description

Surgical compression stockings are designed to reduce edema and enhance circulation with graduated compression. Graduated compression means that each stocking has the greatest amount of compression at the ankle and gradually decreases as the garment comes up the leg toward the heart. Graduated compression ensures that the garment will not have a constricting or strangulation affect on the leg. Surgical stockings should be properly fit to the individual patient. A surgical compression stocking will have at least 20 mmHg of compression at the ankle, which is the minimum compression considered therapeutic. Ulcerations of the legs, edema of the legs, varicose veins, and lymphedema are some of the problems aided by surgical stockings. There are many different surgical stocking lengths available, such as above the knee, thigh length, below the knee, and full length. There are also many types of surgical stockings ranging in size and custom made. Use HCPCS Level II code A4490 for each above the knee length surgical stocking, A4495 for each thigh length surgical stocking, A4500 for each below the knee length surgical stocking, and A4510 for each full length surgical stocking. These HCPCS Level II codes do not include antiembolism stocking (TED hose) as these only have a minimal gradient compression.

A4520

A4520 Incontinence garment, any type, (e.g., brief, diaper), each

Lay Description

Incontinence garments of any type are reported with A4520. Incontinence garments may be disposable or reusable and may be a flat diaper or a brief. Disposable garments include those commonly found at supermarkets. Flat reusable cloth diapers are generally rectangular with the same thickness throughout. Fit is accomplished by folding. Reusable briefs come in many varieties and may vary from slightly contoured to fully fitted briefs. There are also fully fitted briefs made of patented materials that are designed to be used with internal pads. Report A4520 for each incontinence garment provided.

A4550

A4550 Surgical trays

Lay Description

A surgical tray comprises procedure-specific instruments, devices, and dressings within a ready-to-use sterilized package. The trays are prepared and inventoried for any of a variety of anticipated procedures (e.g., suture removal). The instruments may be sterilized and repackaged; however, a recent trend is toward the use of disposable surgical trays. In the past, Medicare defined three levels of surgical trays: minor, major, and specialized. The term is generally recognized by Medicare today as the minor variety used for routine procedures in office and outpatient settings.

A4554

A4554 Disposable underpads, all sizes

Lay Description

Disposable underpads are designed for incontinent patients to protect bedding and furniture from leakage. Most have a soft quick-drying cover layer, an absorbent center core, and a waterproof bottom layer.

A4556-A4558

A4556 Electrodes (e.g., apnea monitor), per pair
A4557 Lead wires (e.g., apnea monitor), per pair
A4558 Conductive gel or paste, for use with electrical device (e.g., TENS, NMES), per oz

Lay Description

Apnea monitors and transcutaneous electrical nerve stimulation (TENS) units consist of several components: the apnea monitor or TENS unit, lead wires, electrodes, and for some devices, an electrode belt and conductive paste or gel. Electrodes for devices such as TENS units and apnea monitors are reported with A4556. Electrodes are dispensed in pairs and may be stick-on electrodes or, in the case of an apnea monitor, contained within an electrode belt. Electrodes are placed on the proper site to deliver stimulation (in the case of a TENS unit) or to monitor breathing (in the case of an apnea monitor). Lead wires are reported with A4557 and are also dispensed in pairs. They are usually color coded because each wire must be attached to the correct electrode. For example, an apnea monitoring system will usually have one black and one white lead wire. The white lead wire is attached to the electrode on the right side of the chest and the black one is attached to the electrode on the left. The lead wires are then attached to the TENS unit or apnea monitor via a cable. Conductive paste or gel may be used on the skin at the site where the electrodes are placed to improve conduction of electrical impulses.

Medicare Information

See chapter titled "Medicare Guidelines," under "TENS," for Medicare billing and documentation information.

A4559

A4559   Coupling gel or paste, for use with ultrasound device, per oz

Lay Description

Coupling gels and pastes are used with ultrasonic probes and devices. The gel and/or paste acts as an agent to keep the probe from sticking to the patient's skin, probe cover, or other covers. The probes temperature can range from cool to hot and may require specific, high-heat gels or pastes. Ultrasound conductive coupling gel may be covered and separately payable if an ultrasonic osteogenesis stimulator is covered.

A4561-A4562

A4561   Pessary, rubber, any type
A4562   Pessary, nonrubber, any type

Lay Description

A pessary is a hard rubber, plastic, or silicon device that is inserted into the vagina, often to support the uterus and/or bladder from prolapse. The device may be ring-shaped, similar to the outer structure of a cervical cap or diaphragm. Other designs are also seen. The device may be prescribed for extended use or for short-term treatment. Regardless, the device should be removed regularly for hygienic considerations. Report A4561 for a rubber pessary, any type; and A4562 for a non-rubber pessary, any type.

A4565

A4565   Slings

Lay Description

Typically constructed of canvas-type material or other materials such as cotton or nylon (including mesh-type products), an arm sling usually uses the shoulder/neck as the primary anchor, suspending the upper limb as needed, supporting the shoulder, upper arm, elbow, and, to a limited degree, the wrist and hand. Arm slings can be used with a cast or splint for any of these body areas, providing an added measure of support and protection. Arm slings may protect against reinjury.

Documentation Standards

If the item is furnished secondary to a fracture (traumatic or nontraumatic [such as due to severe osteoporosis]), a copy of the x-ray study confirming the fracture should be easily accessible within the medical record. If the device is furnished post-surgery, a copy of the operative report should be contained in the medical record. This information should be available to the payer upon request.

Medicare Information

Splints and casting supplies are separately payable and should be reported with the appropriate HCPCS Level II codes. For Medicare patients, CPT code 99070 *Supplies and materials (except spectacles), provided by the physician over and above those usually included with the office visit of other services rendered (list drugs, trays, supplies, or materials provided)* may not be used to bill separately for supplies.

A4570

A4570   Splint

Lay Description

A splint is an orthotic medical device used to immobilize a limb or the spine. A splint is usually composed of two pieces held in place by some type of cotton or nylon material. It may be used to temporarily immobilize a suspected fracture or dislocation until additional medical help can be obtained. Code A4570 is an undefined splint. Report this code only if a more appropriate HCPCS code is not available.

A4575

A4575   Topical hyperbaric oxygen chamber, disposable

Lay Description

A topical hyperbaric oxygen chamber is a device that applies oxygen at a high atmospheric pressure to a skin or surface wound. It is noninvasive and used in the home. The topical application of a limited supply of pressurized oxygen is purported to promote the healing of various acute and chronic wounds. The topical application has frequently been prescribed for decubitus ulcers and other chronic wounds of the skin and its underlying structures.

A4580-A4590

A4580 Cast supplies (e.g., plaster)
A4590 Special casting material (e.g., fiberglass)

Lay Description
Casting materials are made of plaster-imbedded strips or bandages or fiberglass wraps or strips, available in varieties pertinent to the type of fracture or post-surgical state requiring the support and protection of a cast. Some of these materials are initially dry and are water-activated, while others come premoistened for immediate application. Plaster varieties can be embedded with strength-adding chemical compounds such as polyurethane. Splints are used when a cast is not necessary but the injury or condition requires immobilization. Casts and casting materials support and protect fractured or strained extremities or other body areas. They hold manipulated (set) fractures in place or can assist other devices (pins, wires, screws) in doing so and protect against reinjury. Codes Q4001-Q4051 identify the different casting materials (e.g., fiberglass or plaster) for physicians, the type of immobilization provided (e.g., splint or cast for adult or pediatric patients), and the length or shape of casts for the different types of injuries or conditions (e.g., shoulder or body cast, long or short leg or arm cast).

Medicare Information
These codes are not recognized by Medicare. Non-OPPS facilities should report Q4001–Q4050.

Casting supplies used in conjunction with covered services are considered incidental supplies in a hospital or skilled nursing facility. Separate payment is not made. Reimbursement is considered to be included in the payment for the procedure.

A4595

A4595 Electrical stimulator supplies, 2 lead, per month, (e.g., TENS, NMES)

Lay Description
This code reports electrical stimulator supplies, two leads, per month (e.g., TENS, NMES). A transcutaneous electrical nerve stimulator (TENS) is a device that uses electrical current delivered through electrodes placed on the surface of the skin to decrease the patient's perception of pain, by inhibiting the transmission of afferent pain nerve impulses, and/or by stimulating the release of endorphins. The TENS unit can be applied in a variety of settings (in the patient's home, a physician's office, or in an outpatient clinic). A TENS unit alleviates or palliates acute postoperative pain, as well as chronic or intractable pain, depending on the etiology of the patient's condition. A four-lead TENS unit may be used with either two leads or four leads, depending on the characteristics of the patient's pain. The leads direct the current from the stimulator to the electrodes to the area in which pain control is needed.

Medicare Information
See the chapter titled "Medicare Guidelines," under "TENS," for Medicare information.

A4600

A4600 Sleeve for intermittent limb compression device, replacement only, each

Lay Description
Intermittent limb compression devices are used to inflate and deflate a compression sleeve. The sleeve is inflated to apply compressive pressure gradient against the limb which will decrease from a lower to upper portion of the limb to enhance the accelaeration of the flow of blood through the limb.

A4601

A4601 Lithium ion battery for nonprosthetic use, replacement

Lay Description
These battery systems fall into two major categories: primary or single-use batteries, which are cells containing lithium-metal anodes; and secondary or rechargeable batteries, which are systems utilizing lithium-ion chemistry. Primary lithium batteries have been used for implantable devices such as cardiac pacemakers, drug pumps, neurostimulators, and cardiac defibrillators. Rechargeable batteries have been used with left ventricular assist devices and total artificial hearts. All of these cells share the characteristics of high safety, reliability, energy density, and predictability of performance.

A4604

A4604 Tubing with integrated heating element for use with positive airway pressure device

Lay Description
Supply of tubing with an integrated heating element to be used with a positive airway pressure device is reported with A4604. The heating element is embedded in the outer spiral of the inspiratory limb of the tubing and has a smooth inner surface. This allows delivery of positive airway pressure with optimal humidity that does not condense in the tubing. This device is used primarily for individuals with obstructive sleep apnea who require heated humidification with positive airway pressure.

Medicare Information

An enrolled DME supplier must supply this item. The device will be covered when medically necessary to treat the patient's medical condition.

A4605

A4605 Tracheal suction catheter, closed system, each

Lay Description

A closed system tracheal suction catheter is designed to remove bronchial secretions in intubated patients. Closed suction catheters allow suctioning without requiring the patient to be disconnected from the ventilator. The advantage of a closed system is the prevention of hypoxemia during suctioning because ventilation is maintained during the suctioning process.

A4606

A4606 Oxygen probe for use with oximeter device, replacement

Lay Description

Oximetry is a noninvasive method to measure blood hemoglobin (Hb), usually to determine oxygen saturation. A probe is attached to the patient's earlobe or a fingertip. The probe emits a light source. The hemoglobin absorbs a percentage of the light, depending upon its oxygen saturation level, and the results are digitally recorded, sometimes in addition to other data, such as pulse. This code reports a replacement unit for the oxygen probe.

A4608

A4608 Transtracheal oxygen catheter, each

Lay Description

This code reports supply of a transtracheal oxygen (TTO) catheter, a small-diameter flexible tube that is fitted directly into the trachea. A stoma is surgically created to accommodate the catheter. The system is designed to directly deliver oxygen to the lungs at high efficiency. The catheter is inserted to a level several centimeters above the carinal junction. Compared to nasal cannulas, more oxygen is conserved, flow is largely uninterrupted, and arterial blood oxygen levels are better maintained. Additionally, speech is unimpeded and eating routines are unaffected. Generally, cleaning of the catheter is required several times per day. Durable catheters may require change-out about every 90 days, or earlier as needed. Other systems may feature disposable catheter components. Report A4608 for supply of each transtracheal oxygen catheter.

A4611-A4613

A4611 Battery, heavy-duty; replacement for patient-owned ventilator
A4612 Battery cables; replacement for patient-owned ventilator
A4613 Battery charger; replacement for patient-owned ventilator

Lay Description

This range of codes reports supply of batteries and related components for patient-owned ventilators. Patient-owned ventilators are likely to be conventional AC-powered devices with supplemental internal and external sealed lead acid (SLA) batteries for emergency use and portability. A 12 V or 24 V external battery and charging system with a direct current to alternating current inverter are common features of many ventilator systems. Typically, the external battery charges a 24 V internal battery, as does the AC system while in use. The internal battery always remains fully charged and is the power source of last resort. In emergencies, these systems can run on conventional 12 V car batteries. The SLA batteries are generally notable for price, reliability, charge retention, and relatively long life. Disadvantages include slow recharge time and the need to keep the charge topped off while the battery is not in use. Some patients prefer deep cycle marine batteries that stand up better to near-complete discharge and recharge. Most systems require special cables. Nickel cadmium (NiCad) batteries are usually acceptable for air travel and have other advantages, but they tend to lose charge over time while not in use.

A4614

A4614 Peak expiratory flow rate meter, hand held

Lay Description

A peak expiratory flow rate meter measures the maximum amount of air an individual can forcibly exhale. Hand held units are commonly used by asthmatics to determine a need for bronchodilation medications and to record regular readings in a daily journal. Hand held units vary in design, but many feature an air resistance cylinder that freezes a needle at the point of peak exhalation.

A4615
A4615 Cannula, nasal

Lay Description
A cannula is a hollow tube or sheath inserted into a vessel, duct, or cavity to facilitate passage of another instrument, such as a trocar or flexible tubing, fluid, or air. Use this code to report a nasal cannula, one that sits in the nostrils to facilitate the delivery of therapeutic oxygen, also called nasal prongs.

A4616
A4616 Tubing (oxygen), per foot

Lay Description
Oxygen tubing is reported by the foot but is usually supplied in lengths of 25 and 50 feet. Tubing is crush resistant to prevent interruptions in the flow of oxygen and may be supplied with tubing connectors.

Medicare Information
See chapter titled "Medicare Guidelines," under "Oxygen and Oxygen Equipment," for Medicare billing and documentation information.

A4617
A4617 Mouthpiece

Lay Description
Mouthpieces for nebulizers may be purchased separately. They are available in pediatric and adult sizes. Mouthpieces are used to deliver inhalant medications dispensed via small volume nebulizers.

Medicare Information
An enrolled DME supplier must bill this item to the DME MAC.

Small-volume nebulizers, accessories, and supplies are covered when used to administer medically necessary inhalation therapy in the following specific instances:

- Beta-adrenergics, corticosteroids, and cromolyn for the management of obstructive pulmonary disease
- Gentamicin, tobramycin, amikacin, or dornase alfa for patients with cystic fibrosis
- Gentamicin for patients with bronchiectasis
- Pentamidine for patients with HIV pneumocystosis or posttransplant patients who experience complications
- Mucolytics, other than dornase alfa, for patients with thick or tenacious pulmonary secretions

Large-volume nebulizers, accessories, and supplies are covered when used to administer medically necessary humidified inhalation therapy to patients with thick, tenacious secretions with:

- Cystic fibrosis
- Bronchiectasis
- A tracheostomy
- A tracheobronchial stent
- HIV pneumocystosis

Nebulizers used to administer inhalation therapy for other than the above indications are not covered. Nebulizers used to administer noncovered drugs are not covered.

A4618
A4618 Breathing circuits

Lay Description
A breathing circuit is a component array used to connect an intubated patient's airway to a gas anesthesia delivery system. The circuit creates an artificial atmosphere that the patient both draws air from as well as breathes exhaled air into. Components include: a port to deliver various anesthetic and other gases to the breathing circuit; a port to the patient's intubated airway; a reservoir bag for gas; an expiration port to release and control exhaled gas into room air; a carbon dioxide absorbing system for total rebreathing circuit; and tubes to connect the various components. A breathing circuit can be set so that no rebreathing of air is allowed (fresh gas is not mixed with exhaled gas). A partial rebreathing setting allows for a portion of exhaled gas to be mixed with fresh gas. Total rebreathing settings require that exhaled gas be purged of carbon dioxide. A variety of breathing circuit features is available, including an interface with ventilation assist and alarms.

A4619
A4619 Face tent

Lay Description
A face tent is a soft plastic facemask type of device for the delivery of oxygen or combination of gases. The device differs from a facemask in that the perimeter of the device does not come in contact with the patient's skin. Face tents are useful for individuals who have had facial surgery or who otherwise cannot tolerate the contact of a facemask or nasal cannulas. Disadvantages include difficulty in delivering therapeutic quantities of gas due to the imperfect air seal.

A4620

A4620   Variable concentration mask

Lay Description
Variable concentration masks are also known as low flow masks and deliver oxygen at variable rates depending upon how the patient is breathing. The device is usually a simple facemask with tubing and is used in instances where a fixed concentration of oxygen is not required.

A4623

A4623   Tracheostomy, inner cannula

Lay Description
Inner cannulas are used inside of outer cannulas after a tracheostomy. A small opening is made through the stoma and a breathing tube is placed directly into the trachea (windpipe). There are three parts to the placement of a trach tube. The obturator is used to pass the trach tube into the trachea and a portion is removed leaving the outer cannula in place. The outer cannula has a plate that sits against the skin of the neck and holds the trach in place. The inner cannula fits inside the outer cannula and locks it into place.

A4624

A4624   Tracheal suction catheter, any type other than closed system, each

Lay Description
Tracheal suction catheters are used to clear the airways of excessive secretions. Catheters are made of soft rubber or hard plastic material. The diameter of each catheter is measured according to the French catheter scale, and they vary in length. Catheter tips may be a two-eye whistle tip design reducing the chance of damage to the mucosal tissue, or softer rounded style, which can be gentler on the mucosal lining. This code is for a tracheal suction catheter, any type.

Documentation Standards
ICD-9-CM diagnosis code V44.0 should be entered on the claims form when billing.

Medicare Information
Supplies are covered when they are medically necessary and used with a medically necessary suction pump.

When a suction pump is covered, tracheal suction catheters are separately reportable supplies. Sterile catheters are usually only medically necessary for tracheostomy suctioning. Three catheters per day are covered for medically necessary tracheal suctioning, unless additional documentation is provided. If a tracheal suction catheter is used to suction the oropharynx, the catheter can be reused if properly cleansed and/or disinfected (the oropharynx is not sterile). When tracheal suction catheters are used to suction the oropharynx, only three catheters per week are allowed unless additional documentation is submitted showing medical necessity.

A4625-A4626, A4629

A4625   Tracheostomy care kit for new tracheostomy
A4626   Tracheostomy cleaning brush, each
A4629   Tracheostomy care kit for established tracheostomy

Lay Description
A tracheostomy care kit for a new tracheostomy is used following an open surgical tracheostomy that is expected to remain open for at least three months. These kits are composed of supplies that are used to routinely clean and care for tracheostomy tubes, accessories, and the area around the tracheostomy. Tracheostomy care is necessary to reduce the chance of inflammation and infection around the tracheostomy site. Cleaning the tracheostomy tube allows air to move freely through the tube. Report A4625 for each tracheostomy care or cleaning starter kit that is used following an open surgical tracheostomy; A4626 for a tracheostomy cleaning brush; and A4629 for a care kit for an established tracheostomy.

Consolidated Billing

All tracheostomy care supplies dispensed to a nursing home resident or home health recipient are included in the procedure.

Documentation Standards
ICD-9-CM diagnosis code V44.0 should be entered on the claims form when billing.

Medicare Information
Gloves, cups, basins, solutions, and other items are included in the tracheal care kit code A4625 when a suction pump is used for tracheal suctioning, and should not be reported separately.

Supplies are covered when they are medically necessary and used with a medically necessary suction pump.

A tracheostomy care or cleaning starter kit (A4625) is covered following an open surgical tracheostomy.

One tracheostomy care kit (A4625, A4629) per day is necessary for routine care of a tracheostomy.

Tracheostomy care kits provided in the first two postoperative weeks should be coded as A4625.

Tracheostomy care kits provided after the first two postoperative weeks should be coded as A4629.

A4627

A4627 Spacer, bag or reservoir, with or without mask, for use with metered dose inhaler

Lay Description

A spacer, bag, or reservoir used with a metered dose inhaler increases the space between the metered dose inhaler and the mouth. It helps the patient inhale more medication into the lungs and decreases the amount of medication that is deposited at the back of the throat. Spacers, bags, and reservoirs are particularly useful for children, particularly those with asthma, due to the difficulty some children have in inhaling slowly while depressing the inhaler at the same time. Report A4627 for a spacer, bag, or reservoir with or without a mask.

A4628

A4628 Oropharyngeal suction catheter, each

Lay Description

An oropharyngeal suction catheter is used to remove secretions from the oral cavity and pharynx. Report A4628 for each catheter.

Medicare Information

See chapter titled "Medicare Guidelines," under "Oxygen and Oxygen Equipment," for Medicare billing and documentation information.

A4629

A4629 Tracheostomy care kit for established tracheostomy

Lay Description

Please refer to codes A4625–A4626 for the description, coding, and billing information.

A4630

A4630 Replacement batteries, medically necessary, transcutaneous electrical stimulator, owned by patient

Lay Description

Transcutaneous electrical nerve stimulator (TENS) units require the use of a 9-volt, standard battery or a rechargeable cell. The initial purchase of a TENS unit generally includes a battery. When the battery for a patient-owned, medically necessary TENS unit requires replacement, report A4630.

Medicare Information

See chapter titled "Medicare Guidelines," under "TENS," for Medicare billing and documentation information.

A4633-A4634

A4633 Replacement bulb/lamp for ultraviolet light therapy system, each
A4634 Replacement bulb for therapeutic light box, tabletop model

Lay Description

Lightbox therapy is used in the treatment of seasonal affective disorder (SAD), diurnal disorders, or sometimes to mitigate the sedating effect of medications. Although bulbs are rated for 20,000 hours of use, they generally begin to lose intensity after four to five years of use and require replacement. When long-term ultraviolet light or lightbox therapy is required, the bulbs must be periodically replaced. Report A4633 for each replacement bulb or lamp for an ultraviolet light therapy system and A4634 for replacement of each tabletop lightbox bulb.

Medicare Information

The replacement bulb is covered only when the device itself is covered. The device may be covered when medically necessary to treat the patient's medical condition.

A4635-A4637

A4635 Underarm pad, crutch, replacement, each
A4636 Replacement, handgrip, cane, crutch, or walker, each
A4637 Replacement, tip, cane, crutch, walker, each

Lay Description

Underarm pads, hand grips, and tips for patient-owned crutches, canes, and walkers periodically require replacement. Report replacement of underarm pads with A4635, hand grips with A4636, and tips with A4637.

Medicare Information

Underarm pads, handgrips, and tips are covered when the crutch, cane, or walker is covered. The *Medicare National Coverage Determinations Manual*, Pub. 100-3, chap. 1, part 4, sec. 280.3, *Mobility Assistance Equipment* details coverage criteria for the crutch, cane, or walker.

A4638

A4638 Replacement battery for patient-owned ear pulse generator, each

Lay Description

Replacement battery for patient-owned ear pulse generator used in the tympanic treatment of inner ear endolymphatic fluid, also known as Ménière's disease, is reported with A4638.

A4639

Medicare Information
An enrolled DME supplier must bill this item to the DME MAC. Coverage is at the contractor's discretion.

A4639

A4639 Replacement pad for infrared heating pad system, each

Lay Description
An infrared heating pad system consists of a pad or pads containing mechanisms (e.g., luminous gallium aluminum arsenide diodes) that generate infrared (or near infrared) light and a power source. Use this code for each replacement pad.

A4640

A4640 Replacement pad for use with medically necessary alternating pressure pad owned by patient

Lay Description
An alternating pressure pad is designed to distribute the patient's body weight more effectively, preventing pressure points from developing. The pressure pad is attached to a pump that alternately inflates and deflates air cells in the pressure pad. Air cycling through the air cells provides patient lift and pressure reduction that assists in reducing pressure on skin and tissues and facilitates blood flow to all areas of the body that come in contact with the mattress. Alternating pressure pads are used to prevent and/or treat pressure ulcers and lesions, such as decubitus ulcers. Report A4640 for a replacement pad used with a patient-owned alternating pressure pad system.

Medicare Information
See chapter titled "Medicare Guidelines," under "Pressure Reducing Support surfaces," for Medicare billing and documentation information.

A4641

A4641 Radiopharmaceutical, diagnostic, not otherwise classified

Lay Description
This code is used to report the supply of radiopharmaceutical diagnostic imaging agents that do not have another specific HCPCS Level II code. Radiopharmaceuticals are radioactive isotopes, such as radioactive iodine or radioactive cobalt. They are often attached to carrier molecules and used in diagnostic nuclear medicine procedures.

Medicare Information
Report A4641 only when another more specific code does not exist for the radiopharmaceutical diagnostic agent administered. Coverage is at the contractor's discretion.

A4642

A4642 Indium In-111 satumomab pendetide, diagnostic, per study dose, up to 6 millicuries

Lay Description
Satumomab pendetide is a murine monoclonal antibody that binds to a glycoprotein, a cell surface antigen, produced in large amounts by colorectal and ovarian tumors. This monoclonal antibody does not generally react with normal adult tissue, but it may react with salivary gland ducts, normal post-ovulatory endometria, some benign ovarian tumors, and fetal gastrointestinal tissue. Indium 111 is a radioactive form of the metallic element indium. It has a half-life of approximately 56 hours and decays by electron capture and gamma emission. The monoclonal antibody is combined with indium 111 chloride so that it can be readily identified in images. Indium 111 satumomab pendetide is administered intravenously. It rapidly attaches itself to colorectal adenocarcinomas and common epithelial ovarian carcinomas. Optimal images are obtained 48 to 72 hours following administration. Since satumomab pendetide may attach itself to nonmalignant tissue, use of this diagnostic agent is not recommended for screening purposes. Indium 111 satumomab pendetide is indicated for patients with known colorectal or ovarian cancer to determine the extent and location of disease. HCPCS Level II code A4642 represents a study dose of up to 6 millicuries of indium 111 satumomab pendetide.

A4648

A4648 Tissue marker, implantable, any type, each

Lay Description
An implantable tissue marker is a small, non-absorbable piece of material, usually metal, that is used to mark an area of concern within soft tissue. The tissue marker is usually visible with multiple types of imaging and can be used to mark an area that needs continued follow-up. The marker can also be used to indicate an area to be removed or biopsied. Code A4648 represents one implantable tissue marker.

A4649

A4649 Surgical supply; miscellaneous

Lay Description
This code is used to report miscellaneous surgical supplies and should only be used if a more specific HCPCS Level II or CPT code is not available.

A4650

A4650 Implantable radiation dosimeter, each

Lay Description

An implantable radiation dosimeter is a permanent, small, non-absorbable device that is inserted into the target area that is to be irradiated with external beam ionizing radiation. The device measures the amount of radiation reaching the targeted area and serves as a marker. This allows the physician to better track and calibrate the location and amount of radiation delivered.

A4651

A4651 Calibrated microcapillary tube, each

Lay Description

This code reports the supply of each calibrated microcapillary tube. These are glass laboratory tubes designed to measure and contain extremely small quantities of liquid. Some may have a coating of heparin on the inside surface to maintain blood in liquid storage. Others may be tempered to withstand extreme temperature variations. Most can be sealed for centrifuging or mechanical agitation. Report A4651 for supply of each tube.

Medicare Information

Microcapillary tubes and sealant used to administer or perform covered services are considered incidental supplies in a hospital, skilled nursing facility, or physician office. Separate payment is not made. Reimbursement is considered to be included in the payment for the procedure.

Under certain circumstances supplies necessary for home dialysis may be paid separately. In those specific instances, billing and coverage is determined by the specific circumstances (e.g., the DME supplier bills supplies for home dialysis patients covered under Method II).

When a calibrated microcapillary tube (A4651) is furnished in conjunction with home dialysis supplies and equipment, modifier AX *Items furnished in conjunction with home dialysis services*, should be appended.

A4652

A4652 Microcapillary tube sealant

Lay Description

Microcapillary tubes are glass laboratory tubes used to measure and contain small quantities of liquid. Most can be sealed for centrifuging or mechanical agitation. Report A4652 for supply of sealant used to seal microcapillary tubes.

Medicare Information

Microcapillary tubes and sealant used to administer or perform covered services are considered incidental supplies in a hospital, skilled nursing facility, or physician office. Separate payment is not made. Reimbursement is considered to be included in the payment for the procedure.

Under certain circumstances supplies necessary for home dialysis may be paid separately. In those specific instances, billing and coverage is determined by the specific circumstances (e.g., the DME supplier bills supplies for home dialysis patients covered under Method II).

When microcapillary tube sealant (A4642) is furnished in conjunction with home dialysis supplies and equipment, modifier AX *Items furnished in conjunction with home dialysis services*, should be appended.

A4653

A4653 Peritoneal dialysis catheter anchoring device, belt, each

Lay Description

Peritoneal dialysis is an alternative to hemodialysis. Peritoneal dialysis requires that a peritoneal catheter be inserted into the abdominal (peritoneal) cavity. The catheter consists of a 15-inch tube with two cuffs in the middle of the catheter. One section of tubing is placed into the peritoneal cavity. The cuffs in the middle section are placed just outside the peritoneal cavity in the fatty tissue and protect the catheter site from infection and leakage. The outer portion of tubing is used to connect the dialysis solution. Dialysis solution is then instilled through the catheter into the peritoneal cavity where it removes impurities, waste products, and extra fluid when this function can no longer be performed by the kidneys due to disease or injury. Patients on peritoneal dialysis sometimes require additional supplies to protect the catheter, such as an anchoring device that helps to protect the catheter from becoming dislodged. Report A4653 for supply of a peritoneal dialysis catheter anchoring device, such as a belt.

Medicare Information

Dialysis supplies used in conjunction with covered dialysis services are covered. All necessary supplies and equipment used in the dialysis facility are reimbursed under the composite payment rate. For patients who elect Method II of home dialysis, the DME supplier bills for supplies.

A4657

A4657 Syringe, with or without needle, each

Lay Description
A sterile syringe is used for injecting or withdrawing fluid from any vessel or cavity. Syringes may vary in size and may be supplied with or without a needle. Report A4657 for a syringe of any size with or without a needle.

A4660

A4660 Sphygmomanometer/blood pressure apparatus with cuff and stethoscope

Lay Description
This code reports the supply of a sphygmomanometer with cuff and stethoscope. This is the traditional blood pressure measuring device still in common use. A cuff and rubber bag are wrapped around the upper arm and secured with Velcro. Tubing connects the bag to a mercury manometer, which measures pressure within the cuff. The bag is inflated, usually by squeezing an air bulb, until pressure on the arm exceeds arterial pressure. A stethoscope over the brachial artery below the cuff confirms that no blood movement is heard. A valve slowly releases pressure on the bag. The artery first emits sound upon peak pressure from the heart, or systolic pressure. This is noted by the observer and the manometer reading is taken. As pressure on the cuff continues to drop, arterial occlusion fails even upon lowest pressure from the heart, the diastolic pressure. This characteristic sound heard through the stethoscope is also noted by the trained observer and the second manometer reading is taken. The two pressures, systolic and diastolic, are recorded as the patient's blood pressure. Report A4660 for supply of a sphygmomanometer with cuff and stethoscope.

A4663

A4663 Blood pressure cuff only

Lay Description
This code reports the supply of a traditional sphygmomanometer blood pressure cuff only. The cuff is the portion of the apparatus that wraps around the upper arm and is secured with Velcro. The traditional cuff contains a rubber bag that is connected to a manometer or other device to measure pressure. The bag is inflated, usually by squeezing an air bulb, placing pressure on the arteries of the arm. Report A4663 for supply of each blood pressure cuff.

A4670

A4670 Automatic blood pressure monitor

Lay Description
An automatic blood pressure monitor consists of a digital gauge and a stethoscope in one unit. Automatic blood pressure monitors are powered by batteries. The cuff may be inflated manually or automatically depending on the model. The blood pressure recording is displayed on a digital screen that will also display error messages. The error messages help ensure accurate blood pressure readings. Deflation of the cuff is automatic. Some models of automatic blood pressure monitors will also provide a paper printout of blood pressure recordings.

A4671

A4671 Disposable cycler set used with cycler dialysis machine, each

Lay Description
During automated peritoneal dialysis, also called continuous cycling peritoneal dialysis (CCPD) or nocturnal cyclical peritoneal dialysis, a sterile mixture of sugar and minerals dissolved in water (dialysis solution) flows through a catheter into the peritoneal cavity using a cycler machine. Using osmosis, the solution draws wastes, impurities, chemicals, and extra water from the tiny blood vessels in the peritoneal membrane into the solution. The cycler machine automatically infuses the dialysis solution and then drains it several times during the night. Disposable cycler kits are available that contain supplies required for CCPD. Report A4671 for each cycler kit used.

Medicare Information
Dialysis supplies used in conjunction with covered dialysis services are covered. All necessary supplies and equipment used in the dialysis facility are reimbursed under the composite payment rate. For patients who elect Method II of home dialysis, the DME supplier bills for supplies.

A4672-A4673

A4672 Drainage extension line, sterile, for dialysis, each
A4673 Extension line with easy lock connectors, used with dialysis

Lay Description
Extension lines for dialysis provide added length to catheters, which can assist in patient comfort and mobility. Report A4672 for a sterile drainage extension line and A4673 for an extension line with easy lock connectors.

HCPCS Lay Descriptions

Medicare Information
Dialysis supplies used in conjunction with covered dialysis services are covered. All necessary supplies and equipment used in the dialysis facility are reimbursed under the composite payment rate. For patients who elect Method II of home dialysis, the DME supplier bills for supplies.

A4674

A4674 Chemicals/antiseptics solution used to clean/sterilize dialysis equipment, per 8 oz

Lay Description
There are two types of dialysis, hemodialysis and peritoneal dialysis. Hemodialysis removes excess fluids, wastes, impurities, and chemicals from the blood by use of a dialyzer. Hemodialysis requires the use of a dialysis machine, dialyzer, dialysis solution, treated water, and disposable supplies. Peritoneal dialysis is an alternative to hemodialysis. Peritoneal dialysis uses the thin lining in the abdomen that coats the outer surface of the intestines (peritoneal membrane) to remove waste products and balance fluids. The dialysis solution is instilled through a catheter placed through the skin into the peritoneal cavity. The dialysis solution removes waste products and excess fluid and is then drained from the abdomen and discarded. Dialysis equipment must be properly cleaned and sterilized to prevent infection. Report A4674 for chemicals and antiseptic solutions used to clean or sterilize dialysis equipment, per 8 ounces.

Medicare Information
Dialysis supplies used in conjunction with covered dialysis services are covered. All necessary supplies and equipment used in the dialysis facility are reimbursed under the composite payment rate. For patients who elect Method II of home dialysis, the DME supplier bills for supplies.

A4680

A4680 Activated carbon filter for hemodialysis, each

Lay Description
Report A4680 for each activated carbon filter used for hemodialysis as a component of a water purification system to remove unsafe concentrations of chloride or chloramines.

A4690

A4690 Dialyzer (artificial kidneys), all types, all sizes, for hemodialysis, each

Lay Description
This code reports the supply of a dialyzer, the portion of a hemodialysis machine that cleanses blood in patients with end-stage renal disease (ESRD). Dialysis is a physicochemical and filtration process. The dialyzer portion of a hemodialysis unit is typically a two-chambered clear plastic cylinder. The cylinder is packed with hollow fiber strands that form a membrane between the chambers. One chamber circulates blood drawn from the patient. The second circulates a solution known as dialysate in the opposite direction from movement of the blood. This semipermeable membrane between the chambers allows accumulated uremic toxins, excess ions, and water in the blood to pass into the dialysate. A similar dialyzer design, known as the parallel plate process, separates the chambers by a cellophane-type membrane. With either process, cleansed blood is returned to the patient as the dialysate is constantly refreshed. The dialyzer is generally changed out between patients, although the same patient may use a single dialyzer repeatedly. Report A4690 for supply of any type or size of dialyzer for hemodialysis purposes.

A4706-A4707

A4706 Bicarbonate concentrate, solution, for hemodialysis, per gallon
A4707 Bicarbonate concentrate, powder, for hemodialysis, per packet

Lay Description
These codes report the supply of bicarbonate concentrate for hemodialysis. Hemodialysis is a physicochemical and filtration process. The dialyzer portion of a hemodialysis unit is typically two-chambered. One chamber circulates blood drawn from the patient. The second circulates a solution known as dialysate in the opposite direction from movement of the blood. A semipermeable membrane between the chambers allows accumulated uremic toxins, excess ions, and water in the blood to pass into the dialysate. Cleansed blood is returned to the patient as the dialysate is constantly refreshed. Bicarbonate concentrate is added to treated water and acetic acid in a fixed proportion to form the dialysate base. Low concentrations of bicarbonate in the dialysate can result in metabolic acidosis. Ordinarily, a sensor and alarm on the hemodialysis unit alert the operator of an imbalance in the dialysate solution. Report A4706 for supply of each gallon of bicarbonate concentrate in solution. Report A4707 for supply of each packet of bicarbonate concentrate in powder form.

A4708-A4709

A4708 Acetate concentrate solution, for hemodialysis, per gallon
A4709 Acid concentrate, solution, for hemodialysis, per gallon

Lay Description

These codes report the supply of acetate concentrate and acid concentrate solutions for hemodialysis. Hemodialysis is a physicochemical and filtration process. The dialyzer portion of a hemodialysis unit is typically two chambered. One chamber circulates blood drawn from the patient. The second circulates a solution know as dialysate in the opposite direction from movement of the blood. A semipermeable membrane between the chambers allows accumulated uremic toxins, excess ions, and water in the blood to pass into the dialysate. Cleansed blood is returned to the patient as the dialysate is constantly refreshed. Acetate and/or acid concentrate, as well as bicarbonate concentrate, must be mixed with dialysate in specific ratios depending on the type of dialysis equipment being used to achieve the proper chemical balance in the dialysis solution. Report A4708 per gallon of acetate concentrate solution and A4709 per gallon of acid concentrate.

Medicare Information

Dialysis supplies used in conjunction with covered dialysis services are covered. All necessary supplies and equipment used in the dialysis facility are reimbursed under the composite payment rate. For patients who elect Method II of home dialysis, the DME supplier bills for supplies.

A4714

A4714 Treated water (deionized, distilled, or reverse osmosis) for peritoneal dialysis, per gallon

Lay Description

Peritoneal dialysis is an alternative to hemodialysis. Peritoneal dialysis uses the thin lining in the abdomen that coats the outer surface of the intestines (peritoneal membrane) to remove waste products and balance fluids. The dialysis solution is instilled through a catheter placed through the skin into the peritoneal cavity. The dialysis solution removes waste products and excess fluid and is then drained from the abdomen and discarded. Treatments are generally performed by the patient. Peritoneal dialysis requires the use of dialysis solution, treated water, and disposable supplies. Report A4714 per gallon for deionized, distilled, or reverse osmosis treated water for peritoneal dialysis.

Medicare Information

Dialysis supplies used in conjunction with covered dialysis services are covered. All necessary supplies and equipment used in the dialysis facility are reimbursed under the composite payment rate. For patients who elect Method II of home dialysis, the DME supplier bills for supplies.

A4719

A4719 "Y set" tubing for peritoneal dialysis

Lay Description

This code reports the supply of y-set tubing for peritoneal dialysis. Peritoneal dialysis (PD) is the main alternative to hemodialysis for patients with end-stage renal disease (ESRD). In PD, used dialysate is exchanged for fresh product, usually once or twice per day. The patient will have a surgically created stoma and an indwelling peritoneal catheter. A special y-tube with clamps is connected to the PD catheter. A clamp on the y-tube is opened and used dialysate is drained from the cavity and collected. Upon completion, the drain tube is clamped and about 1.5 to 3 liters of fresh dialysate is gravity infused through the other lead of the y-tube catheter into the peritoneal cavity. The dialysate may be left in place for one to eight hours, depending on the patient's requirements. Y-set tubing is reusable for up to several months.

A4720-A4726

A4720 Dialysate solution, any concentration of dextrose, fluid volume greater than 249 cc, but less than or equal to 999 cc, for peritoneal dialysis

A4721 Dialysate solution, any concentration of dextrose, fluid volume greater than 999 cc but less than or equal to 1999 cc, for peritoneal dialysis

A4722 Dialysate solution, any concentration of dextrose, fluid volume greater than 1999 cc but less than or equal to 2999 cc, for peritoneal dialysis

A4723 Dialysate solution, any concentration of dextrose, fluid volume greater than 2999 cc but less than or equal to 3999 cc, for peritoneal dialysis

A4724 Dialysate solution, any concentration of dextrose, fluid volume greater than 3999 cc but less than or equal to 4999 cc, for peritoneal dialysis

A4725 Dialysate solution, any concentration of dextrose, fluid volume greater than 4999 cc but less than or equal to 5999 cc, for peritoneal dialysis

A4726 Dialysate solution, any concentration of dextrose, fluid volume greater than 5999 cc, for peritoneal dialysis

Lay Description

This range of codes reports various sized supplies of dialysate solution for peritoneal dialysis. The codes are differentiated by volume of solution supplied. Peritoneal dialysis (PD) is the main alternative to hemodialysis for patients with end-stage renal disease (ESRD). In PD, used dialysate is exchanged for fresh product, usually once or twice per day. The patient will have a surgically created stoma and an indwelling peritoneal catheter. A special y-tube with clamps is connected to the PD catheter. A clamp on the y-tube is opened and used dialysate is drained from the cavity and collected. Upon completion, the drain tube is clamped and about 1.5 to 3 liters of fresh dialysate is gravity infused through the other lead of the y-tube catheter into the peritoneal cavity. The fresh solution contains dextrose (sugar) that helps to withdraw wastes and excess fluids. This range of codes is independent of dextrose concentrations in the dialysate.

Medicare Information

Dialysis supplies used in conjunction with covered dialysis services are covered. All necessary supplies and equipment used in the dialysis facility are reimbursed under the composite payment rate. For patients who elect Method II of home dialysis, the DME supplier bills for supplies.

A4728

A4728 Dialysate solution, nondextrose containing, 500 ml

Lay Description

There are two types of dialysis, hemodialysis and peritoneal dialysis. Both make use of a solution called dialysate to draw waste products out of the blood. Hemodialysis removes excess fluids, wastes, impurities, and chemicals from the blood by use of a dialyzer. Hemodialysis requires the use of a dialysis machine, dialyzer, dialysis solution (dialysate), treated water, and disposable supplies. Peritoneal dialysis is an alternative to hemodialysis. Peritoneal dialysis uses the thin lining in the abdomen that coats the outer surface of the intestines (peritoneal membrane) to remove waste products and balance fluids. The dialysis solution (dialysate) is instilled through a catheter placed through the skin into the peritoneal cavity. The dialysis solution removes waste products and excess fluid and is then drained from the abdomen and discarded. Report each 500 ml of nondextrose containing dialysate solution used with A4728.

Medicare Information

Dialysis supplies used in conjunction with covered dialysis services are covered. All necessary supplies and equipment used in the dialysis facility are reimbursed under the composite payment rate. For patients who elect Method II of home dialysis, the DME supplier bills for supplies.

A4730

A4730 Fistula cannulation set for hemodialysis, each

Lay Description

This code reports the supply of each fistula cannulation set for hemodialysis. In most cases, patients will have had a surgically created arterial-venous fistula in the wrist or elbow region, and several configurations are seen. A synthetic graft of soft plastic tubing between the artery and the vein may be chosen. The plastic graft portion of the fistula, which may lie exteriorly, can then be repeatedly accessed for hemodialysis. The cannula set is designed to interface between the fistula and the hemodialysis unit. Report A4730 for supply of each cannulation set for hemodialysis.

A4736-A4737

A4736 Topical anesthetic, for dialysis, per g
A4737 Injectable anesthetic, for dialysis, per 10 ml

Lay Description
These codes report local anesthetics used during dialysis. Local anesthetics reduce sensation or feeling in the area of the body where they are applied or injected. Report A4736 for 1 gram of topical anesthetic used during dialysis; report A4737 for 10 ml of injectable anesthetic.

Medicare Information
Dialysis supplies used in conjunction with covered dialysis services are covered. All necessary supplies and equipment used in the dialysis facility are reimbursed under the composite payment rate. For patients who elect Method II of home dialysis, the DME supplier bills for supplies.

A4740

A4740 Shunt accessory, for hemodialysis, any type, each

Lay Description
A hemodialysis shunt is an artificial, external blood route that provides access to the blood supply. Shunt accessories such as connectors and adapters are attached to the hemodialysis shunt to perform dialysis. Report A4740 for any type of hemodialysis shunt accessory. Examples of items that would be reported with A4740 include shunt connectors, universal connectors, Teflon connectors, shunt adapters, universal adapters, and Teflon adapters.

A4750-A4755

A4750 Blood tubing, arterial or venous, for hemodialysis, each
A4755 Blood tubing, arterial and venous combined, for hemodialysis, each

Lay Description
Hemodialysis tubing consists of a plastic tube or tubes that is attached to a fistula needle or shunt connector and allows blood to flow to and from the patient and dialyzer. Blood tubing for hemodialysis may be separate arterial and venous tubing or combined arteriovenous tubing. Report A4750 for each separate arterial and venous tubing set; report A4755 for each combined arteriovenous set.

Medicare Information
Dialysis supplies used in conjunction with covered dialysis services are covered. All necessary supplies and equipment used in the dialysis facility are reimbursed under the composite payment rate. For patients who elect Method II of home dialysis, the DME supplier bills for supplies.

A4760

A4760 Dialysate solution test kit, for peritoneal dialysis, any type, each

Lay Description
Dialysate is an electrolyte solution containing elements such as potassium, sodium, chloride, etc. Dialysate that is supplied in solution or powder concentrate form must be mixed with purified water prior to use. The mixed solution requires testing to verify that electrolyte levels are correct. Test kits that include supplies such as reagents, test strips, and chloride indicators are reported with A4760.

Medicare Information
Dialysis supplies used in conjunction with covered dialysis services are covered. All necessary supplies and equipment used in the dialysis facility are reimbursed under the composite payment rate. For patients who elect Method II of home dialysis, the DME supplier bills for supplies.

A4765-A4766

A4765 Dialysate concentrate, powder, additive for peritoneal dialysis, per packet
A4766 Dialysate concentrate, solution, additive for peritoneal dialysis, per 10 ml

Lay Description
Dialysate is an electrolyte solution containing elements such as potassium, sodium, chloride, etc. Dialysate that is supplied in solution or powder concentrate form must be mixed with purified water prior to use. Report A4765 for each packet of dialysate concentrate powder for peritoneal dialysis; report A4766 for each 10 ml of dialysate concentrate solution.

Medicare Information
Dialysis supplies used in conjunction with covered dialysis services are covered. All necessary supplies and equipment used in the dialysis facility are reimbursed under the composite payment rate. For patients who elect Method II of home dialysis, the DME supplier bills for supplies.

A4770-A4771

A4770 Blood collection tube, vacuum, for dialysis, per 50
A4771 Serum clotting time tube, for dialysis, per 50

Lay Description
These codes report blood collection tubes for dialysis. Vacuum tubes have a precisely controlled vacuum that allows the correct amount of blood to be collected for each specimen required and are reported with A4770 for each 50 tubes supplied. Serum clotting time tubes are designed specifically to

test blood samples for clotting time and are reported with A4771 for each 50 tubes supplied.

Medicare Information
Dialysis supplies used in conjunction with covered dialysis services are covered. All necessary supplies and equipment used in the dialysis facility are reimbursed under the composite payment rate. For patients who elect Method II of home dialysis, the DME supplier bills for supplies.

A4772-A4774
A4772   Blood glucose test strips, for dialysis, per 50
A4773   Occult blood test strips, for dialysis, per 50
A4774   Ammonia test strips, for dialysis, per 50

Lay Description
These codes report test strips used to check blood glucose, occult blood, and ammonia levels in patients undergoing dialysis. Report A4772 per 50 blood glucose test strips; A4773 per 50 occult blood test strips; and A4774 per 50 ammonia test strips.

Medicare Information
Dialysis supplies used in conjunction with covered dialysis services are covered. All necessary supplies and equipment used in the dialysis facility are reimbursed under the composite payment rate. For patients who elect Method II of home dialysis, the DME supplier bills for supplies.

A4802
A4802   Protamine sulfate, for hemodialysis, per 50 mg

Lay Description
Protamine sulfate is used to neutralize the effects of heparin. Protamine sulfate is a strong basic polypeptide that when administered alone has an anticoagulant effect. However, when administered with heparin, protamine sulfate complexes with the strongly acidic heparin to form an inactive stable salt and the complex has no anticoagulant activity. Report A4802 for each 50 mg of protamine sulfate administered during hemodialysis.

Medicare Information
Dialysis supplies used in conjunction with covered dialysis services are covered. All necessary supplies and equipment used in the dialysis facility are reimbursed under the composite payment rate. For patients who elect Method II of home dialysis, the DME supplier bills for supplies.

A4860
A4860   Disposable catheter tips for peritoneal dialysis, per 10

Lay Description
This code is used to report supply of 10 disposable catheter tips used during peritoneal dialysis.

Medicare Information
Dialysis supplies used in conjunction with covered dialysis services are covered. All necessary supplies and equipment used in the dialysis facility are reimbursed under the composite payment rate. For patients who elect Method II of home dialysis, the DME supplier bills for supplies.

A4870-A4890
A4870   Plumbing and/or electrical work for home hemodialysis equipment
A4890   Contracts, repair and maintenance, for hemodialysis equipment

Lay Description
These codes are used to report plumbing and electrical modifications required in the patient's home so that the dialysis equipment can be effectively and safely used, as well as contract work performed on hemodialysis equipment. Report A4870 for costs associated with plumbing and electrical modifications. Report A4890 for contract work, repair, and maintenance of hemodialysis equipment that is owned or rented by the patient.

Medicare Information
Dialysis supplies used in conjunction with covered dialysis services are covered. All necessary supplies and equipment used in the dialysis facility are reimbursed under the composite payment rate. For patients who elect Method II of home dialysis, the DME supplier bills for supplies.

A4911-A4932

A4911   Drain bag/bottle, for dialysis, each
A4913   Miscellaneous dialysis supplies, not otherwise specified
A4918   Venous pressure clamp, for hemodialysis, each
A4927   Gloves, nonsterile, per 100
A4928   Surgical mask, per 20
A4929   Tourniquet for dialysis, each
A4930   Gloves, sterile, per pair
A4931   Oral thermometer, reusable, any type, each
A4932   Rectal thermometer, reusable, any type, each

Lay Description

These codes report additional supplies used during dialysis. All codes are for specific supplies except A4913, which should be used to report miscellaneous dialysis supplies when a more specific code is not available. Report A4911 for each drain bag or bottle; A4918 for each venous pressure clamp; A4927 for each box of 100 non-sterile gloves; A4928 for each box of 20 surgical masks; A4929 for each tourniquet, A4930 for each pair of sterile gloves; A4931 for each reusable oral thermometer; and A4932 for each reusable rectal thermometer.

Medicare Information

Dialysis supplies used in conjunction with covered dialysis services are covered. All necessary supplies and equipment used in the dialysis facility are reimbursed under the composite payment rate. For patients who elect Method II of home dialysis, the DME supplier bills for supplies.

A5051-A5054

A5051   Ostomy pouch, closed; with barrier attached (1 piece), each
A5052   Ostomy pouch, closed; without barrier attached (1 piece), each
A5053   Ostomy pouch, closed; for use on faceplate, each
A5054   Ostomy pouch, closed; for use on barrier with flange (2 piece), each

Lay Description

These codes represent ostomy pouches that are for use with patients who have had a surgically created opening for diversion of stool. Ostomy pouches collect the stomal output, in this case feces, and can be drainable or closed. Drainable pouches have an opening at the bottom through which fecal contents can be emptied. Closed pouches have a sealed bottom with no outlet for feces. Ostomy pouches described by A5051-A5054 are closed pouches. There are also one-piece and two-piece systems. One-piece systems are supplied "with barrier attached" or "without barrier attached." Two-piece systems have a locking or non-locking flange that is coupled to a skin barrier with flange. Skin barriers are an interface between the patient's skin and the pouching system and have a variety of different options, such as built-in convexity, filters, locking or nonlocking flanges, and use with or without faceplates. Report A5051 for a one-piece, closed ostomy pouch with barrier attached; A5052 for the same type of device without barrier attached; A5053 for a closed ostomy pouch that is used on a separate faceplate; and A5054 for a two-piece closed ostomy pouch that is used on a barrier with flange.

Medicare Information

See chapter titled "Medicare Guidelines," under "Ostomy Devices and Supplies," for Medicare billing and documentation information.

A5055

A5055   Stoma cap

Lay Description

Stoma caps are designed to retain discharge at the site of the stoma for patients with ostomies. A stoma is an artificial opening into a body passageway or organ. It is performed when the organ cannot function normally. Ostomies are usually permanent openings, created for drainage to the outside of the body, so that fecal or urinary materials can be eliminated. The stoma caps are extremely absorbent, flexible, waterproof covers that may also include odor control features.

Medicare Information

See the chapter titled "Medicare Guidelines," under "Ostomy Devices and Supplies," for Medicare information.

A5061-A5063

A5061   Ostomy pouch, drainable; with barrier attached, (1 piece), each
A5062   Ostomy pouch, drainable; without barrier attached (1 piece), each
A5063   Ostomy pouch, drainable; for use on barrier with flange (2-piece system), each

Lay Description

These codes represent drainable ostomy pouches. Ostomy pouches are used by patients who have had a surgically created opening for diversion of urine. The ostomy pouch with barrier attached is a one-piece system in which a solid barrier serving to create an adhesive seal is part of the ostomy pouch. The barrier may be either pectin-based or karaya-based for normal wear, or pectin-based with special additives for extended wear. A flange or plastic ring on both the pouch and skin barrier secures the barrier and the pouch. Report A5061 for a drainable ostomy pouch with a barrier attached (one piece); A5062 for one without a barrier attached (one piece); and A5063 for a pouch used on a barrier with flange (two piece system).

Medicare Information
Ostomy devices and supplies are covered prosthetics. Hospitals may be paid for these items only when they are dispensed at the time of the surgery that created the ostomy, or at the time of a surgical revision. Routine and replacement supplies are considered DMEPOS and must be billed by the supplier.

A5071-A5073

A5071   Ostomy pouch, urinary; with barrier attached (1 piece), each
A5072   Ostomy pouch, urinary; without barrier attached (1 piece), each
A5073   Ostomy pouch, urinary; for use on barrier with flange (2 piece), each

Lay Description
These codes represent urinary ostomy pouches. Urinary ostomy pouches are for use with patients who have had a surgically created opening for diversion of the urine. There are one-piece and two-piece systems. In one-piece appliances, the collection pouch and barrier cannot be separated from one another; whereas the two-piece appliance is designed so that the barrier and collection pouch are separated by a locking mechanism. An ostomy faceplate is a solid interface between the patient's skin and the pouch. It is usually made of plastic, rubber, or encased metal. It can be taken off the skin and reattached repeatedly. It is held on by means of a separate adhesive and/or an elastic belt. Report A5071 for a urinary ostomy pouch with barrier attached (one piece); A5072 for one without barrier attached (one piece); and A5073 for a pouch used on barrier with flange (two piece).

Medicare Information
Ostomy devices and supplies are covered prosthetics. Hospitals may be paid for these items only when they are dispensed at the time of the surgery that created the ostomy, or at the time of a surgical revision. Routine and replacement supplies are considered DMEPOS and must be billed by the supplier.

A5081-A5083

A5081   Continent device; plug for continent stoma
A5082   Continent device; catheter for continent stoma
A5083   Continent device, stoma absorptive cover for continent stoma

Lay Description
These codes report specific supplies for continent stomas. A continent stoma usually involves a surgically fashioned "neobladder" that allows for natural voiding capability. In some instances the pouch is created from a section of ileum, cecum, or other portions of the colon. Part of the bladder may be preserved and the intestinal graft attached to it. Nerves and blood vessels of the graft are usually preserved. The ileocecal sphincter may be preserved and used as a valve. The stoma is managed by a plug and catheter system, and these codes report the supply of these products. Report A5081 for supply of a plug for a continent stoma. Report A5082 for supply of a catheter for a continent stoma. Report A5083 for an absorptive cover for a continent stoma.

A5093

A5093   Ostomy accessory; convex insert

Lay Description
A convex insert is an ostomy accessory that fits between the ostomy pouch and the ostomy pad surrounding the stoma opening. The convex insert helps to provide the ostomy pouch with a tighter fit. An ostomy convex insert is reported with A5093.

Medicare Information
See chapter titled "Medicare Guidelines," under "Ostomy Devices and Supplies," for Medicare billing and documentation information.

A5102

A5102   Bedside drainage bottle with or without tubing, rigid or expandable, each

Lay Description
Patients with urinary ostomies may use a bedside drainage bottle. The bedside drainage bottle is reusable and collects urinary output from a pouch. It is sometimes necessary, especially at night, for the bottle to be connected to the pouch to prevent urinary overflow and excessive weight in the pouch, which could cause urinary leakage and disruption of the pouch seal. The bottle is made of a high-density polyethylene and can hold up to 2,000 cc. Report this code for rigid or expandable bedside bottle with or without tubing.

Medicare Information

See the chapter titled "Medicare Guidelines," under "Urological Supplies," for Medicare information.

A5105

A5105 Urinary suspensory with leg bag, with or without tube, each

Lay Description

This code reports the supply of an external urinary suspensory garment. This garment is usually designed for males and is worn like a jockey strap. A urinal sheath is attachable to a portion that fits around the penis. This in turn is attachable to a tube and leg bag to drain urine. Report A5105 for each urinary suspensory, with or without leg bag, with or without tube.

A5112

A5112 Urinary drainage bag, leg or abdomen, latex, with or without tube, with straps, each

Lay Description

Urinary leg bags are used with male external urinary catheters. At the top is an anti-reflux flutter valve that attaches to the urinary catheter and allows urine to drain from the bladder into the leg bag. At the bottom is a drainage valve that allows the catheter to be emptied as needed. Leg bags may be constructed of a variety of materials. Latex leg bags are reported with A5112.

Medicare Information

See chapter titled "Medicare Guidelines," under "Urological Supplies," for Medicare billing and documentation information.

A5113-A5114

A5113 Leg strap; latex, replacement only, per set

A5114 Leg strap; foam or fabric, replacement only, per set

Lay Description

Codes A5113 and A5114 are for replacement leg straps used with a urinary leg bag. Report A5113 for each set of latex straps and A5114 for each set of foam or fabric straps used. These codes are not used for a leg strap for an indwelling catheter.

Medicare Information

See the chapter titled "Medicare Guidelines," under "Urological Supplies," for Medicare information.

A5120

A5120 Skin barrier, wipes or swabs, each

Lay Description

Skin barrier wipes and swabs are used to clean and protect the stoma site. Wipes and swabs are formulated with soothing, nonsting cleanser that also provides a protective film around the stoma to prevent irritation of the stoma between pouch changes. Wipes and swabs may also be medicated to provide further protection to the stoma site. Report each swab or wipe with A5120.

Medicare Information

See chapter titled "Medicare Guidelines," under "Ostomy Devices and Supplies," for Medicare billing and documentation information.

A5121-A5122

A5121 Skin barrier; solid, 6 x 6 or equivalent, each

A5122 Skin barrier; solid, 8 x 8 or equivalent, each

Lay Description

Please refer to code A4362 for the description, coding, and billing information.

A5126

A5126 Adhesive or nonadhesive; disk or foam pad

Lay Description

Please refer to code A4364 for the description, coding, and billing information.

A5131

A5131 Appliance cleaner, incontinence and ostomy appliances, per 16 oz

Lay Description

Appliance cleaners are used to deodorize, remove crystallized deposits, and clean the inside of rubber, latex, and plastic incontinence or ostomy collection devices. Report this code for every 16 oz. of cleaner.

Medicare Information

See the chapter titled "Medicare Guidelines," under "Ostomy Devices and Supplies," for Medicare information.

A5200

A5200 Percutaneous catheter/tube anchoring device, adhesive skin attachment

Lay Description
A percutaneous catheter/tube anchoring device is a dressing with adhesive that is designed to be applied directly over the cutaneous opening through which the catheter/tube passes. This dressing has a hole through which the catheter/tube passes and a mechanism for firmly anchoring the catheter/tube to the dressing.

Medicare Information
See chapter titled, "Medicare Guidelines," under "Enteral Nutrition," for Medicare billing and documentation information.

A5500-A5501

A5500 For diabetics only, fitting (including follow-up), custom preparation and supply of off-the-shelf depth-inlay shoe manufactured to accommodate multidensity insert(s), per shoe

A5501 For diabetics only, fitting (including follow-up), custom preparation and supply of shoe molded from cast(s) of patient's foot (custom molded shoe), per shoe

Lay Description
These items include fitting with follow-up, custom preparation, and supply of off-the-shelf or custom made shoes that will accommodate various shoe inserts. Shoes and shoe inserts assist the diabetic patient with ambulation, decrease pressure points that may be present in non-prescription shoes, and help prevent ulcerative conditions of the feet. They are used in patients with partial or complete amputation (opposite foot). Previous foot ulcerations and current pre-ulcerative conditions may be present. Circulation may be impaired, and deformity and/or peripheral neuropathy may be present. Report A5500 for off-the-shelf depth shoes, which are custom prepared and have multi-density (varying depths) of insert. They usually are full-length. In A5501, a molded cast of the patient's foot may be performed or may be heat-molded to fit almost any foot. They also have removable inserts that can be altered, with some form of shoe closure. Each code is reported per shoe.

Medicare Information
Diabetic shoes, inserts, and/or modifications to the shoes are covered, when eligible, under the DME benefit if all of the following criteria are met:

- The patient has diabetes mellitus
- The patient has one of the following conditions:
  - peripheral neuropathy with evidence of callus formation of either foot
  - history of previous foot ulceration
  - history of pre-ulcerative calluses
  - previous amputation of the other foot, or part of either foot
  - foot deformity
  - poor circulation

The certifying physician managing the patient's diabetic-systemic condition must certify:

- The physician is treating the patient under a comprehensive plan of care for diabetes
- The patient needs diabetic shoes
- A podiatrist or other qualified physician performs prescription of the footwear
- The footwear must be fitted and furnished by a podiatrist or other qualified person, such as a pedorthist, orthotist, or a prosthetist. The certifying physician cannot furnish the diabetic shoes unless they are qualified

For patients meeting the previously listed criteria, coverage is limited to one of the following within one calendar year:

- One pair of custom-molded shoes (A5501) (including inserts provided with the shoes) and two additional pairs of inserts (A5502)
- One pair of depth shoes (A5500) and three pairs of inserts (A5502) (not including the non-customized removable inserts provided with the shoes)

Separate inserts may be covered and dispensed independently of diabetic shoes, if the supplier of the shoes verifies in writing that the patient has appropriate footwear in which to place the insert. However, the footwear must meet the definitions for in-depth or custom-molded shoes.

A custom-molded shoe is covered when the patient's foot deformity will not allow the use of a depth shoe.

When a patient qualifies for both diabetic shoes and a leg brace, the items are covered separately. Certification for the need for diabetic shoes, prescription of the shoes, and fitting are include in the payment for the visit or consultation, unless the physician documents that these services were not the sole purpose of the visit or consultation.

A5503-A5506

A5503 For diabetics only, modification (including fitting) of off-the-shelf depth-inlay shoe or custom molded shoe with roller or rigid rocker bottom, per shoe

A5504 For diabetics only, modification (including fitting) of off-the-shelf depth-inlay shoe or custom molded shoe with wedge(s), per shoe

A5505 For diabetics only, modification (including fitting) of off-the-shelf depth-inlay shoe or custom molded shoe with metatarsal bar, per shoe

A5506 For diabetics only, modification (including fitting) of off-the-shelf depth-inlay shoe or custom molded shoe with off-set heel(s), per shoe

Lay Description

These items include fitting with follow-up, custom preparation, and supply of off-the-shelf or custom made shoes with special added features. A molded cast of the patient's foot may be performed. Shoes and shoe inserts assist the diabetic patient with ambulation, decrease pressure points that may be present in non-prescription shoes, and help prevent ulcerative conditions of the feet. They are used in patients with partial or complete amputation (opposite foot). Previous foot ulcerations and current pre-ulcerative conditions may be present. Circulation may be impaired, and deformity and/or peripheral neuropathy may be present. Rigid rocker bottoms (A5503) are exterior elevations. The apex (a narrowed or pointed end) is measured from the back end of the heel and is positioned behind the metatarsal heads and tapers off sharply to the front tip of the sole. Apex height helps to eliminate pressure at the metatarsal heads. The heel tapers off in back to cause the shoe heel to strike in the middle of the heel. The steel in a patient's shoe ensures rigidity. Roller bottoms (sole or bar) (A5503) are the same as rocker bottoms, but the heel is tapered from the apex to the front tip of the sole. A Shoe with wedges that are either of the hind foot, fore foot, or both and may be in the middle or to the side is reported with A5504. The function is to shift or transfer weight bearing upon standing or during ambulation to the opposite side for added support, stabilization, equalized weight distribution, or balance. In A5505, an exterior bar is placed behind the metatarsal heads in order to remove pressure from the metatarsal heads. The bars are of various shapes, heights, and construction depending on the purpose it serves. Report A5506 for an offset heel flanged at its base either in the middle, to the side, or a combination, that is then extended upward to the shoe in order to stabilize extreme positions of the hind foot.

Medicare Information

Diabetic shoes, inserts, and/or modifications to the shoes are covered, when eligible, under the DME benefit if all of the following criteria are met:

- The patient has diabetes mellitus
- The patient has one of the following conditions:
  - peripheral neuropathy with evidence of callus formation of either foot
  - history of previous foot ulceration
  - history of pre-ulcerative calluses
  - previous amputation of the other foot, or part of either foot
  - foot deformity
  - poor circulation

The certifying physician managing the patient's diabetic-systemic condition must certify:

- The physician is treating the patient under a comprehensive plan of care for diabetes
- The patient needs diabetic shoes
- A podiatrist or other qualified physician performs prescription of the footwear.
- The footwear must be fitted and furnished by a podiatrist or other qualified person, such as a pedorthist, orthotist, or a prosthetist. The certifying physician cannot furnish the diabetic shoes unless they are qualified

For patients meeting the previously listed criteria, coverage is limited to one of the following within one calendar year:

- One pair of custom-molded shoes (A5501) (including inserts provided with the shoes) and two additional pairs of inserts (A5502)
- One pair of depth shoes (A5500) and three pairs of inserts (A5502) (not including the non-customized removable inserts provided with the shoes)

Separate inserts may be covered and dispensed independently of diabetic shoes, if the supplier of the shoes verifies in writing that the patient has appropriate footwear in which to place the insert. However, the footwear must meet the definitions for in-depth or custom-molded shoes.

A custom-molded shoe is covered when the patient's foot deformity will not allow the use of a depth shoe.

When a patient qualifies for both diabetic shoes and a leg brace, the items are covered separately. Certification for the need for diabetic shoes, prescription of the shoes, and fitting are include in the payment for the visit or consultation, unless the physician documents that these services were not the sole purpose of the visit or consultation.

A5507-A5508

A5507 For diabetics only, not otherwise specified modification (including fitting) of off-the-shelf depth-inlay shoe or custom molded shoe, per shoe
A5508 For diabetics only, deluxe feature of off-the-shelf depth-inlay shoe or custom molded shoe, per shoe

Lay Description
Code A5507 is only to be used for not otherwise specified therapeutic modifications to an off-the-shelf depth-inlay or custom-made shoe for a diabetic patient. Report A5508 for a deluxe feature of an off-the-shelf depth-inlay or custom-made shoe that does not contribute to the therapeutic function of the diabetic shoe. It may include, but is not limited to style, color, or type of leather.

Medicare Information
Diabetic shoes, inserts, and/or modifications to the shoes are covered, when eligible, under the DME benefit if all of the following criteria are met:

- The patient has diabetes mellitus
- The patient has one of the following conditions:
  - peripheral neuropathy with evidence of callus formation of either foot
  - history of previous foot ulceration
  - history of pre-ulcerative calluses
  - previous amputation of the other foot, or part of either foot
  - foot deformity
  - poor circulation

The certifying physician managing the patient's diabetic-systemic condition must certify:

- The physician is treating the patient under a comprehensive plan of care for diabetes
- The patient needs diabetic shoes
- A podiatrist or other qualified physician performs prescription of the footwear
- The footwear must be fitted and furnished by a podiatrist or other qualified person, such as a pedorthist, orthotist, or a prosthetist. The certifying physician cannot furnish the diabetic shoes unless they are qualified

For patients meeting the previously listed criteria, coverage is limited to one of the following within one calendar year:

- One pair of custom-molded shoes (A5501) (including inserts provided with the shoes) and two additional pairs of inserts (A5502)
- One pair of depth shoes (A5500) and three pairs of inserts (A5502) (not including the non-customized removable inserts provided with the shoes)

Separate inserts may be covered and dispensed independently of diabetic shoes, if the supplier of the shoes verifies in writing that the patient has appropriate footwear in which to place the insert. However, the footwear must meet the definitions for in-depth or custom-molded shoes.

A custom-molded shoe is covered when the patient's foot deformity will not allow the use of a depth shoe.

When a patient qualifies for both diabetic shoes and a leg brace, the items are covered separately. Certification for the need for diabetic shoes, prescription of the shoes, and fitting are include in the payment for the visit or consultation, unless the physician documents that these services were not the sole purpose of the visit or consultation.

A5510-A5513

A5510 For diabetics only, direct formed, compression molded to patient's foot without external heat source, multiple-density insert(s) prefabricated, per shoe
A5512 For diabetics only, multiple density insert, direct formed, molded to foot after external heat source of 230 degrees Fahrenheit or higher, total contact with patient's foot, including arch, base layer minimum of 1/4 inch material of shore a 35 durometer or 3/16 inch material of shore a 40 durometer (or higher), prefabricated, each
A5513 For diabetics only, multiple density insert, custom molded from model of patient's foot, total contact with patient's foot, including arch, base layer minimum of 3/16 inch material of shore a 35 durometer or higher), includes arch filler and other shaping material, custom fabricated, each

Lay Description
A diabetic shoe insert is a total contact, removable inlay that is directly molded to the patient's foot or a model of the patient's foot and that is made of a suitable material with regard to the patient's condition. There are several methods of fabrication including compression molded without the use of a heat source, direct formed with the use of a heat source, and custom molded from a model of the patient's foot. In A5510, the insert is prefabricated, multiple density, and formed using a compression mold of the patient's foot without the use of a heat source. In A5512, the insert is prefabricated and direct formed to the foot using an external heat source and total contact with the patient's foot. In A5513, the insert is custom-fabricated from a model

of the patient's foot. Codes A5512 and A5513 contain additional specific requirements for the insert. The inserts must provide total contact including arch support with a base layer minimum of 1/4 inch material of shore A dermometer or 3/16 inch material of shore A 40 dermometer or higher. Codes A5510-A5513 are reported for each insert.

Medicare Information

Diabetic shoes, inserts, and/or modifications to the shoes are covered, when eligible, under the DME benefit if all of the following criteria are met:

- The patient has diabetes mellitus
- The patient has one of the following conditions:
  - peripheral neuropathy with evidence of callus formation of either foot
  - history of previous foot ulceration
  - history of pre-ulcerative calluses
  - previous amputation of the other foot or part of either foot
  - foot deformity
  - poor circulation

The certifying physician managing the patient's diabetic-systemic condition must certify:

- The physician is treating the patient under a comprehensive plan of care for diabetes
- The patient needs diabetic shoes
- A podiatrist or other qualified physician prescribes the footwear
- The footwear must be fitted and furnished by a podiatrist or other qualified person, such as a pedorthist, orthotist, or a prosthetist. The certifying physician cannot furnish the diabetic shoes unless qualified

For patients meeting the previously listed criteria, coverage is limited to one of the following within one calendar year:

- One pair of custom-molded shoes (A5501) (including inserts provided with the shoes) and two additional pairs of inserts (A5502)
- One pair of depth shoes (A5500) and three pairs of inserts (A5502) (not including the non-customized removable inserts provided with the shoes)

Separate inserts may be covered and dispensed independently of diabetic shoes, if the supplier of the shoes verifies in writing that the patient has appropriate footwear in which to place the insert. However, the footwear must meet the definitions for in-depth or custom-molded shoes.

A custom-molded shoe is covered when the patient's foot deformity will not allow the use of a depth shoe.

When a patient qualifies for both diabetic shoes and a leg brace, the items are covered separately. Certification for the need for diabetic shoes, prescription for the shoes, and fitting are included in the payment for the visit or consultation, unless the physician documents that these services were not the sole purpose of the visit or consultation.

A6000

A6000 Noncontact wound-warming wound cover for use with the noncontact wound-warming device and warming card

Lay Description

Wound healing occurs best in a warm, moist environment that enhances subcutaneous oxygen tension and increases blood flow to the wound. A noncontact wound warming device, also referred to as noncontact normothermic wound therapy (NNWT), is a wound treatment device designed to create an optimal environment to promote wound healing. A non-contact wound warming device includes a non-contact bandage and a warming unit designed to maintain 100 percent relative humidity and to produce optimal temperatures in the wound and surrounding tissues. The bandage consists of a sterile foam collar that adheres to the skin surrounding the wound and a sterile, transparent film that covers the top of the wound without touching it. An infrared warming card or flexible heat unit is inserted into a pocket in the film covering. Supply of the noncontact bandage is reported with A6000.

A6010-A6011

A6010 Collagen based wound filler, dry form, sterile, per g of collagen
A6011 Collagen based wound filler, gel/paste, per g of collagen

Lay Description

Collagen based wound filler is a natural hydrolyzed protein available in a dry powder (A6010) or a gel/paste (A6011). Collagen based wound filler may be used for chronic wounds and dermal ulcers including pressure ulcers, stasis ulcers, diabetic ulcers, first and second degree burns, surgical wounds, and traumatic wounds. Collagen based wound fillers provide a platform for new cell growth, supply a nutritive protein to the wound site, and protect the wound from bacteria. The powder type forms a gel when it combines with the wound exudate to provide a moist healing environment. The gel/paste type is a hydrogel that contains collagen.

Medicare Information
See chapter titled "Medicare Guidelines," under "Dressings," for Medicare billing and documentation information.

A6021-A6023
A6021 Collagen dressing, sterile, pad size 16 sq in or less, each
A6022 Collagen dressing, sterile, pad size more than 16 sq in but less than or equal to 48 sq in, each
A6023 Collagen dressing, sterile, pad size more than 48 sq in, each

Lay Description
Surgical dressings include both primary dressings (i.e., therapeutic or protective coverings applied directly to wounds or lesions either on the skin or caused by an opening to the skin) and secondary dressings (i.e., materials needed to secure a primary dressing). Collagen dressings are sterile dressings used for moderate to heavily draining wounds to enhance healing and tissue repair. These dressings can be used on burns, pressure ulcers, scrapes, cuts, and for dermatologic conditions. They also come in wet form for burns and other wounds. In general, these products are used for direct wound care, including protecting a wound from infection, absorbing wound exudate (drainage), filtering into the wound, and/or cleansing the wound. Dressings also reduce inflammation and edema and allow for gas exchange. Report A6021 for a collagen dressing, pad size 16 sq inches or less; A6022 for more than 16 sq inches, but less than or equal to 48 sq inches; and A6023 for a dressing more than 48 sq inches.

Medicare Information
See the chapter titled "Medicare Guidelines," under "Dressings," for Medicare information.

A6024
A6024 Collagen dressing wound filler, sterile, per 6 in

Lay Description
Usually made from a bovine collagen, sterile collagen dressing wound filler is a hydrolysate powder that interacts with the wound site and forms a gel that provides a moist wound-healing environment when mixed with the wounds exudate. Collagen promotes new cell growth and provides protein to the wound site. The collagen wound filler is typically used for the management of chronic wounds such as pressure ulcers, diabetic ulcers, and venous insufficiency ulcers, as well as surgically or trauma induced wounds.

A6025
A6025 Gel sheet for dermal or epidermal application, (e.g., silicone, hydrogel, other), each

Lay Description
Gel sheets help create and maintain a moist environment. Increasing moisture to a wound helps keep the wound clean and assists in debridement of necrotic tissue. Gel sheets are used mainly for wounds with minimal or no exudate.

A6154
A6154 Wound pouch, each

Lay Description
A wound pouch is a waterproof collection device with a drainable port that adheres to the skin around a wound. Use this code for each wound pouch supplied.

A6196-A6199
A6196 Alginate or other fiber gelling dressing, wound cover, sterile, pad size 16 sq in or less, each dressing
A6197 Alginate or other fiber gelling dressing, wound cover, sterile, pad size more than 16 sq in but less than or equal to 48 sq in, each dressing
A6198 Alginate or other fiber gelling dressing, wound cover, sterile, pad size more than 48 sq in, each dressing
A6199 Alginate or other fiber gelling dressing, wound filler, sterile, per 6 in

Lay Description
Alginate or other fiber gelling sterile dressing covers and fillers are used for moderately to highly exudative full thickness wounds (e.g., stage III or IV ulcers). Usual dressing change is up to once per day. One wound cover sheet of the approximate size of the wound or up to two units of wound filler (one unit = 6 inches of alginate or other fiber gelling dressing rope) is usually used at each dressing change. It is usually inappropriate to use alginates or other fiber gelling dressings in combination with hydrogels.

Medicare Information
See chapter titled "Medicare Guidelines," under "Dressings," for additional Medicare billing and documentation information.

A6203-A6205

A6203 Composite dressing, sterile, pad size 16 sq in or less, with any size adhesive border, each dressing
A6204 Composite dressing, sterile, pad size more than 16 sq in, but less than or equal to 48 sq in, with any size adhesive border, each dressing
A6205 Composite dressing, sterile, pad size more than 48 sq in, with any size adhesive border, each dressing

Lay Description

Composite dressings are products combining physically distinct components into a single dressing that provides multiple functions. These functions must include, but are not limited to (a) a bacterial barrier, (b) an absorptive layer other than an alginate or other fiber gelling dressing, foam, hydrocolloid, or hydrogel, and (c) either a semi-adherent or nonadherent property over the wound site. Usual composite dressing change is up to three times per week, one wound cover per dressing change.

Medicare Information

See chapter titled "Medicare Guidelines," under "Dressings," for additional Medicare billing and documentation information.

A6206-A6208

A6206 Contact layer, sterile, 16 sq in or less, each dressing
A6207 Contact layer, sterile, more than 16 sq in but less than or equal to 48 sq in, each dressing
A6208 Contact layer, sterile, more than 48 sq in, each dressing

Lay Description

Contact layers are thin, non-adherent sheets placed directly on an open wound bed to protect the wound tissue from direct contact with other agents or dressings applied to the wound. They are porous to allow wound fluid to pass through for absorption by an overlying dressing. Contact layer dressings are used to line the entire wound; they are not intended to be changed with each dressing change. Usual dressing change is up to once per week. Report A6206 for each contact layer that is 16.0 sq. inches or smaller. Report A6207 for each contact layer dressing that is larger than 16.0 sq. inches but smaller than or equal to 48.0 sq. inches. Report A6208 for each contact layer dressing that is larger than 48.0 sq. inches.

Medicare Information

See chapter titled "Medicare Guidelines," under "Dressings," for additional Medicare billing and documentation information.

A6209-A6215

A6209 Foam dressing, wound cover, sterile, pad size 16 sq in or less, without adhesive border, each dressing
A6210 Foam dressing, wound cover, sterile, pad size more than 16 sq in but less than or equal to 48 sq in, without adhesive border, each dressing
A6211 Foam dressing, wound cover, sterile, pad size more than 48 sq in, without adhesive border, each dressing
A6212 Foam dressing, wound cover, sterile, pad size 16 sq in or less, with any size adhesive border, each dressing
A6213 Foam dressing, wound cover, sterile, pad size more than 16 sq in but less than or equal to 48 sq in, with any size adhesive border, each dressing
A6214 Foam dressing, wound cover, sterile, pad size more than 48 sq in, with any size adhesive border, each dressing
A6215 Foam dressing, wound filler, sterile, per g

Lay Description

Foam dressings are used on full thickness wounds (e.g., stage III or IV ulcers) with moderate to heavy exudate. Usual dressing change for a foam wound cover used as a primary dressing is up to three times per week. When a foam wound cover is used as a secondary dressing for wounds with heavy exudate, dressing change may also be up to three times per week. Usual dressing change for foam wound fillers is up to once per day. Report A6209 for each foam dressing wound cover pad that is 16.0 sq. inches or smaller without an adhesive border. Report A6210 for each dressing pad that is larger than 16.0 sq. inches but smaller than 48.0 sq. inches and has no adhesive border. Report A6211 for each dressing pad that is larger than 48.0 sq. inches without an adhesive border. Report A6212 for each foam dressing pad that has an adhesive border and is 16.0 sq. inches or smaller in size. Report A6213 for each dressing pad that is larger than 16.0 sq. inches but smaller than 48.0 sq. inches and has an adhesive border. Report A6214 for each foam dressing pad that is larger than 48.0 sq. inches and has an adhesive border. Report A6215 for every gram of foam wound filler being reported.

Medicare Information

See chapter titled "Medicare Guidelines," under "Dressings," for additional Medicare billing and documentation information.

A6216-A6221

A6216 Gauze, nonimpregnated, nonsterile, pad size 16 sq in or less, without adhesive border, each dressing

A6217 Gauze, nonimpregnated, nonsterile, pad size more than 16 sq in but less than or equal to 48 sq in, without adhesive border, each dressing

A6218 Gauze, nonimpregnated, nonsterile, pad size more than 48 sq in, without adhesive border, each dressing

A6219 Gauze, nonimpregnated, sterile, pad size 16 sq in or less, with any size adhesive border, each dressing

A6220 Gauze, nonimpregnated, sterile, pad size more than 16 sq in but less than or equal to 48 sq in, with any size adhesive border, each dressing

A6221 Gauze, nonimpregnated, sterile, pad size more than 48 sq in, with any size adhesive border, each dressing

Lay Description

Usual non-impregnated gauze dressing change is up to three times per day for a dressing without a border and once per day for a dressing with a border. It is usually not necessary to stack more than two gauze pads on top of each other in any one area. Report A6216 for each non-sterile, non-impregnated gauze pad 16.0 sq. inches or smaller without an adhesive border. Report A6217 for each pad without an adhesive border that is larger than 16.0 sq. inches but smaller than 48.0 sq. inches. Report A6218 for each gauze pad that is larger than 48.0 sq. inches and has no adhesive border. Report A6219 for each pad that has an adhesive border and is 16.0 sq. inches or smaller. Report A6220 for each pad that is larger than 16.0 sq. inches but smaller than 48.0 sq. inches and has an adhesive border. Report A6221 for each gauze pad that is larger than 48.0 sq. inches and has an adhesive border.

Medicare Information

See chapter titled "Medicare Guidelines," under "Dressings," for additional Medicare billing and documentation information.

A6222-A6233

A6222 Gauze, impregnated with other than water, normal saline, or hydrogel, sterile, pad size 16 sq in or less, without adhesive border, each dressing

A6223 Gauze, impregnated with other than water, normal saline, or hydrogel, sterile, pad size more than 16 sq in, but less than or equal to 48 sq in, without adhesive border, each dressing

A6224 Gauze, impregnated with other than water, normal saline, or hydrogel, sterile, pad size more than 48 sq in, without adhesive border, each dressing

A6228 Gauze, impregnated, water or normal saline, sterile, pad size 16 sq in or less, without adhesive border, each dressing

A6229 Gauze, impregnated, water or normal saline, sterile, pad size more than 16 sq in but less than or equal to 48 sq in, without adhesive border, each dressing

A6230 Gauze, impregnated, water or normal saline, sterile, pad size more than 48 sq in, without adhesive border, each dressing

A6231 Gauze, impregnated, hydrogel, for direct wound contact, sterile, pad size 16 sq in or less, each dressing

A6232 Gauze, impregnated, hydrogel, for direct wound contact, sterile, pad size greater than 16 sq in, but less than or equal to 48 sq in, each dressing

A6233 Gauze, impregnated, hydrogel, for direct wound contact, sterile, pad size more than 48 sq in, each dressing

Lay Description

Impregnated gauze dressings are woven or non-woven materials into which substances such as iodinated agents, petrolatum, zinc paste, crystalline sodium chloride, chlorhexidine gluconate (CHG), bismuth tribromophenate (BTP), water, aqueous saline, hydrogel, or other agents have been incorporated into the dressing material by the manufacturer. Report A6222 for each gauze pad 16.0 sq. inches or smaller that has no adhesive border and is impregnated with other than water, normal saline, or hydrogel. Report A6223 for each pad impregnated with other than water, normal saline, or hydrogel that is larger than 16.0 sq. inches but smaller than 48.0 sq. inches and does not have an adhesive border. Report A6224 for each pad impregnated with other than water, normal saline, or hydrogel that is larger than 48.0 sq. inches and does not have an adhesive border. Report A6228 for each pad impregnated with water or normal saline that is 16.0 sq. inches or smaller without an adhesive border. Report A6229 if the pad is impregnated with water or normal saline, has no adhesive border, and is larger than 16.0 sq. inches but less than or equal to 48.0 sq.

inches. Report A6230 for each pad impregnated with water or normal saline that is larger than 48.0 sq. inches and has no adhesive border. Report A6231 for each gauze pad impregnated with hydrogel for direct wound contact that is 16.0 sq. inches or smaller. Report A6232 for each pad impregnated with hydrogel that is larger than 16.0 sq. inches but smaller than or equal to 48.0 sq. inches. Report A6233 for each gauze pad larger than 48.0 sq. inches that is impregnated with hydrogel.

Medicare Information

See chapter titled "Medicare Guidelines," under "Dressings," for additional Medicare billing and documentation information.

A6234-A6241

A6234 Hydrocolloid dressing, wound cover, sterile, pad size 16 sq in or less, without adhesive border, each dressing

A6235 Hydrocolloid dressing, wound cover, sterile, pad size more than 16 sq in but less than or equal to 48 sq in, without adhesive border, each dressing

A6236 Hydrocolloid dressing, wound cover, sterile, pad size more than 48 sq in, without adhesive border, each dressing

A6237 Hydrocolloid dressing, wound cover, sterile, pad size 16 sq in or less, with any size adhesive border, each dressing

A6238 Hydrocolloid dressing, wound cover, sterile, pad size more than 16 sq in but less than or equal to 48 sq in, with any size adhesive border, each dressing

A6239 Hydrocolloid dressing, wound cover, sterile, pad size more than 48 sq in, with any size adhesive border, each dressing

A6240 Hydrocolloid dressing, wound filler, paste, sterile, per oz

A6241 Hydrocolloid dressing, wound filler, dry form, sterile, per g

Lay Description

Hydrocolloid dressings are covered for use on wounds with light to moderate exudate. Usual dressing change for hydrocolloid wound covers or hydrocolloid wound fillers is up to three times per week. Report A6234 for each hydrocolloid wound cover pad 16.0 sq. inches or smaller without an adhesive border. Report A6235 if the dressing pad is larger than 16.0 sq. inches but smaller than or equal to 48.0 sq. inches without an adhesive border. Report A6236 if the dressing pad is larger than 48.0 sq. inches with no adhesive border. Report A6237 for each wound cover 16.0 sq. inches or smaller that has an adhesive border. Report A6238 for each wound cover that is larger than 16.0 sq. inches but smaller than or equal to 48.0 sq. inches with an adhesive border. Report A6239 for each hydrocolloid wound cover larger than 48.0 sq. inches with an adhesive border. Report A6240 for each fluid ounce of paste used for a hydrocolloid dressing wound filler. Report A6241 for each gram if the wound filler is a dry form.

Medicare Information

See chapter titled "Medicare Guidelines," under "Dressings," for additional Medicare billing and documentation information.

A6242-A6248

A6242 Hydrogel dressing, wound cover, sterile, pad size 16 sq in or less, without adhesive border, each dressing

A6243 Hydrogel dressing, wound cover, sterile, pad size more than 16 sq in but less than or equal to 48 sq in, without adhesive border, each dressing

A6244 Hydrogel dressing, wound cover, sterile, pad size more than 48 sq in, without adhesive border, each dressing

A6245 Hydrogel dressing, wound cover, sterile, pad size 16 sq in or less, with any size adhesive border, each dressing

A6246 Hydrogel dressing, wound cover, sterile, pad size more than 16 sq in but less than or equal to 48 sq in, with any size adhesive border, each dressing

A6247 Hydrogel dressing, wound cover, sterile, pad size more than 48 sq in, with any size adhesive border, each dressing

A6248 Hydrogel dressing, wound filler, gel, per fl oz

Lay Description

Hydrogel dressings are used on full thickness wounds with minimal or no exudate (e.g., stage III or IV ulcers). Hydrogel dressings are not usually medically necessary for stage II ulcers. Report A6242 for each hydrogel dressing wound cover pad 16.0 sq. inches or smaller without an adhesive border. Report A6243 if the dressing pad is larger than 16.0 sq. inches but smaller than or equal to 48.0 sq. inches without an adhesive border. Report A6244 if the dressing pad is larger than 48.0 sq. inches with no adhesive border. Report A6245 for each wound cover 16.0 sq. inches or smaller that has an adhesive border. Report A6246 for each cover that is larger than 16.0 sq. inches but smaller than or equal to 48.0 sq. inches with an adhesive border. Report A6247 for each hydrogel wound dressing cover larger than 48.0 sq. inches with an adhesive border. Report A6248 for each fluid ounce of wound filler gel.

Medicare Information

See chapter titled "Medicare Guidelines," under "Dressings," for additional Medicare billing and documentation information.

A6250

A6250 Skin sealants, protectants, moisturizers, ointments, any type, any size

Lay Description

Skin sealants and protectants are liquid barrier films made of polymers and solvents. The solvent evaporates after the sealant or protectant is applied to the skin, leaving behind a protective film. A moisturizer is a water and oil mixture. Ointments are oil in water emulsions. This code is used to report any type or size of skin sealant, protectant, moisturizer, or ointment when a more specific code is not available.

Medicare Information

See chapter titled "Medicare Guidelines," under "Dressings," for Medicare billing and documentation information.

A6251-A6256

A6251 Specialty absorptive dressing, wound cover, sterile, pad size 16 sq in or less, without adhesive border, each dressing

A6252 Specialty absorptive dressing, wound cover, sterile, pad size more than 16 sq in but less than or equal to 48 sq in, without adhesive border, each dressing

A6253 Specialty absorptive dressing, wound cover, sterile, pad size more than 48 sq in, without adhesive border, each dressing

A6254 Specialty absorptive dressing, wound cover, sterile, pad size 16 sq in or less, with any size adhesive border, each dressing

A6255 Specialty absorptive dressing, wound cover, sterile, pad size more than 16 sq in but less than or equal to 48 sq in, with any size adhesive border, each dressing

A6256 Specialty absorptive dressing, wound cover, sterile, pad size more than 48 sq in, with any size adhesive border, each dressing

Lay Description

Specialty absorptive dressings are unitized multi-layer dressings that provide either a semi-adherent quality or nonadherent layer and highly absorptive layers of fibers, such as absorbent cellulose, cotton, or rayon. These may or may not have an adhesive border. Report A6251 for each specialty absorptive dressing wound cover pad 16.0 sq. inches or smaller without an adhesive border. Report A6252 for each pad without an adhesive border that is larger than 16.0 sq. inches but smaller than or equal to 48.0 sq. inches. Report A6253 for each pad larger than 48.0 sq. inches without an adhesive border. Report A6254 for each dressing pad 16.0 sq. inches or smaller with an adhesive border. Report A6255 for each pad with an adhesive border that is larger than 16.0 sq. inches but smaller than or equal to 48.0 sq. inches. Report A6256 for each specialty absorptive dressing wound cover pad larger than 48.0 sq. inches with an adhesive border.

Medicare Information

See chapter titled "Medicare Guidelines," under "Dressings," for additional Medicare billing and documentation information.

A6257-A6259

A6257 Transparent film, sterile, 16 sq in or less, each dressing

A6258 Transparent film, sterile, more than 16 sq in but less than or equal to 48 sq in, each dressing

A6259 Transparent film, sterile, more than 48 sq in, each dressing

Lay Description

Transparent film dressings are used on closed wounds or open partial thickness wounds with minimal exudate. Usual dressing change is up to three times per week. Report A6257 for each transparent film dressing 16.0 sq. inches or smaller; A6258 for a transparent film dressing larger than 16.0 sq. inches but smaller than or equal to 48.0 sq. inches for each dressing; and A6259 for each transparent film dressing that is larger than 48.0 sq. inches.

Medicare Information

See chapter titled "Medicare Guidelines," under "Dressings," for additional Medicare billing and documentation information.

A6260

A6260 Wound cleansers, any type, any size

Lay Description

This code reports wound cleansers of any type and any size that do not a have more specific code listed. Wound cleansers remove wound debris as the wound is cleansed and washed. Wound cleansers are often over-the-counter products that can be used as a rinse or can be sprayed on the wound.

Medicare Information

See chapter titled "Medicare Guidelines," under "Dressings," for Medicare billing and documentation information.

A6261-A6262

A6261 Wound filler, gel/paste, per fl oz, not otherwise specified
A6262 Wound filler, dry form, per g, not otherwise specified

Lay Description

Wound fillers are dressing materials that are placed into open wounds to eliminate dead space and absorb exudate, or maintain a moist wound surface. Use these codes for wound fillers, gel/paste, or dry form not specifically listed elsewhere. Usual dressing change is up to once per day. Report A6261 for each fluid ounce of a gel or paste filler and A6262 for each gram of dry form filler.

Medicare Information

The units of service for wound fillers are 1 gram, 1 fluid ounce, or 6-inch length depending on the product. If the individual product is packaged as a fraction of a unit (e.g., 1/2 fluid ounce), determine the units billed by multiplying the number dispensed times the individual product size, and rounding to the nearest whole number. For example, if 11 1/2 oz. tubes of a wound filler are dispensed, bill six units (11 X 1/2 = 5.5; round to 6).

Note: See chapter titled "Medicare Guidelines," under "Dressings," for additional Medicare billing and documentation information.

A6266

A6266 Gauze, impregnated, other than water, normal saline, or zinc paste, sterile, any width, per linear yd

Lay Description

Impregnated gauze dressings are woven or non-woven materials in which substances such as iodinated agents, petrolatum, zinc compounds, crystalline sodium chloride, chlorhexidine gluconate (CHG), bismuth tribromophenate (BTP), water, aqueous saline, or other agents have been incorporated into the dressing material by the manufacturer. Report A6266 per linear yard of impregnated gauze when the impregnating substance used is other than water, normal saline, or zinc paste.

Medicare Information

See chapter titled "Medicare Guidelines," under "Dressings," for additional Medicare billing and documentation information.

A6402-A6404

A6402 Gauze, nonimpregnated, sterile, pad size 16 sq in or less, without adhesive border, each dressing
A6403 Gauze, nonimpregnated, sterile, pad size more than 16 sq in, less than or equal to 48 sq in, without adhesive border, each dressing
A6404 Gauze, nonimpregnated, sterile, pad size more than 48 sq in, without adhesive border, each dressing

Lay Description

Usual non-impregnated gauze dressing change is up to three times per day for a dressing without a border and once per day for a dressing with a border. It is usually not necessary to stack more than two gauze pads on top of each other in any one area. Report A6402 for each sterile, non-impregnated gauze pad dressing 16.0 sq. inches or smaller without an adhesive border. Report A6403 if the pad is larger than 16.0 sq. inches but smaller than or equal to 48.0 sq. inches and without an adhesive border. Report A6404 if the pad is larger than 48.0 sq. inches without a border.

Medicare Information

See chapter titled "Medicare Guidelines," under "Dressings," for Medicare billing and documentation information.

A6407

A6407 Packing strips, nonimpregnated, sterile, up to 2 in in width, per linear yd

Lay Description

Packing strips are placed in open wounds and are often used in wet-to-dry type of wound treatment. They are sterile supplies that are usually made of fine mesh cotton gauze. Some are impregnated with antiseptics, such as iodoform. Report A6407 for packing strips, up to two inches in width, per linear yard.

Medicare Information

See chapter titled "Medicare Guidelines," under "Dressings," for Medicare billing and documentation information.

A6410-A6412

A6410 Eye pad, sterile, each
A6411 Eye pad, nonsterile, each
A6412 Eye patch, occlusive, each

Lay Description

Eye pads are used to protect an injured eye from further injury by keeping the eyelid closed. Eye pads are usually constructed of soft absorbent cotton covered by fine mesh gauze and contoured to fit the eye. They may be sterile (A6410) or nonsterile (A6411) supplies. An occlusive eye patch may be used to protect an injured eye or to treat a condition such as amblyopia. Light occlusive eye patches, in addition to providing a soft absorbent pad, contain a film on the outer surface that blocks specific wavelengths of light. Report A6412 for each occlusive eye patch.

Medicare Information

See chapter titled "Medicare Guidelines," under "Dressings," for Medicare billing and documentation information.

A6413

A6413 Adhesive bandage, first aid type, any size, each

Lay Description

An adhesive bandage is a sterile piece of gauze or other absorptive material affixed to a fabric or film that has been coated with a pressure-sensitive adhesive. Report A6413 for each adhesive bandage.

A6441

A6441 Padding bandage, nonelastic, nonwoven/nonknitted, width greater than or equal to 3 in and less than 5 in, per yd

Lay Description

A nonelastic, nonwoven/nonknitted padding bandage is used to pad and protect the wound surface. Report A6441 for each yard of padding bandage with a width greater than or equal to 3 inches and less than 5 inches.

Medicare Information

See chapter titled "Medicare Guidelines," under "Dressings," for Medicare billing and documentation information.

A6442-A6447

A6442 Conforming bandage, nonelastic, knitted/woven, nonsterile, width less than 3 in, per yd
A6443 Conforming bandage, nonelastic, knitted/woven, nonsterile, width greater than or equal to 3 in and less than 5 in, per yd
A6444 Conforming bandage, nonelastic, knitted/woven, nonsterile, width greater than or equal to 5 in, per yd
A6445 Conforming bandage, nonelastic, knitted/woven, sterile, width less than 3 in, per yd
A6446 Conforming bandage, nonelastic, knitted/woven, sterile, width greater than or equal to 3 in and less than 5 in, per yd
A6447 Conforming bandage, nonelastic, knitted/woven, sterile, width greater than or equal to 5 in, per yd

Lay Description

Nonelastic conforming bandages are made of a knitted, crocheted, or woven material that allows them to stretch. Nonelastic conforming bandages are supplied in rolls that are then used to wrap the wound. Other dressings such as 2 X 2's or 4 X 4's may be layered under and held in place by the conforming bandage. Report A6442 for each yard of non-sterile conforming bandage with a width less than 3 inches; A6443 for a width greater than or equal to 3 inches but less than 5 inches; and A6444 for a width greater than or equal to 5 inches. Report A6445 for each yard of sterile conforming bandage with a width less than 3 inches; A6446 for a width greater than or equal to 3 inches but less than 5 inches; and A6447 for a width greater than or equal to 5 inches.

Medicare Information

See chapter titled "Medicare Guidelines," under "Dressings," for Medicare billing and documentation information.

A6448-A6452

A6448 Light compression bandage, elastic, knitted/woven, width less than 3 in, per yd
A6449 Light compression bandage, elastic, knitted/woven, width greater than or equal to 3 in and less than 5 in, per yd
A6450 Light compression bandage, elastic, knitted/woven, width greater than or equal to 5 in, per yd
A6451 Moderate compression bandage, elastic, knitted/woven, load resistance of 1.25 to 1.34 ft lbs at 50% maximum stretch, width greater than or equal to 3 in and less than 5 in, per yd
A6452 High compression bandage, elastic, knitted/woven, load resistance greater than or equal to 1.35 ft lbs at 50% maximum stretch, width greater than or equal to 3 in and less than 5 in, per yd

Lay Description

Elastic, knitted/woven compression bandages are used as support wraps for conditions such as sprains, strains, and venous ulcers. They come in a variety of types including variable stretch, limited stretch, and high stretch that provide varying degrees of compression. The type used depends on the condition or injury being treated. Report A6448 per yard for a light compression bandage, width less than 3 inches; A6449 for a width greater than or equal to 3 inches but less than 5 inches; and A6450 for a width greater than or equal to 5 inches. Report A6451 per yard for a moderate compression bandage, defined as a load resistance of 1.25 to 1.34 foot pounds at 50 percent maximum stretch for a width greater than or equal to 3 inches but less than 5 inches. Report A6452 per yard for a high compression bandage, defined as a load resistance of greater than or equal to 1.35 foot pounds at 50 percent maximum stretch for a width greater than or equal to 3 inches but less than 5 inches.

Medicare Information

See chapter titled "Medicare Guidelines," under "Dressings," for Medicare billing and documentation information.

A6453-A6455

A6453 Self-adherent bandage, elastic, nonknitted/nonwoven, width less than 3 in, per yd
A6454 Self-adherent bandage, elastic, nonknitted/nonwoven, width greater than or equal to 3 in and less than 5 in, per yd
A6455 Self-adherent bandage, elastic, nonknitted/nonwoven, width greater than or equal to 5 in, per yd

Lay Description

Elastic, self-adherent, nonknitted/nonwoven bandages are composed of laminated non-woven and elastic materials. The wrap is made of a material that will stick to itself, but will not adhere to other fabrics, materials, or the skin. It is supplied in rolls in a variety of widths. Report A6453 per yard of self-adherent bandage with a width of less than 3 inches; A6454 for a width greater than or equal to 3 inches but less than 5 inches; and A6455 for a width greater than or equal to 5 inches.

Medicare Information

See chapter titled "Medicare Guidelines," under "Dressings," for Medicare billing and documentation information.

A6456

A6456 Zinc paste impregnated bandage, nonelastic, knitted/woven, width greater than or equal to 3 in and less than 5 in, per yd

Lay Description

A nonelastic, knitted/woven zinc paste-impregnated bandage may be used as a wrap for venous insufficiency or other conditions. Zinc oxide paste-impregnated bandages stay soft and flexible and conform to the leg to promote healing. A zinc oxide paste-impregnated bandage is typically used under a compression bandage, which is reported separately. Report A6456 per yard for bandages that are greater than or equal to 3 inches but less than 5 inches in width.

Medicare Information

See chapter titled "Medicare Guidelines," under "Dressings," for Medicare billing and documentation information.

A6457

A6457 Tubular dressing with or without elastic, any width, per linear yard

Lay Description

Tubular dressing is a secondary dressing used to secure the primary dressing. It is used as an alternative to a gauze wrap or adhesive tape. Tubular dressings are available in a variety of materials including synthetic materials such as nylon or natural materials such as cotton. Some types of tubular dressings require application using a metal cage device while others can be placed by hand. Report A6457 per linear yard for any width of tubular dressing with or without elastic.

Medicare Information

See chapter titled "Medicare Guidelines," under "Dressings," for Medicare billing and documentation information.

A6501-A6513

A6501	Compression burn garment, bodysuit (head to foot), custom fabricated
A6502	Compression burn garment, chin strap, custom fabricated
A6503	Compression burn garment, facial hood, custom fabricated
A6504	Compression burn garment, glove to wrist, custom fabricated
A6505	Compression burn garment, glove to elbow, custom fabricated
A6506	Compression burn garment, glove to axilla, custom fabricated
A6507	Compression burn garment, foot to knee length, custom fabricated
A6508	Compression burn garment, foot to thigh length, custom fabricated
A6509	Compression burn garment, upper trunk to waist including arm openings (vest), custom fabricated
A6510	Compression burn garment, trunk, including arms down to leg openings (leotard), custom fabricated
A6511	Compression burn garment, lower trunk including leg openings (panty), custom fabricated
A6512	Compression burn garment, not otherwise classified
A6513	Compression burn mask, face and/or neck, plastic or equal, custom fabricated

Lay Description

Compression burn garments are used to reduce hypertrophic scarring and joint contractures following a burn injury. Report A6501 for a custom fabricated body suit, A6502 for a custom fabricated chin strap, A6503 for a custom fabricated facial hood, A6504 for a custom fabricated glove up to the wrist, A6505 for a glove up to the elbow, and A6506 for a glove to the axilla. Report A6507 for a custom burn garment from the foot to the knee, A6508 for a garment from the foot to the thigh, and A6509 for a custom garment for the upper trunk to the waist including arm openings. Report A6510 for a custom fabricated burn garment for the trunk (leotard), including arms down to the leg openings. Report A6511 for a burn garment for the lower trunk (panty) including leg openings. Report A6512 for a burn garment not otherwise specified. Report A6513 for a custom fabricated burn mask for the face and/or neck.

Medicare Information

See chapter titled "Medicare Guidelines," under "Dressings," for Medicare billing and documentation information.

A6530-A6535

A6530	Gradient compression stocking, below knee, 18-30 mm Hg, each
A6531	Gradient compression stocking, below knee, 30-40 mm Hg, each
A6532	Gradient compression stocking, below knee, 40-50 mm Hg, each
A6533	Gradient compression stocking, thigh length, 18-30 mm Hg, each
A6534	Gradient compression stocking, thigh length, 30-40 mm Hg, each
A6535	Gradient compression stocking, thigh length, 40-50 mm Hg, each

Lay Description

This range of codes reports the supply of below-the-knee and thigh length compression stockings. These stockings may be prescribed for a variety of conditions, such as prevention of deep vein thrombosis (DVT) or postoperative prevention of venous thromboembolisms. Gradient compression refers to the difference in pressure exerted over the length of the stocking. For example, the squeezing pressure at the ankle is usually greatest, gradually diminishing proximally toward the calf area. The pressure is expressed in millimeters of mercury (mmHg). The patient's anatomical dimensions and the presence of edema can affect sizing of these stockings. Pressures less than 15 mmHg are generally considered less than therapeutic. Pressures in the 18 to 20 mmHg range are considered mildly therapeutic for minor varicosity. Pressures in the 20 to 30 mmHg range are considered firm while those above 30 mmHg are considered extra firm.

Medicare Information

Medicare may cover compression stockings of 30–40 mmHg and 40–50 mmHg when used as a dressing. See chapter titled "Medicare Guidelines," under "Dressings," for Medicare billing and documentation information.

A6533-A6535

A6533 Gradient compression stocking, thigh length, 18-30 mm Hg, each
A6534 Gradient compression stocking, thigh length, 30-40 mm Hg, each
A6535 Gradient compression stocking, thigh length, 40-50 mm Hg, each

Lay Description

This range of codes reports the supply of thigh length compression stockings. These stockings may be prescribed for a variety of conditions, such as prevention of deep vein thrombosis (DVT) or postoperative prevention of venous thromboembolisms. Gradient compression refers to the difference in pressure exerted over the length of the stocking. For example, the squeezing pressure at the ankle is usually greatest, gradually diminishing proximally toward the thigh area. The pressure is expressed in millimeters of mercury (mmHg). The patient's anatomical dimensions and the presence of edema can affect sizing of these stockings. Pressures less than 15 mmHg are generally considered less than therapeutic. Pressures in the 18 to 20 mmHg range are considered mildly therapeutic for minor varicosity. Pressures in the 20 to 30 mmHg range are considered firm while those above 30 mmHg are considered extra firm. Report A6533 for supply of thigh length compression stockings rated in the 18-30-mmHg range; A6534 for supply of thigh length compression stockings rated in the 30-40 mmHg range; and A6535 for supply of thigh length compression stockings rated in the 40-50 mmHg range.

A6536-A6538

A6536 Gradient compression stocking, full-length/chap style, 18-30 mm Hg, each
A6537 Gradient compression stocking, full-length/chap style, 30-40 mm Hg, each
A6538 Gradient compression stocking, full-length/chap style, 40-50 mm Hg, each

Lay Description

This range of codes reports the supply of full length, chap style compression stockings. These stockings may be prescribed for a variety of conditions, such as prevention of deep vein thrombosis (DVT) or postoperative prevention of venous thromboembolisms. Gradient compression refers to the difference in pressure exerted over the length of the stocking. For example, the squeezing pressure at the ankle is usually greatest, gradually diminishing proximally toward the thigh and waist region. The pressure is expressed in millimeters of mercury (mmHg). The patient's anatomical dimensions and the presence of edema can affect sizing of these stockings. Pressures less than 15 mmHg are generally considered less than therapeutic. Pressures in the 18 to 20 mmHg range are considered mildly therapeutic for minor varicosity. Pressures in the 20 to 30 mmHg range are considered firm while those above 30 mmHg are considered extra firm. Report A6536 for supply of a full length, chap style compression stocking rated in the 18-30 mmHg range; A6537 for supply of full length, chap style compression stockings rated in the 30-40 mmHg range; and A6538 for supply of full length, chap style compression stockings rated in the 40-50 mmHg range.

A6539-A6544

A6539 Gradient compression stocking, waist length, 18-30 mm Hg, each
A6540 Gradient compression stocking, waist length, 30-40 mm Hg, each
A6541 Gradient compression stocking, waist length, 40-50 mm Hg, each
A6544 Gradient compression stocking, garter belt

Lay Description

This range of codes reports the supply of waist length compression stockings and related supplies for compression garments, as well as other supplies and accessories used with compression stockings. These stockings may be prescribed for a variety of conditions, such as prevention of deep vein thrombosis (DVT) or postoperative prevention of venous thromboembolisms. Gradient compression refers to the difference in pressure exerted over the length of the stocking. For example, the squeezing pressure at the ankle is usually greatest, gradually diminishing proximally toward the thigh and waist region. The pressure is expressed in millimeters of mercury (mmHg). The patient's anatomical dimensions and the presence of edema can affect sizing of these stockings. Pressures less than 15 mmHg are generally considered less than therapeutic. Pressures in the 18 to 20 mmHg range are considered mildly therapeutic for minor varicosity. Pressures in the 20 to 30 mmHg range are considered firm, while those above 30 mmHg are considered extra firm.

A6545

A6545 Gradient compression wrap, nonelastic, below knee, 30-50 mm Hg, each

Lay Description

This code reports the supply of a below knee gradient compression wrap. It uses adjustable bands to provide therapeutic compression levels. Compression wraps may be prescribed for a variety of conditions, such as lymphedema, and to treat venous disease and active venous stasis ulcers. Surgical removal of lymph nodes can cause lymphedema, a condition hallmarked by fluid retention and swelling in the affected extremity. Gradient compression refers to the difference in pressure exerted over the length of the wrap. For example, the squeezing pressure at the ankle is usually greatest, gradually diminishing proximally toward the thigh and waist region. The pressure is expressed in millimeters of mercury (mmHg). The components of the gradient wrap are a nonelastic binder that is fitted at the prescribed compression level using markers on the neoprene strip and a built in pressure system that runs posterior length of the device.

A6549

A6549   Gradient compression stocking/sleeve, not otherwise specified

Lay Description

Please refer to codes A6542-A6544 for the description, coding, and billing information.

A6550

A6550   Wound care set, for negative pressure wound therapy electrical pump, includes all supplies and accessories

Lay Description

Negative pressure wound therapy (NPWT), also called vacuum assisted closure (VAC), uses subatmospheric pressure to assist in treatment of acute, subacute, and chronic wounds. NPWT promotes healing by increasing local vascularity and oxygenation of the wound bed, evacuating wound fluid thereby reducing edema, and removing exudates and bacteria. The subatmospheric pressure is generated using an electrical pump that is reported as a separate supply (E2402). The electrical pump conveys intermittent or continuous subatmospheric pressure through connecting tubing to a specialized wound dressing. A specialized wound dressing includes porous foam dressing that covers the entire wound surface and an airtight adhesive dressing that seals the wound and contains the subatmospheric pressure at the wound site. Each wound care set inclusive of all supplies and accessories is reported with A6550.

A7000-A7002

A7000   Canister, disposable, used with suction pump, each
A7001   Canister, nondisposable, used with suction pump, each
A7002   Tubing, used with suction pump, each

Lay Description

Canisters to be used with suction pumps can be disposable or non-disposable. Canisters are made of a hard plastic and are used for collecting aspirated materials. Although they vary in size, they usually hold approximately 800 cc to 1200 cc, have a lid and splash guard. Tubing runs from the suction catheter to the canister to deliver the aspirated material. Report A7000 for a disposable canister used with a suction pump; A7001 for a non-disposable one, and A7002 for tubing used with a suction pump.

Documentation Standards

ICD-9-CM diagnosis code V44.0 should be entered on the claims form when billing.

Medicare Information

Supplies are covered when they are medically necessary and used with a medically necessary suction pump.

A7003-A7006

A7003   Administration set, with small volume nonfiltered pneumatic nebulizer, disposable
A7004   Small volume nonfiltered pneumatic nebulizer, disposable
A7005   Administration set, with small volume nonfiltered pneumatic nebulizer, nondisposable
A7006   Administration set, with small volume filtered pneumatic nebulizer

Lay Description

Nebulizer base equipment is comprised of an air compressor for airflow nebulization or a generator for nebulization of liquid by means of ultrasonic vibrations. The actual nebulizer is the chamber in which the nebulization of the liquid medication or solution for inhalation occurs. The nebulizing chamber is attached to the aerosol compressor or an ultrasonic generator. Nebulization therapy is considered beneficial to patients with a variety of respiratory and/or pulmonary conditions and diseases, including cystic fibrosis, bronchiectasis, chronic obstructive pulmonary disease, emphysema, severe asthma (when metered dose inhalers are ineffective), as well as other conditions such as AIDS, which requires the administration of medications like pentamidine. Small volume nebulizers are designed primarily to deliver inhalation medications. Nebulization occurs when

Coders' Desk Reference for HCPCS

the medication and/or solution to be administered is vaporized and subsequently inspired by the patient via the lungs, through which the medication enters the patient's system, or the medication has a direct effect on mucus retained by the lungs and bronchi (known as mucolytic action). Various accessory supplies may be required for use with the nebulizer. Report A7003 for a disposable or A7005 for a nondisposable administration set with small volume nonfiltered pneumatic nebulizer. Report A7006 for an administration set for a small volume filtered pneumatic nebulizer. Administration sets represented by A7003, A7005, and A7006 include the lid, jar baffles, tubing, T-piece, and mouthpiece. Report A7004 for a disposable small volume nonfiltered pneumatic nebulizer, which includes only the lid, jar, and baffles.

Medicare Information

Small-volume nebulizers, accessories, and supplies are covered when used to administer medically necessary inhalation therapy in the following specific instances:

- Beta-adrenergics, corticosteroids, and cromolyn for the management of obstructive pulmonary disease
- Gentamicin, tobramycin, amikacin, or dornase alfa for patients with cystic fibrosis
- Gentamicin for patients with bronchiectasis
- Pentamidine for patients with HIV pneumocystosis or posttransplant patients who experience complications
- Mucolytics, other than dornase alfa, for patients with thick or tenacious pulmonary secretions

Large-volume nebulizers, accessories, and supplies are covered when used to administer medically necessary humidified inhalation therapy to patients with thick, tenacious secretions with:

- Cystic fibrosis
- Bronchiectasis
- A tracheostomy
- A tracheobronchial stent
- HIV pneumocystosis

Nebulizers used to administer inhalation therapy for other than the above indications are not covered. Nebulizers used to administer noncovered drugs are not covered.

A7007-A7012

A7007   Large volume nebulizer, disposable, unfilled, used with aerosol compressor
A7008   Large volume nebulizer, disposable, prefilled, used with aerosol compressor
A7009   Reservoir bottle, nondisposable, used with large volume ultrasonic nebulizer
A7010   Corrugated tubing, disposable, used with large volume nebulizer, 100 ft
A7011   Corrugated tubing, nondisposable, used with large volume nebulizer, 10 ft
A7012   Water collection device, used with large volume nebulizer

Lay Description

Nebulizer base equipment is comprised of an air compressor for airflow nebulization or a generator for nebulization of liquid by means of ultrasonic vibrations. The actual nebulizer is the chamber in which the nebulization occurs. The nebulizing chamber is attached to the aerosol compressor or an ultrasonic generator. Large volume nebulizers are designed to deliver humidified gas, such as oxygen, in concentrations ranging from 28 percent to 98 percent along with medications. Large volume nebulizers are useful in the treatment of conditions such as cystic fibrosis, bronchiectasis, and tracheostomy where humidified gas assists in thinning respiratory secretions. Large volume nebulizers are also useful for administration of pentamidine in the treatment of HIV. Various accessory supplies may be required for use with the nebulizer. Report A7007 for an unfilled or A7008 for a prefilled, disposable large volume nebulizer to be used with aerosol compressor. Report A7009 for a nondisposable reservoir bottle; A7010 for each 100 feet of corrugated tubing; A7011 for each 10 feet of corrugated tubing; and A7012 for a water collection device.

Medicare Information

Small-volume nebulizers, accessories, and supplies are covered when used to administer medically necessary inhalation therapy in the following specific instances:

- Beta-adrenergics, corticosteroids, and cromolyn for the management of obstructive pulmonary disease
- Gentamicin, tobramycin, amikacin, or dornase alfa for patients with cystic fibrosis
- Gentamicin for patients with bronchiectasis
- Pentamidine for patients with HIV pneumocystosis or posttransplant patients who experience complications
- Mucolytics, other than dornase alfa, for patients with thick or tenacious pulmonary secretions

Large-volume nebulizers, accessories, and supplies are covered when used to administer medically necessary humidified inhalation therapy to patients with thick, tenacious secretions with:

- Cystic fibrosis
- Bronchiectasis
- A tracheostomy
- A tracheobronchial stent
- HIV pneumocystosis

Nebulizers used to administer inhalation therapy for other than the above indications are not covered. Nebulizers used to administer noncovered drugs are not covered.

A7013-A7016

A7013 Filter, disposable, used with aerosol compressor or ultrasonic generator
A7014 Filter, nondisposable, used with aerosol compressor or ultrasonic generator
A7015 Aerosol mask, used with DME nebulizer
A7016 Dome and mouthpiece, used with small volume ultrasonic nebulizer

Lay Description

Nebulizer base equipment is comprised of an air compressor for airflow nebulization or a generator for nebulization of liquid by means of ultrasonic vibrations. The actual nebulizer is the chamber in which the nebulization occurs. The nebulizing chamber is attached to the aerosol compressor or an ultrasonic generator. Various accessory supplies may be required for use with the nebulizer. Report A7013 for a disposable filter used with an aerosol compressor; A7014 for a nondisposable filter used with an aerosol compressor or ultrasonic generator; A7015 for an aerosol mask; and A7016 for a dome and mouthpiece to be used with a small volume ultrasonic nebulizer.

Medicare Information

An enrolled DME supplier must bill this item to the DME MAC.

Small-volume nebulizers, accessories, and supplies are covered when used to administer medically necessary inhalation therapy in the following specific instances:

- Beta-adrenergics, corticosteroids, and cromolyn for the management of obstructive pulmonary disease
- Gentamicin, tobramycin, amikacin, or dornase alfa for patients with cystic fibrosis
- Gentamicin for patients with bronchiectasis
- Pentamidine for patients with HIV pneumocystosis or posttransplant patients who experience complications
- Mucolytics, other than dornase alfa, for patients with thick or tenacious pulmonary secretions

Large-volume nebulizers, accessories, and supplies are covered when used to administer medically necessary humidified inhalation therapy to patients with thick, tenacious secretions with:

- Cystic fibrosis
- Bronchiectasis
- A tracheostomy
- A tracheobronchial stent
- HIV pneumocystosis

Nebulizers used to administer inhalation therapy for other than the above indications are not covered. Nebulizers used to administer noncovered drugs are not covered.

A7017

A7017 Nebulizer, durable, glass or autoclavable plastic, bottle type, not used with oxygen

Lay Description

A nebulizer is an apparatus for producing a fine spray or mist. This may be made by rapidly passing air through a liquid or by vibrating a liquid at a high frequency so that the particles produced are extremely small. Use this code to report a durable, bottle-type nebulizer made of glass or plastic that can be sterilized in an autoclave and is not used with oxygen.

Medicare Information

Small-volume nebulizers, accessories, and supplies are covered when used to administer medically necessary inhalation therapy in the following specific instances:

- Beta-adrenergics, corticosteroids, and cromolyn for the management of obstructive pulmonary disease
- Gentamicin, tobramycin, amikacin, or dornase alfa for patients with cystic fibrosis
- Gentamicin for patients with bronchiectasis
- Pentamidine for patients with HIV pneumocystosis or posttransplant patients who experience complications
- Mucolytics, other than dornase alfa, for patients with thick or tenacious pulmonary secretions

Large-volume nebulizers, accessories, and supplies are covered when used to administer medically necessary humidified inhalation therapy to patients with thick, tenacious secretions with:

- Cystic fibrosis
- Bronchiectasis
- A tracheostomy

© 2010 Ingenix

- A tracheobronchial stent
- HIV pneumocystosis

Nebulizers used to administer inhalation therapy for other than the above indications are not covered. Nebulizers used to administer noncovered drugs are not covered.

A7018

A7018 Water, distilled, used with large volume nebulizer, 1000 ml

Lay Description

Nebulizer base equipment is comprised of an air compressor for airflow nebulization or a generator for nebulization of liquid by means of ultrasonic vibrations. The actual nebulizer is the chamber in which the nebulization occurs. The nebulizing chamber is attached to the aerosol compressor or an ultrasonic generator. Large volume nebulizers are designed to deliver humidified gas, such as oxygen, in concentrations ranging from 28 percent to 98 percent along with medications. Large volume nebulizers are useful in the treatment of conditions such as cystic fibrosis, bronchiectasis, and tracheostomy where humidified gas assists in thinning respiratory secretions. Large volume nebulizers are also useful for administration of pentamidine in the treatment of HIV. Various accessory supplies may be required for use with the nebulizer. Distilled water (1,000 cc) supplied for use with a large volume nebulizer is reported with A7018.

Medicare Information

Small-volume nebulizers, accessories, and supplies are covered when used to administer medically necessary inhalation therapy in the following specific instances:

- Beta-adrenergics, corticosteroids, and cromolyn for the management of obstructive pulmonary disease
- Gentamicin, tobramycin, amikacin, or dornase alfa for patients with cystic fibrosis
- Gentamicin for patients with bronchiectasis
- Pentamidine for patients with HIV pneumocystosis or posttransplant patients who experience complications
- Mucolytics, other than dornase alfa, for patients with thick or tenacious pulmonary secretions

Large-volume nebulizers, accessories, and supplies are covered when used to administer medically necessary humidified inhalation therapy to patients with thick, tenacious secretions with:

- Cystic fibrosis
- Bronchiectasis

- A tracheostomy
- A tracheobronchial stent
- HIV pneumocystosis

Nebulizers used to administer inhalation therapy for other than the above indications are not covered. Nebulizers used to administer noncovered drugs are not covered.

A7025-A7026

A7025 High frequency chest wall oscillation system vest, replacement for use with patient-owned equipment, each

A7026 High frequency chest wall oscillation system hose, replacement for use with patient-owned equipment, each

Lay Description

These codes report replacement supplies that are used with a patient owned, high-frequency chest wall oscillation (HFCWO) system. The vest component consists of an inflatable vest connected by tubes to an air-pulse generator. The air-pulse generator rapidly inflates and deflates the vest, compressing and releasing the chest wall. HFCWO allows the patient to clear mucus by generating increased airflow velocities that create repetitive cough-like shear forces and decrease the viscosity of secretions. Report A7025 for replacement of a high frequency chest wall oscillation system vest and A7026 for replacement of a system hose.

Medicare Information

Medicare may cover these devices when medically necessary to treat well-documented failure of standard treatment to adequately mobilize secretions in:

- Patients with cystic fibrosis
- Patients with bronchiectasis characterized by daily productive cough for at least six continuous months, or more than two exacerbations a year requiring antibiotic treatment, and confirmed by high resolution spiral or standard CT scan.

Coverage is at the contractor's discretion.

A7027-A7029

A7027 Combination oral/nasal mask, used with continuous positive airway pressure device, each

A7028 Oral cushion for combination oral/nasal mask, replacement only, each

A7029 Nasal pillows for combination oral/nasal mask, replacement only, pair

Lay Description

Code A7027 describes a combination oral/nasal mask used with a continuous positive airway pressure device (CPAP). The mask is connected to tubing and a swivel connector, which is then connected to the continuos positive pressure device. Report A7028 for replacement of the oral cushion used for the combination oral/nasal mask. Report A7029 for replacement of the nasal pillows used for the combination oral/nasal mask.

A7030-A7039

A7030 Full face mask used with positive airway pressure device, each
A7031 Face mask interface, replacement for full face mask, each
A7032 Cushion for use on nasal mask interface, replacement only, each
A7033 Pillow for use on nasal cannula type interface, replacement only, pair
A7034 Nasal interface (mask or cannula type) used with positive airway pressure device, with or without head strap
A7035 Headgear used with positive airway pressure device
A7036 Chinstrap used with positive airway pressure device
A7037 Tubing used with positive airway pressure device
A7038 Filter, disposable, used with positive airway pressure device
A7039 Filter, nondisposable, used with positive airway pressure device

Lay Description

CPAP is a noninvasive method of providing air pressure through the patient's nostrils, usually through a nasal mask or flow generator system. These devices are used primarily in conservative therapy (vs. surgery) for patients with documented sleep apnea; however, not all patients benefit from this conservative approach because some cannot tolerate the CPAP device during sleep. The CPAP device assists the patient in nocturnal respiration (during sleep), particularly when the patient's oropharyngeal tissues relax, collapse, and/or otherwise obstruct the normal airflow during inspiration and expiration, causing a variety of symptoms including hypersomnolence during the day, loss of concentration, headache, agitation, depression, fatigue, and many others. Report A7030 for a full facemask. Report A7031 for a facemask interface, a replacement for the full facemask. Report A7032 for a replacement cushion for a nasal application device; A7033 for a pair of replacement pillows for a nasal application device; A7034 for a mask or cannula type nasal interface used with CPAP, with or without head strap; A7035 for headgear; A7036 for a chin strap; A7037 for tubing; A7038 for a disposable filter; and A7039 for a nondisposable filter used with a CPAP device.

Documentation Standards

Initial coverage is based upon documentation that proves that coverage criteria have been met. The initial coverage is for three months. Continued coverage will be provided if the supplier can ascertain from the patient or physician that the patient is continuing to use the CPAP device. This determination of use cannot be made any sooner than the 61st day after therapy has been initiated.

Claims for more than the anticipated maximum accessory amounts will be denied as not medically necessary, unless accompanied by additional documentation that justifies why the greater-than-anticipated quantity is being claimed for reimbursement.

Effective with dates of service on or after July 1, 2002, a CMN is no longer required for CPAP. Claims for dates of service prior to July 1, 2002, still require that a CMN be completed and filed with the initial claim.

The formal or separate physician order for the CPAP device is required.

Copies of the patient's sleep lab evaluation, including polysomnogram, pulmonary function tests, and oxygen saturations, must be retained in the provider's record.

Polysomnography, as recognized by the Medicare program, is the continuous and simultaneous monitoring and recording of various physiological and pathophysiological parameters of sleep for six or more hours with provider review, interpretation, and report. The study must include sleep staging, defined as a one-to-four lead electroencephalogram (EEG), electro-oculogram (EOG), and submental electromyogram (EMG). The study must also include at least these characteristics of sleep: airflow, respiratory effort, and O2 saturation by oximetry.

The polysomnogram must be performed in a facility-based sleep study laboratory. Sleep studies performed in the home, a mobile facility, or performed by the DME MAC are not considered acceptable proof for coverage criteria. The facility laboratory must be a qualified Medicare provider and must comply with all federal and state regulations.

Medicare Information

Continuous positive airway pressure (CPAP) devices and accessories are covered for patients with a diagnosis of obstructive sleep apnea (OSA). Services furnished between January 1987 and March 31, 2002 were covered if there was documentation of at least 30 episodes of apnea, each lasting a minimum of 10 seconds, during six to seven hours of recorded sleep. Medicare provided coverage for patients with moderate or severe OSA for whom surgery was a likely alternative. Effective with services furnished on or after April 1, 2002, criteria were changed to include the Apnea-Hypopnea Index (AHI). Coverage for a CPAP to be used for adult patients with OSA is available when ordered and prescribed by the licensed treating physician, and if one of the following is documented:

- The AHI is greater than or equal to 15 events per hour
- The AHI is greater than or equal to five and less than or equal to 14 events per hour, with documented symptoms of excessive daytime sleepiness, impaired condition, mood disorders or insomnia; or documented hypertension, ischemic heart disease, or a history of stroke
- The AHI is equal to the average number of episodes per hour of apnea or hypopnea. It must be based upon a minimum of two hours of sleep recorded by a polysomnogram. It must be based upon actual recorded hours of sleep and cannot be extrapolated or projected

The supplier must take steps to determine if the device is being used. If at any time the patient stops using the CPAP, the supplier must stop billing for the equipment and related supplies.

The following table outlines the usual maximum amount of accessories that are anticipated as medically necessary when a base CPAP device is prescribed. Accessories used with CPAP devices should be billed separately, whether the device is rented or purchased. Accessories are reimbursable at the time of the original provision and as they are placed. The following accessories may be eligible for Medicare coverage:

Accessories	Medicare Coverage
A7034	1 per 3 months
A7032, A7033	2 every month
A7035	1 per 6 months
A7036	1 per 6 months
A7037	1 every month
A7038	2 every month
A7039	1 per 6 months

Medicare modifiers
The following modifier may need to be reported on Medicare claims, when appropriate:

KX — Specific required documentation on file

A7040-A7041
A7040 One way chest drain valve
A7041 Water seal drainage container and tubing for use with implanted chest tube

Lay Description
Chest tubes are inserted into the pleural space to drain blood, fluid, or air from the pleural cavity and to allow full expansion of the lungs. The chest tube is inserted through an incision between the ribs into the pleural space and connected to a water seal system to prevent air from being sucked into the chest cavity and to allow the continuous or intermittent removal of fluid. A water seal thoracic drainage unit for removal of fluids from the thoracic cavity of a patient can use one, two, or three containers. A single-container water seal consists of a drainage collection container that also serves as the water seal. The container is initially filled with 100 ml of sterile water to form the seal. A two-container water seal is comprised of a collection chamber for receiving fluids from the patient and a second container that provides the underwater seal. Generally, the water or other liquid for the seal is provided with the collection chamber and water seal container as a complete unit ready for use. A three-container water seal system uses a collection chamber, a water seal container, and a third container that provides suction control. Report A7041 for the supply of a water seal drainage container and the tubing required to connect the container to the chest tube. A one-way chest drain valve (A7040) may be used to prevent backflow of fluid into the chest.

Medicare Information
This device may be covered when medically necessary to treat the patient's medical condition. Coverage is at the contractor's discretion.

A7042-A7043
A7042 Implanted pleural catheter, each
A7043 Vacuum drainage bottle and tubing for use with implanted catheter

Lay Description
An implantable pleural catheter and drainage kit is used for long-term treatment of symptomatic, chronic/recurrent, malignant, pleural effusion. This type of implantable catheter allows intermittent drainage of the effusion. The small-bore catheter consists of three sections: internal, middle, and external. The internal section has a fenestrated end that is placed into the pleural space. The middle section is tunneled through the skin for several inches. The external section includes an exposed length of catheter with a one-way valve. A separate

drainage kit is required that includes a lightweight, plastic, vacuum drainage bottle and tubing. Each day or as needed the patient or caregiver drains the pleural fluid by temporarily attaching the external length of catheter to the tubing, which is connected to the pre-evacuated (vacuum) drainage bottle. Report the implantable pleural catheter supply with A7042 and the drainage kit (drainage bottle and tubing) with A7043.

Medicare Information

These devices may be covered when medically necessary to treat the patient's medical condition. Coverage is at the contractor's discretion.

A7044

A7044   Oral interface used with positive airway pressure device, each

Lay Description

This code reports the supply of each oral interface used with a positive airway pressure (PAP) device. Such devices may also be prescribed for use on a continuous basis (CPAP). The oral interface may be a removable tube-like component that the patient uses during treatment. The interface for CPAP is likely to be of the nasal mask or cannula variety reported by A7034, although either CPAP or PAP systems may require a more customized device for access to the oral airway. Report A7044 for supply of each oral interface used with a positive airway pressure device.

A7045

A7045   Exhalation port with or without swivel used with accessories for positive airway devices, replacement only

Lay Description

Some masks used with positive pressure airway devices require the use of an accessory supply called an exhalation port to function properly. An exhalation port allows predetermined amounts of exhaled air to "leak" through the exhalation port. This is necessary to properly exhaust exhaled CO_2 from the mask so the patient does not rebreathe the CO_2. Some masks have a swivel device that allows the circuit tubing to move freely. Report A7045 for an exhalation port with or without swivel used with accessories for positive airway devices, replacement only.

Medicare Information

Positive pressure airway devices, accessories, and related supplies may be covered when used to treat the following conditions:

- Restrictive thoracic disorders, such as neuromuscular diseases, that restrict respiration and create reduced oxygen flow
- Severe chronic obstructive pulmonary disease
- Central sleep apnea diagnosed after a complete facility-based attended polysomnogram
- Obstructive sleep apnea diagnosed after a complete facility-based attended polysomnogram

A7046

A7046   Water chamber for humidifier, used with positive airway pressure device, replacement, each

Lay Description

Some humidifiers used with positive airway pressure devices have separate water chambers. The water chamber holds the water used in the humidifier. Removable water chambers are more easily cleaned. This code reports replacement of a removable water chamber.

Medicare Information

Positive pressure airway devices, accessories, and related supplies may be covered when used to treat the following conditions:

- Restrictive thoracic disorders, such as neuromuscular diseases, that restrict respiration and create reduced oxygen flow
- Severe chronic obstructive pulmonary disease
- Central sleep apnea diagnosed after a complete facility-based attended polysomnogram
- Obstructive sleep apnea diagnosed after a complete facility-based attended polysomnogram

A7501-A7502

A7501   Tracheostoma valve, including diaphragm, each
A7502   Replacement diaphragm/faceplate for tracheostoma valve, each

Lay Description

This code reports the supply of a tracheostoma valve, including diaphragm. These devices are typically used by laryngectomees who retain a level of potential voice function. Designs such as the prototypical Blom-Singer provide the user a means to speak without first manually occluding the stoma with a finger. Tracheostoma valves are often two-unit devices. A faceplate inserts over the tracheostoma. A disposable diaphragm in the valve can be adjusted to control airflow through the stomal opening. When the diaphragm is closed, or near closed, speech can be accomplished. The diaphragm may be set to allow one-way airflow upon expiration. Report A7501 for supply of each tracheostoma valve, including diaphragm. Report A7502 for replacement of the diaphragm and/or faceplate of the tracheostoma valve.

Medicare Information

See chapter titled "Medicare Guidelines," under "Ostomy Devices and Supplies," for Medicare billing and documentation information.

A7503-A7506

A7503 Filter holder or filter cap, reusable, for use in a tracheostoma heat and moisture exchange system, each
A7504 Filter for use in a tracheostoma heat and moisture exchange system, each
A7505 Housing, reusable without adhesive, for use in a heat and moisture exchange system and/or with a tracheostoma valve, each
A7506 Adhesive disc for use in a heat and moisture exchange system and/or with tracheostoma valve, any type each

Lay Description

A tracheostoma heat and moisture exchange system is used by some tracheostomy patients to add warmth and water vapor to the air when they inhale. A heat and moisture exchange system can retain up to 60 percent of the humidity in the patient's airway, greatly reducing coughing and mucus production. It consists of a reusable plastic holder or cap (A7503), also referred to as a cassette, that contains a filter (A7504) made of foam, paper, or other material. The holder fits into reusable plastic housing (A7505) that is held in place over the tracheostoma by an adhesive disc (A7506). A heat and moisture exchanger may be used by itself or in addition to a tracheostoma valve.

Medicare Information

See chapter titled "Medicare Guidelines," under "Ostomy Devices and Supplies," for Medicare billing and documentation information.

A7507-A7509

A7507 Filter holder and integrated filter without adhesive, for use in a tracheostoma heat and moisture exchange system, each
A7508 Housing and integrated adhesive, for use in a tracheostoma heat and moisture exchange system and/or with a tracheostoma valve, each
A7509 Filter holder and integrated filter housing, and adhesive, for use as a tracheostoma heat and moisture exchange system, each

Lay Description

A tracheostoma heat and moisture exchange system is used by some tracheostomy patients to add warmth and water vapor to the air when they inhale. A heat and moisture exchange system can retain up to 60 percent of the humidity in the patient's airway, greatly reducing coughing and mucus production. Some heat and moisture exchange systems use integrated components. A filter holder with integrated filter without adhesive is reported with A7507; housing with integrated adhesive is reported with A7508; and a filter holder with integrated filter housing and adhesive is reported with A7509.

Medicare Information

See chapter titled "Medicare Guidelines," under "Ostomy Devices and Supplies," for Medicare billing and documentation information.

A7520-A7522

A7520 Tracheostomy/laryngectomy tube, noncuffed, polyvinylchloride (PVC), silicone or equal, each
A7521 Tracheostomy/laryngectomy tube, cuffed, polyvinylchloride (PVC), silicone or equal, each
A7522 Tracheostomy/laryngectomy tube, stainless steel or equal (sterilizable and reusable), each

Lay Description

A tracheostomy/laryngectomy tube, also called a trach tube, is a curved tube that is inserted into a tracheostomy stoma (the surgically created hole made in the neck and windpipe). Tracheostomy tubes can be made of a variety of materials including metal, plastic, or silicone. Plastic and silicone tubes have the advantage of being lighter weight with less crusting of secretions than with metal tubes. Tracheostomy tubes come in cuffed and uncuffed models. A cuff is a soft balloon around the distal (far) end of the tube. The cuff is inflated with air, foam, or sterile water to allow for mechanical ventilation in patients with respiratory failure. Cuffs can be low or high volume. The low volume cuff is round while a high volume cuff is barrel-shaped. The high volume cuff spreads the pressure out over a larger surface area and may be better at averting complications such as stenosis than the low volume cuff that tends to push on one spot in the airway. When the balloon is deflated, the tube allows air around the tube for vocalization. Report A7420 for a cuffed and A7421 for a noncuffed tracheostomy tube constructed of polyvinylchloride (PVC), silicone, or other plastic. Stainless steel or other metal tracheostomy tubes are reported with A7522.

Medicare Information

See chapter titled "Medicare Guidelines," under "Ostomy Devices and Supplies," for Medicare billing and documentation information.

A7523

A7523 Tracheostomy shower protector, each

Lay Description

A tracheostomy shower protector is used to protect the tracheostomy stoma (the surgically created hole made in the neck and windpipe) from water, soaps, and shampoos when showering. Tracheostomy shower protectors are made of waterproof materials such as latex and fit like a bib over the stoma site to shield and deflect the water from the stoma site when showering.

Medicare Information

See chapter titled "Medicare Guidelines," under "Ostomy Devices and Supplies," for Medicare billing and documentation information.

A7524

A7524 Tracheostoma stent/stud/button, each

Lay Description

A tracheostoma stent, stud, or button is a rigid cannula that is placed into the tracheostoma after removal of a tracheostomy tube. These devices are used primarily for conditions such as obstructive sleep apnea where the patient requires the tracheostoma for breathing at night, but does not need it for breathing during the day. A stent, stud, or button allows the stoma to be closed and the patient to breathe through the nose and mouth instead of through the tracheostoma site during the day. These devices do not extend into the tracheal lumen so patients are able to breath and talk normally when these types of devices are in place.

Medicare Information

See chapter titled "Medicare Guidelines," under "Ostomy Devices and Supplies," for Medicare billing and documentation information.

A7525

A7525 Tracheostomy mask, each

Lay Description

Tracheostomy masks are used in conjunction with nebulizers. They are composed of a flexible mask-shaped plastic covering that fits securely over the tracheostomy tube. The outer portion has an opening that connects with the nebulizer tubing. Masks are used for ventilation and to humidify inspired air.

Medicare Information

See chapter titled "Medicare Guidelines," under "Ostomy Devices and Supplies," for Medicare billing and documentation information.

A7526

A7526 Tracheostomy tube collar/holder, each

Lay Description

A tracheostomy tube collar or holder attaches to each side of the tracheostomy tube and then loosely wraps around the back of the neck. A tracheostomy tube holder or collar is used to secure the tracheostomy tube in place. Collars and holders are made of a variety of materials that include stainless steel metal chains, laminates of foam and nylon, plastics, and other materials.

Medicare Information

See chapter titled "Medicare Guidelines," under "Ostomy Devices and Supplies," for Medicare billing and documentation information.

A7527

A7527 Tracheostomy/laryngectomy tube plug/stop, each

Lay Description

This code reports the specialized plug or stopper for use with a tracheostomy, fenestration, or laryngectomy tube, which the patient has in place. The plug, also called a decannulation plug, is used to obstruct the proximal end of the tube and permit breathing through the fenestration and the upper airway. Using the plug with the tube facilitates weaning in preparation for extubation and aids in speaking.

A8000-A8004

A8000 Helmet, protective, soft, prefabricated, includes all components and accessories
A8001 Helmet, protective, hard, prefabricated, includes all components and accessories
A8002 Helmet, protective, soft, custom fabricated, includes all components and accessories
A8003 Helmet, protective, hard, custom fabricated, includes all components and accessories
A8004 Soft interface for helmet, replacement only

Lay Description

Protective helmets are head coverings used to prevent or lessen injury or damage to the head. The helmets may be composed of hard material such as hard plastic or soft material such as nylon or fabric. Protective helmets may be used to protect patients prone to falling or hitting their head. Prefabricated helmets are pre-made and are usually purchased off the shelf. Custom-fabricated helmets are constructed specifically for a patient using the patient's physical measurements and needs. Helmets may contain straps or belts to hold the helmet on the head. Report

HCPCS Level II code A8000 for a prefabricated soft helmet, A8001 for a prefabricated hard helmet, A8002 for a custom-fabricated soft helmet, and A8003 for a custom-fabricated hard helmet. Codes A8000-A8003 include all components and accessories. HCPCS Level II code A8004 represents a replacement soft interface.

A9150

A9150 Nonprescription drugs

Lay Description

This code reports drugs that do not require a prescription, also referred to as over-the-counter (OTC) drugs. Identify the specific drug provided, as well as the strength, amount, and condition being treated.

Medicare Information

See chapter titled "Medicare Guidelines," under "Drugs, Biologicals, and Radiopharmaceuticals," for Medicare billing and documentation information.

A9152-A9153

A9152 Single vitamin/mineral/trace element, oral, per dose, not otherwise specified
A9153 Multiple vitamins, with or without minerals and trace elements, oral, per dose, not otherwise specified

Lay Description

Code A9152 reports one oral dose of a single vitamin, mineral, or trace element. Code A9153 reports one oral dose of multiple vitamins, which may or may not contain minerals and trace elements. Vitamins are organic substances found in small amounts within foods. Minerals are nonorganic solid substances found in the earth's crust. Trace mineral elements occur in very small amounts. These are essential nutrients needed by the body in varying, small amounts for proper metabolic function.

A9155

A9155 Artificial saliva, 30 ml

Lay Description

Natural saliva is more than 99 percent water, with some buffering agents, enzymes, and minerals. Saliva coats, lubricates, and helps cleanse the tissues in the mouth. It also begins the digestive process as we chew. When the saliva glands do not produce enough saliva, the mouth becomes dry. Artificial saliva is intended to replace natural saliva. Artificial saliva usually contains water, a mixture of buffering agents, cellulose derivatives, and flavoring agents. However, it does not contain the digestive and antibacterial enzymes, other proteins, or minerals present in real saliva. Artificial saliva is used to treat xerostomia, or dry mouth, which results from an inadequate flow of saliva. Drying irritates the soft tissues in the mouth, which can make them inflamed and more susceptible to infection. HCPCS Level II code A9155 represents 30 ml. of artificial saliva.

A9180

A9180 Pediculosis (lice infestation) treatment, topical, for administration by patient/caretaker

Lay Description

A pediculicide is a topical medication applied to hair used to treat lice infestations. Pediculicides are available in both over-the-counter (OTC) formulas and by prescription. OTC formulas include pyrethrins, a natural extract from the chrysanthemum flower, sometimes in combination with piperonyl butoxide. Another OTC formula is permethrin. Prescription medications include malathion and lindane. Treatment is the same regardless of whether an OTC or prescription medication is used. The pediculicide is applied to unwashed hair. After approximately eight to 12 hours, the hair should be checked for live lice. The hair should be combed to remove dead lice and any remaining live lice. The hair should be combed daily with a fine tooth or nit comb and checked every two to three days for the presence of live lice. The hair should be retreated seven to 10 days after the first treatment. HCPCS Level II code A9180 represents this self-administered drug.

A9270

A9270 Noncovered item or service

Lay Description

Noncovered services are services that are billed to the patient. In many cases, the beneficiary is already aware that the services are noncovered because they are included in the information given in the Medicare handbook (e.g., oral medications, screening mammograms in less than the designated waiting period, etc.) or by their insurance provider. At other times, the services are listed as noncovered because they are considered either experimental or investigational in nature.

A9273

A9273 Hot water bottle, ice cap or collar, heat and/or cold wrap, any type

Lay Description

An ice cap or collar is a cold therapy application to deliver treatment to affected tissues, usually following a surgical procedure or trauma. Cold therapy is generally used in the immediate postoperative or post-trauma period to reduce edema and control pain. An ice cap or collar is a passive method to deliver cold therapy. A hot water bottle is a container, usually made of plastic or rubber, that may be filled with hot or cold water and applied to an injured or painful body part.

A9274

A9274   External ambulatory insulin delivery system, disposable, each, includes all supplies and accessories

Lay Description

External ambulatory insulin delivery systems, also called insulin pumps, are computerized, battery-powered delivery devices with programming capabilities. These devices are used as a treatment for people with insulin-dependent diabetes mellitus. A sterile reservoir is filled with rapid-acting insulin. The sterile reservoir is connected to the patient by a thin plastic tube that has a small catheter needle attached. The needle is usually inserted into the subcutaneous tissue of the abdomen. The device continuously delivers micro-doses of insulin at a programmed rate. HCPCS Level II code A9274 represents one system, including all supplies and accessories.

A9275

A9275   Home glucose disposable monitor, includes test strips

Lay Description

Glucometers are used for patients with all types of diabetes mellitus to monitor blood glucose and are available in a variety of models with various features, including disposable home glucose monitors. Whether or not the patient is on insulin, many diabetics require frequent, if not daily, blood glucose monitoring. For Type I diabetes mellitus patients who require insulin (the patient's body does not manufacture insulin and therefore it must come from an external source, such as injections), blood glucose monitoring is a life-sustaining requirement. Disposable types of home glucose monitors are provided with test strips that are inserted into the monitor to provide a glucose reading. When all of the test strips have been used or upon the expiration date of the meter, whichever comes first, the patient discards the entire unit (meter and any remaining test strips). Report A9275 for a disposable home glucose monitor with test strips.

A9276-A9278

A9276   Sensor; invasive (e.g., subcutaneous), disposable, for use with interstitial continuous glucose monitoring system, 1 unit = 1 day supply

A9277   Transmitter; external, for use with interstitial continuous glucose monitoring system

A9278   Receiver (monitor); external, for use with interstitial continuous glucose monitoring system

Lay Description

Continuous glucose monitoring systems make continuous measurements of glucose levels. Many of these devices take measurements from subcutaneous tissue rather than from blood. Most systems consist of a sensor that is attached to the back of the arm or abdomen. The sensor has a very thin wire that is inserted subcutaneously. The wire then measures the glucose level in interstitial fluid that exits between the cells. The sensor is attached to a transmitter that sends the glucose readings to a wireless receiver. The receiver is a small computerized device that records and stores the glucose readings. The following HCPCS Level II codes represent replacement components for a continuous glucose monitoring system: A9276 represents the sensor that is partially implanted into the subcutaneous tissue (one sensor is one day's supply); A9277 is the external transmitter; and A9278 is the receiver.

A9279

A9279   Monitoring feature/device, stand-alone or integrated, any type, includes all accessories, components and electronics, not otherwise classified

Lay Description

This code may be applied to numerous technologies and is nonspecific. HCPCS Level II code A9279 represents an entire system, whether stand-alone or integrated into a delivery system. It includes all accessories, components and electronics. Report a more specific code if there is one available.

A9280

A9280   Alert or alarm device, not otherwise classified

Lay Description

This code reports alert or alarm devices that do not have a more specific code available. Provide a detailed description of the device when reporting A9280.

A9281

A9281 Reaching/grabbing device, any type, any length, each

Lay Description

A reaching/grabbing device is used to pick up objects without twisting the wrist. It typically lifts objects that are 5 lbs. or less. It is often used by people who have difficulty lifting objects due to arthritic conditions, small hands, or who have restrictive movement.

A9282

A9282 Wig, any type, each

Lay Description

A hairpiece of human or artificial hair worn as personal adornment or to conceal baldness. A wig or hairpiece is a supply for hair loss.

A9283

A9283 Foot pressure off loading/supportive device, any type, each

Lay Description

This code reflects various devices used to reduce pressure on the foot to help prevent ulcers. The device usually has an antibacterial layer and an inner layer that may contain gel, foam, small beads, or other pressure reducing material that help support and redistribute the pressure of the foot. The patient can usually adjust the device as needed.

A9284

A9284 Spirometer, nonelectronic, includes all accessories

Lay Description

A spirometer measures pulmonary function. It measures the lung output on both inspiration and expiration and is used to track and diagnose a number of respiratory and cardiac conditions. It may also be used to keep the lungs clear and functioning.

A9300

A9300 Exercise equipment

Lay Description

Report this code for exercise equipment used for rehabilitation therapy (e.g., stimulation balls, theraputty, and therabands).

A9500

A9500 Technetium tc-99m sestamibi, diagnostic, per study dose

Lay Description

Sestamibi is a chemical complex that principally congregates in the heart, breast tissue, and parathyroid. Technetium is a radioactive metallic element that is a byproduct of uranium decay. It may also be produced by bombarding another metal, molybdenum, with specific atoms. Technetium 99m is a widely used radionuclide with a half-life of approximately six hours, which is long enough to examine metabolic processes, but short enough to minimize the radiation dose received by the patient. It decays by gamma emission, which is measured by scintillation or gamma cameras. Sestamibi is combined with technetium 99m to produce functional and physiological images of the breast, heart, or parathyroid. The radiopharmaceutical is administered by intravenous injection. Technetium Tc-99m sestamibi is used to diagnose heart disease, parathyroid diseases, and thyroid disorders. It may also be used as a second line diagnostic tool in breast imaging after a mammography to evaluate breast lesions in patients with an abnormal mammogram or a palpable breast mass. HCPCS Level II code A9500 represents a study dose of technetium Tc-99m sestamibi.

Medicare Information

See chapter titled "Medicare Guidelines," under "Drugs, Biologicals, and Radiopharmaceuticals," for Medicare billing and documentation information.

A9501

A9501 Technetium Tc-99m teboroxime, diagnostic, per study dose

Lay Description

Teboroxime is a chemical complex that principally congregates in the heart. Technetium is a radioactive metallic element that is a byproduct of uranium decay. It may also be produced by bombarding another metal, molybdenum, with specific atoms. Technetium 99m is a widely used radionuclide with a half-life of approximately six hours, which is long enough to examine metabolic processes, but short enough to minimize the radiation dose received by the patient. It decays by gamma emission, which is then measured by scintillation or gamma cameras. Teboroxime is combined with technetium 99m to produce functional and physiological images of the heart. Technetium Tc-99m teboroxime is used to diagnose reversible myocardial ischemia in the presence or absence of an infarction, for myocardial perfusion studies in patients with known or suspected coronary artery disease, and for the assessment of patients being evaluated for heart disease. HCPCS Level II code A9501 represents one study dose.

A9502

A9502 Technetium Tc-99m tetrofosmin, diagnostic, per study dose

Lay Description

Tetrofosmin is a chemical complex that principally congregates in the heart. Technetium is a radioactive metallic element that is a byproduct of uranium decay. It may also be produced by bombarding another metal, molybdenum, with specific atoms. Technetium 99m is a widely used radionuclide with a half-life of approximately six hours, which is long enough to examine metabolic processes, but short enough to minimize the radiation dose received by the patient. It decays by gamma emission, which is then measured by scintillation or gamma cameras. Tetrofosmin is combined with technetium 99m to produce functional and physiological images of the heart. The radiopharmaceutical is administered by intravenous injection. Technetium Tc-99m tetrofosmin is used to diagnose reversible myocardial ischemia in the presence or absence of an infarction, for myocardial perfusion studies in patients with known or suspected coronary artery disease, and for the assessment of left ventricular function (ejection fraction and wall motion) in patients being evaluated for heart disease. HCPCS Level II code A9502 represents a study dose of Technetium Tc-99m tetrofosmin.

A9503

A9503 Technetium Tc-99m medronate, diagnostic, per study dose, up to 30 millicuries

Lay Description

Medronate is a chemical complex that principally congregates in the bone. Technetium is a radioactive metallic element that is a byproduct of uranium decay. It may also be produced by bombarding another metal, molybdenum, with specific atoms. Technetium 99m is a widely used radionuclide with a half-life of approximately six hours, which is long enough to examine metabolic processes, but short enough to minimize the radiation dose received by the patient. It decays by gamma emission, which is then measured by scintillation or gamma cameras. Medronate is combined with technetium 99m to delineate areas of altered osteogenesis. The radiopharmaceutical is administered by intravenous injection. Optimal imaging is obtained from one to four hours after administration. Technetium Tc-99m medronate is used to diagnose disorders of bone formation. HCPCS Level II code A9503 represents a study dose of up to 30 millicuries of technetium Tc-99m medronate.

A9504

A9504 Technetium Tc-99m apcitide, diagnostic, per study dose, up to 20 millicuries

Lay Description

Apcitide is a synthetic peptide that binds to receptors on the surface of platelets. Technetium is a radioactive metallic element that is a byproduct of uranium decay. It may also be produced by bombarding another metal, molybdenum, with specific atoms. Technetium 99m is a widely used radionuclide with a half-life of approximately six hours, which is long enough to examine metabolic processes, but short enough to minimize the radiation dose received by the patient. It decays by gamma emission, which is then measured by scintillation or gamma cameras. Apcitide is combined with technetium 99m to locate areas of thrombus. The radiopharmaceutical is administered by intravenous injection. Optimal imaging is obtained from 10 to 60 minutes after administration. HCPCS Level II code A9504 represents a study dose of up to 20 millicuries of technetium Tc-99m apcitide.

A9505

A9505 Thallium Tl-201 thallous chloride, diagnostic, per millicurie

Lay Description

Thallium is a toxic heavy metal found within various rare ores. It is usually recovered from the byproducts of lead and zinc ores by dissolving the ore in hydrochloric acid and precipitating out the thallous chloride. Thallium-201 is a radioactive isotope of thallous chloride that is used as a diagnostic imaging agent. It is administered by intravenous injection. Thallous chloride TL-201 is indicated for use in myocardial perfusion studies and localization of sites of parathyroid hyperactivity, as well as diagnosing and staging of head and neck cancer. Thallous chloride TL-201 has a half-life of 72 hours and decays by electron capture. HCPCS Level II code A9505 represents 1 millicurie of thallous chloride 201.

Medicare Information

See chapter titled "Medicare Guidelines," under "Drugs, Biologicals, and Radiopharmaceuticals," for Medicare billing and documentation information.

A9507

A9507 Indium In-111 capromab pendetide, diagnostic, per study dose, up to 10 millicuries

Lay Description

Capromab pendetide is a murine monoclonal antibody that binds to a glycoprotein, a cell surface antigen that attaches itself to the sites of prostate specific membrane antigen (PSMA). PSMA is associated with prostatic adenocarcinoma cells and is useful in diagnosing metastatic disease. Indium 111 is a radioactive form of the metallic element indium. It has a half-life of approximately 56 hours and decays by electron capture and gamma emission. The monoclonal antibody is combined with indium 111 chloride so that it can be readily identified in images. Indium In-III capromab pendetide is administered intravenously over five minutes. Optimal imaging is obtained from 72 to 120 hours after administration. HCPCS Level II code A9507 represents a study dose up to 10 millicuries of indium In-III capromab pendetide.

Medicare Information

See chapter titled "Medicare Guidelines," under "Drugs, Biologicals, and Radiopharmaceuticals," for Medicare billing and documentation information.

A9508

A9508 Iodine I-131 iobenguane sulfate, diagnostic, per 0.5 millicurie

Lay Description

Iobenguane sulfate is an analogue of norepinephrine that binds to receptors in the sympathetic nervous system and to related tumors. Iodine 131 is a radioactive isotope of the common element iodine. Iodine 131 has a half-life of eight days and decays by beta and gamma emissions. Iobenguane sulfate combined with Iodine 131, also known as MIBG, is a radiopharmaceutical used as a diagnostic imaging agent for neuroendocrine tumors and disorders of the adrenal medulla. It is also used for local radiation therapy in the treatment of carcinoid syndrome, pheochromocytoma, and neuroblastoma. Iodine I-131 iobenguane sulfate is injected intravenously. Multiple scans are usually performed for up to four days post administration. HCPCS Level II code A9508 represents 0.5 millicuries of iobenguane sulfate I-131 used for diagnostic purposes only.

Medicare Information

See chapter titled "Medicare Guidelines," under "Drugs, Biologicals, and Radiopharmaceuticals," for Medicare billing and documentation information.

A9509

A9509 Iodine I-123 sodium iodide, diagnostic, per millicurie

Lay Description

Iodine is a common nonmetallic element necessary for the proper function of the thyroid gland. Iodine 123 sodium iodide is a radioactive isotope of iodine produced in a cyclotron. It decays by electron capture and gamma emission with a half-life of 13 hours. Iodine 123 sodium iodide is administered orally in capsule form. It is readily absorbed from the gastrointestinal tract and congregates primarily in the thyroid gland. Optimal images may be initiated six hours after administration. Sodium iodide I-123 is indicated for diagnostic use in the evaluation of thyroid function and/or morphology. HCPCS Level II code A9509 represents one millicurie of I-123 sodium iodide.

A9510

A9510 Technetium Tc-99m disofenin, diagnostic, per study dose, up to 15 millicuries

Lay Description

Disofenin is a derivative of an iminodiacetic acid that is a form of acetoacetic acid, a byproduct of metabolism that congregates in the gallbladder. Technetium is a radioactive metallic element that is a byproduct of uranium decay. It may also be produced by bombarding another metal, molybdenum, with specific atoms. Technetium 99m is a widely used radionuclide with a half-life of approximately six hours, which is long enough to examine metabolic processes, but short enough to minimize the radiation dose received by the patient. It decays by gamma emission, which is then measured by scintillation or gamma cameras. Disofenin is combined with technetium 99m to provide images of the gallbladder and surrounding ducts. The radiopharmaceutical is administered by intravenous injection. Dosage is based upon patient's body weight. Optimal imaging is obtained from one to four hours after administration. Technetium Tc-99m disofenin is used to diagnose acute cholecystitis and may be used to rule out this disease in patients with right upper quadrant pain or tenderness and jaundice. HCPCS Level II code A9510 represents a study dose of up to 15 millicuries of technetium Tc-99m disofenin.

Medicare Information

See chapter titled "Medicare Guidelines," under "Drugs, Biologicals, and Radiopharmaceuticals," for Medicare billing and documentation information.

A9512

A9512 Technetium Tc-99m pertechnetate, diagnostic, per millicurie

Lay Description

Technetium Tc-99m pertechnetate is an ionized acid of technetium. Technetium is a radioactive metallic element that is a byproduct of uranium decay. It may also be produced by bombarding another metal, molybdenum, with specific atoms. Technetium 99m is a widely used radionuclide with a half-life of approximately six hours, which is long enough to examine metabolic processes, but short enough to minimize the radiation dose received by the patient. It decays by gamma emission, which is then measured by scintillation or gamma cameras. The pertechnetate form of technetium rapidly diffuses into the blood stream and localizes in the thyroid gland, gastric mucosa, salivary glands, certain areas of the brain, sweat glands, and other mucosal tissues. The radiopharmaceutical is administered primarily by intravenous injection, but it may be administered orally, as an ophthalmic solution, or by instillation into the urinary bladder. The dosage administered depends upon the body area being imaged. Technetium Tc-99m pertechnetate is used to provide images of the thyroid, salivary glands, and nasolacrimal drainage system. It is also used for placental localization, brain imaging including cerebral angiography, blood pool imaging including angiography, and urinary bladder imaging for detection of vesicoureteral reflux. Technetium Tc-99m pertechnetate may also be used to prepare other technetium 99m imaging agents. HCPCS Level II code A9512 represents 1 millicurie of technetium Tc-99m pertechnetate.

A9516

A9516   Iodine I-123 sodium iodide, diagnostic, per 100 microcuries, up to 999 microcuries

Lay Description

Iodine is a common nonmetallic element necessary for the proper function of the thyroid gland. Iodine 123 sodium iodide is a radioactive isotope of iodine produced in a cyclotron. It decays by electron capture and gamma emission with a half-life of 13 hours. Iodine 123 sodium iodide is administered orally in capsule form. It is readily absorbed from the gastrointestinal tract and congregates primarily in the thyroid gland. Optimal images may be initiated six hours after administration. Sodium iodide I-123 is indicated for diagnostic use in the evaluation of thyroid function and/or morphology. HCPCS Level II code A9516 represents 100 microcuries of I-123 sodium iodide.

Medicare Information

See chapter titled "Medicare Guidelines," under "Drugs, Biologicals, and Radiopharmaceuticals," for Medicare billing and documentation information.

A9517

A9517   Iodine I-131 sodium iodide capsule(s), therapeutic, per millicurie

Lay Description

Iodine is a common nonmetallic element necessary for the proper function of the thyroid gland. Iodine 131 sodium iodide is a radioactive isotope of iodine produced in a cyclotron. It decays by beta and gamma emission with a half-life of eight hours. Iodine 131 sodium iodide is administered orally in capsule or solution form. It is readily absorbed from the gastrointestinal tract and congregates primarily in thyroid tissue. Therapeutic doses of sodium iodide I-131 capsules are indicated for the treatment of hyperthyroidism and selected cases of thyroid cancer. Palliative effects may be seen in patients with papillary and/or follicular carcinoma of the thyroid. Sodium iodide I-131 is not usually used for the treatment of hyperthyroidism in patients younger than 30 years of age unless circumstances preclude other methods of treatment. HCPCS Level II code A9517 represents 1 millicurie of therapeutic I-131 sodium iodide in capsule form.

Medicare Information

See the chapter titled "Medicare Guidelines," under "Drugs, Biologicals, and Radiopharmaceuticals," for Medicare information.

A9521

A9521   Technetium Tc-99m exametazime, diagnostic, per study dose, up to 25 millicuries

Lay Description

Exametazime, also known as hexamethylpropyleneamine oxime, is a chemical complex that is taken up by leukocytes and selectively retained in neutrophils. Technetium is a radioactive metallic element that is a byproduct of uranium decay. It may also be produced by bombarding another metal, molybdenum, with specific atoms. Technetium 99m is a widely used radionuclide with a half-life of approximately six hours, which is long enough to examine metabolic processes, but short enough to minimize the radiation dose received by the patient. It decays by gamma emission, which is then measured by scintillation or gamma cameras. Tc-99m exametazime is used to label autologous leukocytes. The labeled leukocytes are then used in imaging to localize or identify areas of intra-abdominal infection or inflammation. Optimal imaging with labeled leukocytes is two to four hours after administration. When technetium Tc-99m pertechnetate is added to the exametazime, the resulting radiopharmaceutical is taken up by lipids that can cross the blood-brain barrier. The technetium Tc-99m pertechnetate/exametazime is useful for only 30 minutes. Its useful life can be extended by the addition of methylene blue. Tc-99m pertechnetate/exametazime is used in cerebral perfusion imaging to detect regions altered by stroke. The radiopharmaceutical is administered by intravenous injection. Optimal imaging for cerebral perfusion studies may begin immediately after administration and can continue up to six hours after administration. HCPCS Level II code A9521 represents a study dose up to 25 millicuries of technetium Tc-99m exametazime.

Medicare Information
See chapter titled "Medicare Guidelines," under "Drugs, Biologicals, and Radiopharmaceuticals," for Medicare billing and documentation information.

A9524

A9524 Iodine I-131 iodinated serum albumin, diagnostic, per 5 microcuries

Lay Description
Serum albumin is a protein component of blood. Iodine 131 is a radioactive isotope of the common element iodine. Iodine 131 has a half-life of eight days and decays by beta and gamma emissions. Serum albumin is combined with iodine 131 to provide images of the blood pool and its movement. The radiopharmaceutical is administered by intravenous injection and is dispersed within the intravascular pool within 10 minutes. Full distribution throughout the body takes from two to four days after administration. Dosage depends upon the imaging to be performed. Iodinated I-131 serum albumin is indicated for use in determinations of total blood and plasma volumes, cardiac output, cardiac and pulmonary blood volumes and circulation times, and in protein turnover studies, heart and great vessel delineation, localization of the placenta, and localization of cerebral neoplasms. HCPCS Level II code A9524 represents a study dose up to 5 microcuries of iodinated I-131 serum albumin.

Medicare Information
See chapter titled "Medicare Guidelines," under "Drugs, Biologicals, and Radiopharmaceuticals," for Medicare billing and documentation information.

A9526

A9526 Nitrogen N-13 ammonia, diagnostic, per study dose, up to 40 millicuries

Lay Description
Nitrogen N-13 ammonia is a radioisotope composed of ammonia molecules combined with nitrogen N-13 that is widely used in cardiac imaging. Nitrogen N-13 is a radioactive isotope of nitrogen produced within a cyclotron. Nitrogen 13 has a half-life of approximately 10 minutes and decays by positron emission. The positrons are used to produce positron emission tomography (PET) images. Due to its short half-life, nitrogen N-13 ammonia must be produced shortly before use. Nitrogen N-13 ammonia is injected intravenously and is rapidly distributed to all organs of the body. Optimal imaging of the myocardium is generally obtained 15 to 20 minutes after administration. Nitrogen N-13 ammonia is currently approved only for myocardial perfusion for the diagnosis and management of patients with known or suspected coronary artery disease. The perfusion study may be performed at rest or with pharmacological stress. HCPCS Level II code A9526 represents a study dose up to 40 millicuries of nitrogen N-13 ammonia.

Medicare Information
Ammonia N-13 is covered by Medicare when used in a covered positron emission tomography (PET) scan for myocardial perfusion for the diagnosis and management of patients with known or suspected coronary artery disease. The perfusion study may be performed at rest or with pharmacological stress.

The PET scan and the ammonia N-13 is covered only when it is performed in place of, but not in addition to, a single photon emission computed tomography (SPECT); or it is used following a SPECT that was found to be inconclusive. When the SPECT is found to be inconclusive, the PET scan must have been considered necessary in order to determine what medical or surgical intervention is required to treat the patient. For Medicare coverage requirements, an inconclusive test is a test whose results are equivocal, technically not interpretable, or discordant with a patient's other clinical data and must be documented in the patient's medical record.

Report the ammonia N-13 on the same claim as the PET scan.

A9527

A9527 Iodine I-125, sodium iodide solution, therapeutic, per millicurie

Lay Description
Iodine 125 sodium iodide is a radioactive isotope of iodine produced by the neutron irradiation of xenon-124. It decays by electron capture and gamma emission with a half-life of 60 days. Therapeutic iodine 125 sodium iodide is administered in solution form. It is used to treat hyperthyroidism, and prostate and brain cancers. HCPCS Level II code A9527 represents one millicurie of I-125 sodium iodide solution used as a therapeutic dose.

A9528-A9531

A9528 Iodine I-131 sodium iodide capsule(s), diagnostic, per millicurie
A9529 Iodine I-131 sodium iodide solution, diagnostic, per millicurie
A9530 Iodine I-131 sodium iodide solution, therapeutic, per millicurie
A9531 Iodine I-131 sodium iodide, diagnostic, per microcurie (up to 100 microcuries)

Lay Description
Iodine is a common nonmetallic element necessary for the proper function of the thyroid gland. Iodine 131 sodium iodide is a radioactive isotope of iodine produced in a cyclotron. It decays by beta and gamma emission with a half-life of eight hours. Iodine 131 sodium iodide is administered orally in capsule or solution form. It is readily absorbed from the gastrointestinal tract and congregates primarily in thyroid tissue. Therapeutic doses of sodium iodide I-131 capsules are indicated for the treatment of hyperthyroidism and selected cases of thyroid cancer. Palliative effects may be seen in patients with papillary and/or follicular carcinoma of the thyroid. Sodium iodide 1-131 is not usually used for the treatment of hyperthyroidism in patients younger than 30 years of age unless circumstances preclude other methods of treatment. HCPCS Level II code A9528 represents 1 millicurie of diagnostic I-131 sodium iodide in capsule form; A9529 represents 1 millicurie of diagnostic I-131 sodium iodide in solution form; A9530 represents 1 millicurie of therapeutic I-131 sodium iodide in solution form; and A9531 represents 1 microcurie of diagnostic I-131 sodium iodide. HCPCS Level II code A9531 should be reported only up to 100 microcuries.

Medicare Information
See chapter titled "Medicare Guidelines," under "Drugs, Biologicals, and Radiopharmaceuticals," for Medicare billing and documentation information.

A9532

A9532 Iodine I-125 serum albumin, diagnostic, per 5 microcuries

Lay Description
Serum albumin is a protein component of blood. Iodine 125 is a radioactive isotope of the common element iodine. Iodine 125 has a half-life of 60 days and decays by beta and gamma emissions. Serum albumin is combined with iodine 125 to provide measures of the blood and plasma pool. The radiopharmaceutical is administered by intravenous injection. Dosage depends upon body weight and can vary from 5 to 50 microcuries. At five and 15 minutes after administration, blood samples are drawn from the arm that was not injected. The radioactivity of the blood samples is measured and a calculation of the patient's blood volume is determined. For plasma volume, the samples are first centrifuged and the red blood cells removed. Iodinated I-125 serum albumin is indicated for use in determinations of total blood and plasma volumes. HCPCS Level II code A9532 represents 5 microcuries of iodinated I-125 serum albumin.

Medicare Information
See chapter titled "Medicare Guidelines," under "Drugs, Biologicals, and Radiopharmaceuticals," for Medicare billing and documentation information.

A9536

A9536 Technetium Tc-99m depreotide, diagnostic, per study dose, up to 35 millicuries

Lay Description
Depreotide is a synthetic peptide that binds to somatostatin receptors in cells. Somatostatin is a peptide that regulates the release of hormones by many different neuroendocrine cells in the brain, pancreas, and gastrointestinal tract. Technetium is a radioactive metallic element that is a byproduct of uranium decay. It may also be produced by bombarding another metal, molybdenum, with specific atoms. Technetium 99m is a widely used radionuclide with a half-life of approximately six hours, which is long enough to examine metabolic processes, but short enough to minimize the radiation dose received by the patient. It decays by gamma emission, which is then measured by scintillation or gamma cameras. Depreotide is combined with technetium 99m to determine the nature of pulmonary masses in patients who have known or suspected malignancy. The radiopharmaceutical is administered by intravenous injection. Dosage is 15 to 20 mCi. Optimal imaging is obtained from two to four hours after administration. HCPCS Level II code A9536 represents a study dose of up to 35 millicuries of technetium Tc-99m depreotide.

Medicare Information
See chapter titled "Medicare Guidelines," under "Drugs, Biologicals, and Radiopharmaceuticals," for Medicare billing and documentation information.

A9537

A9537 Technetium Tc-99m mebrofenin, diagnostic, per study dose, up to 15 millicuries

Lay Description
Mebrofenin is a derivative of an iminodiacetic acid that is a form of acetoacetic acid, a byproduct of metabolism that congregates in the gallbladder. Technetium is a radioactive metallic element that is a

byproduct of uranium decay. It may also be produced by bombarding another metal, molybdenum, with specific atoms. Technetium 99m is a widely used radionuclide with a half-life of approximately six hours, which is long enough to examine metabolic processes, but short enough to minimize the radiation dose received by the patient. It decays by gamma emission, which is then measured by scintillation or gamma cameras. Mebrofenin is combined with technetium 99m to provide images of the gallbladder and surrounding ducts. Technetium Tc-99m mebrofenin is rapidly cleared and has a short useful life. The radiopharmaceutical is administered by intravenous injection. Dosage is based upon patient's body weight. Optimal imaging is obtained from 10 to 60 minutes after administration. Technetium Tc-99m mebrofenin is used for hepatobiliary system imaging and hepatic function studies. HCPCS Level II code A9537 represents a study dose of up to 15 millicuries of technetium Tc-99m mebrofenin.

Medicare Information

See chapter titled "Medicare Guidelines," under "Drugs, Biologicals, and Radiopharmaceuticals," for Medicare billing and documentation information.

A9538

A9538   Technetium Tc-99m pyrophosphate, diagnostic, per study dose, up to 25 millicuries

Lay Description

Pyrophosphate is a form of phosphorus formed by the breakdown of adenosine triphosphate (ATP) into adenosine monophosphate (AMP). Technetium is a radioactive metallic element that is a byproduct of uranium decay. It may also be produced by bombarding another metal, molybdenum, with specific atoms. Technetium 99m is a widely used radionuclide with a half-life of approximately six hours, which is long enough to examine metabolic processes, but short enough to minimize the radiation dose received by the patient. It decays by gamma emission, which is then measured by scintillation or gamma cameras. Pyrophosphate combined with technetium 99m seems to be attracted to certain crystals found in bone and damaged heart cells. The radiopharmaceutical is administered by intravenous injection. Dosage and optimal imaging depend on the area being imaged. Technetium Tc-99m pyrophosphate is used in skeletal imaging to identify areas of altered bone, such as occurs in metastatic disease, Paget's disease, arthritis, osteomyelitis, and fractures. It is used in cardiac imaging to aid in the diagnosis of an acute myocardial infarction. Technetium Tc-99m pyrophosphate may also be used in conjunction with Technetium Tc-99m pertechnetate for the labeling of red blood cells. HCPCS Level II code A9538 represents a study dose of up to 25 millicuries of technetium Tc-99m pyrophosphate.

Medicare Information

See chapter titled "Medicare Guidelines," under "Drugs, Biologicals, and Radiopharmaceuticals," for Medicare billing and documentation information.

A9539

A9539   Technetium Tc-99m pentetate, diagnostic, per study dose, up to 25 millicuries

Lay Description

The pentetate here refers to calcium trisodium pentetate, which is a chelating agent that forms stable bounds with metals, which are then excreted in the urine. Technetium is a radioactive metallic element that is a byproduct of uranium decay. It may also be produced by bombarding another metal, molybdenum, with specific atoms. Technetium 99m is a widely used radionuclide with a half-life of approximately six hours, which is long enough to examine metabolic processes, but short enough to minimize the radiation dose received by the patient. It decays by gamma emission, which is then measured by scintillation or gamma cameras. Pentetate combined with technetium 99m is rapidly distributed throughout the body and is excreted from the body by glomerular filtration. The images of the kidneys obtained in the first few minutes after administration will show the blood pool within the kidney. Subsequent images show kidney function. Technetium Tc-99m pentetate also tends to accumulate in intracranial lesions with many new blood vessels or with an altered blood-brain barrier. The radiopharmaceutical is administered by intravenous injection. Dosage and optimal imaging depend on the area being imaged. Technetium Tc-99m pentetate is used for kidney and brain imaging and to assess renal function and estimate the glomerular filtration rate. When in aerosol form, it is administered by inhalation. The aerosol form is used to assess airway patency, especially in conjunction with perfusion lung imaging to evaluate for a pulmonary embolism. HCPCS Level II code A9539 represents a study dose of up to 25 millicuries of injected technetium Tc-99m pentetate.

Medicare Information

See chapter titled "Medicare Guidelines," under "Drugs, Biologicals, and Radiopharmaceuticals," for Medicare billing and documentation information.

A9540

A9540　Technetium Tc-99m macroaggregated albumin, diagnostic, per study dose, up to 10 millicuries

Lay Description

Macroaggregated albumin, also called aggregated albumin, is an unusually large amount of albumin, a protein component of blood. Technetium is a radioactive metallic element that is a byproduct of uranium decay. It may also be produced by bombarding another metal, molybdenum, with specific atoms. Technetium 99m is a widely used radionuclide with a half-life of approximately six hours, which is long enough to examine metabolic processes, but short enough to minimize the radiation dose received by the patient. It decays by gamma emission, which is then measured by scintillation or gamma cameras. Macroaggregated albumin combined with technetium 99m pertechnetate rapidly accumulates in pulmonary alveolar capillaries. The radiopharmaceutical is administered by intravenous injection. Dosage depends upon body weight. Optimal imaging can be obtained immediately after administration. Technetium Tc-99m macroaggregated albumin is used for a lung imaging agent and may be used as an adjunct in the evaluation of pulmonary perfusion in adults and pediatric patients. It may be used in adults for evaluation of peritoneovenous (LeVeen) shunt patency. HCPCS Level II code A9540 represents a study dose of up to 10 millicuries of technetium Tc-99m macroaggregated or aggregated albumin.

A9541

A9541　Technetium Tc-99m sulfur colloid, diagnostic, per study dose, up to 20 millicuries

Lay Description

Sulfur colloid is sulfur, a nonmetallic element, in very fine particulars. Technetium is a radioactive metallic element that is a byproduct of uranium decay. It may also be produced by bombarding another metal, molybdenum, with specific atoms. Technetium 99m is a widely used radionuclide with a half-life of approximately six hours, which is long enough to examine metabolic processes, but short enough to minimize the radiation dose received by the patient. It decays by gamma emission, which is then measured by scintillation or gamma cameras. Sulfur colloid combined with technetium 99m is rapidly eliminated by the reticuloendothelial system, which is a group of cells within the immune system. The radiopharmaceutical is administered by intravenous or intra-peritoneal injection or orally. Dosage and optimal imaging depends upon body weight and intended area study. Technetium Tc-99m sulfur colloid injected intravenously is used for imaging of the liver, spleen, and bone marrow. Administered orally it is used for the evaluation of swallowing functions, gastroesophageal reflux studies, and to detect pulmonary aspiration of gastric contents. Technetium Tc-99m sulfur colloid injected intra-peritoneally may be used in adults for evaluation of peritoneovenous (LeVeen) shunt patency. HCPCS Level II code A9541 represents a study dose of up to 20 millicuries of technetium Tc-99m sulfur colloid.

Medicare Information

See chapter titled "Medicare Guidelines," under "Drugs, Biologicals, and Radiopharmaceuticals," for Medicare billing and documentation information.

A9542-A9543

A9542　Indium In-111 ibritumomab tiuxetan, diagnostic, per study dose, up to 5 millicuries

A9543　Yttrium Y-90 ibritumomab tiuxetan, therapeutic, per treatment dose, up to 40 millicuries

Lay Description

Ibritumomab is a murine monoclonal antibody produced in Chinese hamster ovary cells. This antibody is specifically directed against the CD20 antigen, which is found on the surface of normal and malignant B lymphocytes. Tiuxetan is a chelating agent that allows ibritumomab to form stable bonds with metals. Indium 111 is a radioactive form of the metallic element indium. It has a half-life of approximately 56 hours and decays by electron capture and gamma emission. Indium 111 ibritumomab tiuxetan is used to determine the biodistribution pattern in preparation for the administration of yttrium 90 of ibritumomab tiuxetan. The usual dose for diagnostic purposes is 5 millicuries injected intravenously. Yttrium 90 is a radioactive form of the metallic element yttrium found in rare earth minerals. Ibritumomab tiuxetan combined with yttrium 90 is used for the treatment of relapsed or refractory low-grade, follicular, or transformed B cell non-Hodgkin's lymphoma, including rituximab-refractory follicular non-Hodgkin's lymphoma. The dosage for therapeutic yttrium 90 ibritumomab tiuxetan depends upon body weight. It is administered by intravenous injection. Both forms of ibritumomab tiuxetan are administered in conjunction with rituximab. HCPCS Level II code A9542 represents a study dose of up to 5 millicuries of indium 111 ibritumomab tiuxetan. HCPCS Level II code A9543 represents a therapeutic treatment dose of up to 40 millicuries of yttrium 90 ibritumomab tiuxetan.

Medicare Information

See chapter titled "Medicare Guidelines," under "Drugs, Biologicals, and Radiopharmaceuticals," for Medicare billing and documentation information.

A9544-A9545

A9544   Iodine I-131 tositumomab, diagnostic, per study dose
A9545   Iodine I-131 tositumomab, therapeutic, per treatment dose

Lay Description

Tositumomab is a murine monoclonal antibody produced in mammalian cells. This antibody is specifically directed against the CD20 antigen, which is found on the surface of normal and malignant B lymphocytes. Iodine 131 is a radioactive isotope of the common element iodine. It decays by beta and gamma emission with a half-life of eight hours. The diagnostic dosage of tositumomab is used to determine the biodistribution pattern in preparation for the administration of the therapeutic dosage. The usual dose for diagnostic purposes is 450 mg of tositumomab infused intravenously over one hour followed by 5 mCi of iodine 131 tositumomab infused intravenously over 20 minutes. The therapeutic dosage depends on the patient's body weight and condition and is infused intravenously over 20 minutes. Iodine I-131 tositumomab is used for the treatment of relapsed or refractory CD20 positive follicular, non-Hodgkin's lymphoma, including rituximab-refractory follicular non-Hodgkin's lymphoma. HCPCS Level II code A9544 represents a study dose of diagnostic iodine I-131 tositumomab. HCPCS Level II code A9545 represents a therapeutic treatment dose of iodine I-131 tositumomab.

Medicare Information

See chapter titled "Medicare Guidelines," under "Drugs, Biologicals, and Radiopharmaceuticals," for Medicare billing and documentation information.

A9546

A9546   Cobalt Co-57/58, cyanocobalamin, diagnostic, per study dose, up to 1 microcurie

Lay Description

Cyanocobalamin Co-57/58 is a radioactive form of vitamin B12 in which portions of the molecules contain cobalt 57 or cobalt 58. The drug is administered orally and used to diagnose pernicious anemia and intestinal defects of vitamin B12 absorption. HCPCS Level II code A9546 represents up to 1 microcurie of cyanocobalamin Co-57/58.

A9547

A9547   Indium In-111 oxyquinoline, diagnostic, per 0.5 millicurie

Lay Description

Indium 111 oxyquinoline is a radioisotope used to label autologous white blood cells. These labeled cells are then administered intravenously and used to scan for abscesses and other inflammatory processes where the white cells would usually congregate. Indium 111 oxyquinoline is not the preferred technique for the initial evaluation of patients with a suspected abscess in an unknown location. It should be considered only if other methods prove unsuccessful or ambiguous. Imaging is performed approximately two hours postinjection. Indium 111 decays by electron capture with a half-life of 67.2 hours. HCPCS Level II code A9547 represents 0.5 millicuries of indium 111 oxyquinoline.

A9548

A9548   Indium In-111 pentetate, diagnostic, per 0.5 millicurie

Lay Description

Pentetate, also known as pentetic acid or DTPA, is a chelating agent that binds with iron. Indium 111 is a radioactive form of indium, a metallic element. Indium 111 has a half-life of 2.8 days and decays by electron capture and gamma emission. Pentetate combined with indium In-111 is used to provide images of the cerebrospinal fluid (CSF) flow. It is indicated for use in radionuclide cisternography to study the flow of CSF in the brain for identification of CSF abnormalities and sites of CSF leakage, and for evaluation of CSF shunt patency. Indium In-111 pentetate is administered by intrathecal injection into the lumbar intrathecal space. It flows up the spinal canal with the CSF to the brain. Under normal flow patterns, it does not penetrate into the ventricles. Indium In-111 pentetate is supplied as a unit dose. Each unit dose vial contains 0.7 mCi of sterile indium In-111 pentetate. The maximum recommended dose for an adult (average weight 70 kg) is 10.5 mCi. Any unused portion must be discarded. HCPCS Level II code A9548 represents 0.5 millicurie (mCi) of indium In-111 pentetate.

A9550

A9550   Technetium Tc-99m sodium gluceptate, diagnostic, per study dose, up to 25 millicurie

Lay Description

Sodium gluceptate is a carbohydrate derivative. Technetium is a radioactive metallic element that is a byproduct of uranium decay. It may also be produced by bombarding another metal, molybdenum, with specific atoms. Technetium 99m is a widely used radionuclide with a half-life of approximately six hours, which is long enough to examine metabolic processes, but short enough to minimize the radiation dose received by the patient. It decays by gamma emission, which is then measured by scintillation or gamma cameras. Sodium gluceptate combined with technetium 99m pertechnetate is rapidly eliminated from the body by the kidneys. It tends to accumulate in intracranial lesions with many new blood vessels or with an altered blood-brain barrier. Technetium 99m sodium gluceptate is used for kidney and brain imaging and to assess renal and brain perfusion. The radiopharmaceutical is administered by intravenous injection. The recommended adult dosage is 10 to 15 mCi for renal imaging and 15 to 20 mCi for brain imaging. Dynamic imaging may begin immediately after administration and static images can be obtained up to several hours after administration. HCPCS Level II code A9550 represents a study dose of up to 25 millicuries of technetium Tc-99m sodium gluceptate.

Medicare Information
See chapter titled "Medicare Guidelines," under "Drugs, Biologicals, and Radiopharmaceuticals," for Medicare billing and documentation information.

A9551

A9551   Technetium Tc-99m succimer, diagnostic, per study dose, up to 10 millicuries

Lay Description
Succimer, also known as DMSA, is a chelating agent that is similar to dimercaprol and is used in the treatment of heavy metal poisoning. Technetium is a radioactive metallic element that is a byproduct of uranium decay. It may also be produced by bombarding another metal, molybdenum, with specific atoms. Technetium 99m is a widely used radionuclide with a half-life of approximately six hours, which is long enough to examine metabolic processes, but short enough to minimize the radiation dose received by the patient. It decays by gamma emission, which is then measured by scintillation or gamma cameras. Succimer combined with technetium 99m pertechnetate is rapidly eliminated from the body by the kidneys. The radiopharmaceutical is administered by intravenous injection. Technetium 99m succimer is used in the evaluation of renal parenchymal disorders. The recommended adult dosage is 2 to 6 mCi. Optimal imaging may be obtained one to two hours after administration. HCPCS Level II code A9551 represents a study dose of up to 10 millicuries of technetium Tc-99m succimer.

Medicare Information
See chapter titled "Medicare Guidelines," under "Drugs, Biologicals, and Radiopharmaceuticals," for Medicare billing and documentation information.

A9552

A9552   Fluorodeoxyglucose F-18 FDG, diagnostic, per study dose, up to 45 millicuries

Lay Description
Glucose is a sugar actively taken up by cells. Fludeoxyglucose F18 (FDG) is a radioisotope widely used in positron emission tomography (PET imaging). FDG is a radioactive version of glucose that is administered intravenously. Peak imaging is at 30 to 40 minutes after injection. FDG is indicated for identifying regions of abnormal glucose metabolism that can be associated with foci of epileptic seizures or evaluation of malignancy in patients who have an existing diagnosis or who have known or suspected abnormalities identified by other methods. FDG may also be used to assess coronary artery disease and left ventricular dysfunction when used together with myocardial perfusion. It must be produced from cyclotron bombardment of fluorine F18, which is itself produced from proton bombardment of enriched water. FDG decays by positron emission and has a half-life of 109.8 minutes. HCPCS Level II code A9552 represents a study dose up to 45 millicuries of FDG.

A9553

A9553   Chromium Cr-51 sodium chromate, diagnostic, per study dose, up to 250 microcuries

Lay Description
Chromium CR 51 is a radioisotope of sodium chromate, which binds to red blood cells. Chromium 51 is used to label red blood cells and the labeled cells are administered intravenously. Labeled red blood cells are used for determining red blood cell volume or mass, evaluating blood loss, and studying red blood cell survival time for conditions such as hemolytic anemia. Chromium 51 decays by electron capture and gamma emission. It has a half-life of 27.7 days. HCPCS Level II code A9553 represents a study dose up to 250 microcuries of chromium CR 51.

A9554

A9554 Iodine I-125 sodium iothalamate, diagnostic, per study dose, up to 10 microcuries

Lay Description

Sodium iothalamate is a solution of iodine and sodium hydroxide that is used as a contrast agent. Iodine I-125 is a radioactive version of iodine that has a half-life of 60 days and decays by electron capture and gamma emission. Sodium iothalamate combined with iodine I-125 is used for the evaluation of renal glomerular filtration in the diagnosis or monitoring of patients with renal disease. The compound is cleared by renal glomerular filtration without tubular secretion or reabsorption. The suggested dose range employed in an adult patient (average weight 70 kg) is dependent on infusion method. For continuous intravenous infusion the dose is 20 to 100 uCi. For single intravenous injection the dose is 10 to 30 uCi. Blood and urine sample are collected from the patient at varying intervals post administration. The concentration of iodine I-125 in each specimen is then measured using scintillation counters. These figures are used to compute clearance factors, which provide an indication of renal function. HCPCS Level II code A9554 represents up to 10 microcuries of iodine I-125 sodium iothalamate.

A9555

A9555 Rubidium Rb-82, diagnostic, per study dose, up to 60 millicuries

Lay Description

Rubidium-82 is a radioisotope that is widely used in cardiac imaging, as it is a chemical analog to potassium. Potassium ions are metabolized by muscle tissue including the heart. Once in the heart, the beta decay of the rubidium-82 is used to help produce a PET image. The half-life of rubidium-82 is 1.273 minutes. Due to its short half-life, rubidium-82 must be produced shortly before use by a rubidium-82 generator. Rubidium-82 is produced by the beta decay of strontium-82. Strontium-82 is an isotope that can readily be made in an accelerator and has a half-life of 25.5 days. The relatively long-lived strontium-82 in the form of a solution is loaded into the rubidium-82 generator. As the strontium-82 decays, rubidium-82 is produced. A solvent is then selectively used to remove the rubidium-82 from the solution. As the strontium-82 is continually decaying and producing rubidium-82, one can allow the rubidium to accumulate and remove the rubidium-82 as needed. HCPCS Level II code A9555 represents a study dose up to 60 millicuries of rubidium-82.

Medicare Information

See chapter titled "Medicare Guidelines," under "Drugs, Biologicals, and Radiopharmaceuticals," for Medicare billing and documentation information.

A9556

A9556 Gallium Ga-67 citrate, diagnostic, per millicurie

Lay Description

Gallium is a rare metal that is liquid at room temperature. Gallium GA 67 citrate is a radioactive version of gallium used to identify the presence and extent of Hodgkin's disease, lymphomas, and bronchogenic carcinomas. It may also be useful in detecting some inflammatory lesions. Gallium GA 67 citrate is administered intravenously and peak imaging is often 48-120 hours after injection. It must be produced from cyclotron proton bombardment of Zinc ZN 68 enriched metal. Gallium GA 67 decays by electron capture and gamma emission. It has a half-life of 78.3 hours. HCPCS Level II code A9556 represents 1 millicurie of gallium GA 67 citrate.

Medicare Information

See chapter titled "Medicare Guidelines," under "Drugs, Biologicals, and Radiopharmaceuticals," for Medicare billing and documentation information.

A9557

A9557 Technetium Tc-99m bicisate, diagnostic, per study dose, up to 25 millicuries

Lay Description

Bicisate, also known as ethyl cysteinate dimer (ECD), is a lipophilic amine having the ability to cross the blood-brain barrier and localize in the brain. Technetium is a radioactive metallic element that is a byproduct of uranium decay. It may also be produced by bombarding another metal, molybdenum, with specific atoms. Technetium 99m is a widely used radionuclide with a half-life of approximately six hours, which is long enough to examine metabolic processes, but short enough to minimize the radiation dose received by the patient. It decays by gamma emission, which is then measured by scintillation or gamma cameras. Bicisate combined with technetium 99m pertechnetate is used in single photon emission computerized tomography (SPECT) imaging as an adjunct to conventional CT or MRI imaging in the localization of stroke in patients in whom stroke has already been diagnosed. The radiopharmaceutical is injected intravenously. The recommended adult dosage is 10 to 30 mCi. Optimal imaging may be obtained 30 to 60 minutes after administration. HCPCS Level II code A9557 represents a study dose of up to 25 millicuries of technetium Tc-99m bicisate.

Medicare Information

See chapter titled "Medicare Guidelines," under "Drugs, Biologicals, and Radiopharmaceuticals," for Medicare billing and documentation information.

A9558

A9558 Xenon Xe-133 gas, diagnostic, per 10 millicuries

Lay Description

Xenon is a gaseous element that is not chemically reactive. Xenon Xe133 gas is a mixture of radioactive xenon gas and carbon dioxide inhaled by the patient for use in diagnostic evaluations of pulmonary functions, pulmonary imaging, and in the assessment of cerebral blood flow. The gas is a reactor-produced by-product of uranium U235 fission. Xenon Xe133 gas decays by beta and gamma emissions with a half-life of 5.245 days. HCPCS Level II code A9558 represents 10 millicuries of xenon Xe133.

Medicare Information

See chapter titled "Medicare Guidelines," under "Drugs, Biologicals, and Radiopharmaceuticals," for Medicare billing and documentation information.

A9559

A9559 Cobalt Co-57 cyanocobalamin, oral, diagnostic, per study dose, up to 1 microcurie

Lay Description

Cyanocobalamin Co-57 is a radioactive forms of vitamin B12 in which portions of the molecules contain cobalt 57. The drug is administered orally and used to diagnose pernicious anemia and intestinal defects of vitamin B12 absorption. HCPCS Level II code A9559 represents 1 microcurie of cyanocobalamin Co-57.

Medicare Information

See chapter titled "Medicare Guidelines," under "Drugs, Biologicals, and Radiopharmaceuticals," for Medicare billing and documentation information.

A9560

A9560 Technetium Tc-99m labeled red blood cells, diagnostic, per study dose, up to 30 millicuries

Lay Description

Technetium is a radioactive metallic element that is a byproduct of uranium decay. It may also be produced by bombarding another metal, molybdenum, with specific atoms. Technetium 99m is a widely used radionuclide with a half-life of approximately six hours, which is long enough to examine metabolic processes, but short enough to minimize the radiation dose received by the patient. It decays by gamma emission, which is then measured by scintillation or gamma cameras. Technetium 99m pertechnetate is used to label autologous red blood cells. The labeled red blood cells are injected intravenously. The recommended adult dosage is 10 to 20 mCi. Technetium Tc-99m labeled red blood cells are used for blood pool imaging, including cardiac first pass and gated equilibrium imaging, and for detection of sites of gastrointestinal bleeding. HCPCS Level II code A9560 represents a study dose of up to 30 millicuries of technetium Tc-99m labeled red blood cells.

Medicare Information

See chapter titled "Medicare Guidelines," under "Drugs, Biologicals, and Radiopharmaceuticals," for Medicare billing and documentation information.

A9561

A9561 Technetium Tc-99m oxidronate, diagnostic, per study dose, up to 30 millicuries

Lay Description

Oxidronate, also known as HDP and HMDP, is a chemical compound that is attracted to sites of bone mineralization. Technetium is a radioactive metallic element that is a byproduct of uranium decay. It may also be produced by bombarding another metal, molybdenum, with specific atoms. Technetium 99m is a widely used radionuclide with a half-life of approximately six hours, which is long enough to examine metabolic processes, but short enough to minimize the radiation dose received by the patient. It decays by gamma emission, which is then measured by scintillation or gamma cameras. Oxidronate combined with technetium 99m is used for skeletal imaging to identify areas of altered bone growth. The radiopharmaceutical is injected intravenously. The recommended adult dosage is 10 to 20 mCi. Optimal imaging is three to four hours after administration. HCPCS Level II code A9561 represents a study dose of up to 30 millicuries of technetium Tc-99m oxidronate.

Medicare Information

See chapter titled "Medicare Guidelines," under "Drugs, Biologicals, and Radiopharmaceuticals," for Medicare billing and documentation information.

A9562

A9562 Technetium Tc-99m mertiatide, diagnostic, per study dose, up to 15 millicuries

Lay Description

Mertiatide is a chemical compound that binds to plasma protein. Technetium is a radioactive metallic element that is a byproduct of uranium decay. It may also be produced by bombarding another metal, molybdenum, with specific atoms. Technetium 99m is a widely used radionuclide with a half-life of approximately six hours, which is long enough to examine metabolic processes, but short enough to minimize the radiation dose received by the patient. It decays by gamma emission, which is then measured by scintillation or gamma cameras. Mertiatide combined with technetium 99m pertechnetate is used for renal imaging to diagnose congenital and acquired abnormalities, renal failure, urinary tract obstruction, and calculi in adults and children. It is a diagnostic aid in providing renal function, split function, renal angiograms, and renogram curves for whole kidney and renal cortex. The radiopharmaceutical is injected intravenously. The recommended adult dosage is 5 to 10 mCi. HCPCS Level II code A9562 represents a study dose of up to 15 millicuries of technetium Tc-99m mertiatide.

Medicare Information

See chapter titled "Medicare Guidelines," under "Drugs, Biologicals, and Radiopharmaceuticals," for Medicare billing and documentation information.

A9563

A9563 Sodium phosphate P-32, therapeutic, per millicurie

Lay Description

Phosphorus is a common nonmetallic element essential to the human body. It is a major component of bone, is abundant in all tissues, and is involved in some form in almost all metabolic processes. Phosphorus 32 is a radioactive form of phosphorus. It has a half-life of approximately 14.28 days and decays by beta emission. Sodium is a common metallic element, an electrolyte necessary for the proper functioning of the body. Sodium phosphate P-32 is a compound of sodium and phosphorus P-32. It concentrates largely in rapidly proliferating tissue, accumulating in the liver, spleen, and bone marrow. Sodium phosphate P-32 is used for the therapeutic treatment of polycythemia vera, chronic myelocytic leukemia, and chronic lymphocytic leukemia. It may also be used for the palliative treatment of bone pain associated with multiple areas of skeletal metastases. HCPCS Level II code A9563 represents 1 millicurie of sodium phosphate P-32.

Medicare Information

See chapter titled "Medicare Guidelines," under "Drugs, Biologicals, and Radiopharmaceuticals," for Medicare billing and documentation information.

A9564

A9564 Chromic phosphate P-32 suspension, therapeutic, per millicurie

Lay Description

Phosphorus is a common nonmetallic element essential to the human body. It is a major component of bone, is abundant in all tissues, and is involved in some form in almost all metabolic processes. Phosphorus 32 is a radioactive form of phosphorus. It has a half-life of approximately 14.28 days and decays by beta emission. Chromium is a metallic trace element used in glucose metabolism and is essential to the body in small amounts. Chromic phosphate P-32 is a compound of phosphorus 32 and chromium. It is administered by intraperitoneal or intrapleural instillation or interstitial injection. Chromic phosphate P-32 is used intraperitoneally or intrapleurally for the therapeutic treatment of effusions resulting from metastatic disease and interstitially in the treatment of certain ovarian and prostate carcinomas. Dosages vary from 0.1 to 20 millicuries depending on the disease being treated and method of administration. HCPCS Level II code A9564 represents 1 millicurie of chromic phosphate P-32.

Medicare Information

See chapter titled "Medicare Guidelines," under "Drugs, Biologicals, and Radiopharmaceuticals," for Medicare billing and documentation information.

A9566

A9566 Technetium Tc-99m fanolesomab, diagnostic, per study dose, up to 25 millicuries

Lay Description

Fanolesomab is a murine monoclonal antibody that binds to the CD15 antigen. The CD15 antigen is found on the surface of some neutrophils, eosinophils, and monocytes, which are types of leukocytes or white blood cells. Technetium is a radioactive metallic element that is a byproduct of uranium decay. It may also be produced by bombarding another metal, molybdenum, with specific atoms. Technetium 99m is a widely used radionuclide with a half-life of approximately six hours, which is long enough to examine metabolic processes, but short enough to minimize the radiation dose received by the patient. It decays by gamma emission, which is then measured by scintillation or gamma cameras. Fanolesomab combined with technetium 99m pertechnetate labels the leukocytes or white blood cells. Leukocytes gather at the site of an infection. Technetium 99m fanolesomab is used to confirm appendicitis in patients with the signs and symptoms associated with appendicitis. The radiopharmaceutical is injected intravenously. The recommended adult dosage is 10 to 200 mCi. Imaging may begin immediately after administration. HCPCS Level II code A9566 represents a study dose of up to 25 millicuries of technetium Tc-99m fanolesomab.

Medicare Information
See chapter titled "Medicare Guidelines," under "Drugs, Biologicals, and Radiopharmaceuticals," for Medicare billing and documentation information.

A9567
A9567 Technetium Tc-99m pentetate, diagnostic, aerosol, per study dose, up to 75 millicuries

Lay Description
The pentetate here refers to calcium trisodium pentetate, which is a chelating agent that forms stable bounds with metals, which are then excreted in the urine. Technetium is a radioactive metallic element that is a byproduct of uranium decay. It may also be produced by bombarding another metal, molybdenum, with specific atoms. Technetium 99m is a widely used radionuclide with a half-life of approximately six hours, which is long enough to examine metabolic processes, but short enough to minimize the radiation dose received by the patient. It decays by gamma emission, which is then measured by scintillation or gamma cameras. Pentetate combined with technetium 99m is rapidly distributed throughout the body and is excretion from the body by glomerular filtration. The images of the kidneys obtained in the first few minutes after administration will show the blood pool within the kidney. Subsequent images show kidney function. Technetium Tc-99m pentetate also tends to accumulate in intracranial lesions with many new blood vessels or with an altered blood-brain barrier. The radiopharmaceutical is administered by intravenous injection. Dosage and optimal imaging depend on the area being imaged. Technetium Tc-99m pentetate is used for kidney and brain imaging and to assess renal function and estimate the glomerular filtration rate. When in aerosol form, it is administered by inhalation. The aerosol form is used to assess airway patency, especially in conjunction with perfusion lung imaging to evaluate for a pulmonary embolism. HCPCS Level II code A9567 represents a study dose of up to 75 millicuries of inhaled technetium Tc-99m pentetate.

Medicare Information
See chapter titled "Medicare Guidelines," under "Drugs, Biologicals, and Radiopharmaceuticals," for Medicare billing and documentation information.

A9568
A9568 Technetium Tc-99m arcitumomab, diagnostic, per study dose, up to 45 millicuries

Lay Description
Arcitumomab is murine monoclonal antibody directed to the carcinoembryonic antigen (CEA), a tumor-associated antigen the expression of which is increased in a variety of carcinomas, particularly of the gastrointestinal tract, and in certain inflammatory states (e.g., Crohn's disease, inflammatory bowel disease, post-radiation therapy to the bowel). Technetium is a radioactive metallic element that is a byproduct of uranium decay. It may also be produced by bombarding another metal, molybdenum with specific atoms. Technetium 99m is a widely used radionuclide with a half-life of approximately six hours, which is long enough to examine metabolic processes, but short enough to minimize the radiation dose received by the patient. It decays by gamma emission which is then measured by scintillation or gamma cameras. Arcitumomab combined with technetium 99m pertechnetate is indicated, in conjunction with standard diagnostic evaluations, for detection of the presence, location and extent of recurrent and/or metastatic colorectal carcinoma involving the liver, extrahepatic abdomen and pelvis in patients with a histologically confirmed diagnosis of colorectal carcinoma. The radiopharmaceutical is administered by intravenous injection. The recommended adult dosage is 1 mg labeled with 20-30 millicuries of technetium TC 99m arcitumomab. Optimal imaging is at two to five hours after administration. HCPCS Level II code A9549 represents a study dose of up to 45 millicuries of technetium TC 99m arcitumomab.

Medicare Information
See chapter titled "Medicare Guidelines," under "Drugs, Biologicals, and Radiopharmaceuticals," for Medicare billing and documentation information.

A9569
A9569 Technetium Tc-99m exametazime labeled autologous white blood cells, diagnostic, per study dose

Lay Description
Exametazime, also known as hexamethylpropyleneamine oxime, is a chemical complex that is taken up by leukocytes and selectively retained in neutrophils. Technetium is a radioactive metallic element that is a byproduct of

uranium decay. It may also be produced by bombarding another metal, molybdenum, with specific atoms. Technetium 99m is a widely used radionuclide with a half-life of approximately six hours, which is long enough to examine metabolic processes but short enough to minimize the radiation dose received by the patient. It decays by gamma emission, which is then measured by scintillation or gamma cameras. Tc-99m exametazime is used to label autologous leukocytes. The labeled leukocytes are then used in imaging to localize or identify areas of intra-abdominal infection or inflammation. Optimal imaging with labeled leukocytes is two to four hours after administration. When technetium Tc-99m pertechnetate is added to the exametazime, the resulting radiopharmaceutical is taken up by lipids that can cross the blood-brain barrier. The technetium Tc-99m pertechnetate/exametazime is useful for only 30 minutes. Its useful life can be extended by the addition of methylene blue. Tc-99m pertechnetate/exametazime is used in cerebral perfusion imaging to detect regions altered by stroke. The radiopharmaceutical is administered by intravenous injection. Optimal imaging for cerebral perfusion studies may begin immediately after administration and can continue up to six hours after administration. HCPCS Level II code A9569 represents one diagnostic study dose.

A9570

A9570 Indium In-111 labeled autologous white blood cells, diagnostic, per study dose

Lay Description

Indium 111 is a radioactive form of indium, a metallic element. Indium 111 has a half-life of 2.8 days and decays by electron capture and gamma emission. Indium 111 is used to label autologous white blood cells. These labeled cells are then reinfused into the patient intravenously and used to scan for abscesses and other inflammatory processes where the white cells would usually congregate. Imaging is performed approximately two hours postinjection. HCPCS Level II code A9570 represents one diagnostic study dose.

A9571

A9571 Indium In-111 labeled autologous platelets, diagnostic, per study dose

Lay Description

Indium 111 is a radioactive form of indium, a metallic element. Indium 111 has a half-life of 2.8 days and decays by electron capture and gamma emission. Indium 111 is used to label autologous platelets. These labeled cells are then reinfused into the patient intravenously. Platelets tend to aggregate at areas of thrombosis or active bleeding.

Indium-labeled platelets are used to scan for deep vein thrombosis, vascular integrity, and platelet survival. Imaging is performed approximately two hours postinjection. HCPCS Level II code A9571 represents one diagnostic study dose.

A9572

A9572 Indium In-111 pentetreotide, diagnostic, per study dose, up to 6 millicuries

Lay Description

Pentetreotide is a mixture of pentetic acid and octreotide. Pentetic acid, also known as pentetate or DTPA, is a chelating agent that binds with iron. Octreotide is a synthetic version of somatostatin, which is a peptide that inhibits the release of growth hormone, thyrotropin, and corticotropin. Indium 111 is a radioactive form of indium, a metallic element. Indium 111 has a half-life of 2.8 days and decays by electron capture and gamma emission. Indium In-111 pentetreotide binds somatostatin receptors on cell surfaces throughout the body. After approximately an hour following intravenous injection most of the indium In-111 pentetreotide is distributed throughout the body and is seen concentrated in tumors containing a high density of somatostatin receptors. Indium In-111 pentetreotide allows imaging that identifies the presence and location of primary and metastatic neuroendocrine tumors bearing somatostatin receptors. Indium In-111 pentetreotide is administered by intravenous injection. The recommended dose for planar imaging is 3.0 mCi. The recommended dose for SPECT imaging is 6.0 mCi.

A9576-A9579

A9576 Injection, gadoteridol, (ProHance multipack), per ml
A9577 Injection, gadobenate dimeglumine (MultiHance), per ml
A9578 Injection, gadobenate dimeglumine (MultiHance multipack), per ml
A9579 Injection, gadolinium-based magnetic resonance contrast agent, not otherwise specified (NOS), per ml

Lay Description

Magnetic resonance imaging (MRI) is a radiation-free, noninvasive technique to produce high-quality sectional images of the inside of the body in multiple planes. MRI uses the natural magnetic properties of the hydrogen atoms in our bodies that emit radiofrequency signals when exposed to radio waves within a strong electromagnetic field. These signals are then processed and converted by the computer into high-resolution, three-dimensional, tomographic images. Gadolinium is a rare earth metal that is strongly magnetic at room temperature. Various forms of the metal are used to enhance an MRI. The gadolinium is administered intravenously and circulates within the cardiovascular system allowing greater detail to be captured by the MRI. Gadolinium highlights disruptions of the blood-brain barrier and enhances areas of abnormal vascularization that is common in neoplasms, abscesses, or subacute infarcts. It is indicated for use in MRIs of the brain, spine, head and neck; thoracic, abdominal, and pelvic cavities; and retroperitoneal space. It is not indicated for use in cardiac imaging. Dosage depends on patient body weight with a recommended dose of 0.2 ml per kg.

A9580

A9580 Sodium fluoride F-18, diagnostic, per study dose, up to 30 millicuries

Lay Description

Sodium fluoride F-18 is a radiopharmaceutical used with PET scans. It is a positron emitting substance used to detect abnormal bone activity in the patient. Abnormal activity can be a result of cancer, Paget's disease, or osteomyelitis. Sodium fluoride is injected through an IV line and allowed to circulate. It accumulates in the areas of bone activity. Those areas are visible with the PET scan. The normal dose of sodium fluoride F-18 is 5 mCi to 15 mCi. HCPCS Level II code A9580 is per dose study up to 30 mCi.

A9581

A9581 Injection, gadoxetate disodium, 1 ml

Lay Description

Gadoxetate disodium is a paramagnetic, gadolinium-based contrast agent for MRI that creates a magnetic field. It provides a brightening of blood and tissue. It is used for liver MRIs to look for lesions or liver disease. The recommended dose of gadoxetate disodium is 0.1 mL/kg based on the patient's body weight. It is administered by IV injection. HCPCS Level II code A9581 represents a 1 milliliter dose.

A9582

A9582 Iodine I-123 iobenguane, diagnostic, per study dose, up to 15 millicuries

Lay Description

Iobenguane sulfate is an analogue of norepinephrine that binds to receptors in the sympathetic nervous system and to related tumors. Iodine 123 is a radioactive isotope of the common element iodine produced in a cyclotron. It decays by electron capture and gamma emission with a half life of 13 hours. Iobenguane sulfate combined with Iodine 123, also known as MIBG, is a radiopharmaceutical used as a diagnostic imaging agent for neuroendocrine tumors and disorders of the adrenal medulla. Iodine I-123 iobenguane sulfate is injected intravenously. Multiple scans are usually performed for up to four days post administration. HCPCS Level II code A9582 represents a study dose up to 15 millicuries.

A9583

A9583 Injection, gadofosveset trisodium, 1 ml

Lay Description

Gadofosveset trisodium is a contrast agent used to evaluate vascular structures with magnetic resonance angiography (MRA). The recommended dose is based on body weight and is administered intravenously.

A9600

A9600 Strontium Sr-89 chloride, therapeutic, per millicurie

Lay Description

Strontium is a metallic earth element that is similar to calcium, soft, and decomposes readily in water. Strontium 89 is a radioactive version of strontium. Strontium 89 has a half-life of 50.5 days and decays by beta emissions. Since strontium behaves like calcium, it is concentrated in the bone and in areas of calcium uptake. Strontium 89 is used as a source in radiation therapy. In the form of strontium 89 chloride, it is injected intravenously or delivered by catheter into a large vein. Strontium 89 chloride is indicated as a palliative treatment for debilitating bone pain in patients whose cancer has metastasized to bone. The bone metastasis should be confirmed prior to use of strontium 89. The recommended dosage is 4 mCi. Repeat treatments may be performed at 90-day intervals. HCPCS Level II code A9600 represents 1 millicurie of strontium 89 chloride.

A9604

A9604 Samarium sm-153 lexidronam, therapeutic, per treatment dose, up to 150 millicuries

Lay Description

Samarium is a metallic rare earth element found in other rare earth mineral ores. Samarium 153 is a radioactive form of samarium that has a half-life of 46.7 hours and decays by beta and gamma emissions. Lexidronam, also known as ethylene diamine tetramethylene phosphonate or EDTMP, is a chemical complex that concentrates in the bone and in areas of calcium uptake. Samarium 153 lexidronam is indicated as a palliative treatment for debilitating bone pain in patients whose cancer has metastasized to bone. The bone metastasis should be confirmed prior to use of samarium 153. The recommended dosage is 1 mCi per kg of body weight. It is administered intravenously through an indwelling catheter. HCPCS Level II code A9604 represents a treatment dose up to 150 millicuries.

A9698

A9698 Nonradioactive contrast imaging material, not otherwise classified, per study

Lay Description

Use this code when a HCPCS code for a contrast imaging material utilized has not been issued by CMS.

A9699

A9699 Radiopharmaceutical, therapeutic, not otherwise classified

Lay Description

This code is used to report the supply of radiopharmaceutical therapeutic imaging agents that do not have another specific HCPCS Level II code. Radiopharmaceuticals are radioactive isotopes, such as radioactive iodine or radioactive cobalt. They are often attached to carrier molecules and used in therapeutic nuclear medicine procedures.

Medicare Information

Report A9699 only when another code does not exist for the radiopharmaceutical therapeutic agent administered. Coverage is at the contractor's discretion.

A9700

A9700 Supply of injectable contrast material for use in echocardiography, per study

Lay Description

This code is used to report the supply of injectable contrast material used in echocardiography that does not have another specific HCPCS Level II code. There are HCPCS Level II codes for perflexane lipid microspheres (Q9955), octafluoropropane microspheres (Q9956), and perflutren lipid microspheres (Q9957). Report HCPCS Level II code A9700 once per echocardiography study.

Medicare Information

Report A9700 only when another code does not exist for the echocardiographic agent administered. Coverage is at the contractor's discretion. OPPS hospitals cannot report A9700.

B4034-B4036

B4034 Enteral feeding supply kit; syringe fed, per day, includes but not limited to feeding/flushing syringe, administration set tubing, dressings, tape

B4035 Enteral feeding supply kit; pump fed, per day, includes but not limited to feeding/flushing syringe, administration set tubing, dressings, tape

B4036 Enteral feeding supply kit; gravity fed, per day, includes but not limited to feeding/flushing syringe, administration set tubing, dressings, tape

Lay Description

Patients with chronic illness or trauma cannot be sustained through oral feeding and must rely on either enteral or parenteral therapy, depending upon the particular nature of the medical condition. Daily enteral nutrition is necessary for patients with a functioning gastrointestinal (GI) tract but nonfunctioning body structures for allowing food to reach the small bowel, or for patients with small bowel disease that impairs digestion and absorption of nutrients. Enteral nutrition is administered to a patient through a tube into the stomach or small intestine. The solutions may be administered by syringe, gravity, or infusion pump. Enteral feeding supply kits, per day, are reported with B4034 for syringe, B4035 for pump feed, and B4036 for gravity feed.

Consolidated Billing

For patients receiving home health services: Enteral nutrition solutions, equipment, and accessories are not subject to any HHA

Medicare Information

Medicare will pay for no more than one month's supply of enteral nutrients, accessories, or supplies at any one time. Enteral products that can be administered orally are not covered. Claims submitted retroactively, however, can report multiple months (for providers who perform prospective billing).

The feeding supply kit (B4034–B4036) must correspond to the method of administration. If a pump supply kit (B4035) is ordered and the medical necessity of the pump is not documented, payment will be based on the allowance for the least costly alternative, B4036.

When enteral nutrition is covered, dressings used in conjunction with a gastrostomy or enterostomy tube are included in the supply kit code (B4034–B4036) and should not be billed separately using dressing codes.

B4081-B4088

B4081 Nasogastric tubing with stylet
B4082 Nasogastric tubing without stylet
B4083 Stomach tube — Levine type
B4087 Gastrostomy/jejunostomy tube, standard, any material, any type, each
B4088 Gastrostomy/jejunostomy tube, low-profile, any material, any type, each

Lay Description

Patients with chronic illness or trauma cannot be sustained through oral feeding and must rely on either enteral or parenteral therapy, depending upon the particular nature of the medical condition. Enteral nutrition is administered to a patient through a tube (nasogastric, jejunostomy, or gastrostomy) into the stomach or small intestine. There are several types of gastric tubes including Levin type stomach tube, gastric sump, Moss, Sengstaken Blakemore, and Miller-Abbott. Specifically, feeding tubes are generally referred to as G tubes, J tubes, NG tubes, or surgical feeding tubes. Surgical feeding tubes require intra-operative placement.

Consolidated Billing

For patients receiving home health services:
Enteral nutrition solutions, equipment, and accessories are not subject to any HHA

Medicare Information

Medicare will pay for no more than one month's supply of enteral nutrients, accessories, or supplies at any one time. Enteral products that can be administered orally are not covered. Claims submitted retroactively, however, can report multiple months (for providers who perform prospective billing).

More than three nasogastric tubes (B4081–B4083) or one gastrostomy or jejunostomy tube (B4086) every three months is deemed as rarely medically necessary by Medicare.

Note: See chapter titled, "Medicare Guidelines," under "Enteral Nutrition," for additional Medicare billing and documentation information.

B4100

B4100 Food thickener, administered orally, per oz

Lay Description

Patients who have facial paralysis, due to a stroke, Parkinson's disease, multiple sclerosis, and other conditions, have difficulty swallowing liquids (dysphagia) and often benefit from the use of a food thickener. Thickened food has a pureed consistency necessary to help prevent choking. Commercial instant food thickener has no taste or aftertaste. It mixes with hot or cold foods and liquids and thickens in just 30 seconds. These products allow for normal hydration by releasing available fluid after consumption. The thickened food and liquid does not harden when chilled or cause constipation. Use this code per ounce of food thickener.

B4102-B4104

B4102 Enteral formula, for adults, used to replace fluids and electrolytes (e.g., clear liquids), 500 ml = 1 unit
B4103 Enteral formula, for pediatrics, used to replace fluids and electrolytes (e.g., clear liquids), 500 ml = 1 unit
B4104 Additive for enteral formula (e.g., fiber)

Lay Description

For patients who cannot be sustained through oral feedings, enteral nutrition is administered by means of a nasogastric, jejunostomy, or gastrostomy feeding tube directly into the stomach or small intestine. Report B4102 for a clear liquid enteral formula with electrolyte balance used for fluid replacement and hydration maintenance per 500 ml unit for adults and B4103 for children. B4104 reports an additive for an enteral formula, such as fiber, used to maintain normal bowel function and avoid constipation.

B4149, B4157

B4149 Enteral formula, manufactured blenderized natural foods with intact nutrients, includes proteins, fats, carbohydrates, vitamins and minerals, may include fiber, administered through an enteral feeding tube, 100 calories = 1 unit
B4157 Enteral formula, nutritionally complete, for special metabolic needs for inherited disease of metabolism, includes proteins, fats, carbohydrates, vitamins and minerals, may include fiber, administered through an enteral feeding tube, 100 calories = 1 unit

Lay Description

For patients who cannot be sustained through oral feedings, enteral nutrition is administered by means of a nasogastric, jejunostomy, or gastrostomy feeding tube directly into the stomach or small intestine. Enteral formulas are composed of varying combinations of natural or semi-synthetic proteins, amino acids, fats, carbohydrates, vitamins, and minerals to fulfill different nutritional needs. Code B4149 reports a blenderized natural foods formula of intact nutrients that includes proteins, fats, carbohydrates, vitamins and minerals, and possibly fiber per 100 cal unit. Intact nutrients are not already broken down and remain in a high molecular weight form, which require normal digestive and absorptive ability. Code B4157 reports a nutritionally complete formula designed for the special metabolic needs of inherited metabolism disorders, per 100 cal unit.

B4150-B4152

B4150 Enteral formula, nutritionally complete with intact nutrients, includes proteins, fats, carbohydrates, vitamins and minerals, may include fiber, administered through an enteral feeding tube, 100 calories = 1 unit

B4152 Enteral formula, nutritionally complete, calorically dense (equal to or greater than 1.5 kcal/ml) with intact nutrients, includes proteins, fats, carbohydrates, vitamins and minerals, may include fiber, administered through an enteral feeding tube, 100 calories = 1 unit

Lay Description

These codes report a nutritionally complete enteral formula or nutrient mixture administered to patients who cannot be sustained through oral feedings, given by means of a nasogastric, jejunostomy, or gastrostomy feeding tube directly into the stomach or small intestine. Tube feedings can be administered by bolus feedings, continuous drip feedings, or a combination of the two. Report B4150 for an intact nutrient formula with proteins, fats, carbohydrates, vitamins and minerals, and possibly fiber, per 100 cal unit. Intact nutrients are not already broken down and remain in a high molecular weight form, which require normal digestive and absorptive ability. Report B4152 for a nutritionally complete, calorically dense formula (equal to or greater than 1.5 kcal/ml), per 100 cal unit.

Medicare Information

Medicare will pay for no more than one month's supply of enteral nutrients, accessories, or supplies at any one time. Enteral products that can be administered orally are not covered. Claims submitted retroactively, however, can report multiple months (for providers who perform prospective billing).

Enteral formulas consisting of intact nutrients (B4150) are appropriate for the majority of patients requiring enteral nutrition. Caloric-dense formulas (B4152) are covered if they are ordered and are medically necessary. The medical necessity for special enteral formulas (B4153–B4155) will need to be justified in each patient. If the medical necessity for these formulas is not substantiated, payment will be based on the allowance for the least costly alternative, B4150.

Note: See chapter titled, "Medicare Guidelines," under "Enteral Nutrition," for additional Medicare billing and documentation information.

Medicare modifiers

When enteral nutrients (B4150–B4156) are administered by mouth, modifier BO must be appended to the code.

B4153

B4153 Enteral formula, nutritionally complete, hydrolyzed proteins (amino acids and peptide chain), includes fats, carbohydrates, vitamins and minerals, may include fiber, administered through an enteral feeding tube, 100 calories = 1 unit

Lay Description

This code reports a nutritionally complete enteral formula or nutrient mixture administered to patients who cannot be sustained through oral feedings, given by means of a nasogastric, jejunostomy, or gastrostomy feeding tube directly into the stomach or small intestine. Tube feedings can be administered by bolus feedings, continuous drip feedings, or a combination of the two. This code reports a formula of hydrolyzed proteins of amino acids and peptide chain, including fats, carbohydrates, vitamins and minerals, and possibly fiber, per 100 cal unit. Hydrolyzed proteins have been split down into their smaller building-block forms of amino acids and peptide chains by enzymes, acids, or alkalis and provide the same nutritive equivalent in a more easily digestible form.

Medicare Information

Medicare will pay for no more than one month's supply of enteral nutrients, accessories, or supplies at any one time. Enteral products that can be administered orally are not covered. Claims submitted retroactively, however, can report multiple months (for providers who perform prospective billing).

Enteral formulas consisting of intact nutrients (B4150) are appropriate for the majority of patients requiring enteral nutrition. Caloric-dense formulas (B4152) are covered if they are ordered and are medically necessary. The medical necessity for special enteral formulas (B4153–B4155) will need to be justified in each patient. If the medical necessity for these formulas is not substantiated, payment will be based on the allowance for the least costly alternative, B4150.

Note: See chapter titled, "Medicare Guidelines," under "Enteral Nutrition," for additional Medicare billing and documentation information.

HCPCS Lay Descriptions

Medicare modifiers
When enteral nutrients (B4150–B4156) are administered by mouth, modifier BO must be appended to the code.

B4154-B4155

B4154 Enteral formula, nutritionally complete, for special metabolic needs, excludes inherited disease of metabolism, includes altered composition of proteins, fats, carbohydrates, vitamins and/or minerals, may include fiber, administered through an enteral feeding tube, 100 calories = 1 unit

B4155 Enteral formula, nutritionally incomplete/modular nutrients, includes specific nutrients, carbohydrates (e.g., glucose polymers), proteins/amino acids (e.g., glutamine, arginine), fat (e.g., medium chain triglycerides) or combination, administered through an enteral feeding tube, 100 calories = 1 unit

Lay Description
Code B4154 reports a nutritionally complete enteral formula or nutrient mixture administered to patients who cannot be sustained through oral feedings, given by means of a nasogastric, jejunostomy, or gastrostomy feeding tube directly into the stomach or small intestine. Tube feedings can be administered by bolus feedings, continuous drip feedings, or a combination of the two. This code reports a formula designed for special metabolic needs that are not a consequence of an inherited metabolism disorder. The formula may contain proteins, fats, and carbohydrates in altered composition, and possible fiber, per 100 cal unit. Code B4155 reports a nutritionally incomplete enteral formula of modular nutrients per 100 cal unit. This formula contains specific nutrient forms of carbohydrates, fats, or proteins to cover deficiency needs, such as glucose polymers, glutamine, arginine, and medium chain triglycerides.

Medicare Information
Medicare will pay for no more than one month's supply of enteral nutrients, accessories, or supplies at any one time. Enteral products that can be administered orally are not covered. Claims submitted retroactively, however, can report multiple months (for providers who perform prospective billing).

Enteral formulas consisting of intact nutrients (B4150) are appropriate for the majority of patients requiring enteral nutrition. Caloric-dense formulas (B4152) are covered if they are ordered and are medically necessary. The medical necessity for special enteral formulas (B4153–B4155) will need to be justified in each patient. If the medical necessity for these formulas is not substantiated, payment will be based on the allowance for the least costly alternative, B4150.

Note: See chapter titled, "Medicare Guidelines," under "Enteral Nutrition," for additional Medicare billing and documentation information.

Medicare modifiers
When enteral nutrients (B4150–B4156) are administered by mouth, modifier BO must be appended to the code.

B4157

B4157 Enteral formula, nutritionally complete, for special metabolic needs for inherited disease of metabolism, includes proteins, fats, carbohydrates, vitamins and minerals, may include fiber, administered through an enteral feeding tube, 100 calories = 1 unit

Lay Description
Please refer to code B4149 for the description, coding, and billing information.

B4158-B4159

B4158 Enteral formula, for pediatrics, nutritionally complete with intact nutrients, includes proteins, fats, carbohydrates, vitamins and minerals, may include fiber and/or iron, administered through an enteral feeding tube, 100 calories = 1 unit

B4159 Enteral formula, for pediatrics, nutritionally complete soy based with intact nutrients, includes proteins, fats, carbohydrates, vitamins and minerals, may include fiber and/or iron, administered through an enteral feeding tube, 100 calories = 1 unit

Lay Description
These codes report a pediatric enteral formula or nutrient mixture administered to patients who cannot be sustained through oral feedings, given by means of a nasogastric, jejunostomy, or gastrostomy feeding tube directly into the stomach or small intestine. Tube feedings can be administered by bolus feedings, continuous drip feedings, or a combination of the two in patients who require calorie and protein support. Code B4158 reports a nutritionally complete, intact nutrient, pediatric formula with proteins, fats, carbohydrates, vitamins and minerals, and possibly fiber and/or iron, per 100 cal unit. Intact nutrients are not already broken down and remain in a high molecular weight form, which require normal digestive and absorptive ability. Code

B4159 reports a nutritionally complete, soy-based, pediatric enteral formula, which is used to avoid milk-protein sensitivity, per 100 cal unit.

B4160

B4160 Enteral formula, for pediatrics, nutritionally complete calorically dense (equal to or greater than 0.7 kcal/ml) with intact nutrients, includes proteins, fats, carbohydrates, vitamins and minerals, may include fiber, administered through an enteral feeding tube, 100 calories = 1 unit

Lay Description

This code reports a pediatric enteral formula or nutrient mixture administered to patients who cannot be sustained through oral feedings, given by means of a nasogastric, jejunostomy, or gastrostomy feeding tube directly into the stomach or small intestine. Tube feedings can be administered by bolus feedings, continuous drip feedings, or a combination of the two in patients who require calorie and protein support. This code reports a calorically dense, nutritionally complete formula, with intact nutrients, greater than .7kcal/ml, and possibly including fiber, per 100 cal unit. Intact nutrients are not already broken down and remain in a high molecular weight form, which require normal digestive and absorptive ability.

B4161

B4161 Enteral formula, for pediatrics, hydrolyzed/amino acids and peptide chain proteins, includes fats, carbohydrates, vitamins and minerals, may include fiber, administered through an enteral feeding tube, 100 calories = 1 unit

Lay Description

This code reports a pediatric enteral formula or nutrient mixture administered to patients who cannot be sustained through oral feedings, given by means of a nasogastric, jejunostomy, or gastrostomy feeding tube directly into the stomach or small intestine. Tube feedings can be administered by bolus feedings, continuous drip feedings, or a combination of the two in patients who require calorie and protein support. This code reports a formula of hydrolyzed/amino acids and peptide chain proteins, including fats, carbohydrates, vitamins and minerals, and possibly fiber, per 100 cal unit. Hydrolyzed proteins have been split down into their smaller building-block forms of amino acids and peptide chains by enzymes, acids, or alkalis and provide the same nutritive equivalent in a more easily digestible form.

B4162

B4162 Enteral formula, for pediatrics, special metabolic needs for inherited disease of metabolism, includes proteins, fats, carbohydrates, vitamins and minerals, may include fiber, administered through an enteral feeding tube, 100 calories = 1 unit

Lay Description

This code reports a pediatric enteral formula, or nutrient mixture administered to patients who cannot be sustained through oral feedings, given by means of a nasogastric, jejunostomy, or gastrostomy feeding tube directly into the stomach or small intestine. Tube feedings can be administered by bolus feedings, continuous drip feedings, or a combination of the two in patients who require calorie and protein support. This code reports a nutritionally complete pediatric formula designed for the special metabolic needs of inherited metabolism disorders, per 100 cal unit.

B4164-B4185

B4164 Parenteral nutrition solution: carbohydrates (dextrose), 50% or less (500 ml = 1 unit), home mix
B4168 Parenteral nutrition solution; amino acid, 3.5%, (500 ml = 1 unit) — home mix
B4172 Parenteral nutrition solution; amino acid, 5.5% through 7%, (500 ml = 1 unit) — home mix
B4176 Parenteral nutrition solution; amino acid, 7% through 8.5%, (500 ml = 1 unit) — home mix
B4178 Parenteral nutrition solution: amino acid, greater than 8.5% (500 ml = 1 unit), home mix
B4180 Parenteral nutrition solution: carbohydrates (dextrose), greater than 50% (500 ml = 1 unit), home mix
B4185 Parenteral nutrition solution, per 10 grams lipids

Lay Description

Parenteral nutrition is administered to the patient intravenously. Since the alimentary tract of a patient with severe pathology does not function adequately for ingesting food normally, an indwelling catheter is placed percutaneously in the subclavian vein, and then advanced into the superior vena cava for infusing nutrients intravenously. Parenteral nutrition solutions are based on the composition of ingredients or nutrient source in each product, and whether it is supplied in a home mix or a premix. These codes report home mix solutions of 1 unit equaling 500 ml. Report B4164 for 50 percent or less carbohydrates (dextrose); B4168 for 3.5 percent amino acid; B4172 for 5.5 to 7 percent amino acid; B4176 for 7 to 8.5 percent amino acid, B4178 for amino acid greater than 8.5 percent; and B4180 for greater than 50 percent carbohydrates (dextrose). Report B4185 per 10 grams of lipids.

Medicare Information

If the coverage requirements for PEN therapy are met under the prosthetic device benefit provision, related supplies, equipment, and nutrients are also typically covered.

When home mix parenteral nutrition solutions are used, the component carbohydrates (B4164, B4180), amino acids (B4168–B4178), and lipids (B4184, B4186) are all separately billable.

Note: See chapter titled "Medicare Guidelines," under "Parenteral Nutrition," for additional Medicare billing and documentation information.

B4189-B4216

B4189 Parenteral nutrition solution: compounded amino acid and carbohydrates with electrolytes, trace elements, and vitamins, including preparation, any strength, 10 to 51 g of protein, premix

B4193 Parenteral nutrition solution: compounded amino acid and carbohydrates with electrolytes, trace elements, and vitamins, including preparation, any strength, 52 to 73 g of protein, premix

B4197 Parenteral nutrition solution; compounded amino acid and carbohydrates with electrolytes, trace elements and vitamins, including preparation, any strength, 74 to 100 grams of protein — premix

B4199 Parenteral nutrition solution; compounded amino acid and carbohydrates with electrolytes, trace elements and vitamins, including preparation, any strength, over 100 grams of protein — premix

B4216 Parenteral nutrition; additives (vitamins, trace elements, Heparin, electrolytes), home mix, per day

Lay Description

Parenteral nutrition is administered to the patient intravenously. Since the alimentary tract of a patient with severe pathology does not function adequately for ingesting food normally, an indwelling catheter is placed percutaneously in the subclavian vein, and then advanced into the superior vena cava for infusing nutrients intravenously. Parenteral nutrition solutions are based on the composition of ingredients or nutrient source in each parenteral nutrient product, and whether it is supplied in a home mix or a premix. These codes report premix solutions, including preparation of any strength compounded amino acids and carbohydrates with electrolytes, trace elements, and vitamins. Report B4189 for 10 to 51 grams of protein, B4193 for 52 to 73 grams of protein, B4197 for 74 to 100 grams of protein, and B4199 for more than 100 grams of protein. Report B4216 for parenteral nutrition additives such as vitamins, trace elements, heparin, and electrolytes, in a home mix per day.

Medicare Information

If the coverage requirements for PEN therapy are met under the prosthetic device benefit provision, related supplies, equipment, and nutrients are also typically covered.

When home mix parenteral nutrition solutions are used, the component (B4216) is separately billable. When premix parenteral nutrition solutions are used (B4189–B4199), there must be no separate billing for the carbohydrates, amino acids, or additives (vitamins, trace elements, heparin, electrolytes). However, lipids are separately billable with premix solutions.

In B4189–B4199, one unit of service represents one day's supply of protein and carbohydrate, regardless of the fluid volume and/or the number of bags. For example, if 60 grams of protein are administered per day in two bags of a premix solution, each containing 30 grams of amino acids, correct coding is one unit of B4193, not two units of B4189.

Note: See chapter titled "Medicare Guidelines," under "Parenteral Nutrition," for additional Medicare billing and documentation information.

B4220-B4224

B4220 Parenteral nutrition supply kit; premix, per day

B4222 Parenteral nutrition supply kit; home mix, per day

B4224 Parenteral nutrition administration kit, per day

Lay Description

Patients with chronic illness or trauma cannot be sustained through oral feeding and must rely on either enteral or parenteral therapy, depending upon the particular nature of the medical condition. Parenteral nutrition is administered to the patient intravenously. These codes report the supply and administration kits for parenteral nutrition on a daily basis. Report B4220 for a premix supply kit, B4222 for a home mix supply kit, and B4224 for an administration kit.

Medicare Information

These devices and accessories are coded with the HCPCS Level II code and billed to the DME MAC, not to the Medicare carrier. CMN DME MAC form 10.02A (CMS form 852), Parenteral Nutrition, is required to be completed by the physician and submitted by the supplier for coverage. This form must be submitted with the CMS-1500 claim form. Electronic filers can use the electronic CMN format.

If the coverage requirements for PEN therapy are met under the prosthetic device benefit provision, related supplies, equipment, and nutrients are also typically covered.

Note: See chapter titled, "Medicare Guidelines," under "Enteral Nutrition," for additional Medicare billing and documentation information.

B5000-B5200

B5000   Parenteral nutrition solution: compounded amino acid and carbohydrates with electrolytes, trace elements, and vitamins, including preparation, any strength, renal - Amirosyn RF, NephrAmine, RenAmine - premix

B5100   Parenteral nutrition solution: compounded amino acid and carbohydrates with electrolytes, trace elements, and vitamins, including preparation, any strength, hepatic - FreAmine HBC, HepatAmine - premix

B5200   Parenteral nutrition solution: compounded amino acid and carbohydrates with electrolytes, trace elements, and vitamins, including preparation, any strength, stress - branch chain amino acids - premix

Lay Description

Parenteral nutrition is administered to the patient intravenously. Since the alimentary tract of a patient with severe pathology does not function adequately for ingesting food normally, an indwelling catheter is placed percutaneously in the subclavian vein, and then advanced into the superior vena cava for infusing nutrients intravenously. Parenteral nutrition solutions are based on the composition of ingredients or nutrient source in each parenteral nutrient product, and whether it is supplied in a home mix or a premix. These codes report premix solutions, including preparation of any strength compounded amino acids and carbohydrates with electrolytes, trace elements, and vitamins. Report B5000 for a renal-formulated preparation -amirosyn RF, nephramine, and renamine, B5100 for a hepatic-formulated preparation - freamine HBC and hepatamine, and B5200 for a stress-formulated preparation - branch chain amino acids.

Medicare Information

In B5000-B5200, one unit of service is one gram of amino acid.

If the coverage requirements for PEN therapy are met under the prosthetic device benefit provision, related supplies, equipment, and nutrients are also typically covered.

When premix parenteral nutrition solutions are used (B5000-B5200), there must be no separate billing for the carbohydrates, amino acids, or additives (vitamins, trace elements, heparin, electrolytes). However, lipids are separately billable with premix solutions.

Note: See chapter titled "Medicare Guidelines," under "Parenteral Nutrition," for additional Medicare billing and documentation information.

B9000-B9002

B9000   Enteral nutrition infusion pump — without alarm
B9002   Enteral nutrition infusion pump — with alarm

Lay Description

Infusion pumps are available when enteral nutrition patients experience complications associated with syringe or gravity feedings. An enteral pump is ordered when feeding problems arise such as reflux and/or aspiration, severe diarrhea, dumping syndrome, an administration rate less than 100 ml/hr, blood glucose fluctuations, or circulatory overload. Use B9000 to code an enteral infusion pump with an alarm and B9002 for a pump without an alarm.

Consolidated Billing

For patients receiving home health services:
Enteral nutrition solutions, equipment, and accessories are not subject to any HHA

Medicare Information

Medicare will pay for no more than one month's supply of enteral nutrients, accessories, or supplies at any one time. Enteral products that can be administered orally are not covered. Claims submitted retroactively, however, can report multiple months (for providers who perform prospective billing).

If the claim involves an infusion pump (B9000, B9002), sufficient evidence must be provided to support a determination of medical necessity for the pump (i.e., gravity feeding is not satisfactory due to aspiration, diarrhea, dumping syndrome, and so forth). Medicare program reimbursement for the pump will be based on the reasonable charge for the simplest model that meets the medical needs of the patient as established by medical documentation.

PEN infusion pumps can be either rented or purchased. When rented, they are processed like capped rental items with two notable exceptions: First, they are not subject to the 25 percent reduction payment for the fourth rental month and after. Second, a patient may elect to purchase a PEN pump at any time, but must be offered the opportunity to do so by the 10th month. If the patient decides to purchase the pump once rentals have been paid, the purchase allowance will consist of the used purchase allowance less the amount allowed to date for rentals. Additional rental payments after the 15-month limit has been reached or after the pump has been purchased will only be considered if the attending provider changes the prescription between parenteral and enteral nutrients. A change in suppliers during the 15-month rental period does not begin a new 15-month rental period. The new supplier is entitled to the balance remaining on the 15-month rental period.

The supplier that collects the last month of rental (i.e., the 15th month) is responsible for ensuring that the patient has a pump for as long as it is medically necessary, and for maintenance and servicing of the pump during the period of medical necessity.

Necessary maintenance and servicing of PEN pumps after the 15-month rental limit is reached may include repairs and extensive maintenance that involve the breaking down of sealed components, or performing tests that require specialized testing equipment not available to the patient or nursing home. Payment will only be made for actual incidents of maintenance, servicing, or replacement. For enteral pumps, maintenance and servicing may be considered for payment every six months, beginning six months after the last rental payment for the pump.

Note: See chapter titled, "Medicare Guidelines," under "Enteral Nutrition," for additional Medicare billing and documentation information.

Medicare modifiers

Modifier MS should be appended to the appropriate pump code for maintenance and service claims. Claims for replacement of PEN pumps purchased more than eight years ago will be considered for payment.

B9004-B9999

B9004   **Parenteral nutrition infusion pump, portable**
B9006   **Parenteral nutrition infusion pump, stationary**
B9998   **NOC for enteral supplies**
B9999   **NOC for parenteral supplies**

Lay Description

Permanent conditions of the alimentary tract cause the patient to be unable to maintain weight and strength through normal feeding and require parenteral therapy, the intravenous infusion of nutrients, with the use of a parenteral nutrition infusion pump. Report B9004 for a portable pump and B9006 for a stationary infusion pump. Parenteral supplies that are not otherwise classified, such as nutrition solutions containing less than 10 grams of protein per day, are coded using B9999 (not otherwise classified (NOC) code for parenteral supplies). Report B9998 for enteral supplies not otherwise classified.

Medicare Information

If the claim involves an infusion pump (B9000–B9006), sufficient evidence must be provided to support a determination of medical necessity for the pump. Medicare program reimbursement for the pump will be based on the reasonable charge for the simplest model that meets the medical needs of the patient as established by medical documentation. Only one pump (stationary or portable) will be covered at any one time. Additional pumps will be denied as not medically necessary.

If the coverage requirements for PEN therapy are met under the prosthetic device benefit provision, related supplies, equipment, and nutrients are also typically covered.

Parenteral nutrition solutions containing less than 10 grams of protein per day are coded using the miscellaneous code B9999. When B9999 is billed, the claim must include a clear description of the item, the quantity provided, and the medical necessity of the item for the patient.

Note: See chapter titled, "Medicare Guidelines," under "Enteral Nutrition," for additional Medicare billing and documentation information.

Medicare modifiers

Modifier MS should be appended to the pump code for maintenance and service claims. Claims for replacement of PEN pumps purchased more than eight years ago will be considered for payment.

C1300

C1300 Hyperbaric oxygen under pressure, full body chamber, per 30 minute interval

Lay Description

In hyperbaric oxygen (HBO) therapy, the patient is enclosed in a pressure chamber breathing oxygen at a pressure greater than one's atmosphere. The therapeutic result is hyperoxygenation, with extra oxygen dissolved into the blood plasma. Breathing pure oxygen at three times the normal pressure delivers 15 times as much dissolved oxygen to tissues than room air. This promotes formation of new capillaries into wound areas and sufficient oxygen tensions to meet the needs of the ischemic tissues. Anemias, ischemias, and certain poisonings are effectively treated using hyperoxygenation. HBO therapy also helps free gas bubbles that are trapped in the body. Hyperoxygenation reduces the size of gas bubbles by two-thirds and aids in successful reduction in gas volume to air embolisms and decompression sickness. There is also a "gas wash out" or mass action of gases. This is the flooding of the body with any one gas to wash out all other gases. This treatment occurs quickly under pressure and is excellent as a treatment for carbon monoxide poisoning/intoxication and acute cyanide poisoning. Vasoconstriction is also treated with HBO. High pressure oxygen causes the blood vessels to constrict without creating hypoxia, therefore decreasing edema in affected or injured tissues and decreasing intracranial pressure. This treatment is useful for interstitial bleeding, burns, and crash victims. HBO also restrains the growth of anaerobic and aerobic organisms called Bacteriosis and is useful in conditions where resistance elements are compromised, as in dysvascular conditions. This effect complements the improved action of host disease fighting components. HCPCS Level II code C1300 represents hyperbaric oxygen under pressure, full body chamber, per 30 minute interval.

C1713

C1713 Anchor/screw for opposing bone-to-bone or soft tissue-to-bone (implantable)

Lay Description

An implantable pin and/or screw is used to oppose soft tissue-to-bone, tendon-to-bone, or bone-to-bone. A screw opposes the tissue by means of drilling as follows: soft tissue-to-bone, tendon-to-bone, or bone-to-bone fixation. Pins are inserted or drilled into the bone with the intent to facilitate stabilization or oppose bone-to-bone. In many instances this may include orthopedic plates with accompanying washers and nuts.

C1714

C1714 Catheter, transluminal atherectomy, directional

Lay Description

This code represents a special type of catheter used in transluminal atherectomy procedures. Transluminal atherectomy procedures involve opening the patients blocked arteries or vein grafts by using specialized devices attached to the end of catheters, which assist in the removal of thrombi and plaque material. Rotational atherectomy involves a high speed rotational device that grinds up the plaque material being removed from the vessel. Directional atherectomy scrapes or directs the plaque into in opening on one side of the catheter. Transluminal extraction atherectomy uses a device that cuts plaque off vessel walls and then vacuums it into a bottle. Code C1714 represent the catheter used in directional atherectomy.

C1715

C1715 Brachytherapy needle

Lay Description

This code pertains to needles specifically used in brachytherapy and is utilized per needle not per procedure.

C1716-C1719

C1716 Brachytherapy source, nonstranded, gold-198, per source
C1717 Brachytherapy source, nonstranded, high dose rate iridium-192, per source
C1719 Brachytherapy source, nonstranded, nonhigh dose rate iridium-192, per source

Lay Description

Brachytherapy is a form of radiotherapy in which physicians place the source of irradiation close to the tumor or within a body cavity. Brachytherapy could include placing radioactive sources inside a body cavity (intracavitary brachytherapy) or putting radioactive material directly into body tissue using hollow needles (interstitial brachytherapy). Brachytherapy may be given in addition to external beam radiation, or it may be used as the only form of radiotherapy. In some cases, the radioactive sources may be permanently left in place; in other cases, they are removed after a specified time. Placement of radioactive sources may be repeated several times. The isotope gold-198 (C1716) has a half life of 2.7 days and is used in some cancer treatments and treatments for other diseases. There are two natural isotopes of iridium, and many radioisotopes, the most stable radioisotope being Ir-192 with a half-life of 73.83 days. Ir-192 beta decays into platinum-192, while most of the other radioisotopes decay into osmium. Report C1717 for a nonstranded, high dose rate iridium-192 brachytherapy source and C1718 for a nonstranded, nonhigh dose rate iridium-192 brachytherapy source.

C1721-C1722

C1721   Cardioverter-defibrillator, dual chamber (implantable)
C1722   Cardioverter-defibrillator, single chamber (implantable)

Lay Description

Implantable cardioverter defibrillators are used in patients at risk for recurrent, sustained ventricular tachycardia or fibrillation. The defibrillators are connected to leads that are positioned inside the heart or on the heart surface. These leads deliver electrical shocks, sense the heart's rhythm, and pace the heart as necessary. Various leads are tunneled to the pulse generator, which has been implanted in a pouch made in the skin of the abdomen or chest. When the defibrillator detects ventricular tachycardia or fibrillation, it will automatically shock the heart to restore normal rhythm. Report C1721 for a dual chamber cardioverter defibrillator and C1722 for a single chamber cardioverter defibrillator.

C1724

C1724   Catheter, transluminal atherectomy, rotational

Lay Description

This code represents a special type of catheter used in transluminal atherectomy procedures. Transluminal atherectomy procedures involve opening the patients blocked arteries or vein grafts by using specialized devices attached to the end of catheters, which assist in the removal of thrombi and plaque material. Rotational atherectomy involves a high speed rotational device that grinds up the plaque material being removed from the vessel. Directional atherectomy scrapes or directs the plaque into in opening on one side of the catheter. Transluminal extraction atherectomy uses a device that cuts plaque off vessel walls and then vacuums it into a bottle. Code C1724 represents the catheter being used in rotational atherectomy.

C1725

C1725   Catheter, transluminal angioplasty, nonlaser (may include guidance, infusion/perfusion capability)

Lay Description

A transluminal angioplasty nonlaser catheter is a small hollow tube that is inserted into the central space (or lumen) of an artery or vein .This code refers to a catheter that is not used with a laser, but is used with balloon or other device that is designed to be advanced through the blood vessels to the area of occlusion or blockage. When the catheter is in position, the device is used to compress, break up, or remove the obstruction.

C1726

C1726   Catheter, balloon dilatation, nonvascular

Lay Description

A nonvascular balloon dilatation catheter is a small hollow tube containing a deflated balloon that is inserted into body cavity, duct or other passageway. The catheter is advanced to the area of occlusion or blockage. When the catheter is in position, the balloon is inflated and used to dilate strictures or stenoses. Examples of common sites are the common bile duct, intestines, or ureter.

C1727

C1727   Catheter, balloon tissue dissector, nonvascular (insertable)

Lay Description

A balloon tissue dissector, nonvascular catheter is small hollow tube that contains a deflated balloon. The catheter is guided to the appropriate space, the balloon is inflated and sometimes elongated. It is used to reate a space between soft tissues to improve operative vision and work space.

C1728

C1728   Catheter, brachytherapy seed administration

Lay Description

A brachytherapy seed administration catheter used to temporarily place encapsulated radioactive materials (seeds or sources) in or near the targeted tissue or tumor, or into a body cavity.

C1729

C1729   Catheter, drainage

Lay Description

A drainage catheter is a small hollow tube that is used to drain collected fluids from internal structures out through the skin and subcutaneous tissue. This category does not include Foley catheters or suprapubic catheters.

C1730-C1732

C1730 Catheter, electrophysiology, diagnostic, other than 3D mapping (19 or fewer electrodes)
C1731 Catheter, electrophysiology, diagnostic, other than 3D mapping (20 or more electrodes)
C1732 Catheter, electrophysiology, diagnostic/ablation, 3D or vector mapping

Lay Description

These codes describe catheters that assist in providing anatomic and physiologic information about the heart's electrical activity. Electrophysiology catheters are categorized into two main groups: (1) catheters used for mapping, pacing, and/or recording only, and (2) ablation (therapeutic) catheters that also have diagnostic capability. The electrophysiology ablation catheters are distinct from non-cardiac ablation catheters. Report C1730 for an electrophysiology catheter, diagnostic, used for other than 3D mapping (19 or less electrodes). Report C1731 for 20 or more electrodes. Report C1732 for an electrophysiology catheter, diagnostic/ablation, used for 3D or vector mapping.

C1733

C1733 Catheter, electrophysiology, diagnostic/ablation, other than 3D or vector mapping, other than cool-tip

Lay Description

An electrophysiology, diagnostic/ablation catheter, other than 3D or vector mapping, other than cool-tip, is a small hollow tube that assists in providing anatomic and physiologic information about the cardiac electrical conduction system. Electrophysiology catheters are categorized into two main groups: (1) diagnostic catheters that are used for mapping, pacing, and/or recording only, and (2) ablation (therapeutic) catheters that also have diagnostic capability. The electrophysiology ablation catheters are distinct from non-cardiac ablation catheters. Electrophysiology catheters designated as "cool-tip" refer to catheters with tips cooled by infused and/or circulating saline. Catheters designated as "other than cool-tip" refer to the termister tip catheter with temperature probe that measures temperature at the tissue catheter interface.

C1750, C1752

C1750 Catheter, hemodialysis/peritoneal, long-term
C1752 Catheter, hemodialysis/peritoneal, short-term

Lay Description

These codes describe a catheter that can be a permanent (C1750) or temporary (C1752) placed tube with one or two cuffs. This catheter is surgically placed into the peritoneum in the abdomen via a small incision and works by permitting the exchange of fluid through the catheter, allowing dialysate in and out of the abdominal cavity.

C1751

C1751 Catheter, infusion, inserted peripherally, centrally or midline (other than hemodialysis)

Lay Description

An infusion catheter is a plastic catheter that may have multiple lumens that is inserted into a large vein and ends up in the subclavian, brachiocephalic, or iliac veins, the superior or inferior vena cava, or the right atrium. It can be inserted centrally into the jugular, subclavian, femoral vein or inferior vena cava or peripherally into the basilic or cephalic vein. It can be used to administer medication, hydration, nutrition, and for monitoring and withdrawing blood samples. There are two different types of catheters: tunnelled and non-tunnelled.

C1753

C1753 Catheter, intravascular ultrasound

Lay Description

This code describes a specially designed catheter with a very small ultrasound probe attached to the distal end of the catheter. The proximal end of the catheter is attached to computerized ultrasound equipment. It allows the application of ultrasound technology to see from inside blood vessels out through the surrounding blood column, allowing the visualization of the inner wall of blood vessels.

C1754

C1754 Catheter, intradiscal

Lay Description

An intradiscal catheter is a small hollow tube that is inserted into a vertebral disc through which therapeutic treatments are performed. The flexible catheter is threaded percutaneously using fluoroscopic guidance. The catheter may be used to deliver electrothermal therapy.

C1755

C1755 Catheter, intraspinal

Lay Description

An intraspinal catheter is small hollow tube that is inserted into the spinal column to deliver diagnostic or therapeutic substances within the central nervous system.

C1756

C1756 Catheter, pacing, transesophageal

Lay Description

A transesophageal pacing catheter is a small hollow tube that is inserted into the esophagus and positioned near the posterior aspect of the atria. The catheter contains an electrode that delivers electrical stimulation to the heart and usually includes a device to record an electrocardiogram. The catheter may be used for therapeutic purposes, such as converting an arrythmia during an intraoperative procedure, or for diagnostic purposes, such as in evaluations of sinus node function.

C1757

C1757 Catheter, thrombectomy/embolectomy

Lay Description

A thrombectomy or embolectomy catheter is a small hollow tube that is inserted into a blood vessel and guided to the site of the embolism or thrombus. A device that breaks up or macerates the thromus or embolus may be inserted through the catheter. Usually, the catheter is used to aspirate the thrombus or embolus.

C1758

C1758 Catheter, ureteral

Lay Description

Ureteral catheter is a small hollow tube that is inserted into the ureter to withdraw or introduce fluid. The catheter may be inserted either through the urethra and bladder or posteriorly via the kidney.

C1760

C1760 Closure device, vascular (implantable/insertable)

Lay Description

A vascular closure device seals femoral artery punctures caused by invasive or interventional procedures. The closure or seal is achieved by placing the vessel ends between the device's two primary structures, which are usually an anchor and a biologic substance (e.g., collagen) or suture through the tissue tract.

C1762

C1762 Connective tissue, human (includes fascia lata)

Lay Description

Human connective tissue (includes fascia lata) is natural human cellular collagen or extracellular matrix obtained from autologous rectus fascia, decellularized cadaver fascia lata, or decellularized dermal tissue. The tissue is intended to repair or support damaged or inadequate soft tissue. They are used to treat urinary incontinence resulting from hypermobility or Intrinsic Sphincter Deficiency (ISD), pelvic floor repair, or for implantation to reinforce soft tissues where weakness exists in the urological anatomy. Th category excludes those items that are used to replace skin.

C1763

C1763 Connective tissue, nonhuman (includes synthetic)

Lay Description

Nonhuman connective tissue (includes synthetic) is a natural collagen matrix typically obtained from porcine or bovine small intestinal submucosa, or pericardium. The material is acellular as all cells are removed leaving only a matrix or scaffold. This tissue is intended to promote the growth of the patients cells within the implanted matrix. It is intended to repair or support damaged or inadequate soft tissue. Nonhuman connective tissue is are used to treat urinary incontinence resulting from hypermobility or Intrinsic Sphincter Deficiency (ISD), pelvic floor repair, or for implantation to reinforce soft tissues where weakness exists in the urological or musculoskeletal anatomy. This category excludes those items that are used to replace skin.

C1764

C1764 Event recorder, cardiac (implantable)

Lay Description

Event recorders are implanted in the left front of the chest in a pocket created in the skin. Once implanted, the patient's cardiac events are recorded. Implantable cardiac event monitors are for long-time use, enabling the recorder to capture more infrequent heart rhythms. The device can have auto activation or manual activation depending upon the needs of the patient. If the patient experiences syncopal episodes, the manual activation button can be pressed only after the patient is conscious again. If the device has auto activation, the device records rhythms automatically when the heart rate is in excess or under a preset limit.

C1765

C1765 Adhesion barrier

Lay Description

An adhesion barrier is a bioresorbable substance used on and around neural structures, that minimizes the formation of scar tissue. It is mainly used in spine surgeries such as laminectomies and diskectomies.

C1766

C1766 Introducer/sheath, guiding, intracardiac electrophysiological, steerable, other than peel-away

Lay Description

An intracardiac electrophysiological introducer or sheath, guiding, steerable, other than peel-away, is a small hollow tube that is inserted into the heart and guided to the target area. Elelectrophysiological devices and catheters are then passed through the introducer to the target area.

C1767

C1767 Generator, neurostimulator (implantable), nonrechargeable

Lay Description

An implantable nonrechargeable neurostimulator generator is a device that creates small electrical impulses that are transmitted to electrodes implanted near the spinal cord or a peripheral nerve. The small electrical impulses interrupt pain signals sent to the brain. This type of generator contains a battery that cannot be recharged, but must be removed and replaced.

C1768

C1768 Graft, vascular

Lay Description

A vascular graft is material used to patch a damaged, diseased, or injured area of an artery or for replacement of whole segments of vessels. Vascular grafts may be biological or synthetic. Biological grafts are generally taken from another site in the patient and called autograft. A common autograft is the internal mammary artery generally used in coronary artery bypass surgery. Other biological grafts can come from another member of the same species, such as the use of cadaver grafts. Synthetic grafts are usually made from Dacron or polytetrafluroethylene (PTFE).

C1769

C1769 Guide wire

Lay Description

A guide wire is a thin piece of material that is guided into a desired blood vessel through a trocar. The trocare is then removed and the guideire left in place. Catheters, cannulas or other tubular devices can then be inserted over the guidewire into the blood vessel and the guidewire is withdrawn.

C1770

C1770 Imaging coil, magnetic resonance (insertable)

Lay Description

An insertable magnetic resonance imaging coil is an intracavity probe that is placed in relatively inaccessible or dense body area. The coil emits a magnectic signature that enhances images taken during the MRI.

C1771

C1771 Repair device, urinary, incontinence, with sling graft

Lay Description

Urinary incontinence repair device is a device used to attach or insert body tissue, synthetic material, or mesh for the purpose of strengthening the pelvic floor. The repair material is fashioned into a sling or hammock that supports the urethra. This code represents the device components used to deliver the sling graft and/or fixate (via permanent sutures or bone anchors) the sling graft. HCPCS code C1771 includes the sling graft while C2631does not.

C1772

C1772 Infusion pump, programmable (implantable)

Lay Description

An implantable programmable infusion pump is an electrical device that delivers drugs, nutrients, or fluids into the patient's body. It is surgically placed in a subcutaneous pocket with a catheter that is threaded into a desired position. This code represents a device that has a programmer that can be set to deliver the fuild continuously or at set intervals.

C1773

C1773   Retrieval device, insertable (used to retrieve fractured medical devices)

Lay Description

An insertable retrieval device is used to retrieve fractured medical devices that are lodged within the vascular system. This device can also be used to to exchange intravascular introducers or sheaths.

C1776

C1776   Joint device (implantable)

Lay Description

A joint device is an artificial prosthetic device that is implanted in a patient as a replacement for a natural joint, such as a finger or toe. Generally a joint device is not used to oppose soft tissue-to-bone, tendon-to-bone, or bone-to-bone.

C1777

C1777   Lead, cardioverter-defibrillator, endocardial single coil (implantable)

Lay Description

An endocardial single coil cardioverter-defibrillator lead is an implanted wire with an electrode at its tip that connects a generator to the heart muscle. An electrode detects electrical changes in the heart which are recored by the generator and transmits electrical charges created by the generator to the heart to correct and maintain a steady heart rhythm. A cardioverter-defibrillator is a device designed to detect ventricular tachycardia or fibrillation andto deliver an electrical shock to return the heart to normal rhythm. HCPCS code C1777 represents one lead that attaches to the heart wall of the heart muscle with the other end connected to a cardioverter-defibrillator.

C1778

C1778   Lead, neurostimulator (implantable)

Lay Description

An implantable neurostimulator lead is a wire with an electrode at its tip that connects a generator to the brain or nervous system. An electrode transmits electrical charges created by the neurostimulator. The electrical signal interrupts the brain function or nerve conduction. Neurostimulators can be used to reduce or eliminate pain, activate nerve responses, or control electrical brain discharges.

C1780

C1780   Lens, intraocular (new technology)

Lay Description

This code describes an artificial lens made of plastic, silicone, or acrylic that performs the function of the eye's natural lens, typically a quarter of an inch in diameter. The lens is usually soft enough that it can be folded and placed into the eye through a small incision. This code specifically refers to the intraocular lenses approved by CMS as "new technology IOL."

C1781

C1781   Mesh (implantable)

Lay Description

A mesh implant is a synthetic patch composed of absorbable or nonabsorbable material that is used to repair hernias, support weakened or attenuated tissue, cover tissue defects, etc.

C1782

C1782   Morcellator

Lay Description

A morcellator is a device that cuts, cores, and extracts tissue in laparoscopic procedures. The device uses suction to draw tissue into its tip where it is cut into small piece by a rotating blade. The device then removes the tissue from the feld using suction.

C1784

C1784   Ocular device, intraoperative, detached retina

Lay Description

An intraoperative ocular device for a detached retina is a carbon and flourine (perfluorocarbon) gas that is instilled into the vitreous during a procedure to treat detached retina. The vitreous is a clear collagen gel that fills the eye that helps the retina lie smoothly and firmly against the back wall of the eyeball. The gas is injected to help return the retina to its normal postion or to replace vitreous fluid removed during other retina repair procedures.The gas buble eventually disapates and may be replaced with body fiulds.

C1787

C1787   Patient programmer, neurostimulator

Lay Description

A patient programmer is a handheld device that transmits operational commands to the neurostimulator. A patient may control the amplitude and rate of the electrical impulses delivered by the neurostimulator system

C1814

C1814 Retinal tamponade device, silicone oil

Lay Description

Silicone oil is a silicon analogues of carbon based organic compounds which can form long and complex molecules based on silicon rather than carbon. This HCPCS code represents silicone oil used as a permanent or prolonged retinal tamponade for the treatment of complex retinal detachments. The vitreous is a clear collagen gel that fills the eye and helps the retina lie smoothly and firmly against the back wall of the eyeball. Silicone oil is injected to help return the retina to its normal postion or to replace vitreous fluid removed during other retina repair procedures. The silicone oil eventually disapates and may be replaced with body fiulds

C1817

C1817 Septal defect implant system, intracardiac

Lay Description

An intracardiac septal defect implant system is a an implant placed with the heart for closure of a variety of defects that may occur dividing wall that separates the left and right sides of the heart. The septal defect implant system represented by this code includes a delivery catheter.

C1818

C1818 Integrated keratoprosthesis

Lay Description

An integrated keratoprosthesis is a flexible, one-piece biocompatible polymer lens. It is used to replace diseased native corneas in conditions where traditional corneal transplantation is not indicated or possible.

C1820

C1820 Generator, neurostimulator (implantable), with rechargeable battery and charging system

Lay Description

An implantable rechargeable neurostimulator generator is a device that creates small electrical impulses that are transmitted to electrodes implanted near the spinal cord or a peripheral nerve. The small electrical impulses interrupt pain signals sent to the brain. This type of generator contains a battery that can be recharged. The code represents the generator, rechargeable battery and its charging system.

C1874

C1874 Stent, coated/covered, with delivery system

Lay Description

A stent with delivery system is a small hollow tube made of a biocompatible substances, such as phosphorylcholine, silicone, or metal that is inserted into a natural body passge or conduit. The stent maintains the body passage or conduit allowing less restricted flow. This code represents a stent packaged with a delivery system which generally includes a stent mounted or unmounted on a balloon angioplasty catheter, introducer, and sheath.

C1875

C1875 Stent, coated/covered, without delivery system

Lay Description

A coated or covered stent without a delivery system is a small hollow tube made of a biocompatible substances, such as phosphorylcholine, silicone, or metal that is inserted into a natural body passge or conduit. The stent maintains the body passage or conduit allowing less restricted flow. It is coated with a drug that helps prevent the conduit from becoming narrowed again. This code represents a stent packaged without a delivery system.

C1878

C1878 Material for vocal cord medialization, synthetic (implantable)

Lay Description

Material for vocal cord medialization is a synthetic implantable substance that is not absorbable. The substance is injected or implanted in a vocal cord to move the cord closer to midline to allow a greater strike with the opposite vocal cord.

C1879

C1879 Tissue marker (implantable)

Lay Description

An implantable tissue marker is a material that is placed in the subcutaneous or parenchymal tissue (may also include bone) for radiopaque identification of a target area.

C1883

C1883 Adaptor/extension, pacing lead or neurostimulator lead (implantable)

Lay Description

A pacing or neurostimulator lead adaptor or extension is an implantable device that is placed in between an existing lead and a new generator. The end of the adaptor lead has the appropriate connector pin that will enable the use of the existing lead with a new generator that has a different connecting receptacle. These are required when a generator is replaced or when two leads are connected to the same port in the connector block.

C1884

C1884 Embolization protective system

Lay Description

An embolization protective system is a system designed to trap, macerate, and remove atheromatous or thrombotic debris from the vascular system during an angioplasty, atherectomy, or stenting procedure.

C1885

C1885 Catheter, transluminal angioplasty, laser

Lay Description

A transluminal angioplasty laser catheter is a small hollow tube that is inserted into the central space (or lumen) of an artery or vein. This code refers to a catheter that has a laser at its tip. The catheter is advanced through the blood vessel to the area of occlusion or blockage. When the catheter is in position, the laser emits pulsating beams of light that break up or vaporize the obstruction.

C1887

C1887 Catheter, guiding (may include infusion/perfusion capability)

Lay Description

.A guiding catheter is a small hollow tube used to introduce interventional or diagnostic devices into the coronary or peripheral vascular system. It can be used to inject contrast material, function as a conduit through which other devices pass, and/or provide a mechanism for measuring arterial pressure, and maintain a pathway created by the guide wire during the performance of a procedure.

C1888

C1888 Catheter, ablation, noncardiac, endovascular (implantable)

Lay Description

A noncardiac endovascular ablation catheter is a small hollow tube containing a laser or radiofrequency tip that is inserted into a blood vessel. The catheter is advanced to the target area and a pulse from the laser or radiofrequency device is used to occlude or obliterate the blood vessel.

C1892

C1892 Introducer/sheath, guiding, intracardiac electrophysiological, fixed-curve, peel-away

Lay Description

A guiding, intracardiac electrophysiological, fixed-curve, peel-away introducer or sheath, is a a small hollow tube made of nonabsorbable material. The sheath or introducer that separates into two pieces is guided to the target area. A lead or catheter is then placed through the introducer and the sheath is removed.

C1900

C1900 Lead, left ventricular coronary venous system

Lay Description

A left ventricular coronary venous system lead is an implanted wire with an electrode at its tip that connects a generator to the left ventricule of the heart. It is intended to treat the symptoms associated with heart failure.

C2615

C2615 Sealant, pulmonary, liquid

Lay Description

Liquid pulmonary sealant is an absorable hydrogel formed from two components. Human serum albumin is mixed with a synthetic cross-linking component of polyethylene glycol. It is indicated to seal visceral pleural air leaks during pulmonary resection. The liquid pulmonary sealant is intended for single use . It is not receommeneded that more than 30 ml be used per patient.

C2617

C2617 Stent, noncoronary, temporary, without delivery system

Lay Description

A noncoronary, temporary stent, without a delivery system is a small hollow tube made of a biocompatible substances, such as phosphorylcholine, silicone, or metal that is inserted into a natural body passge or conduit. The stent maintains the body passage or conduit allowing less restricted flow. This code represents a stent packaged without a delivery system. A temporary stent is designed to be removed and is placed for a period of less than one year.

C2617

C2617 Stent, noncoronary, temporary, without delivery system

Lay Description

C2621

C2621 Pacemaker, other than single or dual chamber (implantable)

Lay Description

A pacemaker is an electronic system that monitors the electrical impulses of the heart and delivers an electrical charge when necessary to set normal heart rhythms. The term pacemaker that includes cardiac resynchronization devices. This code represents an implantable pacemaker that is neither a single or dual chamber model..

C2625

C2625 Stent, noncoronary, temporary, with delivery system

Lay Description

A noncoronary, temporary stent, with a delivery system is a small hollow tube made of a biocompatible substances, such as phosphorylcholine, silicone, or metal that is inserted into a natural body passge or conduit. The stent maintains the body passage or conduit allowing less restricted flow. A temporary stent is designed to be removed and is placed for a period of less than one year. This code represents a stent packaged with a delivery system generally including components such as, stent mounted or unmounted on a balloon angioplasty catheter, introducer, and sheath.

C2626

C2626 Infusion pump, nonprogrammable, temporary (implantable)

Lay Description

A nonprogrammable, temporary infusion pump is a short term pain management system which is a component of a permanent implantable system used for the management of chronic pain.

C2630

C2630 Catheter, electrophysiology, diagnostic/ablation, other than 3D or vector mapping, cool-tip

Lay Description

An electrophysiology, diagnostic or ablation, other than 3D or vector mapping, cool-tip catheter is a small hollow tube containing devices that aid in providing anatomic and physiologic information about the cardiac electrical conduction system. This device has temperature sensing capability also contains a cooling mechanism which is a tip cooled by infused, circulating saline.

C2631

C2631 Repair device, urinary, incontinence, without sling graft

Lay Description

Urinary incontinence repair device is a device used to attach or insert body tissue, synthetic material, or mesh for the purpose of strengthening the pelvic floor. The repair material is fashioned into a sling or hammock that supports the urethra. This code represents the device components used to deliver the sling graft and/or fixate (via permanent sutures or bone anchors) the sling graft. HCPCS code C2631 does not include the sling graft while C1771 does. .

C2634-C2643

C2634 Brachytherapy source, nonstranded, high activity, iodine-125, greater than 1.01 mCi (NIST), per source

C2635 Brachytherapy source, nonstranded, high activity, palladium-103, greater than 2.2 mCi (NIST), per source

C2636 Brachytherapy linear source, nonstranded, palladium-103, per 1 mm

C2637 Brachytherapy source, nonstranded, ytterbium-169, per source

C2638 Brachytherapy source, stranded, iodine-125, per source

C2639 Brachytherapy source, nonstranded, iodine-125, per source

C2640 Brachytherapy source, stranded, palladium-103, per source

C2641 Brachytherapy source, nonstranded, palladium-103, per source

C2642 Brachytherapy source, stranded, cesium-131, per source

C2643 Brachytherapy source, nonstranded, cesium-131, per source

Lay Description

Brachytherapy is a form of radiotherapy in which physicians place the source of irradiation close to the tumor or within a body cavity. Brachytherapy could include placing radioactive sources inside a body cavity (intracavitary brachytherapy) or putting radioactive material directly into body tissue using hollow needles (interstitial brachytherapy). Brachytherapy may be given in addition to external beam radiation or it may be used as the only form of radiotherapy. In some cases, the radioactive sources may be permanently left in place; in other cases, they are removed after a specified time. Placement of radioactive sources may be repeated several times. The isotope gold-198 has a half life of 2.7 days and is used in some cancer treatments and treatments for other diseases. There are two natural isotopes of iridium, and many radioisotopes, the most stable radioisotope being Ir-192 with a half-life of 73.83 days. Ir-192 beta decays into platinum-192, while most of the other radioisotopes decay into osmium.

C8900

C8900 Magnetic resonance angiography with contrast, abdomen

Lay Description

Magnetic resonance angiography (MRA) is an application of magnetic resonance imaging (MRI) that provides visualization of blood flow and images of normal and diseased blood vessels. MRA techniques typically are noninvasive because they do not require the use of contrast media. Contrast media may be used to enhance the images in MRA, but use of these agents is not necessary. Report C8900 for an MRA of the abdomen with contrast.

C8901

C8901 Magnetic resonance angiography without contrast, abdomen

Lay Description

Magnetic resonance angiography (MRA) is an application of magnetic resonance imaging (MRI) that provides visualization of blood flow and images of normal and diseased blood vessels. MRA techniques typically are noninvasive because they do not require the use of contrast media. Contrast media may be used to enhance the images in MRA, but use of these agents is not necessary. Report C8901 for an MRA of the abdomen without contrast media.

C8902

C8902 Magnetic resonance angiography without contrast followed by with contrast, abdomen

Lay Description

Magnetic resonance angiography (MRA) is an application of magnetic resonance imaging (MRI) that provides visualization of blood flow and images of normal and diseased blood vessels. MRA techniques typically are noninvasive because they do not require the use of contrast media. Contrast media may be used to enhance the images in MRA, but use of these agents is not necessary. Report C8902 for an MRA of the abdomen with and without contrast.

C8903

C8903 Magnetic resonance imaging with contrast, breast; unilateral

Lay Description

Magnetic resonance imaging (MRI) is a noninvasive, painless test that assists the physician in diagnosing and treating certain medical conditions. MRI uses a powerful magnetic field, radio waves, and a computer to create detailed pictures of bone, organs, soft tissues, and other internal body structures. These detailed pictures allow the physician to better comprehend and evaluate the part of the body in question or diseased areas under scrutiny. An MRI of the breast assists in evaluating abnormalities detected via a mammography, evaluates the integrity of breast implants, differentiates between scar tissue and tumors, assesses multiple tumor locations, determines whether cancer detected by mammography or other radiological tests has spread further into the breast or chest wall pre- or post-surgery, assesses the effect of chemotherapy, and/or provides more information on a diseased breast to make medical treatment decisions. Report C8903 for a unilateral MRI of the breast with contrast.

C8904

C8904 Magnetic resonance imaging without contrast, breast; unilateral

Lay Description

Magnetic resonance imaging (MRI) is a noninvasive, painless test that assists the physician in diagnosing and treating certain medical conditions. MRI uses a powerful magnetic field, radio waves, and a computer to create detailed pictures of bone, organs, soft tissues, and other internal body structures. These detailed pictures allow the physician to better comprehend and evaluate the part of the body in question or diseased areas under scrutiny. An MRI of the breast assists in evaluating abnormalities detected via a mammography, evaluates the integrity of breast implants, differentiates between scar tissue and tumors, assesses multiple tumor locations, determines whether cancer detected by mammography or other radiological tests has spread further into the breast or chest wall pre- or post-surgery, assesses the effect of chemotherapy, and/or provides more information on a diseased breast to make medical treatment decisions. Report C8904 for a unilateral MRI of the breast without contrast.

C8905

C8905 Magnetic resonance imaging without contrast followed by with contrast, breast; unilateral

Lay Description

Magnetic resonance imaging (MRI) is a noninvasive, painless test that assists the physician in diagnosing and treating certain medical conditions. MRI uses a powerful magnetic field, radio waves, and a computer to create detailed pictures of bone, organs, soft tissues, and other internal body structures. These detailed pictures allow the physician to better comprehend and evaluate the part of the body in question or diseased areas under scrutiny. An MRI of the breast assists in evaluating abnormalities detected via a mammography, evaluates the integrity of breast implants, differentiates between scar tissue and tumors, assesses multiple tumor locations, determines whether cancer detected by mammography or other radiological tests has spread further into the breast or chest wall pre- or post-surgery, assesses the effect of chemotherapy, and/or provides more information on a diseased breast to make medical treatment decisions. Report C8905 for a unilateral MRI of the breast with and without contrast.

C8906

C8906 Magnetic resonance imaging with contrast, breast; bilateral

Lay Description

Magnetic resonance imaging (MRI) is a noninvasive, painless test that assists the physician in diagnosing and treating certain medical conditions. MRI uses a powerful magnetic field, radio waves, and a computer to create detailed pictures of bone, organs, soft tissues, and other internal body structures. These detailed pictures allow the physician to better comprehend and evaluate the part of the body in question or diseased areas under scrutiny. An MRI of the breast assists in evaluating abnormalities detected via a mammography, evaluates the integrity of breast implants, differentiates between scar tissue and tumors, assesses multiple tumor locations, determines whether cancer detected by mammography or other radiological tests has spread further into the breast or chest wall pre- or post-surgery, assesses the effect of chemotherapy, and/or provides more information on a diseased breast to make medical treatment decisions. Report C8906 for a bilateral MRI of the breast with contrast.

C8907

C8907 Magnetic resonance imaging without contrast, breast; bilateral

Lay Description

Magnetic resonance imaging (MRI) is a noninvasive, painless test that assists the physician in diagnosing and treating certain medical conditions. MRI uses a powerful magnetic field, radio waves, and a computer to create detailed pictures of bone, organs, soft tissues, and other internal body structures. These detailed pictures allow the physician to better comprehend and evaluate the part of the body in question or diseased areas under scrutiny. An MRI of the breast assists in evaluating abnormalities detected via a mammography, evaluates the integrity of breast implants, differentiates between scar tissue and tumors, assesses multiple tumor locations, determines whether cancer detected by mammography or other radiological tests has spread further into the breast or chest wall pre- or post-surgery, assesses the effect of chemotherapy, and/or provides more information on a diseased breast to make medical treatment decisions. Report C8907 for a bilateral MRI of the breast without contrast.

C8908

C8908 Magnetic resonance imaging without contrast followed by with contrast, breast; bilateral

Lay Description

Magnetic resonance imaging (MRI) is a noninvasive, painless test that assists the physician in diagnosing and treating certain medical conditions. MRI uses a powerful magnetic field, radio waves, and a computer to create detailed pictures of bone, organs, soft tissues, and other internal body structures. These detailed pictures allow the physician to better comprehend and evaluate the part of the body in question or diseased areas under scrutiny. An MRI of the breast assists in evaluating abnormalities detected via a mammography, evaluates the integrity of breast implants, differentiates between scar tissue and tumors, assesses multiple tumor locations, determines whether cancer detected by mammography or other radiological tests has spread further into the breast or chest wall pre- or post-surgery, assesses the effect of chemotherapy, and/or provides more information on a diseased breast to make medical treatment decisions. Report C8908 for a bilateral MRI of the breast with and without contrast.

C8909

C8909 Magnetic resonance angiography with contrast, chest (excluding myocardium)

Lay Description

Magnetic resonance angiography (MRA) is an application of magnetic resonance imaging (MRI) that provides visualization of blood flow and images of normal and diseased blood vessels. MRA techniques typically are noninvasive because they do not require the use of contrast media. This MRA procedure is designed to examine the heart and the blood vessels entering the lungs. Contrast media may be used to enhance the images in MRA, but use of these agents is not necessary. Report C8909 for an MRA of the chest (excluding the myocardium) with contrast.

C8910

C8910 Magnetic resonance angiography without contrast, chest (excluding myocardium)

Lay Description

Magnetic resonance angiography (MRA) is an application of magnetic resonance imaging (MRI) that provides visualization of blood flow and images of normal and diseased blood vessels. MRA techniques typically are noninvasive because they do not require the use of contrast media. This MRA procedure is designed to examine the heart and the blood vessels entering the lungs. Contrast media may be used to enhance the images in MRA, but use of these agents is not necessary. Report C8910 for an MRA of the chest (excluding the myocardium) without contrast.

C8911

C8911 Magnetic resonance angiography without contrast followed by with contrast, chest (excluding myocardium)

Lay Description

Magnetic resonance angiography (MRA) is an application of magnetic resonance imaging (MRI) that provides visualization of blood flow and images of normal and diseased blood vessels. MRA techniques typically are noninvasive because they do not require the use of contrast media. This MRA procedure is designed to examine the heart and the blood vessels entering the lungs. Contrast media may be used to enhance the images in MRA, but use of these agents is not necessary. Report C8911 for an MRA of the chest (excluding the myocardium) with and without contrast.

C8912-C8914

C8912 Magnetic resonance angiography with contrast, lower extremity
C8913 Magnetic resonance angiography without contrast, lower extremity
C8914 Magnetic resonance angiography without contrast followed by with contrast, lower extremity

Lay Description

Magnetic resonance angiography (MRA) of the lower extremity is a minimally invasive medical test that uses a powerful magnetic field, radio waves, and a computer to produce detailed pictures of major blood vessels in the lower extremities. HCPCS code C8912 indicates an MRA of the lower extremity that uses contrast material, C8913 uses no contrast, and C8914 takes images both with and wirthout contrast.

C8918-C8920

C8918 Magnetic resonance angiography with contrast, pelvis
C8919 Magnetic resonance angiography without contrast, pelvis
C8920 Magnetic resonance angiography without contrast followed by with contrast, pelvis

Lay Description

Magnetic resonance angiography (MRA) of the pelvic region is a minimally invasive medical test that uses a powerful magnetic field, radio waves, and a computer to produce detailed pictures of major blood vessels in the lower extremities. HCPCS code C8918 indicates an MRA of the pelvis that uses contrast material, C8919 uses no contrast, and C8920 takes images both with and wirthout contrast.

C8921-C8922

C8921 Transthoracic echocardiography with contrast, or without contrast followed by with contrast, for congenital cardiac anomalies; complete
C8922 Transthoracic echocardiography with contrast, or without contrast followed by with contrast, for congenital cardiac anomalies; follow-up or limited study

Lay Description

Transthoracic echocardiography is performed to detect congenital cardiac anomalies. Contrast is injected into the patient's vein. Transducers are placed on the patient's chest to record an echocardiograph, which uses ultrasound to visualize the heart's function, blood flow, valves, and chambers. Report C8921 for the complete study and C8922 for a follow-up or limited study. Report contrast material separately.

C8923-C8924

C8923 Transthoracic echocardiography with contrast, or without contrast followed by with contrast, real-time with image documentation (2D), includes M-mode recording, when performed, complete, without spectral or color doppler echocardiography

C8924 Transthoracic echocardiography with contrast, or without contrast followed by with contrast, real-time with image documentation (2D), includes M-mode recording when performed, follow-up or limited study

Lay Description

A transthoracic echocardiography is performed with real-time image documentation (2D). Contrast material is injected into the vein. An ultrasound is used to visualize the heart's function, blood flow, valves, and chambers. Two-dimensional echocardiography, also referred to as real-time imaging, is performed using multiple transducers or a rotating transducer, and these images are recorded on videotape. Computer reconstruction provides the two-dimensional image of specific planes of the heart. M-mode, when performed, provides additional detail of specific portions of the heart. A stationary ultrasound beam is directed at the area of the heart requiring additional study. Report C8923 for a complete study and C8924 for a follow-up or limited study. Report contrast material separately.

C8925-C8926

C8925 Transesophageal echocardiography (TEE) with contrast, or without contrast followed by with contrast, real time with image documentation (2D) (with or without M-mode recording); including probe placement, image acquisition, interpretation and report

C8926 Transesophageal echocardiography (TEE) with contrast, or without contrast followed by with contrast, for congenital cardiac anomalies; including probe placement, image acquisition, interpretation and report

Lay Description

Transesophageal echocardiography (TEE) is performed. TEE is an invasive technique whereby contrast material is injected into the vein. The transducer is placed at the tip of an endoscope and introduced into the patient's esophagus to record a two-dimensional echocardiograph. The codes include probe placement, image acquisition, interpretation, and report. Report C8926 when TEE is performed to detect congenital anomalies. Report contrast material separately.

C8927

C8927 Transesophageal echocardiography (TEE) with contrast, or without contrast followed by with contrast, for monitoring purposes, including probe placement, real time 2-dimensional image acquisition and interpretation leading to ongoing (continuous) assessment of (dynamically changing) cardiac pumping function and to therapeutic measures on an immediate time basis

Lay Description

Transesophageal echocardiography (TEE) is performed to assess cardiac pumping function and for therapeutic measures on an immediate time basis. TEE is an invasive technique whereby contrast is injected into the vein. The transducer is placed at the tip of an endoscope and introduced into the patient's esophagus to record a two-dimensional echocardiograph. TEE provides high-quality, real-time images of the beating heart and mediastinal structures. This code reports ongoing hemodynamic monitoring using TEE. TEE may be used to monitor critically ill patients in the intensive care unit, as well as patients in certain operative settings. In both the intensive care unit and the operating room, it is used to monitor cardiac function including cardiac preload, contractility, and valve function in patients with acute hemodynamic decompensation. In addition, TEE may also be used to assess and monitor mediastinal, heart, lung, and aortic injury resulting from blunt chest trauma even in patients undergoing other life-saving procedures. Report contrast material separately.

C8928

C8928 Transthoracic echocardiography with contrast, or without contrast followed by with contrast, real-time with image documentation (2D), includes M-mode recording, when performed, during rest and cardiovascular stress test using treadmill, bicycle exercise and/or pharmacologically induced stress, with interpretation and report

Lay Description

Transthoracic echocardiography is performed while the patient is at rest and exercising on a treadmill or stationary bicycle with or without medication and includes M-mode recording, when performed. TEE is an invasive technique whereby contrast is injected into the vein. Transducers are placed on a patient's chest to record a two-dimensional echocardiograph, which uses ultrasound to visualize the heart's function, blood flow, valves, and chambers. Report contrast material separately.

C8929

C8929 Transthoracic echocardiography with contrast, or without contrast followed by with contrast, real-time with image documentation (2D), includes M-mode recording, when performed, complete, with spectral doppler echocardiography, and with color flow doppler echocardiography

Lay Description

Transthoracic echocardiography (TEE) is performed. TEE is an invasive technique whereby contrast is injected into the vein. Transducers are placed on a patient's chest to record a two-dimensional echocardiograph, which uses ultrasound to visualize the heart's function, blood flow, valves, and chambers. This code is for a complete evaluation that includes spectral and color flow Doppler, which provide information regarding blood flow velocity, direction, type, and hemodynamics. Report contrast material separately.

C8930

C8930 Transthoracic echocardiography, with contrast, or without contrast followed by with contrast, real-time with image documentation (2D), includes M-mode recording, when performed, during rest and cardiovascular stress test using treadmill, bicycle exercise and/or pharmacologically induced stress, with interpretation and report; including performance of continuous electrocardiographic monitoring, with physician supervision

Lay Description

Transthoracic echocardiography (TEE) is performed. TEE is an invasive technique whereby contrast is injected into the vein. Transducers are placed on the patient's chest to record a two-dimensional echocardiograph, which uses ultrasound to visualize the heart's function, blood flow, valves, and chambers. This is completed while the patient is at rest and again while exercising on a treadmill or stationary bicycle, with or without medication, and includes M-mode recording, when performed. It also includes the performance of continuous electrocardiographic monitoring with physician supervision. Supply of the contrast agent and/or the drugs used in pharmacologic stress are reported separately.

C8957

C8957 Intravenous infusion for therapy/diagnosis; initiation of prolonged infusion (more than 8 hours), requiring use of portable or implantable pump

Lay Description

Intravenous infusion for therapy/diagnosis; initiation of prolonged infusion (more than 8 hours), requiring use of portable or implantable pump, is a route of administration in pharmacology and toxicology by which a path in a vein is made allowing the administration of a drug, fluid, or other substance for a period of more than 8 hours. An infusion pump is used for such prolonged infusions.

C9113

C9113 Injection, pantoprazole sodium, per vial

Lay Description

Pantoprazole sodium is a compound that inhibits gastric secretions. Pantoprazole is a proton pump inhibitor (PPI) that suppresses the final step in gastric acid production by forming a covalent bond to two sites of the ATPase enzyme system at the secretory surface of the gastric parietal cell. This effect is dose-related and leads to inhibition of both basal and stimulated gastric acid secretion irrespective of the stimulus. This binding results in a period of antisecretory effect that persists longer than 24 hours for all doses tested. This drug is indicated for short-term treatment (seven to 10 days) for patients with gastroesophageal reflux disease (GERD) and a history of erosive esophagitis, and the hypersecretory conditions that may be associated with Zollinger-Ellison syndrome or other neoplastic conditions. HCPCS Level II code C9113 represents per vial of pantoprazole sodium.

C9121

C9121 Injection, argatroban, per 5 mg

Lay Description

Argatroban is a synthetic direct thrombin inhibitor derived from the amino acid L-arginine. It binds to the active thrombin site and inhibits coagulation including fibrin formation, activation of coagulation factors and protein C, and platelet aggregation. Argatroban is indicated for use as an anticoagulant for prophylaxis and treatment of thrombosis in patients with heparin-induced thrombocytopenia. It is also indicated as an anticoagulant in patients with or at risk for heparin-induced thrombocytopenia undergoing percutaneous coronary interventions. Argatroban is supplied as a concentrate that must be diluted and administered via intravenous infusion. HCPCS Level II code C9121 represents 5 mg of argatroban.

C9248

C9248 Injection, clevidipine butyrate, 1 mg

Lay Description

Clevidipine butyrate is a channel blocker used to treat high blood pressure when other treatments are contraindicated. Channel blockers relax the blood vessels and allow more blood and oxygen get to the heart. The dose varies depending on the patient's condition and blood pressure. Clevevidipine butyrate is administered as an IV infusion. HCPCS level II code C9248 represents 1 mg.

C9250

C9250 Human plasma fibrin sealant, vapor-heated, solvent-detergent (Artiss), 2 ml

Lay Description

Human plasma fibrin sealant, vapor-heated, solvent-detergent (Artiss) is a two-component fibrin sealant used to adhere autologous skin grafts to surgically prepared wounds in burn patients. It is comprised of human sealer protein concentrate and human fibrin. When these two components are combined, the result is a fibrin that seals the graft to the prepared wound site. The solution is applied in a thin layer to the site and the graft is placed. A two ml package coverages approximately 100 square centimeter surface area.

C9254

C9254 Injection, lacosamide, 1 mg

Lay Description

Lacosamide is a functionalized amino acid used as an adjunctive therapy in treating partial-onset seizures for patients 17 years and older who are diagnosed with epilepsy. The exact mechanism by which this drug controls seizures is unknown. The lacosamide is believed to act through voltage-gated sodium channels. Voltage-gated sodium channels help control the electrical activity of the neurons. Lacosamide targets neurons which are depolarized or active for long periods of time, typical of neurons at the focus of an epileptic seizure. The recommended dosage is from 100 mg to 400 mg per day, depending on the patiennt's response. The drug is administered as an IV infusion over 30-60 minutes. HCPCS code C9254 represents 1 mg of the injectible form.

C9257

C9257 Injection, bevacizumab, 0.25 mg

Lay Description

Bevacizumab is a monoclonal antibody produced by recombinant DNA technology in Chinese hamster ovaries. This monoclonal antibody binds to and inhibits the biologic activity of human vascular endothelial growth factor preventing the formation of new blood vessels. Bevacizumab, used in combination with intravenous 5-fluorouracil, is indicated for first-line treatment of patients with metastatic carcinoma of the colon or rectum. The recommended dose is 5 mg per kg of body weight administered once every 14 days disease progression is detected. Bevacizumab is administered by intravenous infusion. The initial dose infusion should be delivered over 90 minutes. If the first infusion is well tolerated, the second infusion may be administered over 60 minutes. If the 60-minute infusion is well tolerated, all subsequent infusions may be administered over 30 minutes. HCPCS Level II code C9257 represents 0.25 mg of bevacizumab.

C9270

C9270 Injection, immune globulin (Gammaplex), intravenous, nonlyophilized (e.g., liquid), 500 mg

Lay Description

Immune globulin (Gammaplex), intravenous, nonlyophilized (e.g., liquid) is an immune globulin liquid used in the treatment of replacement therapy of primary humoral immunodeficiency (PI). Gammaplex may also be used in treatment of a humoral immune defect in common variable immunodeficiency, Wiskott-Aldrich syndrome, X linked agammaglobulinemia, congenital agammaglobulinemia, and severe combined immunodeficiencies. Recommended dose is 300 to 800 mg/kg every three to four weeks. The dose and schedule may vary based on individual response to treatment. Gammaplex is administered by intravenous infusion.

C9272

C9272 Injection, denosumab, 1 mg

Lay Description

Denosumab is a monoclonal antibody used for the treatment of osteoporosis in postmenopausal women with a high risk of bone fractures that were not successful with other osteoporosis therapies. Denosumab reduces the possibility of fractures of the hip and vertebral and non-vertebral fractures because it is a RANK Ligand inhibitor. It works by binding to the Rank Ligand inhibiting osteoclast formation, function, and survival, therefore preventing the osteoclasts from resorbing bone. The recommended dose is 60 mg every six months. Denosumab is administered by subcutaneous injection.

C9273

C9273 Sipuleucel-T, minimum of 50 million autologous CD54+ cells activated with PAP-GM-CSF, including leukapheresis and all other preparatory procedures, per infusion

Lay Description

Sipuleucel T is an autologous cellular immunotherapy used in the treatment of asymptomatic or minimally symptomatic metastic castrate resistant (hormone refractory) prostate cancer. Sipuleucel T consists of autologous peripheral blood mononuclear cells (PBMC) obtained by leukapheresis and cultured or activated using a recombinant human protein (PAP GM CSF) that consists of prostatic acid phosphatase linked to granulocyte macrophage colony stimulating factor. Sipuleucel T is administered by intravenous infusion over a period of approximately 60 minutes.

C9352

C9352 Microporous collagen implantable tube (NeuraGen Nerve Guide), per cm length

Lay Description

A microporous collagen implantable tube, trade name NeuraGen Nerve Guide, is an absorbable collagen tube intended to serve as an interface between a nerve and the tissue around it. The tube creates a channel for axonal growth across a nerve gap. This code specifies a size of per centimeter length.

C9353

C9353 Microporous collagen implantable slit tube (NeuraWrap Nerve Protector), per cm length

Lay Description

A microporous collagen implantable slit tube, trade name NeuraWrap Nerve Protector, is an absorbable collagen implant that provides a nontightening cover for peripheral nerves that are injure. This code specifies a size of per centimeter length.

C9354

C9354 Acellular pericardial tissue matrix of nonhuman origin (Veritas), per sq cm

Lay Description

Acellular pericardial tissue matrix of nonhuman origin, trade name Veritas, is a strong implantable tissue consisting of noncross linked bovine pericardium. This product is acellular meaning all cells have been removed leaving only a collagen matrix. The acellular pericardial tissue matrix is used as a scaffold for tissue repair. This code specifies a size of per square centimeter.

C9355

C9355 Collagen nerve cuff (NeuroMatrix), per 0.5 cm length

Lay Description

A collagen nerve cuff, trade name NeuroMatrix, is a resorbable, semipermeable, collagen tube intended to create a conduit for axon growth across a nerve gap of 2.5 cm or less. This code specifies a size of 0.5 centimeter length.

C9356

C9356 Tendon, porous matrix of cross-linked collagen and glycosaminoglycan matrix (TenoGlide Tendon Protector Sheet), per sq cm

Lay Description

A tendon, porous matrix of cross-linked collagen and glycosaminoglycan matrix, trade name TenoGlide Tendon Protector Sheet, is an absorbable implant made of a porous matrix of cross linked bovine collagen and glycosaminoglycan. This provides a nonconstricting, protective encasement for injured tendons. This item is intended to serve as an interface between the tendon and the tendon sheath or surrounding tissue. This code specifies a size of per square centimeter.

C9358

C9358 Dermal substitute, native, nondenatured collagen, fetal bovine origin (SurgiMend Collagen Matrix), per 0.5 sq cm

Lay Description

A dermal substitute, native, nondenatured collagen, fetal bovine origin, trade name SurgiMend Collagen Matrix, is an oval or square shaped, biocompatible, soft material made of an acellular collagen matrix. All cellular componets are removed from fetal bovine dermis leaving a collagen matrix. This material is intended for soft tissue repair and reconstructive applications. This code specifies the size of 0.5 square centimeters

C9359

C9359 Porous purified collagen matrix bone void filler (Integra Mozaik Osteoconductive Scaffold Putty, Integra OS Osteoconductive Scaffold Putty), per 0.5 cc

Lay Description

Porous purified collagen matrix is a synthetic type of bone void filler that is used for the treatment of gaps or osseous defects of the skeletal system in the extremities, spine, and pelvis. This filler is made from a purified collage matrix, and its chemical composition allows it to be absorbed and replaced with growing host bone during the healing process. The filler is supplied in powder form and mixed with the bone marrow of the host to form a putty-like substance. This putty is often used as a substitute for harvesting bone graft material from the patient's iliac crest. Code C9359 represents 0.5 cc of the bone void filler.

C9360

C9360   Dermal substitute, native, nondenatured collagen, neonatal bovine origin (SurgiMend Collagen Matrix), per 0.5 sq cm

Lay Description

A dermal substitute, native, nondenatured collagen, neonatal bovine origin, trade name SurgiMend Collagen Matrix is an oval or square shaped, biocompatible, soft material made of an acellular collagen matrix. All cellular componets are removed from neonatal bovine dermis leaving a collagen matrix. This material is intended for soft tissue repair and reconstructive applications. This code specifies the size of 0.5 square centimeters

C9363

C9363   Skin substitute (Integra Meshed Bilayer Wound Matrix), per square cm

Lay Description

Integra Meshed Bilayer Wound Matrix is a biologic matrix that provides coverage for partial and full-thickness wounds. It is used to treat chronic and traumatic wounds including pressure ulcers, venous ulcers, diabetic ulcers, chronic and vascular ulcers, tunneled or undermined wounds, surgical wounds, traumatic wounds abrasions, lacerations, and draining wounds. It is a two layer material. It has a silicone outer layer and a second layer created of three-dimensional porous material made from the fibers of a cross-linked bovine tendon collagen. The silicone layer provides protection and moisture control. The matrix provides the framework for tissue and capillary growth. The physician completely debrides the wound site and the wound matrix is applied. it is afixed to the wound site with sutures or staples. Within 14 to 21 days, the tissue is remodeled wth the patient's own cells and the silicone layer is removed.

C9367

C9367   Skin substitute (Endoform Dermal Template) per sq cm

Lay Description

The skin substitute, trade name Endoform Dermal Template, is an extracellular tissue matrix derived from ovine forestomach. This extracellular tissue matrix collagen is bioactive and promotes tissue repair. This code represents a square centimeter.

E0100-E0105

E0100   Cane, includes canes of all materials, adjustable or fixed, with tip
E0105   Cane, quad or 3-prong, includes canes of all materials, adjustable or fixed, with tips

Lay Description

Walking canes provide the legs with some relief for weight bearing in conditions of impaired ambulation. Canes can be single, three, or four prong and add another point or points of ground contact that alter the biomechanics of walking to affect balance, relieve pain, and provide stability. Canes are used on the opposite side of the injury or weakness, regardless of which hand is dominant. The patient puts all of their weight on the unaffected leg, then steps with the affected leg and cane at the same time. Tips provide traction. Report E0100 for a single prong cane. Report E0105 for quad or three-prong canes. Both codes cover adjustable or fixed canes of all materials including tips.

Medicare Information

Canes are covered when prescribed by a provider typically for a patient with a condition causing impaired ambulation or when there is a potential for ambulation.

An enrolled DME supplier must bill these items to the DME MAC.

E0110-E0117

E0110 Crutches, forearm, includes crutches of various materials, adjustable or fixed, pair, complete with tips and handgrips
E0111 Crutch, forearm, includes crutches of various materials, adjustable or fixed, each, with tip and handgrips
E0112 Crutches, underarm, wood, adjustable or fixed, pair, with pads, tips, and handgrips
E0113 Crutch, underarm, wood, adjustable or fixed, each, with pad, tip, and handgrip
E0114 Crutches, underarm, other than wood, adjustable or fixed, pair, with pads, tips, and handgrips
E0116 Crutch, underarm, other than wood, adjustable or fixed, with pad, tip, handgrip, with or without shock absorber, each
E0117 Crutch, underarm, articulating, spring assisted, each

Lay Description

Crutches (wood or aluminum), both standard underarm and forearm crutches that have cuffs encircling the lower portion of the arms, support the body during walking and help protect the injured body limb for patients with impaired ambulation. For forearm crutches of various materials, with tips and handgrips, report E0110 for a pair and E0111 for a single. For underarm wood crutches, with tips, pads, and handgrips, report E0112 for a pair and E0113 for a single. For underarm crutches other than wood, with tips, pads, and handgrips, report E0114 for a pair and E0116 for a single with or without shock absorber. All crutches reported with E0110-E0116 are adjustable or fixed. Report E0117 for each underarm articulating, spring assisted crutch.

Documentation Standards

In E0117, an order for each item billed must be signed and dated by the treating physician, kept on file by the supplier, and made available to the DME MAC upon request. Items billed to the DME MAC before a signed and dated order has been received by the supplier must be submitted with modifier EY added to each affected HCPCS code.

An enrolled DME supplier must bill these items to the DME MAC.

Medicare Information

Crutches are covered when prescribed by a provider typically for a patient with a condition causing impaired ambulation or when there is a potential for impaired ambulation.

The medical necessity for an underarm, articulating, spring-assisted crutch has not been established. If E0117 is ordered, payment will be based on the allowance for the least costly medically appropriate alternative, E0116. A white cane for a blind person is noncovered since it is a self-help item.

E0118

E0118 Crutch substitute, lower leg platform, with or without wheels, each

Lay Description

A crutch substitute is a hands-free device that consists of a long metal bar with a platform attached at knee height at a 90-degree angle. The device has pads on the platform and straps to hold the leg. The patient places the bent knee on the platform and secures the upper leg to the metal bar and the knee to the platform. The device can have a rounded rubber foot or can have wheels attached to the distal end. The device can be used to replace a missing lower leg or to remove weight bearing from an injured lower leg.

Medicare Information

Coverage and payment is at the contractor's discretion.

E0130-E0144

E0130 Walker, rigid (pickup), adjustable or fixed height
E0135 Walker, folding (pickup), adjustable or fixed height
E0140 Walker, with trunk support, adjustable or fixed height, any type
E0141 Walker, rigid, wheeled, adjustable or fixed height
E0143 Walker, folding, wheeled, adjustable or fixed height
E0144 Walker, enclosed, 4 sided framed, rigid or folding, wheeled with posterior seat

Lay Description

Walkers are used by patients with impaired ambulation when there is a need for greater stability and security than can be provided by a cane or crutches. Some walkers are simple "semi-cages," which look like two canes with supporting bars between them. Others are more complicated, and can be rigid or folding, with or without seating, with or without wheels, etc. Walkers may also include a device attached to the walker that provides trunk support. A trunk support device holds the patient upright in a standing position. The device may be flexible and soft padded or may be more rigid. The type of device depends upon the patient's medical condition. For example, a patient with cerebral palsy who has diminished muscle control of the trunk may need a rigid trunk support. Report E0130 for a rigid, pick-up type walker of adjustable or fixed height and E0135 for a folding one. Report E0140 for a walker with trunk support adjustable or fixed height. Report E0141 for a wheeled, rigid walker adjustable or fixed height. Report E0143 for a wheeled, folding walker without a seat. Report E0144 for an enclosed, wheeled, framed folding walker with posterior seat.

Medicare Information

A standard walker (E0130–E0141) and related accessories are covered if both of the following criteria are met:

- It is prescribed by a physician for a patient with a medical condition impairing ambulation and there is a potential for ambulation
- There is a need for greater stability and security than can be provided by a cane or crutches

A wheeled walker (E0141–E0143) is one with two, three, or four wheels. It may be a fixed height or adjustable height. It may or may not include glide-type brakes (or equivalent). The wheels may be fixed or swivel.

Code E0144 describes a folding wheeled walker that has a frame that completely surrounds the patient and an attached seat in the back.

The medical necessity for a walker with an enclosed frame (E0144) compared to a standard folding wheeled walker (E0143) has not been established. If the basic coverage criteria for a walker are met and E0144 is billed, payment will be based on the allowance for the least costly medically appropriate alternative, E0143.

For walkers with a seat and/or crutch attachment, use codes for individual accessories (E0156, E0157), along with a base walker code. For example, a folding wheeled walker with a seat is billed as E0143 plus E0156.

An enrolled DME supplier must bill these items to the DME MAC.

E0147-E0149

E0147 **Walker, heavy duty, multiple braking system, variable wheel resistance**
E0148 **Walker, heavy-duty, without wheels, rigid or folding, any type, each**
E0149 **Walker, heavy-duty, wheeled, rigid or folding, any type**

Lay Description

Walkers are used by patients with impaired ambulation when there is a need for greater stability and security than can be provided by a cane or crutches. Some walkers are simple "semi-cages," which look like two canes with supporting bars between them. Others are more complicated, and can be rigid or folding, with or without seating, with or without wheels, etc. Heavy duty walkers are used by patients with severe neurological disorders or restricted use of one hand, and those who exceed the weight limits of a standard wheeled walker. Report E0147 for a heavy-duty walker with multiple braking system and variable wheel resistance, E0148 for a heavy-duty walker, any type, rigid or folding, without wheels, and E0149 for one with wheels.

Documentation Standards

For Medicare beneficiaries, if a heavy-duty walker (E0148, E0149) is provided and if the supplier has documentation in the records that the patient's weight (within one month of providing the walker) is greater than 300 pounds, modifier KX should be added to the code.

If E0147 is billed to the DME MAC, the claim must include the manufacturer's name, the model name/number, a copy of a note or other documentation from the treating physician giving a detailed description of the functional limitations that preclude the patient using another type of wheeled walker, and the diagnosis causing this limitation.

Medicare Information

A wheeled walker (E0149) is one with two, three, or four wheels. It may be fixed height or adjustable height. It may or may not include glide-type brakes (or equivalent). The wheels may be fixed or swivel.

Code E0147 describes a four-wheeled, adjustable height, folding-walker that has all of the following characteristics:

- Capable of supporting patients who weigh greater than 350 pounds
- Hand operated brakes that cause the wheels to lock when the hand levers are released
- The hand brakes can be set so that either or both can lock both wheels
- The pressure required to operate each hand brake is individually adjustable
- There is an additional braking mechanism on the front crossbar
- At least two wheels have brakes that can be independently set through tension adjustability to give varying resistance

A heavy-duty walker (E0148, E0149) is covered for a patient who meets coverage criteria for a standard walker, and who weighs more than 300 pounds. If one of the walkers represented by codes E0148 or E0149 is provided and the patient does not weigh more than 300 pounds, but does meet coverage criteria for a standard walker, payment will be based on the allowance for the least costly medically appropriate alternative, E0135 or E0143 respectively.

A heavy duty, multiple-braking system, variable wheel resistance walker (E0147) is covered for patients who meet coverage criteria for a standard walker, and who are unable to use a standard walker due to a severe neurologic disorder or other condition causing the restricted use of one hand. Obesity, by itself, is not a sufficient reason for a walker represented by E0147. If this walker is provided and the coverage criteria for a standard walker are met, but the additional coverage criteria for E0147 are not met, payment will be based on the allowance for the least costly medically appropriate alternative, E0143 or E0149 depending on the patient's weight.

The only walkers that may be billed using E0147 are those products listed in the Product Classification List on the SADME MAC web site.

An enrolled DME supplier must bill these items to the DME MAC.

E0153-E0159

E0153   Platform attachment, forearm crutch, each
E0154   Platform attachment, walker, each
E0155   Wheel attachment, rigid pick-up walker, per pair
E0156   Seat attachment, walker
E0157   Crutch attachment, walker, each
E0158   Leg extensions for walker, per set of 4
E0159   Brake attachment for wheeled walker, replacement, each

Lay Description

These codes report the various attachments used with walkers and crutches. Report E0153 for a platform that is attached to a forearm crutch and E0154 for a platform attachment for a walker. Report E0155 for a pair of wheels for attachment to a rigid or pick-up type walker; E0156 for a walker seat attachment; E0157 for a crutch attachment to a walker; and E0158 for leg extensions to a walker. Report one unit of E0158 for every set of four leg extensions. Report E0159 for a replacement brake attachment for a wheeled walker.

Documentation Standards

In E0153, an order for each item billed must be signed and dated by the treating physician, kept on file by the supplier and made available to the DME MAC upon request. Items billed to the DME MAC before a signed and dated order has been received by the supplier must be submitted with modifier EY added to each affected HCPCS code.

Medicare Information

Code A9270 should be used for a white cane used for a blind person.

A glide-type brake (E0159) consists of a spring mechanism (or equivalent), which raises the leg post of the walker off the ground when the patient is not pushing down on the frame.

Leg extensions (E0158) are covered only for patients 6 feet tall or taller.

For walkers with a seat and/or crutch attachment, use codes for individual accessories (E0156, E0157), along with a base walker code. For example, a folding wheeled walker with a seat is billed as E0143 plus E0156.

Codes E0154, E0156, E0157, and E0158 can be used for accessories provided with the initial issue of a walker or for replacement components. Code E0155 can be used for replacements on covered, patient-owned wheeled walkers, or when wheels are subsequently added to a covered, patient-owned nonwheeled walker (E0130, E0135). Code E0155 cannot be used for wheels provided at the time of, or within one month of, the initial issue of a nonwheeled walker. Hemiwalkers must be coded using E0130 or E0135, but not E1399.

Code E0159 is only used to bill for replacement items for covered, patient-owned walkers.

An enrolled DME supplier must bill these items to the DME MAC.

E0160-E0175

E0160   Sitz type bath or equipment, portable, used with or without commode
E0161   Sitz type bath or equipment, portable, used with or without commode, with faucet attachment(s)
E0162   Sitz bath chair
E0163   Commode chair, mobile or stationary, with fixed arms
E0165   Commode chair, mobile or stationary, with detachable arms
E0167   Pail or pan for use with commode chair, replacement only
E0168   Commode chair, extra wide and/or heavy-duty, stationary or mobile, with or without arms, any type
E0170   Commode chair with integrated seat lift mechanism, electric, any type
E0171   Commode chair with integrated seat lift mechanism, nonelectric, any type
E0172   Seat lift mechanism placed over or on top of toilet, any type
E0175   Footrest, for use with commode chair, each

Lay Description

Commodes are generally portable toilets in a chair form that hold a pot under an open toilet seat. Some commodes, known as sitz baths, have large deep pans that also serve as a hip bath to soak the hips, buttocks, or perineal area wounds. There are many types/styles of commodes available on the market. Report E0160 for a portable sitz type bath or equipment, used with or without a commode and E0161 for the same with a faucet attachment. The sitz bath chair is reported with E0162. Report E0163 for a commode chair with fixed arms, mobile or stationary. Report E0165 for a commode chair with detachable arms, mobile or stationary. A replacement pail or pan used with the commode chair is reported with E0167. Extra wide and/or heavy-duty commode chairs are required for large or obese patients and are reported with E0168, whether stationary or mobile, with or without arms. Report E0170 for a commode chair with an integrated electric seat lift mechanism and E0171 for a commode chair with a nonelectric seat lift mechanism. Report E0172 for a seat lift mechanism placed over or on top of a toilet. Report E0175 if a footrest is used with a commode chair.

Medicare Information

For an item to be covered by Medicare, a written signed and dated order must be received by the supplier before a claim is submitted to the DME MAC. If the supplier bills for an item addressed in this policy without first receiving the completed order, the item will be denied as not medically necessary.

A commode is covered when the patient is physically incapable of using regular toilet facilities. This would occur in the following situations:

- The patient is confined to a single room
- The patient is confined to one level of the home environment and there is no toilet on that level
- The patient is confined to the home and there are no toilet facilities in the home

An extra wide/heavy duty commode chair (E0168) is covered for patients who weigh 300 pounds or more. If the patient weighs less than 300 pounds, but the basic coverage criteria for a commode chair are met, payment will be based on the least costly medically appropriate alternative, E0163.

The pail or pan used with the commode chair, represented by E0167, is included in the initial allowance for the commode when provided at the same time.

E0181-E0182

E0181 Powered pressure reducing mattress overlay/pad, alternating, with pump, includes heavy-duty

E0182 Pump for alternating pressure pad, for replacement only

Lay Description

These codes describe power pressure-reducing mattress overlays of alternating pressure or low air loss. These pressure reducing support devices consist of various pads that reduce the pressure of the patient's body weight on any particular area of the body. They are characterized by an air pump or blower that provides either sequential inflation or deflation of air cells or a low interface pressure throughout the overlay. They have inflated cell height of the air cells through which air is being circulated of 2.5 inches or greater. The height of the air chambers, proximity of the air chambers to one another, frequency of air cycling (for alternating pressure overlays), and air pressure provide adequate patient lift, pressure reduction, and prevention of bottoming out. Typically used for patients who are either fully or partially immobile (e.g., paraplegic patient), they assist in reducing the pressure on skin and tissues, allowing blood flow to the focal points in question, to prevent and/or treat pressure ulcers and lesions, such as decubitus ulcers. Report E0181 for alternating pressure pad with pump, including heavy duty; and E0182 for a replacement pump for an alternating pressure pad.

Medicare Information

See chapter titled "Medicare Guidelines," under "Pressure Reducing Support surfaces," for Medicare billing and documentation information.

E0184, E0186-E0187

E0184 Dry pressure mattress
E0186 Air pressure mattress
E0187 Water pressure mattress

Lay Description

These codes report special mattresses that reduce the pressure of the patient's body weight on any particular area of the body. Generally used for patients who are either fully or partially immobile (e.g., paraplegic patient), they assist in reducing the pressure on skin and tissues, allowing blood flow to the focal points in question, to prevent and/or treat pressure ulcers and lesions, such as decubitus ulcers. These codes describe nonpowered pressure-reducing mattresses. A foam, or dry pressure, mattress (E0184) is characterized by a height of 5 inches or greater, with a density and other qualities that provide adequate pressure reduction. It is durable, has a waterproof cover, and can be placed directly on a hospital bed frame. An air pressure (E0186) or water pressure mattress (E0187) is characterized by a height of 5 inches or greater of the air or water contained inside, and has a durable, waterproof cover, and can be placed directly on a hospital bed frame.

E0185, E0197-E0199

E0185 Gel or gel-like pressure pad for mattress, standard mattress length and width
E0197 Air pressure pad for mattress, standard mattress length and width
E0198 Water pressure pad for mattress, standard mattress length and width
E0199 Dry pressure pad for mattress, standard mattress length and width

Lay Description

These codes, identified as "pressure pad for mattress," describe nonpowered pressure reducing mattress overlays. These devices are designed to be placed on top of a hospital or home mattress of standard length and width. Pressure reducing support services consist of various pads for mattresses that reduce the pressure of the patient's body weight on any particular area of the body. Typically used for patient's that are either fully or partially immobile (e.g., paraplegic patient), they assist in reducing the pressure on skin and tissues, allowing blood flow to the focal points in question, to prevent and/or treat pressure ulcers and lesions, such as decubitus ulcers. A gel or gel-like mattress overlay (E0185) is characterized by a gel or gel-like layer contained within the pad reaching a height of 2 inches or greater. An air pressure pad (E0197) is characterized by interconnected air cells having a cell height of 3 inches or greater. A water pressure mattress overlay (E0198) is characterized by a filled height of 3 inches or greater of water contained within the pads cells. A foam mattress overlay (E0199), or dry pressure pad, is characterized by a base thickness of 2 inches or greater and peak height of 3 inches or greater if it is a convoluted overlay (e.g., egg crate-type), or an overall height of at least 3 inches if it is a non-convoluted overlay.

Medicare Information

See chapter titled "Medicare Guidelines," under "Pressure Reducing Support surfaces," for Medicare billing and documentation information.

E0186-E0187

E0186 Air pressure mattress
E0187 Water pressure mattress

Lay Description

Please refer to code E0184 for the description, coding, and billing information.

E0188-E0189, E0191-E0194

E0188 Synthetic sheepskin pad
E0189 Lambswool sheepskin pad, any size
E0191 Heel or elbow protector, each
E0193 Powered air flotation bed (low air loss therapy)
E0194 Air fluidized bed

Lay Description

A decubitus ulcer is also known as a pressure ulcer, pressure sore, or bedsore. Bedsores can range from a mild erythema of the skin to a deep wound extending through bone. Pressure ulcers occur when an incapacitated, bedridden person has constant pressure against the skin, usually over a bony area, which decreases the blood supply, causing tissue death. Use of special pads or beds relieve pressure on the skin. Pads made of synthetic sheepskin (E0188) or lambs wool (E0189) and heel or elbow protectors (E0191) prevent friction against thin fragile skin. Specialized beds such as a powered air flotation bed (E0193) or an air-fluidized bed (E0194) are often used for patients with stage three or four pressure sores that would otherwise require institutionalization. Report E0192 for a low pressure and positioning equalization pad for use in a wheelchair.

Medicare Information

Medicare covers pads if physicians supervise their use in patients who have decubitus ulcers or susceptibility to them. Prior authorization and a written order is required by Medicare for this item.

An air fluidized bed is covered by Medicare if the patient has a stage 3 or stage 4 pressure sore and, without the bed, would require institutionalization. A physician's prescription is required.

See chapter titled "Medicare Guidelines," under "Pressure Reducing Support surfaces," for additional Medicare billing and documentation information.

E0190

E0190 Positioning cushion/pillow/wedge, any shape or size, includes all components and accessories

Lay Description

Positioning cushions/pillows/wedges are typically made of foam or foam-like materials, and come in a variety of densities, shapes, and designs depending on the manufacturer. Most have anatomic-oriented designs so as to provide as much support as possible, although they somewhat limit range of motion. These cushions/pillows/wedges relieve and/or prevent neck tension and may protect against inadvertent reinjury during sleep. HCPCS Level II code E0190 represents any shape or size of positioning cushion/pillow/wedge and includes all components or accesories.

Documentation Standards

The order for the item must be documented in the medical record.

The diagnosis establishing medical necessity for the item must be documented in the medical record.

Medicare Information

If the medical necessity for the item—as determined by the payer—cannot be established due to the nature of the patient's condition, injury, or illness, then the patient should sign a waiver in advance of receiving the item. For Medicare patients, this waiver is called the Advance Beneficiary Notice (ABN). Keep this document on file in case there is a request for proof of the advance notice.

E0191-E0194

E0191 Heel or elbow protector, each
E0193 Powered air flotation bed (low air loss therapy)
E0194 Air fluidized bed

Lay Description

Please refer to codes E0188-E0189 for the description, coding, and billing information.

E0196

E0196 Gel pressure mattress

Lay Description

A gel pressure mattress is a mattress with a top layer of gel that is enclosed in a durable, waterproof bladder. The gel layer must be at least a height of 5 inches. Some gel mattresses have a layer of soft or pillow-top material directly under the gel layer. This is a full mattress that can be placed directly on a bed frame. A gel pressure mattress is designed to distribute weight more evenly across the surface of the mattress and eliminate pressure points. When there is decreased pressure on skin at contact points, such as buttocks and ankles, skin and soft tissue is less likely to break down and form ulcers or other types of open wounds.

Medicare Information

See chapter titled "Medicare Guidelines," under "Pressure Reducing Support surfaces," for Medicare billing and documentation information.

E0197-E0199

E0197 Air pressure pad for mattress, standard mattress length and width
E0198 Water pressure pad for mattress, standard mattress length and width
E0199 Dry pressure pad for mattress, standard mattress length and width

Lay Description

Please refer to code E0185 for the description, coding, and billing information.

E0200, E0205

E0200 Heat lamp, without stand (table model), includes bulb, or infrared element
E0205 Heat lamp, with stand, includes bulb, or infrared element

Lay Description

Heat causes blood vessels to open, creating increased blood flow and allowing tissue purging of debris and by-products of injury. Heat therapy promotes relaxation of collagen tissues within muscle, tendons, and ligaments, which allow them to be stretched. Heat lamps provide dry heat to patients who cannot tolerate pressure of a directly applied heat source, or who may have positioning needs. The heat from a lamp is controlled by the distance between the lamp and the patient. Report E0200 for heat lamps, including bulb or infrared element, for a table model without a stand and E0205 for one with a stand.

E0202

E0202 Phototherapy (bilirubin) light with photometer

Lay Description

A phototherapy (bilirubin) light with photometer is used to treat infants with jaundice caused by elevated levels of bilirubin in the blood. Phototherapy lights provide a specific wavelength of blue fluorescent light that breaks down bilirubin into nontoxic water-soluble components that are excreted by the infant. The photometer or "blue meter" on the lamp measures the intensity of the light emission. Phototherapy lights are available in the form of a lamp, light panel, or special light blanket (wallaby blanket) and all are reported with E0202.

E0203

E0203 Therapeutic lightbox, minimum 10,000 lux, table top model

Lay Description

A therapeutic lightbox with a minimum of 10,000 lux is used to treat seasonal affective disorder (SAD), which is a form of depression; diurnal disorders; or sometimes to mitigate the effects of medications. SAD occurs most frequently in the fall or winter as the daylight hours become shorter and shorter. Therapeutic lightboxes provide cool-white or full spectrum fluorescent light to treat this disorder. The light boxes deliver strong light near the intensity and wavelength of noontime during high summer. Patients expose themselves to the light for a prescribed amount of time per day at set times. Tabletop or desktop lightboxes that emit a minimum of 10,000 lux, which is a measurement of the light intensity, are reported with E0203. Lightboxes that emit lower levels of lux (5,000 or 2,500) should not be reported with E0203.

E0205

E0205 Heat lamp, with stand, includes bulb, or infrared element

Lay Description

Please refer to code E0200 for description, coding, and billing information.

E0210-E0215

E0210 Electric heat pad, standard
E0215 Electric heat pad, moist

Lay Description

Heat causes blood vessels to open, creating increased blood flow and allowing tissue purging of debris and by-products of injury. Heat therapy promotes relaxation of collagen tissues within muscle, tendons, and ligaments, which allow them to be stretched. Electric heating pads are alternatives to hot packs. Because electric heating pads do not cool spontaneously, use should be limited to 20 minutes to avoid the risk of burns.

Medicare modifiers

Code E0210 must be submitted with modifier AX when it is used with home dialysis. If a heating pad (E0210) is not used for home dialysis, it must be billed without modifier AX.

E0217-E0218, E0236, E0249

E0217 Water circulating heat pad with pump
E0218 Water circulating cold pad with pump
E0236 Pump for water circulating pad
E0249 Pad for water circulating heat unit, for replacement only

Lay Description

Heat causes blood vessels to open, creating increased blood flow and allowing tissue purging of debris and by-products of injury. Heat therapy promotes relaxation of collagen tissues within muscle, tendons, and ligaments, which allow them to be stretched. A water circulating heating pad with pump (E0217) is a device that circulates heated water through the pad using a mechanical pump. Cold therapy is the application of cold treatment to affected tissues, generally used in the immediate postoperative or post-trauma period to reduce edema and enhance pain control. Pain sensations are inhibited by cold by reducing the speed of impulses conducted by nerve fibers. Cold therapy reduces muscle spasms and causes constriction of small arteries and veins, which reduces hemorrhage and swelling within injured tissues. A water circulating cold pad with pump (E0218) consists of ice water placed into a reservoir that is circulated through a pad using a mechanical pump. Report E0236 for the pump alone for a water-circulating pad, hot or cold. Report E0249 for the pad replacement alone for a patient owned water circulating heat unit.

E0221

E0221 Infrared heating pad system

Lay Description

An infrared heating pad system consists of a pad or pads containing mechanisms, such as luminous gallium aluminum arsenide diodes, that generate infrared (or near infrared) light and a power source.

Medicare Information

HCPCS code E0221 is in the inexpensive or routinely purchased payment category. This HCPCS code includes both the power source and the infrared therapy pads. Manufacturers or suppliers should contact the SADME MAC for guidance on whether a particular device meets the definition of this HCPCS code.

E0225, E0239

E0225 Hydrocollator unit, includes pads
E0239 Hydrocollator unit, portable

Lay Description

Hydrocollator packs are also known as hot packs and warm tissue by conduction. Usually made of canvas bags filled with silicon dioxide, which absorbs many times its own weight in water, hydrocollator packs are immersed in a hot water bath, removed as needed, then wrapped in layered toweling or padding, or some kind of insulating cover, and applied to the patient. The packs cool slowly and can remain warm for around 30 minutes. Report a hydrocollator unit with pads with E0225. Report E0239 for a portable hydrocollator unit.

E0231-E0232

E0231 Noncontact wound-warming device (temperature control unit, AC adapter and power cord) for use with warming card and wound cover
E0232 Warming card for use with the noncontact wound-warming device and noncontact wound-warming wound cover

Lay Description

Wound healing occurs best in a warm, moist environment that enhances subcutaneous oxygen tension and increases blood flow to the wound. A noncontact wound warming device, also referred to as noncontact normothermic wound therapy (NNWT), is a wound treatment device designed to create an optimal environment to promote wound healing. A noncontact wound warming device includes a noncontact bandage and a warming unit designed to maintain 100 percent relative humidity and to produce optimal temperatures in the wound and surrounding tissues. The bandage consists of a sterile foam collar that adheres to the skin surrounding the wound and a sterile, transparent film that covers the top of the wound without touching it. An infrared warming card or flexible heat unit is inserted into a pocket in the film covering. Supply of the wound warming device is reported with E0231. The warming card is reported with E0232.

E0235

E0235 Paraffin bath unit, portable (see medical supply code A4265 for paraffin)

Lay Description

Paraffin baths are used mainly for treating contractures, occurring in patients with rheumatoid arthritis or scleroderma. The typical paraffin bath is a container that holds and heats a 1:7 mixture of mineral oil and paraffin, maintaining it at around 53¡C into which the patient may either continuously immerse the treated part, such as the hand, for 20-30 minutes, or repetitively dip and remove the treated area from the paraffin. This code is for a portable paraffin bath unit, excluding the paraffin.

E0236

E0236 Pump for water circulating pad

Lay Description

Please refer to codes E0217-E0218 for the description, coding, and billing information.

E0239

E0239 Hydrocollator unit, portable

Lay Description

Please refer to code E0225 for the description, coding, and billing information.

E0240

E0240 Bath/shower chair, with or without wheels, any size

Lay Description

A bath or shower chair is a seat designed to fit into a standard bathtub or walk-in shower that provides stable seating while bathing or showering for those people unsteady on their feet or those unable to stand.

E0241-E0246

E0241 Bathtub wall rail, each
E0242 Bathtub rail, floor base
E0243 Toilet rail, each
E0244 Raised toilet seat
E0245 Tub stool or bench
E0246 Transfer tub rail attachment

Lay Description

Rails are safety items for home use to help a person get in and out of the bathtub or up and down from the toilet by providing a strong hold while securely stepping into the tub, or lowering or raising body weight. Report E0241 for a bathtub rail that mounts on the wall; E0242 for a floor based bathtub rail; and E0246 for a transfer tub rail, which is mounted directly to the tub. Report E0243 for a toilet rail. Other toilet aids for home use include a raised toilet seat (E0244), which is shaped to fit most toilets and a tub stool or bench (E0245).

Medicare Information

Codes E0241–E0245 are not recognized by Medicare.

E0247-E0248

E0247 Transfer bench for tub or toilet with or without commode opening
E0248 Transfer bench, heavy-duty, for tub or toilet with or without commode opening

Lay Description

A transfer bench for tub or toilet is a flat expanded surface without a back that provides stable seating while the person is bathing or showering. These benches may have a commode opening that allows the person to more comfortably maneuver and use a toilet. The benches may be freestanding with legs or attachable to wall or tub. Transfer benches are intended for those people unsteady on their feet or those unable to stand. Heavy-duty benches are generally designed for people who weigh more than 300 lbs.

E0249

E0249 Pad for water circulating heat unit, for replacement only

Lay Description

Please refer to codes E0217–E0218 for the description, coding, and billing information.

E0250-E0256, E0290-E0293

E0250 Hospital bed, fixed height, with any type side rails, with mattress
E0251 Hospital bed, fixed height, with any type side rails, without mattress
E0255 Hospital bed, variable height, hi-lo, with any type side rails, with mattress
E0256 Hospital bed, variable height, hi-lo, with any type side rails, without mattress
E0290 Hospital bed, fixed height, without side rails, with mattress
E0291 Hospital bed, fixed height, without side rails, without mattress
E0292 Hospital bed, variable height, hi-lo, without side rails, with mattress
E0293 Hospital bed, variable height, hi-lo, without side rails, without mattress

Lay Description

Hospital beds for patient home use come in a variety of designs, with a multitude of features and accessories to assist and protect the patient. A hospital bed is generally needed when an ordinary (regular) bed, is not suitable for the patient's medical needs. Hospital beds provide features such as head and leg elevation and height adjustment. Clinical cases generally requiring variable-height hospital bed use include severe arthritis and other injuries to lower extremities (e.g., fractured hip). Report E0250 for a fixed height hospital bed with any type side rails, with mattress; E0251 without mattress; E0290 without side rails, with mattress; and E0291 without side rails or mattress. Variable-height (hi-lo) feature beds assist patients to ambulate by enabling them to place their feet on the floor while sitting on the edge of the bed. Report E0255 for a variable height hospital bed with any type side rails, with mattress; E0256 without mattress; E0292 without side rails, with mattress; and E0293 without side rails or mattress.

Medicare Information

See the chapter titled "Medicare Guidelines," under "Hospital Beds," for Medicare information.

E0260-E0266, E0294-E0297

E0260 Hospital bed, semi-electric (head and foot adjustment), with any type side rails, with mattress
E0261 Hospital bed, semi-electric (head and foot adjustment), with any type side rails, without mattress
E0265 Hospital bed, total electric (head, foot, and height adjustments), with any type side rails, with mattress
E0266 Hospital bed, total electric (head, foot, and height adjustments), with any type side rails, without mattress
E0294 Hospital bed, semi-electric (head and foot adjustment), without side rails, with mattress
E0295 Hospital bed, semi-electric (head and foot adjustment), without side rails, without mattress
E0296 Hospital bed, total electric (head, foot, and height adjustments), without side rails, with mattress
E0297 Hospital bed, total electric (head, foot, and height adjustments), without side rails, without mattress

Lay Description

Hospital beds for patient home use come in a variety of designs, with a multitude of features and accessories to assist and protect the patient. A hospital bed is generally needed when an ordinary, regular bed, is not suitable for the patient's medical needs. Hospital beds provide features such as head and leg elevation and height adjustment. Hospital beds with the semi-electric feature allow for head and foot adjustment, and are used by patients with congestive heart failure, chronic pulmonary disease, or problems with aspiration who require positioning of the body in ways not feasible with an ordinary flat bed. Report E0260 for a semi-electric bed for head and foot adjustment, with any type side rails, with mattress; E0261 without mattress; E0294 without side rails, with mattress; and E0295 without side rails or mattress. Total electric hospital beds enable the patient to lower and raise head and foot adjustments independently as well as adjust the total height of the bed. Report E0265 for a total electric bed with any type side rails, with mattress; E0266 without mattress; E0296 without side rails, with mattress; and E0297 without side rails or mattress.

Medicare Information

See the chapter titled "Medicare Guidelines," under "Hospital Beds," for Medicare information.

E0270

E0270 Hospital bed, institutional type includes: oscillating, circulating and Stryker frame, with mattress

Lay Description

Standard institutional hospital beds typically include a frame for oscillating on a longitudinally extending axis and a patient support which is mounted on the oscillating frame, providing controlled pivoting of the patient support on a transverse axis. A Stryker bed consists of a bed frame that holds the patient and permits turning in various planes without individual motion of parts, allowing medical staff to turn a patient easily. These beds also include securing devices provided on the patient support to hold a patient in place. The mattress is typically made of water resistant vinyl and is durable for long term use while also being fire retardant.

E0271-E0272

E0271 Mattress, innerspring
E0272 Mattress, foam rubber

Lay Description

A foam rubber mattress is used to add comfort to a hospital bed. This device is commonly used in conjunction with other hospital bed components such as bed boards and inner springs. Report E0271 for the supply of one inner spring mattress alone and E0272 for a foam rubber mattress.

Medicare Information

See the chapter titled "Medicare Guidelines," under "Hospital Beds," for Medicare information.

E0273

E0273 Bed board

Lay Description

A bed board is a device placed under a mattress to support the mattress and keep it firm by preventing the mattress from sagging. Bed boards usually consist of wood slats inside a canvas cover or are made of wood with hinges allowing the board to bend with the position of the bed.

E0274, E0315

E0274 Over-bed table
E0315 Bed accessory: board, table, or support device, any type

Lay Description

An over-bed table, board, or support device is a functional convenience item, adjustable in height, or angle, to allow the patient more comfort and ease while writing or eating in bed. An over-the-bed table has a laminate top affixed to a chrome-plated, height-adjustable bar, and casters to ease mobility of the table in any direction.

E0275-E0276

E0275 Bed pan, standard, metal or plastic
E0276 Bed pan, fracture, metal or plastic

Lay Description

Bedpans are used by patients whose conditions require them to remain in bed and not ambulate, even for the purpose of getting to the bathroom. Report E0275 for a standard metal or plastic bedpan and E0276 for a fracture bedpan, which tapers down on one end and can be used as a female urinal, metal or plastic.

E0277

E0277 Powered pressure-reducing air mattress

Lay Description

Code E0277 describes a powered pressure-reducing mattress (alternating pressure, low air loss, or powered flotation without low air loss) that is characterized by the following: an air pump or blower that provides either sequential inflation and deflation of the air cells or a low interface pressure throughout the mattress; an inflated cell height of the air cells through which air is being circulated of 5 inches or greater; air chamber height and proximity and frequency of air circulation (for alternating pressure mattresses), which provides adequate patient lift and pressure reduction to prevent bottoming out; a surface designed to reduce friction; and the ability to be placed directly on a hospital bed frame.

Medicare Information

See chapter titled "Medicare Guidelines," under "Pressure Reducing Support surfaces," for Medicare billing and documentation information.

E0280

E0280 Bed cradle, any type

Lay Description

A bed cradle is used for patients with acute gouty arthritis or burns for whom it is necessary to prevent contact with the bed coverings and any pressure applied to the area. Report this code for any type of bed cradle.

Medicare Information

See the chapter titled "Medicare Guidelines," under "Hospital Beds," for Medicare information.

E0290-E0293

E0290 Hospital bed, fixed height, without side rails, with mattress
E0291 Hospital bed, fixed height, without side rails, without mattress
E0292 Hospital bed, variable height, hi-lo, without side rails, with mattress
E0293 Hospital bed, variable height, hi-lo, without side rails, without mattress

Lay Description

Please refer to codes E0250-E0256 for the description, coding, and billing information.

E0294-E0297

E0294 Hospital bed, semi-electric (head and foot adjustment), without side rails, with mattress
E0295 Hospital bed, semi-electric (head and foot adjustment), without side rails, without mattress
E0296 Hospital bed, total electric (head, foot, and height adjustments), without side rails, with mattress
E0297 Hospital bed, total electric (head, foot, and height adjustments), without side rails, without mattress

Lay Description

Please refer to codes E0260-E0266 for the description, coding, and billing information.

E0300

E0300 Pediatric crib, hospital grade, fully enclosed

Lay Description

A pediatric enclosured crib is an alternative bed for the pediatric patient. It allows the patient full range of motion with no traditional restraints. The crib consists of a mesh like screen that gently contains the patient and prevents wandering. Typically these cribs are available in different sizes and materials.

E0301-E0302

E0301 Hospital bed, heavy-duty, extra wide, with weight capacity greater than 350 pounds, but less than or equal to 600 pounds, with any type side rails, without mattress
E0302 Hospital bed, extra heavy-duty, extra wide, with weight capacity greater than 600 pounds, with any type side rails, without mattress

Lay Description

A hospital bed is generally needed when a home bed, sold as furniture, is not suitable for the patient's medical needs. Heavy duty, extra wide beds are available for individuals weighing more than 350 pounds. These beds have additional support in all parts, including the frame and legs. These beds include side rails as a safety feature. Report E0301 for heavy duty, extra wide beds with a weight capacity from 350 up to and including 600 pounds provided without a mattress, and E0302 for those with a weight capacity greater than 600 pounds.

E0303-E0304

E0303 Hospital bed, heavy-duty, extra wide, with weight capacity greater than 350 pounds, but less than or equal to 600 pounds, with any type side rails, with mattress
E0304 Hospital bed, extra heavy-duty, extra wide, with weight capacity greater than 600 pounds, with any type side rails, with mattress

Lay Description

A hospital bed is generally needed when a home bed, sold as furniture, is not suitable for the patient's medical needs. Extra-wide, heavy-duty hospital beds have side rails and a mattress that has additional support in all parts (e.g., legs) for an individual who weighs anywhere from 350-600 pounds (E0303) or for an individual who weighs more than 600 pounds (E0304).

Medicare Information

See the chapter titled "Medicare Guidelines," under "Hospital Beds," for Medicare information.

E0305-E0310

E0305 Bedside rails, half-length
E0310 Bedside rails, full-length

Lay Description

Bedside rails are used to protect the patient from injury (falling out of the bed). Code E0305 describes half-length bedside rails, which start at the head area of the bed and go down to the mid-point of the bed. These are used when the patient's condition or disease only require minimal protection from falling out of bed. Code E0310 identifies full-length bedside rails, which run the entire length of the bed. These are used when the patient has a higher risk of falling out of bed.

Medicare Information

When mattress or bedside rails are provided at the same time as a hospital bed, use the single code that combines these items.

E0305, E0310: Bedside rails, half-length/full-length:

- When combined with E0290, bill as E0250
- When combined with E0291, bill as E0251
- When combined with E0292, bill as E0255
- When combined with E0293, bill as E0256
- When combined with E0294, bill as E0260
- When combined with E0295, bill as E0261
- When combined with E0296, bill as E0265
- When combined with E0297, bill as E0266

E0271, E0272: Mattress, inner spring/foam rubber plus E0305, E0310: Bedside rails, half-length/full-length:

- When combined with E0291, bill as E0250
- When combined with E0293, bill as E0255
- When combined with E0295, bill as E0260
- When combined with E0297, bill as E0265

E0315

E0315 Bed accessory: board, table, or support device, any type

Lay Description

Please refer to code E0274 for the description, coding, and billing information.

E0316

E0316 Safety enclosure frame/canopy for use with hospital bed, any type

Lay Description

A safety enclosure such as a frame or canopy is used to prevent a patient from leaving the bed. This item encloses the standard hospital bed with a netting attached to a frame and is designed for patients who would need to be restrained. This allows the patient to remain in a safe environment without the need for leg or wrist restraints.

E0325-E0326

E0325 Urinal; male, jug-type, any material
E0326 Urinal; female, jug-type, any material

Lay Description

A urinal is a hand-held container used to collect urine. Some urinals have handles. Urinals are usually usable in a variety of positions. Jug type urinals generally have a lid and can be used multiple times. Urinals provide an option for bed-confined people who cannot use a bedpan. Male urinals are designed to accommodate a penis. Female urinals have various designs that can be used by women to collect urine.

Medicare Information

Urinals may be covered depending upon the reason for their use. When used for convenience or as a temporary measure, they are not covered. When medically necessary for incontinent, bed-confined, or postsurgical patients, urinals may be a covered DME item. See chapter titled "Medicare Guidelines," under "Urological Supplies," for additional information.

E0328-E0329

E0328 Hospital bed, pediatric, manual, 360 degree side enclosures, top of headboard, footboard and side rails up to 24 inches above the spring, includes mattress
E0329 Hospital bed, pediatric, electric or semi-electric, 360 degree side enclosures, top of headboard, footboard and side rails up to 24 inches above the spring, includes mattress

Lay Description

Pediatric hospital beds are surfaces for sleep or rest that are designed for nonadult patients. Different parts of the bed can be adjusted to different levels, angles, and configurations to provide physical relief or ease in comfort. Manual pediatric beds typically include manual cranks by which the patient can be raised or lowered in bed. Electric or semi-electric pediatric beds typically allow back and foot adjustment electronically. Some semi-electric beds allow manual height adjustment. Each type of bed usually includes movable bedside rails. The mattress used for these beds is typically made with a water resistant vinyl cover and is durable for long term use while also being fire retardant.

E0350-E0352

E0350 Control unit for electronic bowel irrigation/evacuation system
E0352 Disposable pack (water reservoir bag, speculum, valving mechanism, and collection bag/box) for use with the electronic bowel irrigation/evacuation system

Lay Description
Pulsed irrigation bowel evacuation is used for bowel management of chronic constipation and fecal impaction in patients with neurogenic bowel dysfunction. Neurogenic bowel dysfunction may be present in patients with spinal cord injury, amyotrophic lateral sclerosis, spina bifida, multiple sclerosis, and diabetes mellitus. Pulsed irrigation bowel evacuation system is an electronic device that delivers small pulses of warm tap water into the rectum to rehydrate feces and promote peristalsis. The system consists of a speculum, tubing, water reservoir bag, valve, a disposable collection container (E0352), and an electrical unit that delivers positive and negative air pressure through the tubing (E0350).

E0370

E0370 Air pressure elevator for heel

Lay Description
Lower extremities are susceptible to pressure ulcers. The heel is a small area that receives a great deal of pressure as it rests on a surface. An air pressure elevator for a heel is a device consisting of one or more air filled chambers that surround the heel and raise it above a hard surface. It may be used with wheelchairs, day chairs, and in bed.

E0371

E0371 Nonpowered advanced pressure reducing overlay for mattress, standard mattress length and width

Lay Description
A nonpowered advanced pressure-reducing mattress overlay is a device composed of separate cells filled with air or fluid that is attached or laid on the top of a mattress. It generally has a height of three inches or more and is covered in a surface that reduces friction. This overlay is designed to raise pressure points. When there is decreased pressure on skin at contact points, such as buttocks and ankles, skin and soft tissue is less likely to break down and form ulcers or other types of open wounds.

Medicare Information
See chapter titled "Medicare Guidelines," under "Pressure Reducing Support surfaces," for Medicare billing and documentation information.

E0372

E0372 Powered air overlay for mattress, standard mattress length and width

Lay Description
A powered pressure-reducing mattress overlay is a device filled with air or fluid that is attached to an electronic device that alternately raises and lowers the air pressure or circulates the air or fluid. The overlay is attached to or laid on top of a mattress. It generally has a height of 3 inches or more and is covered in a surface that reduces friction. This overlay is designed to raise pressure points. When there is decreased pressure on skin at contact points, such as buttocks and ankles, skin and soft tissue is less likely to break down and form ulcers or other types of open wounds.

Medicare Information
See chapter titled "Medicare Guidelines," under "Pressure Reducing Support surfaces," for Medicare billing and documentation information.

E0373

E0373 Nonpowered advanced pressure reducing mattress

Lay Description
A nonpowered, advanced pressure-reducing mattress is a mattress composed of separate cells filled with air or fluid. It generally has a height of 5 inches or more and is covered in a surface that reduces friction. The mattress is designed to raise pressure points. When there is decreased pressure on skin at contact points, such as buttocks and ankles, skin and soft tissue is less likely to break down and form ulcers or other types of open wounds.

Medicare Information
See chapter titled "Medicare Guidelines," under "Pressure Reducing Support surfaces," for Medicare billing and documentation information.

E0424-E0425

E0424 Stationary compressed gaseous oxygen system, rental; includes container, contents, regulator, flowmeter, humidifier, nebulizer, cannula or mask, and tubing
E0425 Stationary compressed gas system, purchase; includes regulator, flowmeter, humidifier, nebulizer, cannula or mask, and tubing

Lay Description
Oxygen is stored in several manners, one of which is as a compressed gas. The compression mandates use of heavy, reinforced tanks that constitute a stationary system. A regulator fits on top of the tank and is an

adjustment device to control the flow of oxygen at the prescribed rate. A flow meter conserves the release of oxygen by turning on and shutting off the regulated flow as the patient inhales and exhales. A nasal cannula is common for lower delivery rates. A mask and/or nebulizer may be used for higher delivery rates and a catheter directly to the trachea is sometimes required. An in-line humidification system may also be used to modulate effects of higher flows. Report E0424 for a rented compresses gaseous oxygen system that includes the contents (oxygen), as well as the regulator, flowmeter, humidifier, nebulizer, cannula or mask, and tubing. Report E0425 for a purchased compressed gas system, which includes the regulator, flowmeter, humidifier, nebulizer, cannula or mask, and tubing, but not the contents (oxygen).

Medicare Information

Suppliers must furnish the units of oxygen contents, except for concentrators and initial rental claims for gas or liquid oxygen delivery systems. For stationary gas system rentals, indicate oxygen contents in unit multiples of 50 cubic feet, rounded to the nearest increment of 50 (e.g., 173 cubic feet of oxygen has been delivered in one rental month, so the units entry on the claim nearest to 50 cubic feet is 03; 100 cubic feet equals two units, and the remaining 73 cubic feet must be rounded down to 50 for an additional cubic foot, amounting to a total of 3 cubic feet).

Note: See chapter titled "Medicare Guidelines," under "Oxygen (O2) and O2 Equipment," for additional Medicare billing and documentation information.

E0430-E0431

E0430 Portable gaseous oxygen system, purchase; includes regulator, flowmeter, humidifier, cannula or mask, and tubing

E0431 Portable gaseous oxygen system, rental; includes portable container, regulator, flowmeter, humidifier, cannula or mask, and tubing

Lay Description

Portable gaseous oxygen systems are typically lightweight aluminum tanks (usually designated as C tanks) containing pressurized gaseous oxygen. The pressurized systems are stable and the product stores well up to time of use. In some instances, these units may be refilled from large stationary gas oxygen tanks. These systems are generally designed for emergency or occasional use. These codes include all delivery hardware associated with use of the system (regulator, flowmeter, mask, tubing, etc.). Report E0430 for a purchased system and E0431 for a rented system.

E0434-E0435

E0434 Portable liquid oxygen system, rental; includes portable container, supply reservoir, humidifier, flowmeter, refill adaptor, contents gauge, cannula or mask, and tubing

E0435 Portable liquid oxygen system, purchase; includes portable container, supply reservoir, flowmeter, humidifier, contents gauge, cannula or mask, tubing and refill adaptor

Lay Description

Portable liquid oxygen tanks are insulated thermos-like units that store comparatively large quantities of oxygen at lower pressures than gaseous systems. Several hundred times more oxygen can be stored as liquid in the same amount of space than in its gaseous form. The liquid oxygen is stored cold and converted to gas as it is warmed through an apparatus at the reservoir. Portable units typically weigh eight to 10 pounds and are designed to be refillable from larger, stationary tanks. Portable liquid systems are prone to evaporation loss and the product should be used shortly after decanting. These codes include all oxygen delivery hardware associated with use of the system (regulator, flowmeter, mask, tubing, etc.), including refill adapters. Report E0434 for a rented system and E0435 for a purchased system.

E0439-E0440

E0439 Stationary liquid oxygen system, rental; includes container, contents, regulator, flowmeter, humidifier, nebulizer, cannula or mask, & tubing

E0440 Stationary liquid oxygen system, purchase; includes use of reservoir, contents indicator, regulator, flowmeter, humidifier, nebulizer, cannula or mask, and tubing

Lay Description

Stationary liquid oxygen systems are insulated thermos-like units that store comparatively large quantities of oxygen at lower pressures than gaseous systems. (Several hundred times more oxygen can be stored as liquid in the same amount of space than in its gaseous form.) The liquid oxygen is stored cold and converted to gas as it is warmed through an apparatus at the reservoir. Stationary units may weigh 75 to 100 pounds and can contain enough liquid oxygen to last patients up to eight days, depending on level of use. In many instances, the stationary system is also used to decant liquid oxygen into smaller, portable systems. These codes include all oxygen delivery hardware associated with use of the stationary system (regulator, flowmeter, mask, tubing, etc.). Report E0439 for a rented system and E0440 for a purchased system.

E0441-E0442

E0441 Stationary oxygen contents, gaseous, 1 month's supply = 1 unit
E0442 Stationary oxygen contents, liquid, 1 month's supply = 1 unit

Lay Description

Traditional oxygen systems are of two general varieties. Compressed gaseous systems, commonly known as "green tanks" or H tanks, are large stationary units that must be secured in place during use. These tanks may be steel, aluminum, or reinforced synthetic material. Smaller units, designated as E tanks and D tanks, are semi-portable units and, in some instances, may be refilled from a larger unit. Gaseous oxygen for stationary systems is typically sold in increments of 50 cubic feet. Report E0441 for a one-month supply of gaseous oxygen product for a purchased system, with or without refillable portable tanks. The second variety consists of liquid oxygen systems. Stationary liquid oxygen systems are insulated thermos-like units that store comparatively large quantities of oxygen at lower pressures than gaseous systems. (Several hundred times more oxygen can be stored as liquid in the same amount of space than in its gaseous form.) The liquid oxygen is stored cold and converted to gas as it is warmed through an apparatus at the reservoir. Stationary units may weigh 75 to 100 pounds and can contain enough liquid oxygen to last patients up to eight days, depending on level of use. In many instances, the stationary system is also used to decant liquid oxygen into smaller, portable systems. Liquid oxygen for stationary systems is typically sold in 10-pound increments. Report E0442 for a one-month supply of liquid oxygen product for a purchased system, with or without refillable portable tanks.

E0443-E0444

E0443 Portable oxygen contents, gaseous, 1 month's supply = 1 unit
E0444 Portable oxygen contents, liquid, 1 month's supply = 1 unit

Lay Description

Traditional portable oxygen systems are of two general varieties. Smaller compressed gaseous systems are designated as E tanks and D tanks and are semi-portable reinforced tanks. Fully portable gaseous oxygen systems are typically lightweight aluminum tanks (usually designated as C tanks) containing the pressurized gaseous oxygen. These pressurized systems are stable and the oxygen product stores well up to time of use. These systems are generally designed for emergency or occasional use. Gaseous oxygen for portable systems is typically sold in increments of five cubic feet. Report E0443 for a one-month supply of gaseous oxygen product for a portable system not refillable from a stationary tank. The second variety consists of liquid oxygen systems. Liquid oxygen is stored cold in low-pressure insulated tanks and converted to gas as it is warmed through an apparatus at the reservoir. Portable units may weigh eight to 10 pounds and can contain enough liquid oxygen to last patients up to four hours, depending on level of use. Liquid oxygen for portable systems is typically sold in one-pound increments. Report E0444 for a one-month supply of liquid oxygen product for a portable system not refillable from a stationary tank.

E0445

E0445 Oximeter device for measuring blood oxygen levels noninvasively

Lay Description

Oximetry is a noninvasive method to measure blood hemoglobin (Hb) oxygen saturation. A probe is attached to the patient's earlobe or a fingertip. The probe emits a light source. The hemoglobin absorbs a percentage of the light, depending upon its oxygen saturation level, and the results are digitally recorded and displayed on a hand-held unit. Additional data, such as pulse, are sometimes recorded and displayed. This code reports supply of the oximeter unit itself. Report A4606 for the oxygen probe replacement unit.

E0450

E0450 Volume control ventilator, without pressure support mode, may include pressure control mode, used with invasive interface (e.g., tracheostomy tube)

Lay Description

Volume control ventilators are typically used to transition patients from fully assisted critical care mechanical ventilation to normal respiration of room air. These systems may fall under the general heading of intermittent positive pressure breathing (IPPB) treatment. Code E0450 reports a volume control ventilator that interfaces with an invasive airway management device, such as a tracheostomy tube or other internal intubation. Code E0461 reports one that interfaces with a noninvasive device, such as a mask. Typically, the patient initiates spontaneous breathing activity that is machine assisted by volume and pressure control. Airflow may be terminated when the airway pressure rises a certain amount above the set pressure criteria. The tidal volume may be controlled by determining the length of inspired breaths. A backup rate feature sounds an alarm should the patient become unable to initiate breathing activity. The machine then automatically takes over breathing functions until the patient once again initiates spontaneous respiratory activity. Numerous settings and alarms are typically featured to monitor respiratory activity and effectiveness.

E0455

E0455   Oxygen tent, excluding croup or pediatric tents

Lay Description

An oxygen tent is a canopy placed over the head and shoulders or over the entire body of a patient to provide oxygen at a higher level than normal. They are made of plastic or other material through which oxygen cannot pass. Oxygen enters the tent through a hose. Physicians seldom use oxygen tents today as newer methods of oxygen delivery provide a better environment and easier patient access. Code E0455 represents oxygen tents that are not pediatric or used to treat croup.

Medicare Information

See chapter titled "Medicare Guidelines," under "Oxygen and Oxygen Equipment," for Medicare billing and documentation information.

E0457-E0459

E0457   Chest shell (cuirass)
E0459   Chest wrap

Lay Description

A chest shell or cuirass is a rigid plastic or metal dome, similar to a tortoise shell, that surrounds the chest and abdomen. The shell has a rubber or foam seal that is attached to the edges of the shell to create a tight seal. A chest wrap is an impermeable nylon jacket suspended by a rigid chest piece that fits over the chest and abdomen. A hose is attached to the center or side of the shell or wrap. The other end of the hose is attached to the ventilator. The ventilator cycles air in and out, creating a vacuum. This causes the chest to raise and air to enter the nose and mouth. A cuirass and a chest wrap are non-invasive methods of negative pressure mechanical ventilation that assist people with paralyzed or weakened diaphragm or intercostal muscles. People with stable or slowly progressing neuromuscular diseases (such as polio or multiple sclerosis), central hypoventilation (e.g., apnea not due to airway obstruction), or chest wall deformities are candidates for the use of negative pressure ventilation.

Medicare Information

This item must be supplied by an enrolled DME supplier. The devices will be covered when medically necessary to treat the patient's medical condition.

E0460

E0460   Negative pressure ventilator; portable or stationary

Lay Description

The "iron lung" was the prototypical negative pressure ventilator device. Fully natural respiration is largely a function of the broad diaphragm muscle that separates the thoracic and abdominal cavities working with intercostals (rib) muscles. Mechanical ventilation may be required when these muscles are paralyzed or otherwise underperforming, as occurs in polio. A patient's thorax is placed in a closed container that can be negatively pressurized and released. As the air pressure surrounding the chest becomes less than atmospheric, the chest expands and the lungs inflate. When the pressure surrounding the chest returns to atmospheric pressure, exhalation occurs as it would naturally. This push-pull action of a negative pressure ventilator can mechanically breathe for the patient. The large stationary iron lung systems are rarely used today. More portable models are still used, however, and E0460 reports the supply of this type of negative pressure ventilator.

E0461

E0461   Volume control ventilator, without pressure support mode, may include pressure control mode, used with noninvasive interface (e.g., mask)

Lay Description

Please refer to code E0450 for the description, coding, and billing information.

E0462

E0462   Rocking bed, with or without side rails

Lay Description

A rocking bed is a bed mounted on a mechanized platform that moves the patient's upper body up and down. This change of positions promotes movement of the diaphragm and thus breathing, particularly for patients who are quadriplegic or have paralysis of the diaphragm. A rocking bed may also be used to improve blood circulation in the treatment of chronic occlusive arterial disease.

Medicare Information

This item must be supplied by an enrolled DME supplier. The devices will be covered when medically necessary to treat the patient's medical condition.

E0463-E0464

E0463 Pressure support ventilator with volume control mode, may include pressure control mode, used with invasive interface (e.g., tracheostomy tube)

E0464 Pressure support ventilator with volume control mode, may include pressure control mode, used with noninvasive interface (e.g., mask)

Lay Description

These codes report a pressure support ventilator used to provide breathing assistance and help maintain open airways. This type of ventilator monitors the patient's breathing efforts and provides the required inspiratory or expiratory airway pressure set by the physician or therapist when the patient's own breathing efforts fall short of the prescribed levels. Airflow may also be terminated when the airway pressure rises a certain amount above the set pressure support level (pressure criteria). The tidal volume may be controlled by the patient when the machine is set in a certain mode by allowing the user to determine the length of inspired breaths. Code E0463 reports a pressure support ventilator for use with an invasive breathing interface, such as a tracheostomy tube, and E0464 reports one used with a noninvasive breathing interface, such as an oxygen mask.

E0470-E0472

E0470 Respiratory assist device, bi-level pressure capability, without backup rate feature, used with noninvasive interface, e.g., nasal or facial mask (intermittent assist device with continuous positive airway pressure device)

E0471 Respiratory assist device, bi-level pressure capability, with back-up rate feature, used with noninvasive interface, e.g., nasal or facial mask (intermittent assist device with continuous positive airway pressure device)

E0472 Respiratory assist device, bi-level pressure capability, with backup rate feature, used with invasive interface, e.g., tracheostomy tube (intermittent assist device with continuous positive airway pressure device)

Lay Description

RADs are noninvasive, spontaneous respiratory assistance devices with positive pressure that use a nasal or facial mask interface, creating a seal. Some of these devices enable the treating physician to avoid the use of more invasive airway access, such as a tracheostomy, and some of these devices are used in conjunction with invasive therapies. A RAD without backup rate (E0470) delivers adjustable, variable levels (within a single respiratory cycle) of positive air pressure by way of tubing and a nasal or oral facial mask to assist in the spontaneous respiratory efforts of the patient, and to supplement the volume of inspired air into the lungs. This is also called noninvasive positive pressure respiratory assistance or NPPRA. A RAD with backup rate (E0471) has, in addition, a timed backup feature to deliver the air pressure whenever sufficient spontaneous patient respiratory efforts fail to occur (i.e., it has a trigger device to deliver a quantity of air into the patient's lungs whenever the patient's spontaneous respiration is insufficient). A RAD with backup rate used in conjunction with invasive therapy (E0472), vs. a noninvasive regimen, delivers adjustable, variable levels (within a single respiratory cycle) of positive air pressure to assist in the spontaneous respiratory efforts of the patient following invasive therapy or surgery, and to supplement the volume of inspired air into the lungs. This RAD also has a timed backup feature to deliver the air pressure whenever sufficient spontaneous patient respiratory efforts fail to occur, i.e., it has a trigger device to deliver a quantity of air into the patient's lungs whenever the patient's spontaneous respiration is insufficient. Noninvasive RADs are different from invasive ventilation, which is administered through a securely intubated airway, generally in patients for whom interruption or failure of the ventilation support would lead to their imminent demise. These devices are not the same as the continuous positive airway pressure (CPAP) devices that are used primarily in the conservative therapy approach (vs. surgery) for patients with documented sleep apnea. CPAP devices provide for continuous amounts of air pressure throughout the oropharynx to prevent the collapse of the oropharyngeal tissues during sleep.

Documentation Standards

The blood gas study results, as well as sleep study results, must be kept on file in the patient's chart.

Polysomnography, as recognized by the Medicare program, is the continuous and simultaneous monitoring and recording of various physiological and pathophysiological parameters of sleep for six or more hours with provider review, interpretation, and report. The study must include sleep staging, defined as a one-to-four lead electroencephalogram (EEG), electro-oculogram (EOG), and submental electromyogram (EMG). The study must also include at least these characteristics of sleep: airflow, respiratory effort, and O2 saturation by oximetry.

Documentation in the patient's chart must be relevant to the patient's clinical progress while engaged in therapy using the RAD device (i.e., improvements, stabilization, or decompensation).

The supplier—not the provider—must obtain the following documentation and retain it on file for RAD use beyond the initial three month period:

- A signed/dated physician statement completed by the physician no sooner than 61 days following initiation of the RAD, declaring the patient is using the device at least four hours per 24-hour period, and that the patient is benefiting from the RAD use
- A signed attestation from the patient (or legal representative).

The patient's attestation must specify that he/she is currently using the device for four or more hours per day (24-hour period), that the device has been in use for at least two months in such fashion, that he/she has seen the treating provider within the month the attestation has been completed and at least within 61 days of initiation of the RAD therapy, and that he/she plans to continue to use the RAD. The attestation must also state that the person who completed the statement was not the supplier of the device.

All of the required documentation specified in this RAD section must be kept on file by the supplier and/or treating physician, but should not be submitted with the claims for the RADs. The DME MAC entity will request copies of the documentation at its discretion.

Medicare Information

Respiratory assist devises (RADs) are eligible for Medicare coverage when the patient's clinical disorder is characterized as and meets the criteria for one of the following clinical conditions:

- Restrictive thoracic disorders (i.e., progressive neuromuscular diseases such as amyotrophic lateral sclerosis or severe thoracic cage abnormalities such as post-thoracoplasty for tuberculosis)
- Severe chronic obstructive pulmonary disease (COPD)
- Central sleep apnea (CSA)
- Obstructive sleep apnea (OSA) (for E0470 only)

These clinical conditions must meet the following criteria:

- Restrictive thoracic disorders:
  - documentation must exist in the medical record that details the progressive neuromuscular disorder or severe thoracic cage abnormality
  - the patient's arterial blood gas reading ($PaCO_2$) must be at least greater than or equal to 45 mmHg. The $PaCO_2$ is obtained while the patient is awake and breathing the usual "FIO_2" (oxygen concentration the patient normally intakes when not undergoing testing; if the patient does not normally use supplemental O_2, his/her FIO_2 is found by breathing room air)
  - sleep oximetry testing demonstrates O_2 saturation less than 88 percent for at least five continuous minutes, obtained while the patient is breathing the usual FIO_2
  - for progressive neuromuscular disease only, the maximum inspiratory pressure is less than 60 cm H_2O or a forced vital capacity of less than 50 percent must be predicted
  - COPD does not contribute to the patient's current pulmonary limitations in a significant manner
- Severe COPD:
  - the $PaCO_2$ is greater than or equal to 52 mmHg
  - sleep oximetry testing indicates that the patient's O_2 saturation is less than 88 percent for at least five continuous minutes, and is performed while the patient is breathing O_2 at 2 liters per minute (LPM) or the patient's usual FIO_2 (whichever is greater)
  - before initiating therapy, the OSA (and treatment with a CPAP apparatus) has been considered and subsequently ruled out as being potentially effective.
- Central Sleep Apnea (CSA) (apnea not due to airway obstruction):
  - A facility-based, attended, polysomnogram study (i.e., a sleep study) must be obtained and documented in the patient's medical record before initiating CSA therapy
  - a formal diagnosis of CSA must be obtained from the sleep study and assigned
  - OSA must be ruled out as the primary cause of the sleep-associated hypoventilation
  - treatment with a CPAP apparatus has been excluded as effective therapy in association with the OSA
  - an O_2 saturation level of less than 88 percent for at least five continuous minutes is documented (obtained while the patient is breathing O_2 at 2 LPM or the usual FIO_2, whichever is higher)
  - significant improvement of the sleep-associated hypoventilation is documented while the patient is using the devices under E0470 or E0471, on settings typically prescribed for home use, while the patient is breathing at the usual FIO_2.
- Obstructive Sleep Apnea (OSA):
  - a facility-based, attended, polysomnogram study (i.e., a sleep study) must be obtained

and documented in the patient's medical record before initiating OSA therapy
- a formal diagnosis of OSA must be obtained from the sleep study and assigned.
- a single level CPAP device (E0601) has been tried and has proven to be clinically ineffective.

A device under E0471 is not medically indicated—under Medicare guidelines—for the primary diagnosis of OSA. If E0471 is billed, but OSA is the primary diagnosis, payment may be made based on the allowance for E0470.

If E0470 is billed, but the criteria for OSA are not met, payment may be based on the allowance for the least costly, but medically appropriate treatment alternative, represented by E0601.

All of the required documentation, in part discussed later in this section, must be kept on file by the supplier and/or treating provider

Medicare modifiers

Do not append modifier KX to the related RAD accessory or supply codes. Suppliers are cautioned not to report this modifier until the necessary documentation has actually been obtained from the physician and/or patient and entered in the supplier's files. Claims with missing or invalid modifiers will be denied as unprocessable when modifiers are required.

Claims for RADs and RAD accessories and supplies are subject to the Medicare DMEPOS fee schedule.

Payment is made if all of the requirements for Medicare reimbursement are met and the applicable DME MAC's medical necessity policies for the RAD are followed. However, when devices are billed without qualifying criteria for E0471, but there are qualifying criteria for E0470, generally payment will be based on the allowance for the least costly, but medically appropriate alternative, in this case, E0470.

At the present time, payment for RADs with bilevel pressure capability and with the backup rate feature (E0471 and E0472) are included in the DME MAC category of DMEPOS items for items requiring frequent and substantial servicing.

Intrapulmonary Percussive Ventilators (IPVs) are devices that provide a mechanized form of chest physical therapy. Instead of a pulmonary therapist cupping the patient's chest wall, the IPV delivers minibursts of respiratory gasses to the lungs, 200 per minute, through a mouthpiece. The IPV's primary function is to mobilize lung and bronchial secretions. Because CMS's clinical information does not support the effectiveness of the IPVs, the devices are not covered in the home setting.

The Medicare program assumes any delivery charges for home RAD equipment is included in the price charged for the equipment. Separate reimbursement for delivery is therefore not typically paid, and, in fact, separate charges are prohibited from being charged. The exception is for rare circumstances in which the Medicare program will allow reimbursement eligibility for separate delivery charges. These cases might entail, for instance, a supplier who must deliver an item of DMEPOS (such as RAD equipment) outside the supplier's normal radius of operation, especially in instances when there are no other suppliers in closer proximity to the patient in need of the RAD equipment. For reimbursement consideration of the delivery charges, the supplier should fully document the information about the case and submit this documentation with the claim.

E0480

E0480 Percussor, electric or pneumatic, home model

Lay Description

A pneumatic or electric percussor is typically a hand-held unit that mimics the hand percussion of the chest traditionally exercised by respiratory therapists to loosen and clear a patient's lungs of mucous and phlegm. Pneumatic models employ a gas driven cylinder to create pulses that reverberate into lung tissues. Electric models create a similar effect through vibration. Either variety will feature adjustments for pulse speed and intensity. Report E0480 for models designed for home use.

E0481

E0481 Intrapulmonary percussive ventilation system and related accessories

Lay Description

An intrapulmonary percussive ventilation system (IPV) is a device that delivers a series of very small bursts of pressurized gas at rates greater than 100 cycles per minute to the respiratory tract. IPV is a mechanized form of chest physical therapy. Instead of a therapist clapping or slapping the patient's chest wall, the IPV delivers small bursts of respiratory gases to the lungs via a mouthpiece. It is intended to mobilize endobronchial secretions and diffuse patchy atelectasis. The patient controls variables such as inspiratory time, peak pressure, and delivery rates. Code E0481 includes the compressor, hand held units, tubing, and all related accessories. This includes both systems in which the very small bursts of air are generated by the compressor and systems in which the very small bursts of air are generated by a hand-held percussive nebulizer used with a standard high-pressure compressor.

E0482

E0482 Cough stimulating device, alternating positive and negative airway pressure

Lay Description

This code reports supply of a specific variety of cough stimulating device. This type of device stimulates the cough reflex by providing alternating positive and negative airway pressure to loosen and clear a patient's lungs of mucous and phlegm. Peak cough ability is important to maintain in patients with diminished pulmonary function. These types of devices are designed to stimulate natural inspiratory and expiratory lung-clearing action. The units are non-invasive, using either a mouthpiece or facemask. Report E0482 for supply of a cough-stimulating device that functions by alternating positive and negative airway pressure.

Documentation Standards

An order for each item billed must be signed and dated by the treating physician, kept on file by the supplier, and made available to the DME MAC upon request. Items billed to the DME MAC before a signed and dated order has been received by the supplier must be submitted with modifier EY added to each affected HCPCS code.

The ICD-9-CM diagnosis code that justifies the need for these items must be included on the claim.

Medicare Information

Mechanical in-exsufflation devices (E0482) are covered for patients who meet all of the following criteria:

- The patient has a neuromuscular disease
- This condition is causing a significant impairment of chest wall and/or diaphragmatic movement, such that it results in an inability to clear retained secretions.

E0483

E0483 High frequency chest wall oscillation air-pulse generator system, (includes hoses and vest), each

Lay Description

High frequency chest wall oscillation (HFCWO) is a therapy strategy to treat patients who suffer from excessive bronchial secretions. It may be used to treat patients with cystic fibrosis and other lung diseases where bronchial secretions can obstruct the airways. Treatments typically involve use of a vest, which is worn while the patient is in an upright position. Tubes connecting the vest to an air-pulse generator provide oscillations, which may be adjustable for intensity and duration. A patient can operate the equipment by use of hand or sometimes foot controls. Treatment intervals last about 10 minutes and may be repeated. The patient clears mobilized bronchial secretions by coughing. Report E0483 for supply of each high frequency chest wall oscillation air-pulse generator system, including hoses and vest.

E0484

E0484 Oscillatory positive expiratory pressure device, nonelectric, any type, each

Lay Description

Oscillatory positive expiratory pressure devices create air vibrations to assist the patient in clearing the airway of mucous and secretions. Non-electric devices are typically hand held units. They manipulate expired air by passing it through or over a vibration-creating apparatus. A vibrating metal ball within a cone is one method. Another involves use of a magnet and counterweight. The oscillation, or flutter, occurs as backpressure is created in the bronchial tract. The natural movement of secretions from the lungs and bronchial tract is assisted, similar to many tiny coughs. Report E0484 for the supply of each oscillatory positive expiratory pressure device of any type.

E0485-E0486

E0485 Oral device/appliance used to reduce upper airway collapsibility, adjustable or nonadjustable, prefabricated, includes fitting and adjustment

E0486 Oral device/appliance used to reduce upper airway collapsibility, adjustable or nonadjustable, custom fabricated, includes fitting and adjustment

Lay Description

An oral device or appliance designed to reduce upper airway soft tissue collapse may be used to treat snoring and/or apnea during sleep. These devices increase the cross-sectional area of the upper airways by moving the mandible and/or the tongue forward. This helps to stabilize the upper airway in patients with obstructive sleep apnea syndrome (OSAS). Report E0485 for an adjustable or nonadjustable, prefabricated oral device and E0486 for a custom fabricated oral device. Fitting and adjustment of the device is included in the payment.

Medicare Information

Coverage and payment is at the contractor's discretion.

E0487

E0487 Spirometer, electronic, includes all accessories

Lay Description

A spirometer is a device used to measure pulmonary function. It measures the lung output on both inspiration and expiration. This is used to track and diagnose a number of respiratory and cardiac conditions. It may also be used to keep the lungs clear and functioning. HCPCS Level II code E0487 is used to report an electronic spirometer and includes all of the accessories.

E0500

E0500 IPPB machine, all types, with built-in nebulization; manual or automatic valves; internal or external power source

Lay Description

This code reports the supply of any type of intermittent positive pressure breathing (IPPB) machine. These units will have a built-in reservoir for medications and neutral liquids. A nebulizer feature atomizes liquid to aerosol spray, which is inhaled by the patient. Control valves may be manual or automatic. Many units have a port to attach an oxygen supply to the mix. These units may be hand-held with a mouthpiece and are used with the nose occluded by a clip. Batteries, an external AC source, or both may power the unit. Although volume ventilators may deliver intermittent positive pressure treatments, these IPPB units are generally classified for use among patients with spontaneous breathing capabilities. The main use of an IPPB machine is for patients with atelectasis (inability to fully expand the lung) or for the delivery of aerosol medication, usually bronchodilators. Report E0500 for supply of any type of IPPB machine, with built-in nebulization, manual or automatic valves, with internal or external power source.

E0550-E0560

E0550 Humidifier, durable for extensive supplemental humidification during IPPB treatments or oxygen delivery
E0555 Humidifier, durable, glass or autoclavable plastic bottle type, for use with regulator or flowmeter
E0560 Humidifier, durable for supplemental humidification during IPPB treatment or oxygen delivery

Lay Description

Intermittent positive pressure breathing (IPPB) treatments may be used for a variety of respiratory conditions. During treatment, machine assisted pressure is delivered upon inspiration to help the patient take large, deep breaths. The IPPB unit features either pressurized gas in tanks or an electric air compressor. Respiratory therapists usually provide treatments. The treatment may be used to deliver medication, to open air passages and loosen mucous, or to increase lung capacity. Humidification is often required for IPPB treatments, particularly when oxygen delivery is involved. Humidifiers reported by this range are durable, reusable containers and the connection devices for a IPPB treatment unit or oxygen system. The containers can be cleaned or autoclaved before refilling with distilled water. Report E0550 for humidifiers used for extensive supplemental humidification and E0560 for supplemental humidification. Report E0555 for glass or autoclavable plastic bottle types of humidifiers.

E0561-E0562

E0561 Humidifier, nonheated, used with positive airway pressure device
E0562 Humidifier, heated, used with positive airway pressure device

Lay Description

A humidifier is a device that increases the amount of moisture in indoor air or in a stream of air. It operates by circulating air over a water-filled pan or wet surface. The water then evaporates and is incorporated into the air stream. Heated humidifiers gently heat the water and the air stream as it comes in contact with the device. This device is used in connection with a continuous positive airway pressure (CPAP) system. Report E0561 for a non-heated humidifier used in connection with a CPAP system. Report E0562 for a heated humidifier used in connection with a CPAP system.

Medicare Information

These items must be supplied by an enrolled DME supplier. A non-heated (E0561) or heated (E0562) humidifier is covered when ordered by the treating physician for use with a covered CAP device (E0601). See E0601 for coverage criteria of CAP devices.

E0565-E0585

E0565	Compressor, air power source for equipment which is not self-contained or cylinder driven
E0570	Nebulizer, with compressor
E0571	Aerosol compressor, battery powered, for use with small volume nebulizer
E0572	Aerosol compressor, adjustable pressure, light duty for intermittent use
E0574	Ultrasonic/electronic aerosol generator with small volume nebulizer
E0575	Nebulizer, ultrasonic, large volume
E0580	Nebulizer, durable, glass or autoclavable plastic, bottle type, for use with regulator or flowmeter
E0585	Nebulizer, with compressor and heater

Lay Description

Nebulizer base equipment is comprised of an air compressor for airflow nebulization or a generator for nebulization of liquid by means of ultrasonic vibrations. The actual nebulizer is the chamber in which the nebulization of the liquid (usually medication) occurs and is considered an accessory to the base equipment. The nebulizing chamber is attached to the aerosol compressor or an ultrasonic generator. Specific accessories, supplies, and medications are used with this equipment. Nebulization therapy is considered beneficial to patients with a variety of respiratory and/or pulmonary conditions and diseases, including cystic fibrosis, bronchiectasis, chronic obstructive pulmonary disease, emphysema, severe asthma (when metered dose inhalers are ineffective), as well as other conditions such as AIDS, which requires the administration of medications like pentamidine. Nebulization occurs when the medication and/or solution to be administered is vaporized and subsequently inspired by the patient via the lungs, through which the medication enters the patient's system, or the medication has a direct effect on mucus retained by the lungs and bronchi (known as mucolytic action). Code E0565 describes an aerosol compressor, which can be set for pressures above 30 pounds per sq inch (psi) at a flow of 6-8 L/m and is capable of continuous operation. A nebulizer with compressor (E0570) is an aerosol compressor delivering a fixed, low pressure, typically used with a small volume nebulizer. A portable compressor (E0571) is an aerosol compressor that delivers a fixed, low pressure, used with a small volume nebulizer. It must have battery or DC power capability, but may have an AC power option. The light duty adjustable pressure compressor described by E0572 is a pneumatic aerosol compressor that can be set for pressures above 30 psi at a flow of 6-8 L/m, but is only capable of intermittent operation. Code E0574 describes an ultrasonic generator used with a small volume chamber for medication delivery, only capable of intermittent operation. It is only AC powered. Code E0575 describes a large volume ultrasonic nebulizer system used for medication and humidification delivery, and is capable of continuous operation. Report E0580 for a durable glass or autoclavable plastic, bottle type, which is used with a regulator or flowmeter. Code E0585 is a combination code describing the compressor, nebulizer component, and a heater.

Consolidated Billing

For patients in a nursing home: If the patient is receiving skilled nursing level care and is covered under Part A benefits, nebulizer equipment may not be billed separately by the SNF or by any other provider or supplier. This would be duplicate billing. The supplies are considered a part of the nursing home's PPS reimbursement. The supplier should bill the nursing home for these items and should probably have an agreement with the home for payment of these items.

If a patient in a nursing home is not receiving a skilled nursing level of care and is not being reimbursed under Part A, then the supplier must bill for nebulizer equipment.

For patients receiving home health services:
Nebulizer equipment is not subject to any HHA

Documentation Standards

For Medicare beneficiaries on inhalation therapy, a new order for the drug to be administered via the nebulizer is required at least every 12 months, even if there is no change in the treatment regimen.

Claims for E0571 must be accompanied by documentation that describes the need for a battery operated (portable) nebulizer.

Medicare Information

There are various coverage criteria for each of these individual nebulizers, usually correlated with the medications administered to the patient while using the equipment. The DME MAC coverage policy should be referenced to determine this region-specific information.

In general, a metered dose inhaler for administration of the medication to the patient must have been considered and ruled out as a feasible means of treatment before the prescription of a nebulizer for the administration of medication. This reasoning must be documented in the patient's medical chart.

A small volume nebulizer and related compressor (E0570 and E0571) are covered when one of the following criteria is met:

- It is medically necessary to administer beta-andrenergics, anticholinergics, corticosteroids, and cromolyn for the management of obstructive pulmonary disease

- It is medically necessary to administer gentamicin, tobramycin, amikacin, or dornase alfa to a patient with cystic fibrosis
- It is medically necessary to administer pentamidine to patients with HIV
- It is medically necessary to administer mucolytics (other than dornase alpha) for persistent thick or tenacious pulmonary secretions

Use of inhalation drugs, other than those listed above, will be denied as not medically necessary.

A large volume nebulizer (A7017), related compressor (E0565 or E0572), and supplies of saline (A7018) are covered when it is medically necessary to deliver humidity to a patient with thick, tenacious secretions, who has cystic fibrosis (ICD-9-CM diagnosis code 277.00), bronchiectasis (ICD-9-CM diagnosis code 494 or 748.61), or a tracheostomy (ICD-9-CM diagnosis code V44.0 or V55.0). Combination code E0585 N*ebulizer, with compressor and heater* will be covered for the same indications. Nebulizer compressors represented by E0565 or E0572 and filtered nebulizer (A7006) are also covered when it is medically necessary to administer pentamidine to patients with HIV.

There is no proven medical benefit to nebulizing particles to diameters smaller than that achievable with a pneumatic model; therefore, if a small volume ultrasonic nebulizer (E0574) is ordered, it will be reimbursed at the least costly alternative equal to that of a comparable pneumatic compressor (E0570). Similarly, a large volume ultrasonic nebulizer (E0575) offers no proven clinical advantage over a comparable pneumatic compressor. According to the Medicare program, a battery-powered compressor (E0571) is rarely medically necessary. If this compressor is provided without accompanying documentation that justifies its medical necessity, and the coverage criteria for code E0570 are met, Medicare payment will be based on the allowance for the least costly medically acceptable alternative of E0570. Disposable large volume nebulizers (A7007, A7008) are not covered; they are categorized as convenience items. A nondisposable unfilled nebulizer (A7017 or E0585) filled with distilled water (A7018 or A7020) is an acceptable alternative. Other uses of compressors/generators will be considered on a case-by-case basis to determine their medical necessity.

Medicare assumes any delivery charges for home nebulization equipment is included in the price charged for the equipment. Separate reimbursement for delivery is not usually paid and separate charges are prohibited from being charged. There may be exceptions to allow reimbursement for separate delivery charges, such as:

- A supplier who must deliver an item of DMEPOS outside the supplier's normal radius of operation, especially in instances when no other suppliers are in closer proximity to the patient in need of the prescribed equipment. For reimbursement consideration of the delivery charges, the supplier should fully document the information about the case and submit this documentation with the claim.

E0600, E2000

E0600   Respiratory suction pump, home model, portable or stationary, electric
E2000   Gastric suction pump, home model, portable or stationary, electric

Lay Description

A portable home model respiratory suction pump is a lightweight, compact, electric aspirator designed for upper respiratory oral pharyngeal and tracheal suction to be used in the home. Use of the device does not require technical or professional supervision. Units are equipped with vacuum regulators to allow variation of vacuum values, varying lamp flow, overflow safety devices, and battery or AC power. Report E0600 for a respiratory, oral pharyngeal, and tracheal suction pump, electric, home model, portable or stationary; E2000 for a gastric suction pump used with gastric tubing only, electric, home model, portable or stationary.

Documentation Standards

ICD-9-CM diagnosis code V44.0 should be entered on the claims form when billing.

Medicare Information

Use of a home model suction machine is covered for patients who have difficulty raising and clearing secretions secondary to:

- Cancer or surgery of the throat or mouth
- Dysfunction of the swallowing muscles
- Unconsciousness or obtunded state
- Tracheostomy

Code E0600 would not be used for a suction pump used in conjunction with a nasogastric tube; use E2000 instead.

E0601

E0601   Continuous airway pressure (CPAP) device

Lay Description

A continuous airway pressure (CPAP) device is a noninvasive method of providing air pressure through the patient's nostrils, usually through a nasal mask or flow generator system. A CPAP device delivers single pressure continuously and assists the patient in nocturnal respiration (breathing during sleep), particularly when the patient's oropharyngeal tissues relax, collapse, and/or otherwise obstruct the normal airflow, causing a variety of symptoms including hypersomnolence during the day, loss of concentration, headache, agitation, depression, fatigue, and many others. These devices are used primarily in conservative therapy (vs. surgery) for patients with documented sleep apnea.

E0602-E0604

E0602 Breast pump, manual, any type
E0603 Breast pump, electric (AC and/or DC), any type
E0604 Breast pump, hospital grade, electric (AC and/or DC), any type

Lay Description

Breast pumps are available in a variety of configurations, all of which are designed to pump human breast milk for short or long-term storage. Some models are simple cylinders that interface with a plastic cone that fits over the areola. A syringe-type piston can then be manually retracted by the user to create and release suction on the nipple. The pumped milk drains by gravity into an attached container. The milk can be decanted into plastic bags for refrigerated storage or freezing. Electric models work by creating pulsating suction, usually by pneumatic action against a diaphragm. Larger facilities may use hospital grade, piston operated electric pumps. With the exception of disposable plastic storage containers, components to all models are generally cleanable and reusable. Report E0602 for supply of any manually operated personal breast pump. Report E0603 for any electric model designed for personal use. Report E0604 for heavy duty, hospital grade models.

E0605

E0605 Vaporizer, room type

Lay Description

This code reports the supply of a room type vaporizer. Humidifiers and moisturizers typically work by absorbing cool water through a wick, which is exposed to a fan. Some models vibrate the cool water (ultrasonic). These devices can effectively raise humidity to larger rooms. Vaporizers heat water to create steam and are usually used for individual treatment of respiratory illness. Extracts can be added to the heated water or steam. Vaporizers are not usually effective to humidify large cubic footage, although room-size models are available and are reported by this code. Report E0605 for supply of a room type vaporizer.

E0606

E0606 Postural drainage board

Lay Description

Postural drainage uses the force of gravity to assist in effectively draining secretions from the lungs and into the central airway where they can be coughed up or suctioned out. The patient is placed in a head or chest down position and turned so that each lung segment can be drained. Percussion and vibration may be performed in conjunction with postural drainage. Postural drainage is used to assist patients with chronic pulmonary conditions or diseases that limit the ability to cough and eliminate secretions, such as cystic fibrosis. A postural drainage board is a smooth, flat, hard surface that supports the patient during postural drainage. Some boards may have foam or other padding that raises the patient's torso above the upper chest.

Medicare Information

This item must be supplied by an enrolled DME supplier. The devices will be covered when medically necessary to treat the patient's medical condition.

E0607, E2100-E2101

E0607 Home blood glucose monitor
E2100 Blood glucose monitor with integrated voice synthesizer
E2101 Blood glucose monitor with integrated lancing/blood sample

Lay Description

Glucometers are used for patients with all types of diabetes mellitus to monitor blood glucose and are available in a variety of models with various features, including digital read-out, memory, result print-out, easy specimen capture, and many others. Glucometers with special features, such as voice-activated or voice-synthesized capabilities, are needed for patients with other concurrent conditions, such as patients with impaired vision. Whether or not the patient is on insulin, many diabetics will require frequent, if not daily, blood glucose monitoring. For Type I diabetes mellitus patients who require insulin (the patient's body does not manufacture insulin and therefore it must come from an external source, such as injections), blood glucose monitoring is a life-sustaining requirement.

Documentation Standards

For Medicare beneficiaries, the order must clearly indicate the following:

- The frequency of testing ("as needed" is not acceptable)
- The patient has insulin-treated or non-insulin-treated diabetes
- Treating physician signature

- Physician's signature date

Suppliers must obtain a new written order from the provider every 12 months with the same information as the original, if no change in the patient's status has occurred in the interim.

Claims for glucometers with special features (E2100, E2101) prescribed for a patient with impaired visual acuity must be documented by a narrative statement from the physician that must include the patient's specific numerical visual acuity (e.g., 20/400) and that this result represents "best corrected" vision.

Similarly, claims for E2101 for patients with impaired manual dexterity must be documented by a narrative statement from the physician that includes an explanation of the patient's medical condition necessitating the monitor with special features. This information does not have to be routinely sent in with the claim, but must be available to the DME MAC on request.

Providers should have a national supplier identification number to allow for billing of the item to the DME MAC.

Medicare Information

Glucometers with special features require substantiation for the need of these specially equipped devices. To be eligible for Medicare benefits for this device, the following criteria must be met:

- The patient has been assigned ICD-9-CM diagnosis codes 250.00–250.93 and is under treatment by a physician
- The treating physician has ordered the glucometer and related accessories/supplies
- The patient (or the patient's caregiver) has successfully completed training or is scheduled to begin training in the use of the device and related accessories and supplies
- The patient (or caregiver) is capable of assessing the test results in order to sustain the patient's glycemic control
- The device is designed for home use

Glucometers with special features, such as voice synthesizers (E2100, E2101), are covered when the basic coverage criteria are met and the treating physician certifies that the patient has a severe visual impairment (i.e., best corrected visual acuity of 20/200 or worse) requiring use of this special monitoring system. Code E2101 is also covered for those with impairment of manual dexterity when the basic coverage criteria are met and the treating physician certifies that the patient has an impairment of manual dexterity severe enough to require the use of this special monitoring system. Coverage of E2101 for patients with manual dexterity impairments is not dependent upon a visual impairment. If all of the coverage criteria are met, but the additional criterion that substantiate the need for a glucometer with special features is not met, then Medicare payment will be based on the least costly, but medically appropriate alternative (E0607).

The medical necessity for a laser skin-piercing device (E0620) has not been established. If E0620 is ordered for use with a covered home blood glucose monitor, payment will be based on the allowance for the least costly medically appropriate alternative (A4258). In addition, since E0620 is not medically necessary, replacement lens shield cartridges (A4257) are also considered not medically necessary. If A4257 is ordered for use with E0620, payment will be based on the allowance for the least costly medically appropriate alternative (A4259).

Medicare modifiers

The following modifier must be reported for patients treated with insulin therapy:

KX   Specific requirements found in the documentation section of the medical policy have been met and evidence of this is available in the supplier's records

If the order indicates that the patient is being treated with insulin injections, modifier KX must be added to the code for the monitor and each related supply on every claim submitted. Modifier KX must not be used for a patient who is not treated with insulin injections.

The following modifier must be reported for patients not treated with insulin therapy, for both the monitor and supplies:

KS   Glucose monitor supply for diabetic patient not treated by insulin

This modifier is not reported on claims for patients treated with insulin. Modifier KS must be added to the code for the monitor and each related supply on every claim submitted. Claims with missing or invalid modifiers will be denied as unprocessable.

Claims for these items are usually subject to the Medicare DMEPOS fee schedule.

E0610-E0615

E0610 Pacemaker monitor, self-contained, (checks battery depletion, includes audible and visible check systems)

E0615 Pacemaker monitor, self-contained, checks battery depletion and other pacemaker components, includes digital/visible check systems

Lay Description

These codes report the supply of self-contained pacemaker monitors. A pacemaker is a device to control cardiac arrhythmias by programmed electrical stimulation of the heart. Pacemaker monitoring equipment detects impending battery failure and checks the overall performance of the pacemaker. Patients with pacemakers, whether permanent or temporary, require periodic examination of battery life and electrical functions. Self-contained units allow patients to perform the evaluation themselves. Some devices collect data that can be transmitted to a provider over a phone line. Battery life is a major factor in many pacemaker malfunctions and is monitored by these units. The conductivity of the pacemaker leads is another major consideration in monitoring. Report E0610 for supply of a self-contained monitor that checks battery depletion using audible and visible signals. Report E0615 for supply of a self-contained monitor that checks battery depletion and other pacemaker components using audible and visible signals.

Documentation Standards

Documentation of the medical necessity for the test must be retained by the ordering physician in the patient medical record. Documentation must state the signs, symptoms, or diagnosis that support the need of the test. Medical records must contain the test results.

Documentation must be made available to Medicare upon request. Failure to do so will result in denial of services.

Medicare Information

The following information must be available for, but need not accompany any claim submitted for, pacemaker monitoring:

- Date of pacemaker implant
- Type of pacer (single or dual chamber)
- Reason for any extenuating circumstances which requires check in excess of parameters. This would include additional diagnosis or symptoms such as but not limited to:
  - hypertrophic obstructive cardiomyopathy that fails medical therapy
  - any rhythm disturbances other than those for which the pacemaker was inserted
  - any signs/symptoms of failure of synchronization of atrial and ventricles, as in cases of dual chamber pacers
  - any noted change in the patient's overall condition

Claims must be submitted with an ICD-9-CM diagnosis code that represents the reason the test was performed.

E0616

E0616 Implantable cardiac event recorder with memory, activator, and programmer

Lay Description

Implantable event recorders are implanted in the left front of the chest in a pocket created in the skin. Once implanted, the patient's cardiac events are recorded. Implantable cardiac event monitors are used for long periods of time, which enables the recorder to capture more infrequent heart rhythms. The device can have autoactivation or manual activation depending upon the needs of the patient. If the patient experiences syncopal episodes, the manual activation button can be pressed after the patient is conscious again. If the device has an autoactivation, the device records rhythms automatically when the heart rate is in excess or under a preset limit.

Documentation Standards

Medical record documentation (e.g., office/progress notes) must be maintained by the ordering/referring physician and must support that all of the conditions for ILR coverage (e.g., the prior testing performed and the results, the patient history of the syncopal or presyncopal incident, and symptomatology) have been met. Additionally, documentation must also support that the service billed was actually performed (e.g., an operative note/report).

Medicare Information

Electrocardiographic (EKG) services are covered under Medicare Part B when provided by a physician (either directly or incident to his/her services), by an approved laboratory, or by an approved supplier of portable EKG services. Since screening services and routine examinations of any type, including EKG services, are not covered under Medicare, the claim must indicate the diagnosis or symptoms for which the service was medically necessary. Coverage Criteria[SUBHEAD LEVEL 1]When medical necessity requirements have been met, a separate charge by an attending or consulting physician for an EKG interpretation is allowed when it is the normal practice to charge for the service in addition to the regular office visit. Payment will not be made for EKG interpretations by any individual other than a physician.

The insertable loop recorder (ILR) itself should be coded as E0616. Code E0616 should be billed to the carrier on a CMS-1500 form if the ILR insertion is performed in a physician's office. Otherwise, claims for E0616 performed in a hospital setting should be submitted to the fiscal intermediary on a UB-92 form.

The ILR device insertion procedure is considered to be a physician service. This major global surgery has a postoperative period of 90 days. The procedure does not require an assistant surgeon.

Electrocardiogram analyses obtained during device insertion for signal quality and amplification purposes are considered part of the implant procedure and should not be reported separately.

Removal of an ILR device on the same day as the insertion of a cardiac pacemaker in any given patient is considered to be part of the pacemaker insertion procedure and will not be reimbursed separately. This limitation applies whether or not the ILR implantation site is used for the pacemaker pocket.

E0617

E0617   External defibrillator with integrated electrocardiogram analysis

Lay Description

Automatic external defibrillators are compact and portable devices that deliver electrical shock to a person who has a sudden cardiac arrest. Automatic external defibrillator units use a microprocessor inside of a portable defibrillator to interpret a person's heart rhythm through electrodes. The computer recognizes ventricular fibrillation or ventricular tachycardia. Once recognized, the computer advises the operator/user that electrical defibrillation is needed or it will automatically deliver a countershock.

E0618-E0619

E0618   Apnea monitor, without recording feature
E0619   Apnea monitor, with recording feature

Lay Description

An apnea monitor is a device designed to detect cessation of breathing, either directly through measurement of respiration and/or indirectly through monitoring of physiological signs such as heart rate, pulse, or blood oxygen concentration. Devices typically feature both visual and audio alarm systems. Some models may differentiate between detection of obstructive apnea (such as is caused by mucous or oropharyngeal membrane) and central apnea (as may be caused by organ system failure). Models are typically connected to AC circuitry with battery power backup. Some may feature remote alarm systems, programmed software, and a monitor. An internal and/or hard copy recording system may also be featured. Report E0618 for provision of an apnea monitor without a recording feature and E0619 for provision of an apnea monitor with a recording feature.

E0620

E0620   Skin piercing device for collection of capillary blood, laser, each

Lay Description

A laser skin-piercing device is a low strength laser that is directed to one area, usually on a finger, and pierces the skin and subcutaneous tissue, allowing blood to be drawn from a capillary or surface blood vessel. This device is used in place of a lancet to draw blood for blood glucose monitoring or similar home blood testing.

Medicare Information

This item must be supplied by an enrolled DME supplier. DME MAC local coverage determinations state that the medical necessity for a laser skin-piercing device has not been established. If a laser skin-piercing device is ordered and purchased for use with a covered home monitor, payment will be based on the allowance for the least costly medically appropriate alternative (A4258). Since the laser skin-piercing device is not medically necessary, replacement lens shield cartridges (A4257) are also considered not medically necessary. If replacement lens shield cartridges are ordered for use with a laser skin-piercing device, payment will be based on the allowance for the least costly medically appropriate alternative (A4259).

If a laser skin-piercing device is ordered and rented for use with a covered home monitor, it will be denied as not medically necessary. Since the laser skin-piercing device is not medically necessary, replacement lens shield cartridges (A4257) are also considered not medically necessary.

E0621-E0625, E0630-E0636

E0621   Sling or seat, patient lift, canvas or nylon
E0625   Patient lift, bathroom or toilet, not otherwise classified
E0630   Patient lift, hydraulic or mechanical, includes any seat, sling, strap(s), or pad(s)
E0635   Patient lift, electric, with seat or sling
E0636   Multipositional patient support system, with integrated lift, patient accessible controls

Lay Description

Patient lift mechanisms are hydraulic or motorized (electric) lifts that enable the patient to transfer from the bed to a chair or other sitting device, or vice versa. The electric patient lifts can be either electric (AC) or battery powered (DC). These lift mechanisms assist patients with varying abnormalities that prevent them from being able to change, unassisted, from a lying down position (in a bed) to a seated position (in a chair, wheelchair, etc.), and vice versa. Trauma, stroke, and chronic diseases are the usual etiologies for the patient's inability to change in these positions. These devices can help during the convalescence period in posttraumatic or postoperative cases, and act as prevention against patient injury or reinjury. Code E0621 represents a seat or sling for a patient lift. It is a reinforced width of nylon or cloth that replaces a similar device used in a patient lift. A seat or sling is considered an accessory item. Code E0625 is a patient lift that is used only in the bathroom to transfer a patient to a toilet, bath, or shower. Code E0630 is a device that uses a manual pumping action to compress a cylinder filled with a fluid, usually oil. Since the oil is thick and molecule dense, it does not absorb the energy or force generated by the pumping action. Instead, the oil amplifies and transfers the energy to the lever used to raise the patient. The hydraulic action allows less energy to be used in the pumping action. Code E0635 is a device that uses electricity to run a motor that raises and moves the patient from one surface (e.g., a bed, chair, or toilet) to another surface. The patient is positioned in a seat or sling and the device performs the work. Electric lifts can be freestanding or ceiling and wall mounted. E0636 is a system that raises and moves the patient. It contains a hinged platform that can be manipulated into various positions. When laid flat and positioned close to the bed, the patient can roll or be lifted onto the platform. The platform can then be positioned so the patient is standing upright or in a seated position. The system can contain both hydraulic and electronic driven mechanisms. The system is padded or cushioned for patient comfort and may contain side rails or straps to securely hold the patient during transfer.

Documentation Standards

The supplier who performs the service should keep documentation of the preauthorization process on file.

Providers should have a national supplier identification number to allow for billing of the item to the DME MAC.

Medicare Information

A patient lift mechanism is covered if transfer of the patient between the bed and a chair, wheelchair, or commode requires the assistance of more than one person and, without the use of a lift, the patient would be bed-confined. This device is covered under the DME payment category.

Code E0621 is covered as an accessory when ordered as a replacement for the original equipment item. The usual payment rules for accessory items apply to this code.

The Column II code (E0621) is included in the allowance for the corresponding Column I code when provided at the same time.

Column I	Column II
E0625	E0621
E0630	E0621
E0635	E0621

E0627-E0629

E0627   Seat lift mechanism incorporated into a combination lift-chair mechanism
E0628   Separate seat lift mechanism for use with patient-owned furniture, electric
E0629   Separate seat lift mechanism for use with patient-owned furniture, nonelectric

Lay Description

Seat lift mechanisms are motorized seat lifts that enable the patient to change from a seated position to a standing position. The lifting mechanism is graded and not based on a catapult or other type of spring system. These mechanisms can be either electric or battery powered. Some mechanisms can be used with the patient's own furniture; others are already built into specially designed chairs, sometimes incorporating the seat lift action with a more total patient lift action, including elevating and pushing the back and arms. Seat lift mechanisms assist patients with varying abnormalities that prevent them from being able to change, unassisted, from a seated to a standing position. Trauma and chronic diseases are the usual etiologies for the patient's inability to change in these positions. These devices can help in posttraumatic or postoperative convalescence, act as adjunctive treatment for chronic diseases, and act as prevention against patient injury or reinjury.

Medicare Information

A seat lift mechanism is covered, when eligible, under the DME benefit if all of the following criteria are met:

- The patient must have severe arthritis of the hip or knee or have a severe neuromuscular disease
- The seat lift mechanism must be a part of the physician's course of treatment and be prescribed to effect improvement or arrest or retard deterioration in the patient's condition
- The patient must be completely incapable of standing up from a regular armchair or any chair in their home. (If a patient has difficulty or is even incapable of getting up from a chair,

particularly a low chair, that is not sufficient justification for a seat lift mechanism. Almost all patients who are capable of ambulating can get out of an ordinary chair if the seat height is appropriate and the chair has arms or other supporting/bracing features)

- Once standing, the patient must have the ability to ambulate

Coverage of seat lift mechanisms is limited to those types that operate smoothly, can be controlled by the patient, and effectively assist a patient in standing up and sitting down without other assistance. Excluded from coverage is the type of lift that operates by spring release mechanism with a sudden, catapult-like motion and jolts the patient from a seated to a standing position.

Medicare Information

A seat lift mechanism is covered, when eligible, under the DME benefit if all of the following criteria are met:

- The patient must have severe arthritis of the hip or knee or have a severe neuromuscular disease
- The seat lift mechanism must be a part of the physician's course of treatment and be prescribed to effect improvement or arrest or retard deterioration in the patient's condition
- The patient must be completely incapable of standing up from a regular armchair or any chair in their home. (If a patient has difficulty or is even incapable of getting up from a chair, particularly a low chair, that is not sufficient justification for a seat lift mechanism. Almost all patients who are capable of ambulating can get out of an ordinary chair if the seat height is appropriate and the chair has arms or other supporting/bracing features)
- Once standing, the patient must have the ability to ambulate

Coverage of seat lift mechanisms is limited to those types that operate smoothly, can be controlled by the patient, and effectively assist a patient in standing up and sitting down without other assistance. Excluded from coverage is the type of lift that operates by spring release mechanism with a sudden, catapult-like motion and jolts the patient from a seated to a standing position.

Coverage is limited to the seat lift mechanism, even if it is incorporated into a chair (E0627). Payment for a seat lift mechanism incorporated into a chair (E0627) is based on the allowance for the least costly, but medically appropriate alternative (E0628, E0629).

The physician ordering the seat lift mechanism must be the attending physician or a consulting physician for the disease or condition resulting in the need for a seat lift. The physician's record must document that all appropriate therapeutic modalities (e.g., medication, physical therapy) have been tried and failed to enable the patient to transfer from a chair to a standing position.

E0630-E0636

E0630   Patient lift, hydraulic or mechanical, includes any seat, sling, strap(s), or pad(s)
E0635   Patient lift, electric, with seat or sling
E0636   Multipositional patient support system, with integrated lift, patient accessible controls

Lay Description

Please refer to codes E0621-E0625 for the description, coding, and billing information.

E0641-E0642

E0641   Standing frame system, multi-position (e.g., 3-way stander), any size including pediatric, with or without wheels
E0642   Standing frame system, mobile (dynamic stander), any size including pediatric

Lay Description

A standing frame system is an assistive device that provides musculoskeletal support for disabled or injured individuals. This device allows an individual to move from a sitting to standing position and provides support when standing. Standing frame systems may include lift devices that assist the patient in moving from a sitting to standing position. Multi-position standing frames allow progressive levels of standing that gradually relieve contractures and spasticity. A standing frame system may be stationary or mobile. Report E0641 for a multiposition standing frame system (e.g., three-way stander) with or without wheels. Report E0642 for a mobile (dynamic) standing frame system. These codes are used to report any size stander including pediatric.

E0650-E0673

- **E0650** Pneumatic compressor, nonsegmental home model
- **E0651** Pneumatic compressor, segmental home model without calibrated gradient pressure
- **E0652** Pneumatic compressor, segmental home model with calibrated gradient pressure
- **E0655** Nonsegmental pneumatic appliance for use with pneumatic compressor, half arm
- **E0656** Segmental pneumatic appliance for use with pneumatic compressor, trunk
- **E0657** Segmental pneumatic appliance for use with pneumatic compressor, chest
- **E0660** Nonsegmental pneumatic appliance for use with pneumatic compressor, full leg
- **E0665** Nonsegmental pneumatic appliance for use with pneumatic compressor, full arm
- **E0666** Nonsegmental pneumatic appliance for use with pneumatic compressor, half leg
- **E0667** Segmental pneumatic appliance for use with pneumatic compressor, full leg
- **E0668** Segmental pneumatic appliance for use with pneumatic compressor, full arm
- **E0669** Segmental pneumatic appliance for use with pneumatic compressor, half leg
- **E0671** Segmental gradient pressure pneumatic appliance, full leg
- **E0672** Segmental gradient pressure pneumatic appliance, full arm
- **E0673** Segmental gradient pressure pneumatic appliance, half leg

Lay Description

Lymphedema is the swelling of subcutaneous tissue due to the accumulation of excessive lymph fluid from an impairment in the normal clearing function of the lymphatic system and/or from excessive lymph production. Lymphedema pumps are segmental or nonsegmental long arm or leg sleeves (similar to a blood pressure cuff) that are placed up around the area of swelling. The device is turned on and the sleeve is periodically inflated to compress the tissues (in segments or in total length), and then deflated. A tube from the compression device (pump) that is attached to the sleeve allows air to be pumped into the sleeve (compression) or air to be removed from the sleeve (decompression). Pneumatic pumps mechanically assist blood and lymph flow through the extremities. This assistance lessens the accumulation of fluids in the affected limb and reduces associated complications such as thrombosis or vessel damage. Codes E0650-E0652 are used for the pneumatic compressor home model. Report E0650 for nonsegmental, E0651 for segmental without calibrated pressure gradient, and E0652 for segmental with calibrated pressure gradient. Codes E0655-E0666 are used for nonsegmental pneumatic appliances for use with a compressor. Report E0655 for a half arm appliance, E0660 for a full leg, E0665 for a full arm, and E0666 for a half leg. Codes E0667-E0669 are used for segmental pneumatic appliances for use with a compressor. Report E0667 for a full leg, E0668 for a full arm, and E0669 for a half leg. Codes E0671-E0673 are used for a segmental gradient pressure pneumatic appliance. Report E0671 for a full leg appliance, E0672 for a full arm, and E0673 for a half leg.

Documentation Standards

The determination by the physician of the medical necessity of a pneumatic compression device must include the following:

- The patient's diagnosis and prognosis
- Symptoms and objective findings, including measurements that establish the severity of the condition
- The reason the device is required, including the treatments that have been tried and failed
- The clinical response to an initial treatment with the device
- Pre-treatment measurements
- Ability to tolerate the treatment session and parameters
- Ability of the patient (or caregiver) to apply the device for continued home use

An order for the compressor and the appliance must be signed and dated by the treating physician and must be kept on file by the supplier. The supplier must keep a CMN on file that has been filled out, signed, and dated by the treating physician. The CMN for pneumatic compression devices/lymphedema pumps is CMS Form 846. If question #3 on the CMN form ("Does the patient have chronic venous insufficiency with venous stasis ulcers?") is answered "Yes," documentation supporting the medical necessity for the device should include a signed and dated statement from the treating physician indicating:

- Location and size of the venous stasis ulcer
- How long each ulcer has been continuously present
- Whether the patient has been treated with a compression bandage system or compression garment, appropriate dressings for the ulcer, exercise, and limb elevation for the past six months
- Whether the patient has been seen regularly by a physician for treatment of venous stasis ulcers during the past six months

If E0652 is billed, additional documentation supporting the medical necessity for this device must include a signed and dated statement from the ordering physician indicating:

- The treatment plan including the pressure in each chamber and the frequency and duration of each treatment episode
- Whether a segmented compressor without calibrated gradient pressure (E0651) or a non-segmented compressor (E0650) with a segmented appliance (E0671–E0673) had been tried and the results
- Why the features of the system that was provided are needed for this patient
- The name, model number, and manufacturer of the device

The claim for a purchase or first month's rental must include a copy of the CMN if filed hard copy.

Medicare Information

Pneumatic compression devices are covered in the home setting for the treatment of lymphedema if the patient has undergone a four-week trial of conservative therapy and the treating physician determines that there has been no significant improvement or if significant symptoms remain after the trial. The trial of conservative therapy must include use of an appropriate compression bandage system or compression garment, exercise, and elevation of the limb. The garment may be prefabricated or custom-fabricated but must provide adequate graduated compression.

Pneumatic compression devices are covered in the home setting for the treatment of chronic venous insufficiency of the lower extremities only if the patient has one or more venous stasis ulcers that have failed to heal after a six-month trial of conservative therapy, directed by the treating physician. The trial of conservative therapy must include a compression bandage system or compression garment, appropriate dressings for the wound, exercise, and elevation of the limb.

A non-segmented device (E0650) or segmented device without manual control of the pressure in each chamber (E0651) is generally sufficient to meet the clinical needs of the patient. A non-segmented compressor (E0650) with a segmented appliance/sleeve (E0671–E0673) is considered functionally equivalent to an E0651 compressor with a segmented appliance/sleeve (E0667–E0669).

A segmented device with manual control of the pressure in each chamber (E0652) when ordered and provided, will be paid based on the allowance for the least costly medically appropriate alternative (E0651) unless there is clear documentation of medical necessity in the individual case. Full payment for E0652 will be made only when there is documentation that the individual has unique characteristics that prevent satisfactory pneumatic compression treatment using a non-segmented device (E0650) with a segmented appliance/sleeve (E0671–E0673) or a segmented device without manual control of the pressure in each chamber (E0651).

A non-segmented pneumatic compressor (E0650) is used with appliances/sleeves coded by E0655–E0666 or E0671–E0673. Segmented pneumatic compressors (E0651 or E0652) are used with appliances/sleeves coded by E0667–E0669.

When a foot or hand segment is used in conjunction with a leg or arm appliance respectively, there should be no separate bill for this segment. It is considered included in the code for the leg or arm appliance.

The devices are covered only when prescribed and managed by a physician under the following criteria:

- Physician evaluation of the patient's condition to determine medical necessity of the device
- Suitable instruction in the operation of the machine
- A treatment plan defining the pressure to be used and the frequency and duration of use
- Ongoing monitoring of use and response to treatment

The use of pneumatic compression devices may be medically appropriate only for patients with generalized, refractory edema from venous insufficiency with lymphatic obstruction, such as:

- Recurrent cellulitis with secondary scarring of the lymphatic system
- Significant ulceration of the lower extremity that has failed to heal after months of continuous treatment

E0675

E0675 Pneumatic compression device, high pressure, rapid inflation/deflation cycle, for arterial insufficiency (unilateral or bilateral system)

Lay Description

Pneumatic compression devices, along with an electrical pneumatic pump, are used to pump compressed air into a garment placed on upper or lower extremities (including feet). The garment is intermittently inflated and deflated with pressure and various time cycles. The use of the pneumatic compression device can greatly reduce the risk of deep venous thrombosis (DVT) and pulmonary embolism (PE) by limiting venous stasis and increasing fibrinolytic activity at both the local and systemic levels.

E0676

E0676   Intermittent limb compression device (includes all accessories), not otherwise specified

Lay Description

An intermittent limb compression device inflates and deflates a compression sleeve that has multiple compression chambers encircling the limb of the patient. The sleeve inflates to apply compressive pressure gradient against the limb of the patient, which decreases from the lower to the upper portion of the limb to enhance the acceleration of blood flow through the limb.

E0691-E0694

E0691   Ultraviolet light therapy system panel, includes bulbs/lamps, timer and eye protection, treatment area 2 sq ft or less
E0692   Ultraviolet light therapy system panel, includes bulbs/lamps, timer and eye protection, 4 ft panel
E0693   Ultraviolet light therapy system panel, includes bulbs/lamps, timer and eye protection, 6 ft panel
E0694   Ultraviolet multidirectional light therapy system in 6 ft cabinet, includes bulbs/lamps, timer, and eye protection

Lay Description

An ultraviolet light therapy system panel is considered durable medical equipment typically consisting of a system panel, ultraviolet bulbs/lamp that emit UVB rays, a timer, and eye protection. It is commonly used for the treatment of skin conditions including psoriasis, pruritic eruptions of HIV, and acne. The system described in E0691 is for treatment of an area 2.0 sq. feet or smaller. The system described in E0692 includes a four-foot panel and E0693 includes a six-foot panel. Use E0694 for a multidirectional light system within a six-foot cabinet that also includes bulbs/lamps, a timer, and eye protection.

E0700

E0700   Safety equipment, device or accessory, any type

Lay Description

Safety equipment such as a belts, harnesses, or vests are used to secure a patient's positioning when the patient is at risk for a fall that could lead to harm or injury. The equipment is comfortably secured around the patient and fastened to a bed or chair to prevent sliding or falling.

E0705

E0705   Transfer device, any type, each

Lay Description

A transfer board is used for ease of moving patients from one stable surface to another (i.e. bed to wheelchair, bed to portable toilet, wheelchair to toilet) and is primarily for seated type transports.

E0710

E0710   Restraints, any type (body, chest, wrist, or ankle)

Lay Description

Restraints are used to contain and control an individual who exhibits behavior that may be harmful to self or others, such as violent behavior or pulling at lifesaving treatments. This code includes body, chest, wrist, or ankle restraints. Each strap is designed with a cuff to be placed around the patient, and a strap that can be threaded through a U bar and secured. Report this code for any type of restraint.

E0720-E0730

E0720   Transcutaneous electrical nerve stimulation (TENS) device, 2 lead, localized stimulation
E0730   Transcutaneous electrical nerve stimulation (TENS) device, 4 or more leads, for multiple nerve stimulation

Lay Description

A transcutaneous electrical nerve stimulator (TENS) is a device that uses electrical current delivered through electrodes placed on the surface of the skin to decrease the patient's perception of pain, by inhibiting the transmission of afferent pain nerve impulses and/or by stimulating the release of endorphins. The TENS unit can be applied in a variety of settings (in the patient's home, a physician's office, or in an outpatient clinic). This device alleviates or palliates acute postoperative pain, as well as chronic or intractable pain, depending on the etiology of the patient's condition. TENS therapy is typically not used for patients with visceral pain or headache, female patients with pelvic pain, and other types of pain considered unresponsive to TENS therapy. Code E0720 describes a two-lead TENS for local stimulation in one generalized area; E0730 identifies a four or more lead TENS for multiple nerve stimulation.

Medicare Information

See the chapter titled "Medicare Guidelines," under "TENS," for Medicare information.

E0731

E0731 Form-fitting conductive garment for delivery of TENS or NMES (with conductive fibers separated from the patient's skin by layers of fabric)

Lay Description
A form-fitting conductive garment has tiny electro-conductive leads and electrodes woven into a stretch fabric. The system offers a great many of easily accessible and interchangeable electrode sites throughout the fabric area. A second layer of conventional fabric lines the garment against the skin. The garment may be worn on an extremity alone or on part or the entire torso. The garment is designed to interface with a transcutaneous electrical nerve stimulation (TENS) generator. The system may be used for patients with conditions that require a great many TENS electrodes for effective therapy and for those with sensitive skin. The system is also sometimes used underneath plaster casting where conventional TENS therapy cannot reach. Report E0731 for each conductive garment supplied.

Medicare Information
See the chapter titled "Medicare Guidelines," under "TENS," for Medicare information.

E0740

E0740 Incontinence treatment system, pelvic floor stimulator, monitor, sensor, and/or trainer

Lay Description
Pelvic floor stimulators are used for the treatment of urinary incontinence to strengthen and exercise the muscles of the pelvic floor. Electrical stimulations targeting the muscles involved are delivered via probes connected to an external pulse generator. The frequency and intensity of the electrical pulse varies based on the patient's needs. Report this code for a pelvic floor stimulator with a monitor, sensor, and/or trainer.

Medicare Information
Section 60–24 *Non-Implantable Pelvic Floor Electrical Stimulator* permits coverage for non-implantable pelvic floor electrical stimulators for the treatment of stress and/or urge urinary incontinence in cognitively intact patients who have failed a documented trial of pelvic muscle exercise (PME) training. A failed trial of PME training is defined as no clinically significant improvement in urinary continence after completing four weeks of an ordered plan of pelvic muscle exercises designed to increase periurethral muscle strength.

Suppliers submitting claims to the DME MAC for pelvic floor electrical stimulator (PFES) should use HCPCS code E0740. This HCPCS code is in the Inexpensive or Routinely Purchased (IRP) reimbursement category. There must be documentation in the patient's medical record that the coverage criteria outlined in the national policy have been met. This documentation does not have to be routinely sent with the claim but must be available to the DME MAC upon request.

E0744

E0744 Neuromuscular stimulator for scoliosis

Lay Description
Neuromuscular stimulators are used to stimulate muscles into activity through an electrical impulse. These devices consist of superficial or implantable electrodes, a modulating output and control circuit, a signal generator, and a battery power supply. Note that E0744 identifies a neuromuscular stimulator for scoliosis.

E0745

E0745 Neuromuscular stimulator, electronic shock unit

Lay Description
Neuromuscular stimulation artificially stimulates muscles that may have atrophied because of damaged nerve pathways, often due to injury, surgery, or infarction. Computer-controlled sequential electrical stimulation of muscles simulates actual use, even when actual muscle contraction is not attained, and may result in a level of muscle tone and strength. Report E0745 for the electronic shock unit itself.

Medicare Information
The Medicare national policy on neuromuscular electrical stimulation (NMES) is published in the *Medicare Coverage Issues Manual,* Section 35–77. This policy states that "coverage of NMES is limited to the treatment of disuse atrophy where nerve supply to the muscle is intact, including brain, spinal cord, and peripheral nerves, and other non-neurological reasons for disuse are causing atrophy." This means that NMES devices are not covered for the treatment of muscle weakness due to the following conditions (not all-inclusive): stroke; spinal cord injury; or peripheral nerve injury; other central nervous system, spinal, or peripheral nerve disease/condition affecting motor and/or sensory pathways to/from the muscles being stimulated.

The national policy gives a few examples of situations in which an NMES device (E0745) may be covered. If there was a situation in which a patient was discharged to the home following hip replacement surgery prior to initiation of gait training and there was documentation of a reasonable expectation that ambulation would eventually occur, then rental of an NMES device would be covered until gait training started (usually within one month). If a patient has disuse atrophy following casting or splinting of the leg after a major knee surgery or injury and the nerve supply is intact, then rental of an NMES device would be covered until the patient was able to begin active rehabilitation (usually within one month). If an NMES device is ordered to treat a contracture in a burn patient where there is reasonable expectation for improvement, rental of the device would be covered as long as significant improvement continued to occur with ongoing use. Coverage for other conditions (where the nerve supply is intact) could be considered on an individual basis if the claim clearly described the patient's condition, what (if any) other therapy had been tried and the results, and included copies of published studies in peer-reviewed journals that clearly document the effectiveness and necessity of NMES devices for these conditions or clear recommendations in major textbooks for use in these conditions.

E0746

E0746 Electromyography (EMG), biofeedback device

Lay Description

An electromyography (EMG) biofeedback device consists of electrodes that are placed over specific muscles, and a recording unit that stores and displays the information from the physiological responses being monitored. Muscle activity can be displayed in real-time or an average over a period of time.

Medicare Information

Biofeedback therapy is covered by Medicare only for re-education of specific muscles or for treatment of incapacitating muscle spasm or weakness.

E0747-E0749

E0747 Osteogenesis stimulator, electrical, noninvasive, other than spinal applications
E0748 Osteogenesis stimulator, electrical, noninvasive, spinal applications
E0749 Osteogenesis stimulator, electrical, surgically implanted

Lay Description

An electrical osteogenesis stimulator is a device that provides electrical stimulation to augment bone repair by stimulating the production of osteocytes (bone cells) and can be invasive or noninvasive. A noninvasive electrical stimulator is characterized by an external power source, which is attached to a coil or electrodes placed on the skin, or placed on a cast or brace over a fracture or surgical bone fusion site. Invasive devices provide electrical stimulation directly at the fracture site, through percutaneous placement of cathodes or by implantation of a coiled cathode wire into the fracture site. The power pack is implanted into soft tissue near the fracture site and subcutaneously connected to the cathode, creating a self-contained system with no external components. With the noninvasive device, opposing pads, wired to an external power supply, are placed over the cast. An electromagnetic field is created between the pads at the fracture site. An ultrasonic osteogenic stimulator emits low intensity, pulsed ultrasound (as opposed to electricity) to stimulate bone repair. The ultrasonic signal is applied to the skin surface at the fracture location via ultrasound conductive coupling gel to accelerate the healing time of the fracture. The device is intended for use with cast immobilization. Code E0747 describes a noninvasive, electrical osteogenesis stimulator that has other than spinal applications; E0748 is an electrical osteogenesis stimulator, noninvasive, with spinal applications; and E0749 represents a surgically implanted, invasive electrical osteogenesis stimulator.

Documentation Standards

The initial claim for an electrical osteogenesis stimulator must include a copy of the CMN if filed hard copy.

When a claim for a spinal electrical osteogenesis stimulator is submitted, some DME MAC entities require both the CMN and additional medical necessity documentation to be included with the claim, in the following situations:

- If it is ordered following a multilevel spinal fusion, the claim must include the date of the surgery and level of the fusion
- If it is ordered when there is a history of a previously failed spinal fusion, the claim must include the date and level of the previous fusion and the fact that the fusion failed

Medicare Information

Medicare covers invasive osteogenic stimulation for nonunion of long bone fractures or as an adjunct to spinal fusion surgery for patients at high risk of pseudoarthroses due to previously failed spinal fusion, or for those undergoing fusion of three or more vertebrae.

This device is billed to the DME MAC, not to the Medicare carrier. CMN form 04.03C (CMS form 847), "Osteogenesis Stimulator," is required to be certified and submitted by the supplier. Payment is made according to DME MAC discretion. Claims for these items are usually subject to the Medicare DMEPOS fee schedule and paid under the DME benefit.

Question #6a on the required CMN for osteogenesis stimulators more clearly defines fracture nonunion, and specifies that suppliers must attach a statement to the CMN, sent to the physician for certification prior to being submitted to the DME MAC, that states the following:

For purposes of answering question #6a on the CMN, a fracture nonunion is considered to exist only when a minimum of two sets of radiographs obtained prior to starting treatment with the osteogenesis stimulator, separated by a minimum of 90 days and each including multiple views of the fracture site, have been interpreted by a physician in writing as showing there is no clinically significant evidence of fracture healing between the two sets of radiographs.

If this definition of fracture nonunion is not met, question #6a must be answered No.

A nonspinal electrical osteogenesis stimulator (E0747) is covered only if any of the following criteria are met:

- Nonunion of a long bone fracture after six or more months have elapsed without healing of the fracture
- Failed fusion of a joint other than in the spine where a minimum of nine months has elapsed since the last surgery
- Congenital pseudarthrosis
- Nonunion, for all types of devices considered existing only after six or more months have elapsed without healing of the fracture

A long bone is limited to a clavicle, humerus, radius, ulna, femur, tibia, fibula, metacarpal, or metatarsal. A nonunion of the long bone fracture is described by ICD-9-CM diagnosis code 733.82 plus the code for the fracture site: 810.00–810.13, 812.00–813.93, 815.00–815.19, 820.00–821.39, 823.00–824.9, 825.25, 825.35.

A spinal electrical osteogenesis stimulator (E0748) is covered only if any of the following criteria are met:

- Failed spinal fusion where a minimum of nine months has elapsed since the last surgery
- Following a multilevel spinal fusion surgery
- Following spinal fusion surgery where there is a history of a previously failed spinal fusion at the same site

A multilevel spinal fusion is one that involves three or more vertebrae (e.g., L3–L5, L4–S1, etc.).

ICD-9-CM diagnosis code V45.4 should be used when billing a spinal electrical osteogenesis stimulator (E0748).

An electrical osteogenesis stimulator will usually be denied as not medically necessary if none of the above criteria is met.

The invasive stimulator (E0749) is covered only for the following indications:

- Nonunion of long bone fractures
- As an adjunct to spinal fusion surgery for patients at high risk of pseudarthrosis due to previously failed spinal fusion at the same site, or for those undergoing multiple level fusion. A multiple level fusion involves three or more vertebrae (e.g., L3BL5, L4BS1, etc.)

The DME MAC does not process claims for an invasive osteogenesis stimulator.

An ultrasonic osteogenesis stimulator (E0760) is covered when all of the following conditions are met:

- Nonunion of a fracture documented by a minimum of two sets of radiographs obtained prior to starting treatment with the osteogenesis stimulator, separated by a minimum of 90 days, each including multiple views of the fracture site and a written interpretation by a physician stating that there has been no clinically significant evidence of fracture healing between the two sets of radiographs
- Documented

E0755

E0755 Electronic salivary reflex stimulator (intraoral/noninvasive)

Lay Description

An electronic salivary reflex stimulator is used to treat xerostomia (dry mouth). Chronic xerostomia may be caused by a number of conditions, including Sjögren's syndrome, certain medications, and radiation therapy. Xerostomia can cause difficulty in eating and swallowing. An electronic salivary reflex stimulator is an intraoral, noninvasive device that emits electrical impulses to the tongue and roof of the mouth. These electrical impulses are distributed to all residual salivary tissues in the oral and pharyngeal regions stimulating salivation.

E0760

E0760 Osteogenesis stimulator, low intensity ultrasound, noninvasive

Lay Description

Please refer to codes E0747-E0749 for the description, coding, and billing information.

E0762

E0762 Transcutaneous electrical joint stimulation device system, includes all accessories

Lay Description

A transcutaneous electrical joint stimulation device used to treat osteoarthritis of the knee and rheumatoid arthritis of the hands. This battery powered device consists of an electrical stimulator with electrical leads that are placed over the affected area. The leads are held in place with a lightweight, flexible wrap and Velcro fasteners. The device delivers electrical impulses of 0.0 to 12.0 volt output to the joint. The device is typically worn for at least six hours per day. The device appears to stimulate development of new hyaline cartilage. Patients using transcutaneous electrical joint stimulation devices report reduced pain and stiffness and improved range of motion and function of the treated joints. This code reports the electrical joint stimulation device and all accessories (wrap, fasteners) needed to use the device.

E0764

E0764 Functional neuromuscular stimulation, transcutaneous stimulation of sequential muscle groups of ambulation with computer control, used for walking by spinal cord injured, entire system, after completion of training program

Lay Description

This code reports a transcutaneous, functional neuromuscular stimulator with computer control used to stimulate muscles of ambulation, which aids patients with spinal cord injuries in walking. A functional neuromuscular stimulator provides sequential electrical stimulation of muscles in the spinal cord injured patient. Use of electrical stimulation to replace stimuli when the nerve pathway has been injured or destroyed may assist in maintaining healthy muscle tone and strength and may enable the spinal cord injured patient to stand or walk independently. Patients are required to complete a training program prior to receiving the device.

E0765

E0765 FDA approved nerve stimulator, with replaceable batteries, for treatment of nausea and vomiting

Lay Description

The FDA approved nerve stimulator for treatment of nausea and vomiting is a battery-powered, noninvasive, portable, stimulation device. It is a small, watch-like device with two metal electrodes that are placed in contact with the skin on the volar aspect of the wrist over the median nerve following application of a hypoallergenic conductive gel to the skin contact site. The device is held in place with a Velcro band. Nerve stimulation therapy is administered by direct skin contact via two metal electrodes. The device has five intensity levels that are controlled by the patient by means of a rotary dial. This device may be used to treat nausea and vomiting secondary to pregnancy, chemotherapy, anesthesia, and motion sickness.

E0769

E0769 Electrical stimulation or electromagnetic wound treatment device, not otherwise classified

Lay Description

This code reports two different types of wound treatment devices that are not otherwise classified. The first type is an electrical stimulation wound treatment device. This type of device uses the application of electrical current through electrodes placed directly on the skin in close proximity to the wound. There are four categories of electrical stimulation devices used for wound healing, including low intensity direct current (LIDC), high voltage pulsed current (HVPC), alternative current (AC), and transcutaneous electrical nerve stimulation (TENS). The second type of device described by this code is an electromagnetic wound treatment device. This type of device employs electromagnetic fields rather than a direct electrical current.

E0776

E0776 IV pole

Lay Description

An intravenous (IV) pole is generally a portable, adjustable stand designed primarily to hang IV solution bags. Most models are mounted on rollers and are adjustable from a base height of about 56 inches up to about 96 inches. Many also feature optional attachments such as urinary bag hooks and clamps to secure oxygen tanks. Report E0776 for provision of each base IV pole.

E0779-E0781

E0779 Ambulatory infusion pump, mechanical, reusable, for infusion 8 hours or greater
E0780 Ambulatory infusion pump, mechanical, reusable, for infusion less than 8 hours
E0781 Ambulatory infusion pump, single or multiple channels, electric or battery operated, with administrative equipment, worn by patient

Lay Description
Ambulatory infusion pumps are portable devices that are typically carried or worn by the patient, often on a belt or strap, to directly infuse medications. The pumps reported by this code range may be electric or mechanical devices that feature reservoirs to hold liquid medication. Pressure is created, either mechanically or electrically, to infuse a regulated flow of medication into the patient over a set period of time. Routes of administration are by cannula and may include intravenous, intra-arterial, intrathecal, or intraperitoneal, among others; however, subcutaneous delivery is perhaps most common. A multiple channel pump allows for several different infusions at one time and will feature a programmable display to enter the prescribed rates. Report E0779 for an ambulatory mechanical pump that is reusable for infusion of eight hours or more; E0780 for an ambulatory infusion pump the is reusable for infusion of less than eight hours; and E0781 for an ambulatory pump with single or multiple channels, battery or electrical, and has administrative equipment.

Medicare Information
Supplies (including dressings) used in conjunction with a durable infusion pump (E0779, E0780, E0781), but excluding external insulin infusion pumps (E0784), are included in A4221 and A4222. Other codes should not be used for the separate billing of these supplies.

Note: See chapter titled "Medicare Guidelines," under "Infusion Pumps, External; Equipment and Supplies," for additional Medicare billing and documentation information.

E0782

E0782 Infusion pump, implantable, nonprogrammable (includes all components, e.g., pump, catheter, connectors, etc.)

Lay Description
An implantable infusion pump is a device carried by the patient in a surgically created subcutaneous pocket to directly infuse medications. Implanted pumps contain a refillable reservoir to hold liquid medication. The units may be used to deliver chemotherapy medications, drugs to address chronic pain, anti-spasmodics, or heparin, among others. Routes may include intravenous, intra-arterial, intrathecal, or intraperitoneal, among others. The reservoir is refilled by needle injection through a self-sealing membrane. Report E0782 for a pump that is not programmable, but includes all components.

Medicare Information
See chapter titled "Medicare Guidelines," under "Infusion Pumps, External; Equipment and Supplies," for Medicare billing and documentation information.

E0783

E0783 Infusion pump system, implantable, programmable (includes all components, e.g., pump, catheter, connectors, etc.)

Lay Description
This code reports the supply of an implantable, programmable infusion pump system. These devices are subcutaneously implanted near the site where the infusion is needed. The system is designed for patients requiring regular or continuous intravenous or intra-arterial infusions of drugs. The system may be used to deliver any of a variety of medicines, particularly those for oncology therapy. Implantable infusion pumps are typically small, biocompatible stainless steel units that are surgically placed subcutaneously near the site of optimal drug delivery. The port and reservoir can be smaller in diameter than a nickel coin. A refillable reservoir delivers a constant, prescribed rate of liquid drug to the target site. Typically, the reservoir features a rubber diaphragm that can be penetrated by a non-coring needle to refill the drug. This code reports the supply of a system that can be programmed to deliver a prescribed quantity of medicine over a given period of time. Report E0783 for supply of an implantable, programmable infusion pump system, including all auxiliary components.

Documentation Standards
For an item to be considered for coverage and payment by Medicare, the information submitted by the supplier must be corroborated by documentation in the patient's medical records indicating that Medicare coverage criteria have been met. The patient's medical records include the provider's office records, hospital records, nursing home records, home health agency records, or records from other health care professionals. This documentation must be available to the DME MAC upon request.

An order for the item that has been signed and dated by the treating provider and a certificate of medical necessity (CMN) that has been filled out, signed, and dated by the treating provider must be kept on file by the supplier. For external infusion pumps, an ICD-9-CM diagnosis code (specific to the fifth digit) describing the condition that necessitates the pump must be included on each order and CMN for the pump, drug/insulin, and/or supplies.

If a patient begins using an infusion for one drug and subsequently the drug is changed or if another drug is added, a revised CMN must be submitted for use of the pump with the new or additional drug. In the case of an additional drug, all drugs for which the pump is used should be included on the revised CMN.

If an inotropic drug is ordered, the initial claim must include a copy of the order (prescription and documentation from the treating physician), which includes information relating to each of the criteria defined in the aforementioned guidelines. This must include the before and after inotropic drug infusion values.

Medical necessity related to specific clinical data may not be completed by the supplier or by anyone in a financial relationship with the supplier. If coverage criteria as stated in the Medicare policy are not met, the claim should be accompanied by a letter from the physician detailing the patient's history (e.g., dates of past hospitalization for heart failure, prior use of parenteral inotropics and the results, etc.). If invasive hemodynamic studies were not performed, a letter and any supporting documentation should accompany the claim explaining the rationale for not performing the tests.

E0784

E0784   External ambulatory infusion pump, insulin

Lay Description

An external ambulatory infusion pump, also known as continuous subcutaneous insulin infusion (CSII), is a portable battery-powered device typically worn on a belt or strap. The device contains a reservoir to hold insulin. An infusion set comprising catheter tubing and a needle delivers microdoses of insulin, usually into subcutaneous tissues of the abdomen. Delivery rates can be closely adjusted to meet changing background needs, such as during strenuous exercise or around meals.

Medicare Information

Supplies (including dressings) used in conjunction with a durable infusion pump (E0779, E0780, E0781, E0791, K0455), but excluding external insulin infusion pumps (E0784), are included in A4221 and A4222. Other codes should not be used for the separate billing of these supplies.

Note: See chapter titled "Medicare Guidelines," under "Infusion Pumps, External; Equipment and Supplies," for additional Medicare billing and documentation information.

E0791

E0791   Parenteral infusion pump, stationary, single, or multichannel

Lay Description

A stationary parenteral infusion pump is a device to deliver liquid nutritional emulsions to patients whose normal gastrointestinal functions are compromised, and for the delivery of certain medications such as chemotherapies and pain management drugs. Proteins, carbohydrates, lipids, and electrolytes are the main components of parenteral nutrition, usually in carefully balanced combinations. The pumps are programmable and multi-channel units allow for several different infusions at one time. Lipids may be introduced separately, for example. Routes of administration include the subclavian, jugular, and femoral veins, as well as smaller vessels and, in some instances, arterial vessels.

Medicare Information

Supplies (including dressings) used in conjunction with a durable infusion pump (E0791), but excluding external insulin infusion pumps (E0784), are included in A4221 and A4222. Other codes should not be used for the separate billing of these supplies.

Note: See chapter titled "Medicare Guidelines," under "Infusion Pumps, External; Equipment and Supplies," for additional Medicare billing and documentation information.

E0830

E0830   Ambulatory traction device, all types, each

Lay Description

An ambulatory traction device uses two supports positioned on the body in such a way that they can lift and provide a decompressive force to the affected body part. In addition to the two supports, a lifting or stretching mechanism must be employed to provide the traction. This code reports any type of ambulatory traction device. If multiple traction devices are employed, each device is reported separately.

E0840-E0860

E0840　Traction frame, attached to headboard, cervical traction
E0849　Traction equipment, cervical, free-standing stand/frame, pneumatic, applying traction force to other than mandible
E0850　Traction stand, freestanding, cervical traction
E0855　Cervical traction equipment not requiring additional stand or frame
E0860　Traction equipment, overdoor, cervical

Lay Description

Cervical traction equipment extends the neck muscles, tissue, and ligaments of the upper portion of the spinal column through a gentle pulling action. Code E0840 reports a cervical traction frame designed to be attached to a headboard. Code E0849 reports cervical traction equipment inclusive of a freestanding stand or frame and pneumatic pump designed to apply traction force to the occiput or any site other than the mandible. Code E0850 reports a freestanding cervical traction stand. Code E0855 reports cervical traction equipment not requiring an additional stand or frame, which typically consists of a foam roll for under the neck, an adjustable head harness, and a weight bag. Code E0860 reports overhead cervical traction, which typically consists of a water-weighted bag suspended from a frame mounted on an overhead door. A cord is threaded through a pulley and attached to a stabilization harness on the patient's head. The traction is designed to relieve gravity pressure on a cervical injury.

E0870-E0900

E0870　Traction frame, attached to footboard, extremity traction (e.g., Buck's)
E0880　Traction stand, freestanding, extremity traction (e.g., Buck's)
E0890　Traction frame, attached to footboard, pelvic traction
E0900　Traction stand, freestanding, pelvic traction (e.g., Buck's)

Lay Description

Traction stands and frames are available in a variety of configurations, depending on the treatment desired. Perhaps most recognizable is the Buck's traction system, which applies gentle, but firm traction (pulling action) to the affected extremity to stabilize the injury. A floor stand or hospital bed is mounted with a frame that curves over the injured arm or leg like a gallows frame. The frame may be fitted with counterweights, pulleys, and cable that connect to traction pins transfixed to the fractured bone or to the casting. It can be a freestanding, floor mechanism or one that is attached using the support of another object for traction. Pelvic fractures may require supports at both ends of the bed or two floor stands at either end. These mechanisms usually comprise a padded sleeve or splint-type product that is applied to the affected extremity, as well as a metal or durable frame affixed to both the sleeve or splint and to the traction-exerting rope and pulley or other system. The benefits from traction use include better extremity circulation, pressure release, separation of bony components, support and protection, and prevention of surrounding ligament and myofascial contracture. Report E0870 for provision of a traction system designed to attach to a bed foot frame for stabilization of fractures of the extremities. Report E0880 for provision of a freestanding traction system designed to attach to a floor frame for stabilization of fractures of the extremities. Report E0890 for provision of a traction system designed to attach to a bed foot frame for stabilization of fractures of the pelvis. Report E0900 for provision of a freestanding traction system designed to attach to a floor frame for stabilization of fractures of the pelvis.

Documentation Standards

If the item is furnished secondary to a fracture (traumatic or nontraumatic, such as due to severe osteoporosis), a copy of the x-ray study confirming the fracture should be easily accessible within the medical record. If the device is furnished postsurgery, a copy of the operative report should be contained in the medical record. This information should be made available to the payer upon request.

No special forms, such as CMNs, are required to be completed for any of these items.

E0910-E0912, E0940

E0910　Trapeze bars, also known as Patient Helper, attached to bed, with grab bar
E0911　Trapeze bar, heavy-duty, for patient weight capacity greater than 250 pounds, attached to bed, with grab bar
E0912　Trapeze bar, heavy-duty, for patient weight capacity greater than 250 pounds, freestanding, complete with grab bar
E0940　Trapeze bar, freestanding, complete with grab bar

Lay Description

A trapeze bar with a grab bar, also referred to as a Patient Helper, is used when a patient needs a device to assist with movement because of a respiratory condition, fracture, or other medical condition. The patient holds onto the bar to maintain control while lifting the body or changing position. Trapeze bars may be attached to the bed or freestanding. Report E0910 for a trapeze bar with a grab bar that is attached to the bed, standard trapeze bar; and E0911 for a heavy-duty trapeze bar for patients weighing more than 250 pounds. Report E0940 for a freestanding standard trapeze bar with a grab bar and E0912 for a freestanding heavy-duty trapeze bar with a grab bar for patients weighing more than 250 pounds.

Medicare Information

When medically indicated, hospital bed accessories can likewise be covered. A trapeze bar is covered when a patient needs this device to sit up because of a respiratory condition, to change body position for other medical reasons, or to get in or out of bed. A bed cradle is covered for a patient with acute gouty arthritis (ICD-9-CM diagnosis code 274.0) or burns (ICD-9-CM diagnosis codes 942.00–943.59, 945.00–945.59) for whom it is necessary to prevent contact with the bed coverings. Side rails are covered, either as an accessory to or as an integral part of a hospital bed, when the patient's conditions require its use.

E0920-E0930

E0920 Fracture frame, attached to bed, includes weights
E0930 Fracture frame, freestanding, includes weights

Lay Description

Fracture frames are over-the-bed support structures from which traction weights and pulley can be mounted for the treatment of serious fractures. The units are available in several configurations. One style attaches to brackets at either end of the bed and another is a freestanding unit, mounting on legged supports. Both feature a strong bar that bridges over the bed and connects to the brackets. Traction weights and pulleys are arrayed along the bar as needed. Most models are modular and can accommodate variations in prescribed traction and weights. Traction counterweights are suspended from an array of cables and pulleys and rarely exceed eight pounds. Fixed, balanced, and sliding traction may be prescribed for treatment. Report E0920 for supply of models mounted on the bed frame, including weights. Report E0930 for supply of a freestanding system, including weights.

E0935

E0935 Continuous passive motion exercise device for use on knee only

Lay Description

Passive motion exercise devices (also known as continuous passive motion or CPM) are rehabilitation treatment strategies that usually follow orthopedic surgery. The knee joint is treated to sessions of continuous motion provided by a mechanical device. Report E0935 for the supply of each passive motion exercise device for use on knee only.

Medicare Information

Use of continuous passive range of motion machines (CPM) is covered by Medicare only after a total knee replacement. CPMs are not covered after any other type of knee or joint surgery. Coverage is limited to 21 days from the date of surgery, and the CPM must be applied within 48 hours of surgery to be eligible for Medicare coverage. The DME MAC should be billed only for those days of CPM treatment after discharge from the hospital.

When billing for a CPM, all of the following documentation must be included with the claim:

- Type of knee surgery performed
- Date of surgery
- Date of application of CPM
- Date of discharge from the hospital.

If any of these four facts are not documented, the claim will be denied for lack of medical necessity.

Medicare modifiers

Suppliers must use modifiers LT and RT when billing for the CPM to indicate the knee to which it was applied.

E0936

E0936 Continuous passive motion exercise device for use other than knee

Lay Description

A continuous passive motion (CPM) device is attached to the patient and moves the affected joint for flexion and/or extension continuously for extended periods of time without patient assistance. The power unit is used to set the variable range of motion and speed. The initial setting for range of motion is based on the patient's comfort level. There may also be other factors used to set motion and speed. Motion and stress play a key role in healing connective tissue. Motion enhances blood flow and decreases pain. CPM can used in postoperative patients to enhance pain relief, improve the circulation of the extremity, reduce edema, improve the cartilage of synovial joints, retard muscular atrophy, reduce stiffness, and prevent contractures and adhesions.

E0940

E0940 Trapeze bar, freestanding, complete with grab bar

Lay Description

Please refer to codes E0910-E0912 for the description, coding, and billing information.

E0941

E0941 Gravity assisted traction device, any type

Lay Description

This code reports the supply of a specialized traction device. Gravity traction devices can range from so-called "tilt tables" to inversion racks and "gravity boots." All of the systems promote spinal or other orthopedic therapy by reversing gravitational forces. Inversion tables and racks turn the user upside-down for a period of time. Gravity boots work in a similar fashion to allow the user to stretch the spine and hips by hanging upside-down from specialized boots. Other gravity traction devices work in a similar fashion. Gravity traction devices may be used to relieve chronic back pain by offering the user a period of suspension from gravitational pressures on the vertebral disk spaces. Report E0941 for supply of any type of gravity assisted traction device.

E0942

E0942 Cervical head harness/halter

Lay Description

This code reports the supply of a specialized head harness for rehabilitation therapy, usually for cervical injuries or disorders. A halo-type apparatus is fitted to the patient's head, sometimes in combination with a chinstrap. This halo is connected to a larger ring attached to a wall surface. Elastic resistance straps or springs connect the patient's halo apparatus to the larger, fixed ring. The patient goes through a variety of range of motion exercises designed to build strength and flexibility in the cervical spine and its supporting musculature. Report E0942 for supply of each cervical head harness or halter device.

E0944

E0944 Pelvic belt/harness/boot

Lay Description

This code reports the supply of a specialized orthopedic device known as a pelvic belt. This is a traction device that may be used intermittently by the patient, usually to relieve chronic pain of the lower back, sacrum, or pelvic regions, or to treat the effects of spondylosis. A wide, padded, form-fitting belt or harness is worn around the lower waist, often with Velcro closures. The belt is connected by elastic resistance straps to provide traction on the belt, relieving lumbosacral pressures. Report E0944 for supply of a pelvic belt or harness or boot.

E0945

E0945 Extremity belt/harness

Lay Description

This code reports supply of a specialized orthopedic device known as an extremity belt or harness. Extremity belts or harness are used with other traction devices to treat fractures of the extremities. The belt or harness is applied distal to the fracture site and is used to suspend the extremity so traction can be applied.

E0946

E0946 Fracture, frame, dual with cross bars, attached to bed, (e.g., Balken, 4 Poster)

Lay Description

A fracture frame with cross bars attached to a bed that consists of an overhead frame supported by upright bars attached to the bedposts or to a separate stand. The fractured limb may be splinted and suspended in a harness that is attached to a rope and pulley with a weight to provide the traction. This type of fracture frame may be referred to as a Balkan or four poster frame. This code reports the frame only.

E0950

E0950 Wheelchair accessory, tray, each

Lay Description

Wheelchair accessory trays are attached securely to the side surface of a conventional wheelchair. There are different tray styles with different functionality, including concealed compartments beneath an extension of an armrest for holding personal items, a cane holder, and a table tray (usually a standard feature).

E0958

E0958 Manual wheelchair accessory, one-arm drive attachment, each

Lay Description

A one-arm drive attachment is a manual wheelchair accessory that allows the patient to propel the wheelchair with only one hand. A patient with hemiplegia or an injury to one extremity might require this option.

E0966

E0966 Manual wheelchair accessory, headrest extension, each

Lay Description

A headrest extension is an accessory for a manual wheelchair that allows the headrest to be raised to a higher position than standard headrest height.

Patients requiring a headrest for support due to weak neck muscles and patients who require reclining back wheelchairs may also require a headrest extension for proper positioning of the headrest.

Medicare Information
Hook-on headrest extension (E0966) is covered if one the following criteria is met:

- The patient has weak neck muscles and needs a headrest for support
- The patient meets the criteria for and has a reclining back on the wheelchair

A fully reclining back option (E1226) is covered if the patient spends at least two hours per day in the wheelchair and has one or more of the following conditions/needs:

- Quadriplegia
- Fixed hip angle
- Trunk or lower extremity casts/braces that require the reclining back feature for positioning
- Excess extensor tone of the trunk muscles
- The need to rest in a recumbent position two or more times during the day, and transfer between wheelchair and bed is difficult

E0971
E0971 Manual wheelchair accessory, antitipping device, each

Lay Description
Anti-tipping devices are common wheelchair accessory options, particularly for pediatric patients. The devices may be paired and clamped onto the front of the chair to prevent forward spills. Report E0971 for each device or set of devices.

Medicare Information
For an item to be covered by Medicare, a written signed and dated order must be received by the supplier before a claim is submitted to the DME MAC. If the supplier bills for an item addressed in this policy without first receiving the completed order, the item will be denied as not medically necessary.

Options and accessories for wheelchairs are covered if the following criteria are met:

- The patient has a wheelchair that meets Medicare coverage criteria
- The patient's condition is such that without the use of a wheelchair, he/she would otherwise be bed or chair confined (an individual may qualify for a wheelchair and still be considered bed confined)
- The options/accessories are necessary for the patient to perform one or more of the following activities:
  - function in the home
  - perform instrumental activities of daily living

An option/accessory that is beneficial primarily in allowing the patient to perform leisure or recreational activities is noncovered.

E0973
E0973 Wheelchair accessory, adjustable height, detachable armrest, complete assembly, each

Lay Description
An adjustable height, detachable armrest is a wheelchair accessory designed for patients who require an armrest height that is not available in standard nonadjustable armrests. This code reports a single armrest and all hardware required for complete assembly. For patients who require adjustable height, detachable armrests for both the right and left arms, the code is reported separately for each side.

Medicare Information
Adjustable arm height option (E0973, K0017–K0018, K0020) is covered if the patient requires an arm height that is different than that available using nonadjustable arms, and the patient spends at least two hours per day in the wheelchair.

E0978
E0978 Wheelchair accessory, positioning belt/safety belt/pelvic strap, each

Lay Description
A positioning belt, safety belt, or pelvic strap is a wheelchair accessory that helps maintain proper positioning in the wheelchair. One or more of these items may be required for a patient with weak upper body muscles, upper body instability, or muscle spasticity. If more than one positioning/safety belt/strap is required, each one is reported separately.

E0986
E0986 Manual wheelchair accessory, push activated power assist, each

Lay Description
A push activated power assist accessory for a manual wheelchair is a device fitted to a rear wheel to sense the force exerted on the wheels. A battery-powered brake and/or propulsion system may then be activated to assist the patient in stopping or advancing the chair.

E0990

E0990 Wheelchair accessory, elevating legrest, complete assembly, each

Lay Description
An elevating legrest is a wheelchair accessory required by patients who have musculoskeletal conditions, casts, or braces that prevent 90-degree flexion at the knee. It may also be required for patients with significant edema of the lower extremities requiring elevation of the legs and for patients who require a reclining back on the wheelchair. This code reports a single elevating legrest and all hardware required for complete assembly. For patients who require elevating legrests for both the right and left legs, the code is reported separately for each side.

E0992

E0992 Manual wheelchair accessory, solid seat insert

Lay Description
A solid seat insert is a wooden or plastic device to bridge the suspension-style seat that comes standard on collapsible wheelchairs.

Medicare Information
A solid seat insert (E0992) is covered when the patient spends at least two hours per day in the wheelchair.

E1002

E1002 Wheelchair accessory, power seating system, tilt only

Lay Description
This code reports a tilt power seating system, a wheelchair accessory that can be added to a power wheelchair. The tilt feature allows the wheelchair to be tilted backward to at least 45 degrees from horizontal. Tilting the chair can increase comfort, reduce fatigue, and relieve pressure points caused by sitting in the same position for long periods of time. Power tilt seating systems include a solid seat platform and solid back; any frame width and depth; arm rests; fixed or swing-away detachable legrests; fixed or flip-up footplates; a motor and related electronics, with or without variable speed programmability; a switch control that is independent of the power wheelchair drive control interface; and any hardware required to attach the seating system to the wheelchair base. In addition to the tilt specifications, tilt systems must have a back height of at least 20 inches, the ability for the supplier to adjust the seat to back angle, and the ability to support a patient weighing up to 250 pounds.

E1003-E1005

E1003 Wheelchair accessory, power seating system, recline only, without shear reduction

E1004 Wheelchair accessory, power seating system, recline only, with mechanical shear reduction

E1005 Wheelchair accessory, power seating system, recline only, with power shear reduction

Lay Description
These codes report a recline power seating system, an accessory that can be added to a power wheelchair. Recline systems must have the ability to recline to at least 150 degrees from horizontal. There are several different types of recline systems. Recline systems differ primarily in their ability to reduce the shearing forces that occur when the wheelchair is reclined. Shearing refers to the shifting of the torso in the chair as it is reclined or raised causing the patient to slide along the back of the chair. Recline systems that reduce the shearing forces allow the patient's back to stay in contact with the chair without sliding. Wheelchair reclining systems that do not have shear reduction capabilities require that the wheelchair user be able to shift position to compensate for the 2- to 3-inch shear that occurs when the wheelchair is reclined or raised. Reclining wheelchairs are categorized as those that do not provide shear reduction (E1003), those that provide mechanical shear reduction (E1004), and those that provide power shear reduction (E1005). A mechanical shear reduction feature consists of two separate back panels. As the posterior back panel reclines or raises, there is a mechanical linkage between the two panels that allows the patient's back to stay in contact with the anterior panel without sliding along that panel. A power shear reduction feature also consists of two back panels. As the posterior back panel reclines or raises, a separate motor controls the linkage between the two panels that allows the patient's back to stay in contact with the anterior panel without sliding along that panel. Power recline seating systems include a solid seat platform and solid back; any frame width and depth; arm rests; fixed or swing-away detachable legrests; fixed or flip-up footplates; a motor and related electronics, with or without variable speed programmability; a switch control that is independent of the power wheelchair drive control interface; and any hardware required to attach the seating system to the wheelchair base. In addition to the recline specifications, recline systems must have a back height of at least 20 inches and the ability to support a patient weighing up to 250 pounds.

E1006-E1008

E1006 Wheelchair accessory, power seating system, combination tilt and recline, without shear reduction
E1007 Wheelchair accessory, power seating system, combination tilt and recline, with mechanical shear reduction
E1008 Wheelchair accessory, power seating system, combination tilt and recline, with power shear reduction

Lay Description

These codes report a combination tilt and recline power seating system, an accessory that can be added to a power wheelchair. The tilt feature allows the wheelchair to be tilted to at least 45 degrees from horizontal. The recline feature allows the chair to recline to at least 150 degrees from horizontal. There are several different types of tilt and recline systems. The systems differ primarily in their ability to reduce the shearing forces that occur when the wheelchair is reclined. Shearing refers to the shifting of the torso in the chair as it is reclined or raised causing the patient to slide along the back of the chair. Recline systems that reduce the shearing forces allow the patient's back to stay in contact with the chair without sliding. Wheelchair reclining systems that do not have shear reduction capabilities require that the wheelchair user be able to shift position to compensate for the 2- to 3- inch shear that occurs when the wheelchair is reclined or raised. Power seating systems with tilt and recline features are categorized as those that do not provide shear reduction (E1006), those that provide mechanical shear reduction (E1007), and those that provide power shear reduction (E1008). A mechanical shear reduction feature consists of two separate back panels. As the posterior back panel reclines or raises, there is a mechanical linkage between the two panels that allows the patient's back to stay in contact with the anterior panel without sliding along that panel. A power shear reduction feature also consists of two back panels. As the posterior back panel reclines or raises, a separate motor controls the linkage between the two panels that allows the patient's back to stay in contact with the anterior panel without sliding along that panel. Power recline seating systems include a solid seat platform and solid back; any frame width and depth; arm rests; fixed or swing-away detachable legrests; fixed or flip-up footplates; a motor and related electronics, with or without variable speed programmability; a switch control that is independent of the power wheelchair drive control interface; and any hardware required to attach the seating system to the wheelchair base. In addition to the tilt/recline specifications, combination tilt and recline systems must have a back height of at least 20 inches and the ability to support a patient weighing up to 250 pounds.

E1009-E1010

E1009 Wheelchair accessory, addition to power seating system, mechanically linked leg elevation system, including pushrod and legrest, each
E1010 Wheelchair accessory, addition to power seating system, power leg elevation system, including legrest, pair

Lay Description

A leg elevation system is a wheelchair accessory that can be added to a power seating system. Two types are available: a mechanically linked leg elevation system (E1009) and a power leg elevation system (E1010). A mechanically linked leg elevation system uses a pushrod that connects the legrest to a power recline seating system. With a mechanically linked leg elevation system, when the back reclines, the legrest elevates; when the back raises, the legrest lowers. A power leg elevation system uses a dedicated motor and related electronics, with or without variable speed programmability, that allows the legrest to be raised and lowered independently of the recline and/or tilt of the seating system. It includes a switch control that may or may not be integrated with the power tilt or recline controls.

E1031

E1031 Rollabout chair, any and all types with castors 5 in or greater

Lay Description

Rollabout chairs, any and all types that have casters of 5 inches or larger, are prescribed for ill, injured, or impaired individuals who require a level of mobility without standing and walking that may be met by the rollabout chair in lieu of a wheelchair. Rollabout chairs are not general use home or office chairs. Rollabout chairs are also referred to as mobile geriatric chairs and geri-chairs.

E1037-E1039

E1037 Transport chair, pediatric size
E1038 Transport chair, adult size, patient weight capacity up to and including 300 pounds
E1039 Transport chair, adult size, heavy-duty, patient weight capacity greater than 300 pounds

Lay Description

Transport chairs come in a variety of sizes with multiple functions, also referred to as a companion wheelchair. Transport chairs are convenient for any type of travel. Transport chairs are usually light weight and can fit into the patient's back seat or trunk. Report E1037 for a pediatric size transport chair; E1038 for an adult size transport chair, with a patient weight capacity up to and including 300 pounds; and E1039 for an adult size transport chair, with a patient weight capacity greater than 300 pounds.

Medicare Information
For more information regarding Medicare Coverage, please see, Medicare National Coverage Determinations Manual Chap 1, Part 4, secs. 280.1 and 280.3 and the Medicare Benefit Policy Manual Chapter 15 – Covered Medical and Other Health Services, sec. 110.

E1050-E1070

E1050 Fully-reclining wheelchair, fixed full-length arms, swing-away detachable elevating legrests
E1060 Fully-reclining wheelchair, detachable arms, desk or full-length, swing-away detachable elevating legrests
E1070 Fully-reclining wheelchair, detachable arms (desk or full-length) swing-away detachable footrest

Lay Description
Fully reclining wheelchairs are indicated for patients who are quadriplegic, have a fixed hip angle, may be currently wearing body or extremity casts or braces that necessitate a reclining position, and for patients who need to rest in their wheelchair in a recumbent position two or more times per day because transfer between wheelchair and bed is difficult. These wheelchairs include a fully reclining backrest with either detachable armrests (desk arm or full-length E0160) or fixed full-length armrests (E1050), and swing-away, detachable, elevating legrests with a pad used to support the calf when the legrest is in an elevated position. Report E1070 for a fully reclining wheelchair with detachable arms, desk or full-length and swing-away, and detachable footrests that are not leg elevating.

E1083-E1086

E1083 Hemi-wheelchair, fixed full-length arms, swing-away, detachable elevating legrest
E1084 Hemi-wheelchair, detachable arms desk or full-length arms, swing-away detachable elevating legrests
E1085 Hemi-wheelchair, fixed full-length arms, swing-away detachable footrests
E1086 Hemi-wheelchair, detachable arms, desk or full-length, swing-away detachable footrests

Lay Description
The hemi-wheelchair is indicated for patients requiring a lower seat height (17 to 18 inches) than the standard 19 to 21 inches from seat to floor because of short stature or the inability to place the feet on the ground for propulsion due to amputation, paralysis, or stroke. Hemi-wheelchairs have a fully reclining backrest. Report E1083 for fixed full-length armrests and E1084 for detachable armrests (desk arm or full-length), both with swing-away, detachable, elevating legrests with a pad used to support the calf when the legrest is in an elevated position. Report E1085 for fixed, full-length armrests and E1086 for detachable armrests (desk arm or full-length) when the hemi-wheelchairs have swing-away, detachable footrests that are not leg elevating.

E1087-E1090

E1087 High strength lightweight wheelchair, fixed full-length arms, swing-away detachable elevating legrests
E1088 High strength lightweight wheelchair, detachable arms desk or full-length, swing-away detachable elevating legrests
E1089 High-strength lightweight wheelchair, fixed-length arms, swing-away detachable footrest
E1090 High-strength lightweight wheelchair, detachable arms, desk or full-length, swing-away detachable footrests

Lay Description
The high-strength lightweight wheelchair is indicated for patients requiring a chair for self-propulsion and/or when the seat height, width, or depth measurements required cannot be accommodated by a standard, hemi, or lightweight wheelchair. This device weighs less than 34 lbs, is fully reclining, and has high-strength side frames and crossbraces. Report E1087 for fixed full-length armrests, E1088 for detachable armrests (desk arm or full-length), both with swing-away, detachable, elevating legrests with a pad used to support the calf when the legrest is in an elevated position. Report E1089 for fixed, full-length armrests and E1090 for detachable armrests (desk or full-length) when the high-strength, lightweight wheelchairs have swing-away, detachable footrests that are not leg elevating.

Medicare Information
For Medicare claims, see K0004.

E1092-E1093

E1092 Wide heavy-duty wheel chair, detachable arms (desk or full-length), swing-away detachable elevating legrests
E1093 Wide heavy-duty wheelchair, detachable arms, desk or full-length arms, swing-away detachable footrests

Lay Description
A wide, heavy-duty wheelchair is indicated for obese patients when the seat measurements required

cannot be accommodated by a standard wheelchair. This device is fully reclining and includes detachable desk or full-length arms. Report E1092 for swing-away, detachable, elevating legrests that have a pad used to support the calf when in the elevated position. Report E1093 for swing-away, detachable footrests that are not elevating.

E1100-E1110

E1100   Semi-reclining wheelchair, fixed full-length arms, swing-away detachable elevating legrests

E1110   Semi-reclining wheelchair, detachable arms (desk or full-length) elevating legrest

Lay Description

A semi-reclining wheelchair provides a backrest that tilts back from the upright position but not into a full-recumbent posture and swing-away, detachable elevating legrests that have a pad used to support the calf when the legrest is in an elevated position. Report E1100 if the armrests are fixed and full-length and E1110 if the armrests are detachable, desk or full-length.

E1130-E1160

E1130   Standard wheelchair, fixed full-length arms, fixed or swing-away detachable footrests

E1140   Wheelchair, detachable arms, desk or full-length, swing-away detachable footrests

E1150   Wheelchair, detachable arms, desk or full-length swing-away detachable elevating legrests

E1160   Wheelchair, fixed full-length arms, swing-away detachable elevating legrests

Lay Description

A standard wheelchair generally has a seat width of 16, 18, or 20 inches, is 16 inches in depth, and 21 inches from seat to floor. It comes with a chrome-plated frame, 24 inch molded rear wheels, 8 inch molded casters, nylon or vinyl upholstery, and arm and footrests. For a standard wheelchair with swing-away, detachable footrests, report E1130 when the armrests are fixed and full-length and E1140 when the armrests are detachable, either desk or full-length. For a standard wheelchair with swing-away, detachable, elevating legrests with a support pad for the calf in an elevated position, report E1150 for detachable armrests, either desk or full-length and E1160 for fixed full-length armrests.

Medicare Information

For Medicare claims, see K0001.

E1220

E1220   Wheelchair; specially sized or constructed, (indicate brand name, model number, if any) and justification

Lay Description

A specially sized or constructed wheelchair is indicated for patients in cases when the measurements of a standard wheelchair will not accommodate the patient's needs. This wheelchair must be justified by reasons such as a patient's physical size or the specific requirements for wheelchair usage in the patient's place of residence, such as narrow doorways that prevent the passage of a standard wheelchair. Report the brand name and model number.

Medicare Information

For Medicare claims indicate brand name, model number, and justification.

E1225-E1226

E1225   Wheelchair accessory, manual semi-reclining back, (recline greater than 15 degrees, but less than 80 degrees), each

E1226   Wheelchair accessory, manual fully reclining back, (recline greater than 80 degrees), each

Lay Description

Manual semi-reclining (E1225) or fully reclining (E1226) wheelchair backs are options that may be required for patients with certain medical conditions including quadriplegia, fixed hip angle, trunk or lower extremity casts/braces, excess extensor tone of the trunk muscles, or the need to rest in a recumbent position periodically during the day. A semi-reclining back is defined as one with a recline capability of greater than 15 degrees, but less than 80 degrees. A fully reclining back is one that can recline to greater than 80 degrees.

E1230

E1230   Power operated vehicle (3- or 4-wheel nonhighway), specify brand name and model number

Lay Description

A POV is a power-operated vehicle with three to four wheels. These may be indoor, outdoor, or both indoor/outdoor models. Indoor models are generally slow-speed with highly maneuverable mechanisms that assist the patient with mobility inside the home. Outdoor models can reach greater speeds and are more durable. POVs usually work from a battery power source. An indoor POV assists patients for whom a wheelchair is unsuitable in the activities of daily living, but POVs are not suited to all types of patients such as stroke victims or some quadriplegic and/or hemiplegic patients who cannot operate the controls nor be left alone while the vehicle is in operation. This code requires specifying the brand name and model number when reporting.

Medicare Information

The power operated vehicle (POV) is covered, when eligible, under the DME benefit. A POV is covered when all of the following criteria are met:

- The patient's condition is such that without the use of a wheelchair, the patient would otherwise be confined to a bed or chair
- The patient is unable to operate a manual wheelchair
- The patient is capable of safely operating the controls for the POV
- The patient can transfer safely in and out of the POV and has adequate trunk stability to be able to safely ride in the POV
- A POV is usually covered only if it is ordered by a physician who is in one of the following medical specialties:
- Physical medicine
- Orthopedic surgery
- Neurology
- Rheumatology

If one of the above specialists is not reasonably accessible (e.g., more than one day's round trip from the patient's home or the patient's condition precludes such travel), a prescription from the patient's treating physician may be acceptable.

Most POVs are ordered for patients who are capable of ambulation within the home, but require a power vehicle for movement outside the home. However, the Medicare program considers this need to be not medically necessary.

A POV that is beneficial primarily in allowing the patient to perform leisure or recreational activities is not medically necessary.

If a POV is covered, a wheelchair provided at the same time or subsequent to the POV is usually not covered for medical necessity reasons.

E1240-E1270

E1240   Lightweight wheelchair, detachable arms, (desk or full-length) swing-away detachable, elevating legrest
E1250   Lightweight wheelchair, fixed full-length arms, swing-away detachable footrest
E1260   Lightweight wheelchair, detachable arms (desk or full-length) swing-away detachable footrest
E1270   Lightweight wheelchair, fixed full-length arms, swing-away detachable elevating legrests

Lay Description

Lightweight wheelchairs are designed for patients who spend a great deal of time in the unit and can take full advantage of the increased mobility a lighter chair offers. Most models weigh 26 to 34 pounds and can be more effectively mobilized by the patient than conventional wheelchairs. Report E1240 for supply of a desk or full-length model that features detachable arms and swing-away elevating legrests. Report E1250 for supply of a model that features fixed full-length arms and swing-away legrests. Report E1260 for supply of a desk or full-length model that features detachable arms and swing-away, detachable footrests. Report E1270 for supply of a model that features fixed full-length arms and swing-away, detachable elevating legrests.

E1280-E1295

E1280   Heavy-duty wheelchair, detachable arms (desk or full-length) elevating legrests
E1285   Heavy-duty wheelchair, fixed full-length arms, swing-away detachable footrest
E1290   Heavy-duty wheelchair, detachable arms (desk or full-length) swing-away detachable footrest
E1295   Heavy-duty wheelchair, fixed full-length arms, elevating legrest

Lay Description

Heavy-duty wheelchairs may be called for to supply patients of extreme size or weight. Most models feature reinforced frames and wheels and can seat patients from 300 to 400 pounds or greater. Some models can accommodate up to 700 pounds. The unit itself may weigh up to 58 pounds. Report E1280 for supply of a desk or full-length heavy-duty wheelchair model with detachable arms and elevating legrests. Report E1285 for supply of a heavy-duty wheelchair model with fixed full-length arms and swing-away, detachable footrests. Report E1290 for supply of a desk or full-length heavy-duty wheelchair model with detachable arms and swing-away, detachable footrests. Report E1295 for supply of a heavy-duty wheelchair with fixed full-length arms and elevating legrests.

E1300-E1310

E1300 Whirlpool, portable (overtub type)
E1310 Whirlpool, nonportable (built-in type)

Lay Description

A therapeutic bath device that uses circulating water and water jets to stimulate circulation, relieve pain, and massage the body. Whirlpools may have a single pump that circulates the water or multiple pumps—one to circulate the water and the others to drive the hydrotherapy jets. A portable, over-tub whirlpool is reported with E1300. A non-portable, built-in whirlpool is reported with E1310.

E1353

E1353 Regulator

Lay Description

An oxygen regulator is a brass (or sometimes aluminum) device that governs the flow of gaseous oxygen from the tank. Some devices may feature an integrated pressure gauge and additional flow ports and safety relief valves. Report E1353 for supply of an oxygen regulator as a stand-alone item.

E1390-E1392

E1390 Oxygen concentrator, single delivery port, capable of delivering 85 percent or greater oxygen concentration at the prescribed flow rate
E1391 Oxygen concentrator, dual delivery port, capable of delivering 85 percent or greater oxygen concentration at the prescribed flow rate, each
E1392 Portable oxygen concentrator, rental

Lay Description

Traditional oxygen systems are of two general varieties: compressed gaseous systems and liquid oxygen systems. In recent years, a third variety has emerged: oxygen concentrators. These units concentrate oxygen from room air by removing nitrogen, which comprises about 80 percent of room air. These units alternately compress ambient air through chambers containing zeolite granules, which absorb nitrogen. While one chamber is pressurized, the second rests and the zeolite release the absorbed nitrogen back into the room air. The concentrated oxygen is filtered and delivered at levels of about five liters per minute at levels approaching 95 percent pure oxygen. Report E1390 for supply of an oxygen concentrator that has a single delivery port that delivers 85 percent or greater concentrations of oxygen at a prescribed flow rate. Report E1391 for an oxygen concentrator that has a dual delivery port that delivers 85 percent or greater concentrations of oxygen at a prescribed flow rate. Report E1392 for a portable oxygen concentrator rental.

E1405-E1406

E1405 Oxygen and water vapor enriching system with heated delivery
E1406 Oxygen and water vapor enriching system without heated delivery

Lay Description

Oxygen delivery systems are units of compressed gaseous, liquid, or concentrated O2 for home use, which are either stationary or portable. In many cases, the units also include the system components required to administer the O2, such as the regulator, flowmeter, contents indicator, nebulizer, humidifier, cannula or mask, and the O2 tubing. The administration of O2 assists in oxygenation of tissues when the patient's cardiopulmonary system is unable to intake sufficient quantities of O2 or is unable to process outside or room air into its elemental components to use the O2 content. For instance, patients with severe chronic obstructive pulmonary disease and emphysema may require O2 therapy. Oxygen also aids in and/or expedites the healing of injured or diseased tissues or organs. Report E1405 for an oxygen and vapor delivery system that is heated; E1406 for an oxygen and vapor delivery system that is not heated.

Medicare Information

The date of the qualifying O2 testing reported on the CMN must be within 30 days before the initial certification, as dated and signed by the prescribing physician.

These items are billed to the DME MAC, not to the Medicare carrier. Payment is made if all of the requirements for Medicare reimbursement are met and the applicable DME MAC's medical necessity policies for the O2 are followed.

Note: See chapter titled "Medicare Guidelines," under "Oxygen (O2) and O2 Equipment," for additional Medicare billing and documentation information.

E1500-E1699

E1500	Centrifuge, for dialysis
E1510	Kidney, dialysate delivery system kidney machine, pump recirculating, air removal system, flowrate meter, power off, heater and temperature control with alarm, IV poles, pressure gauge, concentrate container
E1520	Heparin infusion pump for hemodialysis
E1530	Air bubble detector for hemodialysis, each, replacement
E1540	Pressure alarm for hemodialysis, each, replacement
E1550	Bath conductivity meter for hemodialysis, each
E1560	Blood leak detector for hemodialysis, each, replacement
E1570	Adjustable chair, for ESRD patients
E1575	Transducer protectors/fluid barriers, for hemodialysis, any size, per 10
E1580	Unipuncture control system for hemodialysis
E1590	Hemodialysis machine
E1592	Automatic intermittent peritoneal dialysis system
E1594	Cycler dialysis machine for peritoneal dialysis
E1600	Delivery and/or installation charges for hemodialysis equipment
E1610	Reverse osmosis water purification system, for hemodialysis
E1615	Deionizer water purification system, for hemodialysis
E1620	Blood pump for hemodialysis, replacement
E1625	Water softening system, for hemodialysis
E1630	Reciprocating peritoneal dialysis system
E1632	Wearable artificial kidney, each
E1634	Peritoneal dialysis clamps, each
E1635	Compact (portable) travel hemodialyzer system
E1636	Sorbent cartridges, for hemodialysis, per 10
E1637	Hemostats, each
E1639	Scale, each
E1699	Dialysis equipment, not otherwise specified

Lay Description

These codes describe miscellaneous supplies and equipment needed to accomplish home dialysis. Dialysis is a filtration process that filters impurities from the blood. Dialysis assists malfunctioning kidneys and can replace nonfunctioning kidneys. The functioning of all body parts requires the removal of the various toxins and metabolic byproducts from the blood. If these impurities are allowed to accumulate, death will occur within days. Home dialysis allows the patient to perform this function in home rather than at a facility.

E1700

E1700 Jaw motion rehabilitation system

Lay Description

This code reports the supply of a rehabilitative device for disorders of the temporomandibular joint (TMJ) and restrictive jaw motion. These devices may feature a cushioned mouthpiece that the patient bites against. The patient then squeezes a lever that forces open the mouthpiece and the jaw. Adjustments on the device control the leverage action. The therapy works to improve the range of the TMJ. Patients who have undergone certain radiation treatments often suffer a restrictive and spastic jaw movement known as trismus. Rehabilitation for surgery of the jaw and treatment of conditions that cause "lockjaw" may also warrant use of this type of device.

E1800-E1806

E1800	Dynamic adjustable elbow extension/flexion device, includes soft interface material
E1801	Static progressive stretch elbow device, extension and/or flexion, with or without range of motion adjustment, includes all components and accessories
E1802	Dynamic adjustable forearm pronation/supination device, includes soft interface material
E1805	Dynamic adjustable wrist extension/flexion device, includes soft interface material
E1806	Static progressive stretch wrist device, flexion and/or extension, with or without range of motion adjustment, includes all components and accessories

Lay Description

These codes report the supply of specific rehabilitation devices for the upper limb. These devices are designed to be strapped onto the affected forearm or wrist. The device is designed to alternately stretch and relax muscles in the affected region. A device for rehabilitation of the forearm alternately pronates and supinates at the elbow joint. A similar device on the wrist alternately extends and flexes the wrist. The device is non-motorized and is operated by the patient, sometimes using the unaffected arm to operate controls. Adjustable pads and cuffs are positioned to maximize function. Report E1802 for supply of a dynamic forearm device and E1805 for supply of a dynamic device for the wrist. Both codes include supply of the soft material that interfaces between the skin and the hard structure of the device.

Medicare Information

For claims with dates of service on or after November 1, 1997, codes E1800–E1815, E1825, and

E1830 must be used for the dynamic joint contracture device itself, which includes the joints. These codes are in the capped rental payment category, and payment policy and coding guidelines for capped rental items applies (i.e., modifiers KH, KI, and KJ; 10th month rent/purchase option; maintenance and servicing; etc.). Code E1820 is used for the interface material. It is in the inexpensive or routinely purchased payment category and is billed in addition to the first month's rental of the device.

E2000

E2000 Gastric suction pump, home model, portable or stationary, electric

Lay Description
Please refer to code E0600 for the description, coding, and billing information.

E2100-E2101

E2100 Blood glucose monitor with integrated voice synthesizer

E2101 Blood glucose monitor with integrated lancing/blood sample

Lay Description
Please refer to code E0607 for the description, coding, and billing information.

E2120

E2120 Pulse generator system for tympanic treatment of inner ear endolymphatic fluid

Lay Description
A portable, low-pressure pulse generator system for tympanic treatment of inner ear endolymphatic fluid, also known as Ménière's disease, is reported with E2120. Prior to application of the pulse generator, the patient undergoes a tympanostomy with ventilation tube insertion. The patient must then wait approximately two weeks before treatment with the pressure pulse generator can begin. The device delivers repeated pressure pulses to the ear canal using an air pressure generator and a close-fitting cuff in the ear canal. The treatment is performed several times a day for short intervals (approximately five minutes per treatment session).

Medicare Information
Coverage and payment is at the contractor's discretion.

E2209

E2209 Accessory, arm trough, with or without hand support, each

Lay Description
An arm trough for a manual wheelchair is an accessory designed to support the arm in patients with quadriplegia, hemiplegia, or spasticity of the arms. The arm trough replaces the standard armrest. This code represents an arm trough, with or wirhout hand supports, each.

E2213

E2213 Manual wheelchair accessory, insert for pneumatic propulsion tire (removable), any type, any size, each

Lay Description
An insert for pneumatic propulsion tire consisting of a ring of firm material that is placed inside the pneumatic tire to allow the wheelchair to be used if the pneumatic tire is punctured. This ring of material is distinct from the tire itself. This type of tire insert is sometimes referred to as a flat free insert or a zero pressure tube.

E2300

E2300 Power wheelchair accessory, power seat elevation system

Lay Description
A power seat elevation system allows the seat to be raised and lowered. The system should be able to raise the seat a minimum of 6 inches from its lowest point. A power seat elevation system consists of a motor and related electronics, with or without variable speed programmability; a switch control that is independent of the power wheelchair drive control interface; and hardware needed to attach the seating system to the wheelchair base.

E2301

E2301 Power wheelchair accessory, power standing system

Lay Description
A power standing system wheelchair accessory assists the patient in moving from a sitting to standing position. Power standing systems must have the ability to support a patient weight of at least 250 pounds. A power standing system consists of a solid seat platform and solid back; detachable or flip-up fixed height armrests; hinged legrests; anterior knee supports; fixed or flip-up foot plates; a motor and related electronics, with or without variable speed programmability; a basic switch control that is independent of the power wheelchair drive control interface; and any hardware that is

needed to attach the seating system to the wheelchair base. A headrest is not included and should be reported additionally if supplied.

E2310-E2311

E2310 Power wheelchair accessory, electronic connection between wheelchair controller and one power seating system motor, including all related electronics, indicator feature, mechanical function selection switch, and fixed mounting hardware

E2311 Power wheelchair accessory, electronic connection between wheelchair controller and 2 or more power seating system motors, including all related electronics, indicator feature, mechanical function selection switch, and fixed mounting hardware

Lay Description

These codes describe electronic components that allow the patient to control two or more motors from a single interface using a proportional joystick, touchpad, or nonproportional interface. The motors that can be controlled from the electronic connection include power wheelchair drive, power tilt, power recline, power shear reduction, power leg elevation, power seat elevation, and power standing system. This type of wheelchair accessory includes a function selection switch that allows the patient to select the motor being controlled and an indicator feature to visually show which function has been selected. The indicator feature may also show the direction that has been selected (forward, reverse, left, right). The indicator feature may be in a separate display box or may be integrated into the wheelchair interface. Report E2310 for an electronic connection between wheelchair controller and one power seating system motor and E2320 when there are two or more power seating system motors that must be connected. Both codes include all related electronics, indicator feature, mechanical selection switch, and fixed mounting hardware.

E2321-E2322

E2321 Power wheelchair accessory, hand control interface, remote joystick, nonproportional, including all related electronics, mechanical stop switch, and fixed mounting hardware

E2322 Power wheelchair accessory, hand control interface, multiple mechanical switches, nonproportional, including all related electronics, mechanical stop switch, and fixed mounting hardware

Lay Description

An interface is the mechanism for controlling the movement of the power wheelchair of which there are a number of different types. These codes describe a nonproportional hand control interface that uses a remote joystick (E2321) or multiple mechanical switches (E2322). A remote joystick is one that is separate from the box containing the electronics that connects the interface to the motor and gears (controller box). A mechanical switch system describes a system with three to five mechanical switches that require physical contact to be activated. The switch selected determines the direction of the wheelchair. A mechanical direction change switch, if provided, is included in E2322. A nonproportional interface is a type of interface that allows the patient to control the direction of the wheelchair, but the speed is pre-programmed and cannot be affected by the user. The two nonproportional interface mechanisms described by E2321 and E2322 include all related electronics, mechanical stop switch, and the fixed mounting hardware.

E2323

E2323 Power wheelchair accessory, specialty joystick handle for hand control interface, prefabricated

Lay Description

A prefabricated specialty joystick handle has a shape other than a straight stick. U-shaped and T-shaped handles are reported with this code. Joysticks that have some other nonstandard feature such as a flexible shaft are also reported with E2323.

E2324

E2324 Power wheelchair accessory, chin cup for chin control interface

Lay Description

Wheelchair users who do not have the ability to control a joystick using hand or upper extremity motion can have the joystick modified with a chin cup that allows movement of the wheelchair to be controlled with the chin. The chin cup is attached to the joystick and reported additionally with E2324.

E2325-E2326

E2325 Power wheelchair accessory, sip and puff interface, nonproportional, including all related electronics, mechanical stop switch, and manual swingaway mounting hardware

E2326 Power wheelchair accessory, breath tube kit for sip and puff interface

Lay Description

A sip and puff interface is a nonproportional interface in which the patient holds a tube in the mouth and controls the wheelchair by sucking in (sip) or blowing out (puff). A nonproportional interface is a type of interface that allows the patient to control the direction of the wheelchair, but the speed is pre-programmed and cannot be affected by the user. Code E2325 reports the nonproportional sip and puff interface, all related electronics, a mechanical stop switch, and manual swing-away mounting hardware. The breath tube kit for the sip and puff interface is reported additionally with E2326.

E2327-E2328

E2327 Power wheelchair accessory, head control interface, mechanical, proportional, including all related electronics, mechanical direction change switch, and fixed mounting hardware

E2328 Power wheelchair accessory, head control or extremity control interface, electronic, proportional, including all related electronics and fixed mounting hardware

Lay Description

An interface is the mechanism for controlling the movement of the power wheelchair of which there are a number of different types. Code E2327 describes a mechanical, proportional, head control interface, and E2328 describes an electronic, proportional, head or extremity control interface. A proportional interface is directly controlled by the patient such that both direction and speed is controlled by the patient. A mechanical, proportional, head control interface (E2327) is one in which a headrest is attached to a joystick-like device. The direction and amount of movement of the patient's head pressing on the headrest controls the direction and speed of the wheelchair. An electronic, proportional, head control interface (E2328) is one in which a patient's head movements are sensed by a box placed behind the patient's head, and the direction and speed of the wheelchair are controlled by the sensors. The box does not come into direct contact with the patient's head. An electronic, proportional, extremity control interface, also reported with E2328, is one in which the direction and amount of movement of the patient's arm or leg control the direction and speed of the wheelchair. Interface mechanisms include all related electronics and the fixed mounting hardware. A mechanical direction control switch is included in E2327.

E2329-E2330

E2329 Power wheelchair accessory, head control interface, contact switch mechanism, nonproportional, including all related electronics, mechanical stop switch, mechanical direction change switch, head array, and fixed mounting hardware

E2330 Power wheelchair accessory, head control interface, proximity switch mechanism, nonproportional, including all related electronics, mechanical stop switch, mechanical direction change switch, head array, and fixed mounting hardware

Lay Description

An interface is the mechanism for controlling the movement of the power wheelchair of which there are a number of different types. Code E2329 describes a nonproportional, contact switch, head control interface, and E2330 describes a nonproportional, proximity switch, head control interface. A nonproportional interface is a type of interface that allows the patient to control the direction of the wheelchair, but the speed is preprogrammed and cannot be affected by the user. A nonproportional, contact switch, head control interface (E2329) is one in which the patient activates one of three mechanical switches placed around the back and sides of the head. These switches are activated by pressure of the head against the switch. The switch that is selected determines the direction of the wheelchair. A nonproportional, proximity switch, head control interface (E2330) is one in which the patient activates one of three switches placed around the back and sides of the head. These switches are activated by movement of the head toward the switch, though the head does not touch the switch. The switch that is selected determines the direction of the wheelchair. Both interface mechanisms include all related electronics, mechanical stop switch, mechanical direction change switch, head array, and the fixed mounting hardware.

E2331

E2331 Power wheelchair accessory, attendant control, proportional, including all related electronics and fixed mounting hardware

Lay Description

An attendant control for a power wheelchair allows a caregiver to drive the wheelchair instead of the patient. The attendant control is usually mounted on one of the rear canes of the wheelchair. Attendant control devices are proportional controls, allowing the attendant to control both the direction and the speed of the wheelchair, usually by means of a joystick. All related electronics and fixed mounting hardware are included.

E2373-E2374

E2373 Power wheelchair accessory, hand or chin control interface, compact remote joystick, proportional, including fixed mounting hardware

E2374 Power wheelchair accessory, hand or chin control interface, standard remote joystick (not including controller), proportional, including all related electronics and fixed mounting hardware, replacement only

Lay Description

An interface is the mechanism for controlling the movement of the power wheelchair of which there are a number of different types. This code describes a proportional hand or chin control interface that uses a remote joystick or touchpad. A proportional interface is directly controlled by the patient such that both direction and speed is controlled by the patient moving the joystick or using the touchpad. A remote joystick is separate from the box containing the electronics that connects the interface to the motor and gears (controller box), and encompasses a standard joystick or one that can be controlled by small movements. The latter type may be mini-proportional, compact, or short throw joystick. The second type of interface described by this code is a touchpad similar to the pad-type mouse found on laptop computers. Interface mechanisms include all related electronics and the fixed mounting hardware. Report E2373 for a miniproportional, compact or short interface. Report E7343 for a standard interface. The chin cup is reported separately with E2324.

E2402

E2402 Negative pressure wound therapy electrical pump, stationary or portable

Lay Description

Negative pressure wound therapy (NPWT) is controlled application of subatmospheric pressure to wounds. A pump continuously or intermittently carries subatmospheric pressure through connected tubes directly to a specialized wound dressing. A canister collects the drainage from the wound. NPWT promotes healing of chronic wounds and decubitus ulcers. Controlled pressure of the wound increases vascularity and oxygenation of the wound bed thus reducing edema by getting rid of the wound fluid and removing exudate and bacteria.

E2500-E2510

E2500 Speech generating device, digitized speech, using prerecorded messages, less than or equal to 8 minutes recording time

E2502 Speech generating device, digitized speech, using prerecorded messages, greater than 8 minutes but less than or equal to 20 minutes recording time

E2504 Speech generating device, digitized speech, using prerecorded messages, greater than 20 minutes but less than or equal to 40 minutes recording time

E2506 Speech generating device, digitized speech, using prerecorded messages, greater than 40 minutes recording time

E2508 Speech generating device, synthesized speech, requiring message formulation by spelling and access by physical contact with the device

E2510 Speech generating device, synthesized speech, permitting multiple methods of message formulation and multiple methods of device access

Lay Description

Speech generating devices, also called communication devices, enable an individual to communicate with others more effectively. There are many devices that assist individuals by using speech or voice output and other combinations of assistance. Speech generating devices have been created for individuals who cannot speak, are difficult to understand, or have language retrieval issues. Digitized speech devices are referred to as devices with "whole message" speech output. Digitized speech devices utilize words and phrases that have been pre-recorded by someone other than the user and used for playback by the user. Synthesized speech devices translate a user's input into device-generated speech. Users of synthesized speech devices are not limited to prerecorded messages but can independently create messages as their own communication needs arise. These devices require the user to use a keyboard, touch screen, or other display containing an alphanumeric display. Synthesized speech devices allow the user different methods of message formulation and many methods of access. These methods of message formulation must include the capability for message selection by two or more of the following methods: letters, words, pictures, or symbols. Multiple methods of access must include the capability to access the device by two or more of the following methods: entering information by a keyboard, touch screen, or indirect selection techniques via a specialized access device such as a joystick, a head-mouse, an optical head-pointer, a switch, a light pointer, an infrared pointer, a scanning device, or Morse code.

E2511

E2511 Speech generating software program, for personal computer or personal digital assistant

Lay Description

Speech generating software allows laptops and/or desktop computers or personal digital assistant (PDA) devices to function as a speech generating device. The information can be entered with a pen based system using a stylus and handwriting recognition software, keyboard, downloaded from a computer using special cables, and software.

E2622-E2623

E2622 Skin protection wheelchair seat cushion, adjustable, width less than 22 in, any depth
E2623 Skin protection wheelchair seat cushion, adjustable, width 22 in or greater, any depth

Lay Description

Adjustable wheelchair seat cushions provide skin protection and comfort for individuals who must sit for long periods of time. Adjustable cushions are those that can be adapted to conform to the specific requirements of the individual. Cushions can be constructed of a variety of materials including rubber, foam, gel-foam, and polyester fiber-filled cores with adjustable air pads that allow the user to control the cushion fit. Some cushions have dual air controls that allow the side and center to be inflated to differing levels.

E2624-E2625

E2624 Skin protection and positioning wheelchair seat cushion, adjustable, width less than 22 in, any depth
E2625 Skin protection and positioning wheelchair seat cushion, adjustable, width 22 in or greater, any depth

Lay Description

Adjustable positioning wheelchair seat cushions provide skin protection and positioning for individuals with paralysis, deformities, scoliosis, poor muscle control, or other conditions. Positioning seat cushions can aid in manipulation or control of objects, can assist in the performance of specific activities, and can provide added balance and support. Adjustable cushions are those that can be adapted to conform to the specific requirements of the individual. Cushions can be constructed of a variety of materials including rubber, foam, gel-foam, and polyester fiber-filled cores with adjustable air pads that allow the user to control the cushion fit. Some cushions have dual air controls that allow the sides and center to be inflated to differing levels.

E8000-E8002

E8000 Gait trainer, pediatric size, posterior support, includes all accessories and components
E8001 Gait trainer, pediatric size, upright support, includes all accessories and components
E8002 Gait trainer, pediatric size, anterior support, includes all accessories and components

Lay Description

A gait trainer is a device that allows the patient to move about freely using their own legs. Each gait trainer should be specifically sized for the individual patient and is used in different therapy modalities for gait restoration. Gait trainer supports the patients according to their ability and controls the center of mass in the vertical and horizontal directions.

G0008

G0008 Administration of influenza virus vaccine

Lay Description

Use this code to report the administration of an influenza virus vaccine. Do not bill an office visit if the only reason for the visit was to receive a vaccination.

G0009

G0009 Administration of pneumococcal vaccine

Lay Description
Use this code to report the administration of a pneumococcal vaccine. Do not bill an office visit if the only reason for the visit was to receive a vaccination.

Medicare Information
Medicare will pay 100 percent of the reasonable charge for the vaccine and its administration. Deductibles and coinsurance do not apply.

Roster bills must contain, at a minimum, the following information:

- Provider name and number;
- Date of service;
- Control number for Medicare contractor;
- Patient's health insurance claim number;
- Patient's name;
- Patient's address;
- Date of birth;
- Patient's sex; and
- Beneficiary's signature or stamped "signature on file"

G0010

G0010 Administration of hepatitis B vaccine

Lay Description
Use this code to report the administration of a hepatitis B vaccine on a day when no other service is performed for which there is a physician fee schedule set.

Documentation Standards
Effective with implementation of the national provider identifier (NPI), the NPI must be entered in item 17A of Form CMS-1500 for hepatitis B vaccine since Medicare requires a physician's order or supervision.

Medicare Information
Medicare will provide benefits under Part B for a hepatitis B vaccine and its administration when provided to a patient who is at high or intermediate risk of contracting hepatitis B.

High-risk groups include:

- ESRD patients
- Hemophiliac patients who receive factor VIII or IX concentrates
- Clients of institutions for the mentally retarded
- Persons who live in the same household as a hepatitis B virus (HBV) carrier
- Homosexual men
- Users of illicit injectable drugs

Intermediate-risk groups include:

- ESRD patients
- Staff in institutions for the mentally retarded
- Workers in health care professions who have frequent contact with blood or blood-derived body fluids during routine work
- Individuals in the groups listed above would not be considered to be at high or intermediate risk of contracting hepatitis B if there is laboratory evidence positive for antibodies to hepatitis B.

G0027

G0027 Semen analysis; presence and/or motility of sperm excluding huhner

Lay Description
Semen analysis is the microscopic examination of semen for the presence, quality, and mobility of the sperm contained within the semen. This is usually performed to determine if this is the source of infertility.

G0101

G0101 Cervical or vaginal cancer screening; pelvic and clinical breast examination

Lay Description
This code reports a cervical or vaginal cancer screening and a pelvic and clinical breast examination. The specimen for cancer screening is collected by cervical, endocervical, or vaginal scrapings or by aspiration of vaginal fluid and cells. The pelvic and breast exams are done manually by the physician to check for abnormalities, pain, and/or any palpable lumps or masses.

Medicare modifiers
Modifier 25 may be used to indicate a "significant, separately identifiable evaluation and management (E/M) service by the same physician on the same day of the procedure or service." The modifier is billed with an E/M code that is above and beyond the diagnostic and/or therapeutic procedure performed, that is beyond the usual preoperative and postoperative care associated with the procedure, or when a separate history was taken, a separate physical was performed and a separate medical decision was made.

Modifier 27 is for hospital outpatient reporting purposes. The modifier is used to report the utilization of hospital resources related to separate and distinct E/M encounters performed in multiple

Coders' Desk Reference for HCPCS

outpatient hospital settings on the same date. This modifier is added to each appropriate level of outpatient and/or emergency department E/M codes. It is used to report E/M services provided by physicians in more than one outpatient hospital setting.

G0102

G0102 Prostate cancer screening; digital rectal examination

Lay Description

This code reports a prostate cancer screening performed manually by the physician as a digital rectal exam in order to palpate the prostate and check for abnormalities.

Medicare Information

Screening examinations are applicable only to men who are 50 years of age or older. Both tests are subject to the frequency limitation of no more than once every 12 months and must be performed by a qualified provider such as a physician, nurse practitioner, certified nurse midwife, physician's assistant, or a clinical nurse specialist.

When medically necessary, prostate specific antigen (PSA) testing is allowed once every three months. Not only must the medical documentation support the medical necessity of the procedure, it must also support the frequency of the test. Applicable documentation includes the physician's orders and progress notes, the history and physical, operative report, diagnostic test findings, and consultations.

Carrier guidelines vary with regard to the diagnoses for which this procedure is covered, so it is best to obtain the specific diagnostic coverage criteria from the carriers to which you submit claims regularly.

G0103

G0103 Prostate cancer screening; prostate specific antigen test (PSA)

Lay Description

This code reports a total prostate specific antigen (PSA) test for cancer screening. The specimen collection is by venipuncture. Methods may include radioimmunoassay (RIA) and monoclonal two-site immunoradiometric assay. There are several forms of PSA present in serum. PSA may be complexed with the protease inhibitor alpha-1 antichymotrypsin (PSA-ACT) or found in a free form. Higher levels of free PSA are more often associated with benign conditions than with cancer. Total PSA measures both complexed and free levels to provide a total amount present in the serum. A percentage of each form is sometimes calculated to help distinguish benign from malignant conditions.

Medicare Information

Screening examinations are applicable only to men who are 50 years of age or older. Both tests are subject to the frequency limitation of no more than once every 12 months and must be performed by a qualified provider such as a physician, nurse practitioner, certified nurse midwife, physician's assistant, or a clinical nurse specialist.

When medically necessary, prostate specific antigen (PSA) testing is allowed once every three months. Not only must the medical documentation support the medical necessity of the procedure, it must also support the frequency of the test. Applicable documentation includes the physician's orders and progress notes, the history and physical, operative report, diagnostic test findings, and consultations.

Carrier guidelines vary with regard to the diagnoses for which this procedure is covered, so it is best to obtain the specific diagnostic coverage criteria from the carriers to which you submit claims regularly.

G0104

G0104 Colorectal cancer screening; flexible sigmoidoscopy

Lay Description

A flexible sigmoidoscopy is performed for colorectal cancer screening. After the patient's bowel has been prepped, the physician inserts the flexible sigmoidoscope through the anus and advances the scope into the sigmoid colon. The lumen of the sigmoid colon and rectum are visualized and brushings or washings may be obtained. The sigmoidoscope is withdrawn.

Medicare Information

Medicare covers a flexible sigmoidoscopy once every 48 month for beneficiaries age 50 and older. If, during the course of the screening sigmoidoscopy, a lesion or growth is detected and is biopsied or removed, the physician should bill using the appropriate CPT code for a flexible sigmoidoscopy with biopsy or removal rather than using HCPCS Level II code G0104 for a screening sigmoidoscopy.

Effective for services on and after January 1, 2002, benefits will be provided for flexible screening sigmoidoscopies when performed by a physician assistant, nurse practitioner, or clinical nurse specialist who is authorized under the law of the state in which he/she practices to perform this examination.

G0105

G0105 Colorectal cancer screening; colonoscopy on individual at high risk

Lay Description

A colonoscopy is done on a high-risk patient for colorectal cancer screening. A high-risk patient is one with ulcerative enteritis or a history of malignant neoplasm of the lower gastrointestinal tract. After the patient's bowel has been prepped, the physician inserts the colonoscope through the anus and advances the scope through the colon past the splenic flexure. The lumen of the colon and rectum is visualized. Brushings or washings may be obtained. The colonoscope is withdrawn.

Documentation Standards

Hospital, outpatient, ASC or office records, or procedure reports should clearly state the pertinent history and physical exam, the reason for the procedure, the course of the examination, and the results.

Required documentation should be maintained in the appropriate clinical record and should be submitted only upon request.

Documentation supporting the medical necessity of this item, such as ICD-9-CM codes, must be submitted with each claim. Claims submitted without such evidence will be denied as not medically necessary.

No special requirements are necessary with electronic claim submission.

Medicare Information

Payment may be made for a screening colonoscopy performed on an individual who is at high risk for colorectal cancer if 23 months have passed since the last screening. Payment will not be provided for a screening colonoscopy for an individual who is not at high risk for colorectal cancer.

Those individuals who are at high-risk for colorectal cancer include the following:

- A close relative (sibling, parent, or child) has had colorectal cancer or an adenomatous polyposis
- A family history of familial adenomatous polyposis
- A family history of hereditary nonpolyposis colorectal cancer
- A personal history of colorectal cancer
- A personal history of adenomatous polyps
- A history of inflammatory bowel disease including Crohn's disease or ulcerative colitis.

If, during the course of the screening colonoscopy, a lesion or growth is detected and is biopsied or removed, the physician should bill using the appropriate CPT code for a colonoscopy with biopsy or removal rather than HCPCS Level II code G0105 for a screening colonoscopy.

G0106

G0106 Colorectal cancer screening; alternative to G0104, screening sigmoidoscopy, barium enema

Lay Description

A colorectal screening for cancer is done via barium enema as an alternative to a screening sigmoidoscopy (G0104). This is a radiological exam of the large intestine carried out after the administration of a barium enema to instill the contrast medium into the colon. Fluoroscopy and x-rays are used to observe the images as the contrast fills the colon and helps the physician to diagnose cancer, even colitis, and other diseases. After the patient has emptied the colon, more films are taken.

Medicare Information

Medicare covers colorectal screening for cancer via barium enema once every four years for patients 50 years of age or older.

G0108-G0109

G0108 Diabetes outpatient self-management training services, individual, per 30 minutes
G0109 Diabetes outpatient self-management training services, group session (2 or more), per 30 minutes

Lay Description

These codes are for diabetes self-management training services, either individually as reported with G0108 or in a group of two or more as reported with G0109. Diabetes self-management training is done to teach the diabetic how to control and monitor blood glucose levels with the proper use of the monitoring device, dietary calculations and restrictions, and correct administration of diabetic medications. These codes are reported per 30 minute intervals.

G0117-G0118

G0117 Glaucoma screening for high risk patients furnished by an optometrist or ophthalmologist
G0118 Glaucoma screening for high risk patient furnished under the direct supervision of an optometrist or ophthalmologist

Lay Description

Glaucoma screening is done on a high-risk patient. Glaucoma is a progressive eye disorder, without signs or symptoms in its earlier stages, that leads to irreversible loss of vision. Aqueous pressure in the anterior chamber of a healthy eye remains constant even though it is continually being flushed and renewed. Too little or too much fluid can cause permanent damage. In a test for glaucoma, the patient drinks one quart of water after fasting and then the intraocular pressure of the eye is measured. The patient may also be placed in a dark room, where the eyes are rechecked once they have sufficiently dilated. This determines if fluids in the eyes are at proper levels. High risk factors are related to age, family history, and personal medical history, such as diabetes, previous eye injury, and use of certain medications such as steroids. Report G0117 for glaucoma screening done by an optometrist or ophthalmologist and G0118 for the screening done under the direct supervision of an optometrist or ophthalmologist.

Medicare Information

Medicare covers glaucoma screening exams once every 12 months for high risk individuals. Patients considered high risk under this benefit option include African-Americans age 50 and older, people with diabetes, and people with a family history of glaucoma. Claims should be reported with diagnosis code V80.1 *Special screening for neurological, eye, and ear diseases, glaucoma.*

G0120

G0120   Colorectal cancer screening; alternative to G0105, screening colonoscopy, barium enema

Lay Description

A colorectal screening for cancer is done via barium enema as an alternative to a screening colonoscopy on a high-risk individual (G0105). This is a radiological exam of the large intestine carried out after the administration of a barium enema to instill the contrast medium into the colon. Fluoroscopy and x-rays are used to observe the images as the contrast fills the colon and helps the physician to diagnose cancer, even colitis, and other diseases. After the patient has emptied the colon, more films are taken.

Documentation Standards

Hospital, outpatient, ASC or office records, or procedure reports should clearly state the pertinent history and physical exam, the reason for the procedure, the course of the examination, and the results.

Required documentation should be maintained in the appropriate clinical record and should be submitted only upon request.

Documentation supporting the medical necessity of this item, such as ICD-9-CM codes, must be submitted with each claim. Claims submitted without such evidence will be denied as not medically necessary.

No special requirements are necessary with electronic claim submission.

Medicare Information

Payment may be made for a screening colonoscopy performed on an individual who is at high risk for colorectal cancer if 23 months have passed since the last screening. Payment will not be provided for a screening colonoscopy for an individual who is not at high risk for colorectal cancer.

Those individuals who are at high-risk for colorectal cancer include the following:

- A close relative (sibling, parent, or child) has had colorectal cancer or an adenomatous polyposis
- A family history of familial adenomatous polyposis
- A family history of hereditary nonpolyposis colorectal cancer
- A personal history of colorectal cancer
- A personal history of adenomatous polyps
- A history of inflammatory bowel disease including Crohn's disease or ulcerative colitis.

G0121

G0121   Colorectal cancer screening; colonoscopy on individual not meeting criteria for high risk

Lay Description

A colonoscopy is done for colorectal cancer screening on a patient who does not meet high-risk criteria. This would be a patient without a diagnosis of ulcerative enteritis or without a history of malignant neoplasm of the lower gastrointestinal tract. After the patient's bowel has been prepped, the physician inserts the colonoscope through the anus and advances the scope through the colon past the splenic flexure. The lumen of the colon and rectum is visualized. Brushings or washings may be obtained. The colonoscope is withdrawn.

Documentation Standards

Hospital, outpatient, ASC or office records, or procedure reports should clearly state the pertinent history and physical exam, the reason for the procedure, the course of the examination, and the results.

Required documentation should be maintained in the appropriate clinical record and should be submitted only upon request.

Documentation supporting the medical necessity of this item, such as ICD-9-CM codes, must be submitted with each claim. Claims submitted without such evidence will be denied as not medically necessary.

No special requirements are necessary with electronic claim submission.

Medicare Information

Medicare covers a colonoscopy once every 10 years if the patient is not at high risk for colon cancer. Use code G0121 to indicate the patient is not at high risk.

G0122

G0122   Colorectal cancer screening; barium enema

Lay Description

A colorectal screening for cancer is done via barium enema. This is a radiological exam of the large intestine carried out after the administration of a barium enema to instill the contrast medium into the colon. Fluoroscopy and x-rays are used to observe the images as the contrast fills the colon and helps the physician to diagnose cancer, even colitis, and other diseases. After the patient has emptied the colon, more films are taken.

G0123-G0124

G0123   Screening cytopathology, cervical or vaginal (any reporting system), collected in preservative fluid, automated thin layer preparation, screening by cytotechnologist under physician supervision

G0124   Screening cytopathology, cervical or vaginal (any reporting system), collected in preservative fluid, automated thin layer preparation, requiring interpretation by physician

Lay Description

These cervical or vaginal cytopathology screenings (any reporting system) of specimens collected in preservative fluid may be identified as "thin prep." The specimen is collected by cervical, endocervical, or vaginal scrapings or by aspiration of vaginal fluid and cells. This method saves time by eliminating the need for the physician to prepare a smear; the specimen is placed in a preservative suspension instead. At the laboratory, special instruments take the cells in the preservative suspension and "plate-out" a monolayer for screening, which will carefully review the specimen for abnormal cells. Report G0123 for screening done under physician supervision by a cytotechnologist and G0124 for a thin layer prep screening that requires interpretation by a physician.

Medicare Information

A screening Pap smear is covered by Medicare every two years or annually if there is a high risk for cervical cancer.

G0127

G0127   Trimming of dystrophic nails, any number

Lay Description

A physician trims fingernails or toenails usually with scissors, nail cutters, or other instruments when the nails are defective and dystrophic from nutritional or metabolic abnormalities. Report this code for any number of nails trimmed.

G0128

G0128   Direct (face-to-face with patient) skilled nursing services of a registered nurse provided in a comprehensive outpatient rehabilitation facility, each 10 minutes beyond the first 5 minutes

Lay Description

This code reports direct one-on-one skilled nursing services provided to the patient by a registered nurse in a comprehensive outpatient rehabilitation facility. Report this code as a unit of 10 minutes, for each 10 minutes beyond the initial 5 minutes.

G0129

G0129   Occupational therapy services requiring the skills of a qualified occupational therapist, furnished as a component of a partial hospitalization treatment program, per session (45 minutes or more)

Lay Description

Occupational therapy focuses on helping a person recovering from a serious illness or injury retain movement capabilities for independently managing the activities of daily life. Code G0129 reports occupational therapy services performed by a qualified occupational therapist provided as a component of a partial hospitalization treatment program. Report this code per day that treatment was given.

Documentation Standards

Claims for group therapy services provided under the partial hospitalization program must provide evidence of patient participation and response to psychiatric group therapy services.

Medicare Information

Medicare covers occupational therapy furnished as a component of a partial hospitalization program and pays a per diem rate. Report the number of times the service or procedure, as defined by the HCPCS code, was performed. This HCPCS code cannot be billed with more than one unit of service.

Actual hands-on time is the only allowed time that can be billed. Time for documentation and care conferences is not billable OT time.

G0130

G0130 Single energy x-ray absorptiometry (SEXA) bone density study, one or more sites; appendicular skeleton (peripheral) (e.g., radius, wrist, heel)

Lay Description

Bone mineral density studies are used to evaluate diseases of bone and/or the responses of bone disease to treatment. Densities are measured at the wrist, radius, hip, pelvis, spine, or heel. The studies assess bone mass or density associated with such diseases as osteoporosis, osteomalacia, and renal osteodystrophy. Single energy x-ray absorptiometry (SEXA) utilizes an x-ray tube as the radiation source that is pulsed at a certain energy level. Single energy x-ray absorptiometry is used to scan bone that is in a superficial location with little adjacent soft tissue, such as the wrist or heel. There is a differential attenuation between bone and soft tissue for the energy beam. Excessive soft tissue renders the measurement incorrect. An attenuation profile of the bony components is calculated and the results are given in two scores, which are reported as standard deviations from the normal bone density of a person the same sex, 30 years old, which is the age of peak bone mass, and from the normal bone density of an "age matched" that compares your bone density to what is expected in someone of your age, sex, and size.

G0141, G0147-G0148

G0141 Screening cytopathology smears, cervical or vaginal, performed by automated system, with manual rescreening, requiring interpretation by physician

G0147 Screening cytopathology smears, cervical or vaginal, performed by automated system under physician supervision

G0148 Screening cytopathology smears, cervical or vaginal, performed by automated system with manual rescreening

Lay Description

These cervical or vaginal cytopathology screenings are done on specimens prepared in a smear. The specimen is collected by cervical, endocervical, or vaginal scrapings or by aspiration of vaginal fluid and cells. The screening method is microscopy examination of a spray or liquid fixated smear prepared by the physician collecting the specimen. Screening, defined as the careful review of the specimen for abnormal cells, may then be accomplished by different methods that involve the use of automated systems. Code G0141 should be used to report smears screened by an automated system followed by a manual rescreening and requiring the interpretation of a physician. Code G0147 is reported when the smear is screened by an automated system under physician supervision. Code G0148 is reported when automated screening is followed by manual rescreening and no physician interpretation is required.

Medicare Information

In G0141, the professional component (the interpretation) of abnormal Pap smears furnished to a hospital inpatient by a hospital physician or an independent laboratory is paid according to the physician fee schedule. Payment for Pap smears in all other situations is made under the clinical laboratory fee schedule. The Part B deductible and coinsurance for screening Pap services is not applicable.

Unless the advance notice provision is met, the patient is not liable for services denied as not medically necessary. The patient is also not liable for services that are denied as bundled into another service.

G0143-G0145

G0143 Screening cytopathology, cervical or vaginal (any reporting system), collected in preservative fluid, automated thin layer preparation, with manual screening and rescreening by cytotechnologist under physician supervision

G0144 Screening cytopathology, cervical or vaginal (any reporting system), collected in preservative fluid, automated thin layer preparation, with screening by automated system, under physician supervision

G0145 Screening cytopathology, cervical or vaginal (any reporting system), collected in preservative fluid, automated thin layer preparation, with screening by automated system and manual rescreening under physician supervision

Lay Description

These cervical or vaginal cytopathology screenings (any reporting system) of specimens collected in preservative fluid may be identified as "thin prep." The specimen is collected by cervical, endocervical, or vaginal scrapings or by aspiration of vaginal fluid and cells. This method saves time by eliminating the need for the physician to prepare a smear; the specimen is placed in a preservative suspension instead. At the laboratory, special instruments take the cells in the preservative suspension and "plate-out" a monolayer for screening, which will carefully review the specimen for abnormal cells. Report G0143 for manual screening with rescreening done under physician supervision by a cytotechnologist, G0144 for thin layer prep screening by an automated system under physician supervision, and G0145 for automated screening followed by manual rescreening done under physician supervision.

Medicare Information

In G0143, the professional component (the interpretation) of abnormal Pap smears furnished to a hospital inpatient by a hospital physician or an independent laboratory is paid according to the physician fee schedule. Payment for Pap smears in all other situations is made under the clinical laboratory fee schedule. The Part B deductible and coinsurance for screening Pap services is not applicable.

Unless the advance notice provision is met, the patient is not liable for services denied as not medically necessary. The patient is also not liable for services that are denied as bundled into another service.

G0147-G0148

G0147   Screening cytopathology smears, cervical or vaginal, performed by automated system under physician supervision

G0148   Screening cytopathology smears, cervical or vaginal, performed by automated system with manual rescreening

Lay Description

Please refer to code G0141 for the description, coding, and billing information.

Medicare Information

Please refer to code G0141 for the description, coding, and billing information.

G0151-G0156

G0151   Services performed by a qualified physical therapist in the home health or hospice setting, each 15 minutes

G0152   Services performed by a qualified occupational therapist in the home health or hospice setting, each 15 minutes

G0153   Services performed by a qualified speech-language pathologist in the home health or hospice setting, each 15 minutes

G0154   Direct skilled nursing services of a licensed nurse (LPN or RN) in the home health or hospice setting, each 15 minutes

G0155   Services of clinical social worker in home health or hospice settings, each 15 minutes

G0156   Services of home health/hospice aide in home health or hospice settings, each 15 minutes

Lay Description

These codes are for reporting various services provided by different types of qualified professionals in a home health setting in units of 15 minute increments. Home health includes not only traditional private home settings, but also assisted living quarters, group homes, custodial care facilities, or similar type settings that constitute the patient's place of residence. Report G0151 for services performed by a physical therapist, G0152 for services done by an occupational therapist, G0153 for services of a speech and language pathologist, G0154 for skilled nursing services, G0155 for the services of the clinical social worker, and G0156 for home health services provided by a home health aide.

G0166

G0166   External counterpulsation, per treatment session

Lay Description

External counterpulsation is a therapy for relieving angina and is also beneficial for congestive heart failure patients. The treatment increases blood flow into the arteries and decreases the work load of the heart. The therapy is believed to work by stimulating the growth of new blood vessels around the arteries in the heart that are blocked. The patient has compressive cuffs wrapped around his/her calves and upper and lower thighs. The cuffs inflate when the heart is filling with blood and deflate when the heart is ejecting blood. Treatment sessions last one hour and are usually for a period of five times a week for seven weeks. This code reports one treatment session.

Documentation Standards

The medical record documentation must support that the service was ordered by the physician for a patient with Class III or Class IV angina not amenable to surgical intervention. In addition, the documentation must support that the service was performed. This information is usually found in the history and physical, progress notes, and/or hospital/office notes.

Medicare Information

Medicare coverage is limited to its use in patients with stable anginal pectoris because this use has proven to be effective. The external counterpulsation (ECP) system must have effectively treated patients with severe angina in well-designated clinical trials. The procedure must be performed under the direct supervision of a physician.

G0168

G0168 Wound closure utilizing tissue adhesive(s) only

Lay Description

Wound closure done by using tissue adhesive only, not any kind of suturing or stapling, is reported with G0168. Tissue adhesives, such as Dermabond, are materials that are applied directly to the skin or tissue of an open wound to hold the margins closed for healing.

G0173

G0173 Linear accelerator based stereotactic radiosurgery, complete course of therapy in one session

Lay Description

Stereotactic radiosurgery is a form of computer-assisted radiation therapy for treating tumors or lesions, mainly intracranial, that are not accessible or suitable for open surgery, by high dosage radiation that employs exact three-dimensional location planning. This code reports linear accelerator based stereotactic radiosurgery that directs an extremely narrow x-ray beam from a machine that remains focused on the tumor volume of the lesion while the movement of the machine is carefully coordinated to distribute the beam entry points over a wider radius. Linear accelerators can deliver x-rays (photons) or electrons to a targeted area. Photons can target deeper lying tumor tissue, while electrons are used for the maximum dose of radiation near the skin surface, making the method suitable to treat skin, superficial lesions, and shallow tumor volumes where underlying tissues need to be protected. Use this code for a complete course of linear accelerator based stereotactic radiosurgery therapy in one session.

G0175

G0175 Scheduled interdisciplinary team conference (minimum of 3 exclusive of patient care nursing staff) with patient present

Lay Description

Use this code to report an interdisciplinary team conference with a minimum of three care giving professionals present, not counting the patient care nursing staff. The patient is also present. An interdisciplinary team is composed of professionals who are specialists in different areas and who work together to coordinate the care of patients whose medical condition has multiple diagnoses that require more than one focus of care from different or related fields.

Medicare modifiers

Modifier 27 is for hospital outpatient reporting purposes. The code is used to report the utilization of hospital resources related to separate and distinct E/M encounters performed in multiple outpatient hospital settings on the same date. This modifier is added to each appropriate level of outpatient and/or emergency department E/M code. It is used to report E/M services provided by physicians in more than one outpatient hospital setting.

G0176-G0177

G0176 Activity therapy, such as music, dance, art or play therapies not for recreation, related to the care and treatment of patient's disabling mental health problems, per session (45 minutes or more)

G0177 Training and educational services related to the care and treatment of patient's disabling mental health problems per session (45 minutes or more)

Lay Description

Activities engaging a patient in music, dance, art creations, or any type of play, not as recreation but as therapeutic processes for the care and treatment of a patient with disabling mental health problems, is reported with G0176 for every session of 45 minutes or more. Use G0177 for training and educational services related to the care and treatment of a patient with disabling mental health problems for every session of 45 minutes or more.

Documentation Standards

Claims for therapy services provided under the partial hospitalization program must provide evidence of patient participation and response to psychiatric therapy services.

Medicare Information
Medicare covers activity therapy and training and education services related to the care and treatment of patient's with disabling mental health problems. The payment is per session (45 minutes or more). Report the number of times the service or procedure, as defined by the HCPCS code, was performed.

G0179-G0180

G0179 Physician re-certification for Medicare-covered home health services under a home health plan of care (patient not present), including contacts with home health agency and review of reports of patient status required by physicians to affirm the initial implementation of the plan of care that meets patient's needs, per re-certification period

G0180 Physician certification for Medicare-covered home health services under a home health plan of care (patient not present), including contacts with home health agency and review of reports of patient status required by physicians to affirm the initial implementation of the plan of care that meets patient's needs, per certification period

Lay Description
Code G0179 reports one period of recertification and code G0180 is for one period of certification for a patient's qualifying status for Medicare-covered home health services under a home health plan of care by a physician, without the patient present. This includes all contacts made with the home health agency and reviewing of patient status reports required by physicians to affirm the initial implementation of the care plan designed to meet the patient's needs.

G0181-G0182

G0181 Physician supervision of a patient receiving Medicare-covered services provided by a participating home health agency (patient not present) requiring complex and multidisciplinary care modalities involving regular physician development and/or revision of care plans, review of subsequent reports of patient status, review of laboratory and other studies, communication (including telephone calls) with other health care professionals involved in the patient's care, integration of new information into the medical treatment plan and/or adjustment of medical therapy, within a calendar month, 30 minutes or more

G0182 Physician supervision of a patient under a Medicare-approved hospice (patient not present) requiring complex and multidisciplinary care modalities involving regular physician development and/or revision of care plans, review of subsequent reports of patient status, review of laboratory and other studies, communication (including telephone calls) with other health care professionals involved in the patient's care, integration of new information into the medical treatment plan and/or adjustment of medical therapy, within a calendar month, 30 minutes or more

Lay Description
Code G0181 reports 30 minutes or more of physician supervision of a patient receiving Medicare-covered services provided by a participating home health agency and code G0182 reports the same supervision of a patient under a Medicare-approved hospice. This includes complex and multidisciplinary care modalities involving regular physician development and/or revision of care plans, review of subsequent reports of patient status, review of laboratory and other studies, communication with other health care professionals involved in the patient's care, including all telephone calls, and integration of new information into the medical treatment plan and/or adjustment of medical therapy, within a calendar month. The patient is not present for the physician supervision.

G0186

G0186 Destruction of localized lesion of choroid (for example, choroidal neovascularization); photocoagulation, feeder vessel technique (one or more sessions)

Lay Description
The physician destroys a localized lesion of the choroid, such as choroidal neovascularization (CNV) due to age related macular degeneration, using extrafoveal laser photocoagulation of the feeder vessel providing blood supply to the CNV. The feeder vessel is identified by indocyanine green angiography and looks like a spot in the choroid that is seen to branch off into the CNV as a distinct blood vessel. The physician directs short spots of a laser's beam in a racquet-like pattern at the feeder vessel(s) that have grown beneath the macula to occlude or obliterate the vessel supplying blood flow to the lesion. One or two treatments may be necessary. The patient is followed-up with another angiography to

determine that there has been closure of the feeder vessel after treatment.

G0202-G0206

G0202   Screening mammography, producing direct digital image, bilateral, all views
G0204   Diagnostic mammography, producing direct digital image, bilateral, all views
G0206   Diagnostic mammography, producing direct digital image, unilateral, all views

Lay Description

Mammography is a radiographic technique used to diagnose breast cysts or tumors in women with current symptoms of breast disease or screen for lumps or masses before they are palpable in asymptomatic women. Mammography is done using a different type of x-ray than is used for routine exams that does not penetrate tissue as easily. The breast is compressed firmly between two planes and pictures are taken. This spreads the tissue and allows for a lower x-ray dose. Digital mammography stores the electronic image directly on a computer. Images are recorded digitally, without film, and can be magnified and enhanced, providing better images of the breast tissues. Small tumors and other early signs of cancer can be detected when treatment may be more effective. Use G0202 for digitally imaged mammography done on both breasts in an asymptomatic screening, all views. Report G0204 for digitally imaged mammography, all views, done on both breasts to diagnose any lumps or masses already presenting. Report G0206 for the same diagnostic mammography done on one breast.

Documentation Standards

Documentation must support the ICD-9-CM code submitted with each claim. If the ICD-9-CM code is not documented, the claim may be denied.

A clear, clinical indication for the diagnostic mammogram/breast sonogram/breast MRI/ductogram must be documented in the medical record, as well as in the referral order. A written referral is required for a diagnostic mammogram except when the diagnostic mammogram was initially performed as a screening.

The medical record must include a formal written report describing all of the views completed. The formal written report must include the reason for the test, a description of the test, the interpretation and results of the test, and the name of the physician to whom the report is being sent.

Medicare Information

Code G0202 was statutorily excluded from the Medicare Physician Fee Schedule (MPFS) until January 1, 2002. Payment was equal to the lesser of the actual charge or 150 percent of the locality specific payment for CPT code 76091 (bilateral mammography). On or after January 1, 2002, when G0202 is performed in a hospital outpatient department, a critical access hospital (CAH), or a skilled nursing facility (SNF), payment is to be made under the MPFS for the technical component. Coinsurance is the lesser of the actual charge or the fee schedule amount. The deductible is not applicable.

Prior to January 1, 2002, payment for G0204 and G0206 was based on the MPFS effective April 1, 2001. Payment was equal to the lesser of the actual charge or the locality specific fee schedule amount. On or after January 1, 2002, when G0204 or G0206 is performed in a hospital outpatient department, payment is to be made under the Outpatient Prospective Payment System (OPPS). Coinsurance will be based on the national coinsurance for the ambulatory payment classification (APC), wage adjusted for the specific hospital. When the technical component is performed in a CAH or SNF, payment will be made under the MPFS. Coinsurance will be based on the lower of the actual charge or the fee schedule amount. The deductible does apply to these services.

For dates of service on or after April 1, 2003, this service must be billed with 76090, 76090, G0204, or G0206.

All of the coverage criteria must be met before Medicare can reimburse for this service.

Refer to the Correct Coding Initiative for "bundling" information.

Modifier GG should be used to show that a diagnostic test was performed on the same day as a screening test (used for tracking purposes only; it indicates that the test changed from a screening test to a diagnostic test).

The ICD-9-CM diagnosis code must be present on any claim submitted and must be coded to the highest level of specificity.

Medicare modifiers

If the examination began as a screening mammogram and additional films were ordered based on abnormal results, the specific abnormality must be documented in the record. The GG modifier must be documented on the claim line with the CPT procedure code for a diagnostic mammogram.

G0219

G0219 PET imaging whole body; melanoma for noncovered indications

Lay Description

The whole body is imaged using data received from positron-emitting radionuclides administered to the patient in positron emission tomography (PET) imaging. The imaging relies upon capturing the gamma rays or the positively charged particles and photons, emitted by the decaying radionuclide. The collision of the positrons emitted by the radionuclide with the negatively-charged electrons normally present in body tissue is computer synthesized to produce an image, usually in vivid color, that will show the presence of cancer in tissue through the altered cell function caused by the disease and not simply from anatomical structure changes. PET imaging produces real time functional images of the metabolic processes of body tissue, such as glucose metabolism, and shows precisely where changes induced by a disease are taking place. This code is for whole body imaging the of the entire body seeking regional lymph nodes with increased activity that may indicate that a diagnosed melanoma has metastasized.

G0235

G0235 PET imaging, any site, not otherwise specified

Lay Description

The whole body or body region is imaged using data received from positron-emitting radionuclides administered to the patient in positron emission tomography (PET) imaging. The imaging relies upon capturing the gamma rays or the positively charged particles, photons, emitted by the decaying radionuclide. This detection can be done by using stationary single or double-headed gamma cameras or by rotating a detector, or scanner, around the patient as is done with full and partial-ring bismuth germinate (BGO), sodium iodide (NAI), or crystal detector PET scanner systems. The collision of the positrons emitted by the radionuclide with the negatively-charged electrons normally present in body tissue is computer synthesized to produce an image, usually in vivid color, that will show the presence of cancer in tissue through the altered cell function caused by the disease and not simply from anatomical structure changes. PET imaging produces real time functional images of the metabolic processes of body tissue, such as glucose metabolism, and shows precisely where changes induced by a disease are taking place. This code is for PET imaging of any site not otherwise specified. Not otherwise specified codes are used only when a more specific code is not available to report the service.

G0237-G0239

G0237 Therapeutic procedures to increase strength or endurance of respiratory muscles, face-to-face, one-on-one, each 15 minutes (includes monitoring)

G0238 Therapeutic procedures to improve respiratory function, other than described by G0237, one-on-one, face-to-face, per 15 minutes (includes monitoring)

G0239 Therapeutic procedures to improve respiratory function or increase strength or endurance of respiratory muscles, 2 or more individuals (includes monitoring)

Lay Description

These codes are for therapeutic procedures such as special breathing exercises, performed under the supervision of a therapist, intended to increase the strength or endurance of the respiratory muscles in G0237, and to improve overall respiratory functioning in the patient (other than described in G0237) in G0238. These two codes are reported once for each 15 minutes of individual, one-on-one, face-to-face, therapy time. Report G0239 for special therapeutic exercises intended to increase the strength or endurance of respiratory muscles or improve overall respiratory functioning done under the supervision of a therapist in a group setting of two or more individuals. All codes include monitoring.

Documentation Standards

It may be reasonable and necessary for multiple clinicians to address a patient's particular needs on a physician's order. Each clinician must perform a unique, individualized skilled evaluation within his/her scope of practice and specific area of expertise. Each initial evaluation will identify the problems, develop a specific plan of treatment, and set specific goals.

All documentation must demonstrate clinical rationale for skilled intervention. Clinicians are required to document all activities, tasks, instruction, and treatment provided. This documentation must be done each time the patient receives any pulmonary rehabilitation (PR) service. Team conferences are to occur at the beginning and end of PR. Team conferences may occur during rehabilitation as needed. The patient's progress toward achieving the short-term goals should be assessed at these conferences.

The physician's documentation must be legible and must be maintained in the patient's medical record.

Patients with other severe or chronic pulmonary disorders (e.g., lung cancer, neuromuscular diseases, lung transplant, scoliosis, kyphoscoliosis, etc.) may benefit from PR. Some patients may not meet the medical criteria, yet still be appropriate for PR because of other severe or chronic disorders. All such cases will be reviewed on an individual basis.

The following administrative costs are not line item billable. They are considered indirect costs of providing PR services:

- Teaching and education done by a physician or pharmacist
- Dietary/nutritional counseling
- Social services
- Team and/or family conferences
- Documentation time
- Discharge summaries
- Educational books, pamphlets, audio/video tapes, CDs, DVDs, other computer software, or any other materials not considered medical supplies

Medicare coverage for pulmonary rehabilitation services is limited to services provided by those professionals who meet the Medicare personnel qualifications. These include physicians, registered nurses, licensed practical nurses, occupational therapists, occupational therapy assistants, physical therapists, physical therapy assistants, and respiratory therapists. It does not include services provided by therapy aides, exercise physiologists, or physical trainers. Speech/language pathologists, who may occasionally treat patients to improve respiratory function as part of their treatment of speech and language disorders, should code their services with 92507 *Treatment of speech, language, voice, communication, and/or auditory processing disorder.* Medicare coverage will not be extended to speech/language pathologists who bill for pulmonary rehabilitation services.

Medicare Information

Medicare covers the clinical conditions when positron emission tomography utilizes FDG as a tracer. Carrier billing is on the CMS-1500 form, using appropriate HCPCS G codes on the claim with type of service (TOS) 4, diagnostic radiology.

Medicare modifiers

Modifier GO should be used for services delivered personally by an occupational therapist or under an outpatient occupational therapy Plan of Care.

Modifier GP should be used for services delivered personally by a physical therapist or under an outpatient physical therapy Plan of Care.

G0245-G0246

G0245   Initial physician evaluation and management of a diabetic patient with diabetic sensory neuropathy resulting in a loss of protective sensation (LOPS) which must include: (1) the diagnosis of LOPS, (2) a patient history, (3) a physical examination that consists of at least the following elements: (a) visual inspection of the forefoot, hindfoot, and toe web spaces, (b) evaluation of a protective sensation, (c) evaluation of foot structure and biomechanics, (d) evaluation of vascular status and skin integrity, and (e) evaluation and recommendation of footwear, and (4) patient education

G0246   Follow-up physician evaluation and management of a diabetic patient with diabetic sensory neuropathy resulting in a loss of protective sensation (LOPS) to include at least the following: (1) a patient history, (2) a physical examination that includes: (a) visual inspection of the forefoot, hindfoot, and toe web spaces, (b) evaluation of protective sensation, (c) evaluation of foot structure and biomechanics, (d) evaluation of vascular status and skin integrity, and (e) evaluation and recommendation of footwear, and (3) patient education

Lay Description

Physician evaluation and management is given to a diabetic patient with diabetic sensory neuropathy resulting in a loss of protective sensation, including all of the following in addition to the initial diagnosis of lops: a patient history; patient education; and a physical examination consisting of at least visual inspection of the forefoot, hindfoot, and toe web spaces, evaluation of protective sensation, foot structure, and biomechanics, as well as vascular status and skin integrity, and evaluation and recommendation of footwear. Report G0246 for physician evaluation and management with all of the same criteria as a follow up on a diabetic patient with the established diagnosis of lops.

Documentation Standards

Documentation in the medical record must contain:

- A patient history
- A physical examination that must include at least the following elements:
    - Visual inspection of forefoot and hindfoot (including toe web spaces)
    - Evaluation of protective sensation

- Evaluation of foot structure and biomechanics
- Evaluation of vascular status and skin integrity
- Evaluation of the need for special footwear
• Patient education

Medicare Information
Medicare covers the evaluation services of the feet for people with diabetic peripheral neuropathy with loss of protective sedation. Code G0247 cannot be billed alone. It must be billed with either G0245 or G0246 with the same date of service. The evaluation services are covered no more often than every six months and the patient cannot have seen any other foot care specialist in the interim.

G0247

G0247 Routine foot care by a physician of a diabetic patient with diabetic sensory neuropathy resulting in a loss of protective sensation (LOPS) to include the local care of superficial wounds (i.e., superficial to muscle and fascia) and at least the following, if present: (1) local care of superficial wounds, (2) debridement of corns and calluses, and (3) trimming and debridement of nails

Lay Description
Routine foot care is provided by a physician to a diabetic patient with diabetic sensory neuropathy resulting in a loss of protective sensation and must include, when present, all of the following: local care of superficial wounds, debridement of corns and calluses, and trimming and debridement of nails.

G0248-G0250

G0248 Demonstration, prior to initiation of home INR monitoring, for patient with either mechanical heart valve(s), chronic atrial fibrillation, or venous thromboembolism who meets Medicare coverage criteria, under the direction of a physician; includes: face-to-face demonstration of use and care of the INR monitor, obtaining at least one blood sample, provision of instructions for reporting home INR test results, and documentation of patient's ability to perform testing and report results

G0249 Provision of test materials and equipment for home INR monitoring of patient with either mechanical heart valve(s), chronic atrial fibrillation, or venous thromboembolism who meets Medicare coverage criteria; includes: provision of materials for use in the home and reporting of test results to physician; testing not occurring more frequently than once a week; testing materials, billing units of service include 4 tests

G0250 Physician review, interpretation, and patient management of home INR testing for patient with either mechanical heart valve(s), chronic atrial fibrillation, or venous thromboembolism who meets Medicare coverage criteria; testing not occurring more frequently than once a week; billing units of service include 4 tests

Lay Description
Patients with a mechanical heart valve, chronic atrial fibrillation, or venous thromboembolism are at risk of developing intracardiac or intravascular thrombi and are frequently managed with long-term use of warfarin anticoagulation. Periodic monitoring is necessary to maintain a therapeutic effect of the anticoagulation treatment and reduce thromboembolic and hemorrhagic events. The use of the internationalized normalized ratio (INR) (rather than the prothrombin time) provides a result that is independent of the laboratory reagents used. The INR is the ratio of the patient's prothrombin time compared to the mean prothrombin time for a group of normal individuals. Patient self-testing and self-management through the use of a home INR monitor improve the time in therapeutic rate and hence clinical outcomes. Portable coagulometers that measure the prothrombin time and calculate the INR with the use of a drop of whole blood allow the patient to do self testing. Report G0248 for demonstration of the INR monitor before the first use. Code G0249 reports the provision of test materials and equipment for INR monitoring used in the home, including reporting of test results to the physician for patients who meet Medicare coverage criteria. Code G0250 reports the physician review, interpretation, and patient management for home INR testing, requiring one face-to-face verification by the physician at least once a year (e.g., during an evaluation and management service).

Medicare Information
Home prothrombin time international normalized ratio (INR) monitoring is covered for patients with mechanical heart valves who are on warfarin therapy. A physician must prescribe the monitor and the patient must meet the following criteria:

• Must have been on anticoagulant therapy for at least three months prior to the use of the home INR device

• Must undergo an educational program on anticoagulant management and the use of the device prior to its use in the home

- Must self test with the device only once per week

CMS considers home INR monitoring to be a CLIA-waived diagnostic test. It is not considered DME and cannot be paid by the DME MAC. A hospital or a physician may provide the device, test materials, and education. Claims for home INR monitors will be processed and paid by fiscal intermediaries and physician carriers only. Coverage became effective July 1, 2002.

The cost of the device and supplies are included in the payment for G0249 and are not separately billable to Medicare.

Medicare will allow hospitals to bill up to 3 units of G0249 at a time in order to cover up to 12 tests so that the service is billable on a date when a patient would attend the clinic for a face-to-face visit.

Hospitals may report these services under revenue code 920 or may report G0248 and G0249 under the revenue center where they are performed.

G0251

G0251 Linear accelerator based stereotactic radiosurgery, delivery including collimator changes and custom plugging, fractionated treatment, all lesions, per session, maximum 5 sessions per course of treatment

Lay Description

Linear accelerator based stereotactic radiosurgery is a form of computer-assisted radiation therapy for treating tumors or lesions that are not accessible or suitable for open surgery by high dosage radiation that employs exact three-dimensional location planning. Narrow beams of radiation are directed through a guiding device attached to the patient's head to destroy the appropriate area. When a linear accelerator is used, the extremely narrow x-ray beam from the machine remains focused on the tumor volume of the lesion while the movement of the machine is carefully coordinated to distribute the beam entry points over a wider radius. Linear accelerators can deliver x-rays (photons) or electrons to a targeted area. Photons can target deeper lying tumor tissue, while electrons are used for the maximum dose of radiation near the skin surface, making the method suitable to treat skin, superficial lesions, and shallow tumor volumes where underlying tissues need to be protected. This code is for the delivery of such treatment including collimator changes and custom plugging or blocking, which is a form of shield made from a special energy-absorbing material calculated to protect healthy tissue surrounding the treatment area. Use this code for fractionated treatment, per session, all lesions, up to five sessions for the entire course of treatment.

G0252

G0252 PET imaging, full and partial-ring PET scanners only, for initial diagnosis of breast cancer and/or surgical planning for breast cancer (e.g., initial staging of axillary lymph nodes)

Lay Description

Positron emission tomography (PET) is a noninvasive diagnostic imaging procedure that assesses the level of metabolic activity and perfusion in various organ systems. Initial staging is when a cancers stage remains in question after a standard diagnostic workup, including conventional imaging (computed tomography, magnetic resonance imaging, or ultrasound). PET is used to diagnose cancer when it is expected that conventional imaging is not sufficient for the patient's clinical management and when the patient's clinical management could differ depending on the cancers stage. Report G0252 for PET imaging used for the initial diagnosis of breast cancer and/or surgical planning for breast cancer (e.g., initial staging of axillary lymph nodes).

G0255

G0255 Current perception threshold/sensory nerve conduction test, (SNCT) per limb, any nerve

Lay Description

Current Perception Threshold/Sensory Nerve Conduction Threshold (CPT/SNCT) test diagnosis sensory neurological impairments caused by various pathological conditions or toxic substance exposures. It is a noninvasive test that uses transcutaneous electrical stimulus to evoke a sensation. CPT/SNCT methods quantitate the level of sensory deficit by comparing current output to the nerve conduction threshold, but has the problem, however, that significant variability occurs associated with changing skin resistance. Sensory nerve conduction testing based on the concept that nerves are voltage sensitive can be done to quantitate sensory function with an instrument that provides voltage mediated testing (V-SNCT). It painlessly gathers enough objective data so measurements of subtle changes preceding gross morbidity can be detected. This method measures the actual instigator of nerve conduction - voltage and the results are independent of changes in skin resistance. Report this per limb tested, any nerve.

G0257

G0257 Unscheduled or emergency dialysis treatment for an ESRD patient in a hospital outpatient department that is not certified as an ESRD facility

Lay Description

Dialysis is a process to remove toxins from the blood and to maintain fluid and electrolyte balance when the kidneys no longer function. The patient's blood is removed through a previously placed catheter, pumped through a dialysis machine, and returned to the patient through a second catheter. This code is for an unscheduled or emergency dialysis treatment for a patient with end stage renal disease (ESRD) in a hospital outpatient department that has not been certified as an ESRD facility.

G0259-G0260

G0259 Injection procedure for sacroiliac joint; arthrography
G0260 Injection procedure for sacroiliac joint; provision of anesthetic, steroid and/or other therapeutic agent, with or without arthrography

Lay Description

The physician injects the sacroiliac joint for the purpose of arthrography, which is taking radiographic pictures of the joint internally to visualize the cartilage and ligaments. The contrast material, or gas, is drawn into a syringe and the target structure is localized. Through a posterior approach, the needle is inserted and advanced into the sacroiliac joint, the articulation between the sacrum and ilium in the pelvis, and the contrast injection is visualized under the aid of separately reportable computerized tomography (CT) or fluoroscopic guidance. Report G0260 when an anesthetic, steroid and/or other therapeutic agent is provided in the joint injection for arthrography.

G0268

G0268 Removal of impacted cerumen (one or both ears) by physician on same date of service as audiologic function testing

Lay Description

Under direct visualization, the physician removes impacted cerumen (earwax) using suction, a cerumen spoon, or delicate forceps. If no infection is present, the ear canal may be irrigated. This is done on the same day that the physician performs an audiologic function test.

G0269

G0269 Placement of occlusive device into either a venous or arterial access site, postsurgical or interventional procedure (e.g., angioseal plug, vascular plug)

Lay Description

Incisions into arteries and veins must be closed by suture or a device to stem the loss of blood. Such incisions are frequently made during angioplasties and diagnostic radiological procedures. An occlusive device is a plug or stopper used to close an incision into an artery or vein. This code is intended only for devices such as an angioseal or vascular plug. It should not be used for procedures such as vascular or pseudoaneurysm repair.

G0270-G0271

G0270 Medical nutrition therapy; reassessment and subsequent intervention(s) following second referral in same year for change in diagnosis, medical condition or treatment regimen (including additional hours needed for renal disease), individual, face-to-face with the patient, each 15 minutes
G0271 Medical nutrition therapy, reassessment and subsequent intervention(s) following second referral in same year for change in diagnosis, medical condition, or treatment regimen (including additional hours needed for renal disease), group (2 or more individuals), each 30 minutes

Lay Description

These codes report reassessment and interventions in a patient's medical nutrition therapy when a person has had a change in diagnosis or his/her medical condition and/or treatment regimen, following a second referral in the same year because of the change. Additional hours needed for renal disease cases are included. Report G0270 for each 15-minute block of time spent face to face with an individual patient and G0271 for each unit of 30 minutes spent in a group of two or more.

Documentation Standards

Medical record documentation must include and adhere to all of the following standards:

- The physician managing the beneficiary's diabetes condition must certify in writing that such services are needed, under a comprehensive plan of care related to the beneficiary's diabetes condition, to ensure therapy compliance or to provide the individual with necessary skills and knowledge in the management of his/her condition.

- The development and updating of an individualized assessment for each participant.
- The development of an individualized education plan.
- The assessment, intervention evaluation, and follow-up for each participant documented in progress notes placed in a permanent medical record, by all those directly involved with providing the services (e.g., attending physician, clinical nurse specialist, nurse practitioner, dietitian, social worker, and so forth). This information should be available and generally submitted for reconsideration only (or with the claim if the services are unusual or if a rejection is anticipated).
- Documentation supporting the medical necessity of this item, such as ICD-9-CM diagnostic codes, must be submitted with each claim. Claims submitted without such evidence will be denied as not medically necessary.

No special requirements are necessary with electronic claims submission.

Medicare Information

Medicare covers additional medical nutrition therapy (MNT) if there is a documented change in the beneficiary's medical condition and a referral is provided. The patient must have a diagnosis of either diabetes or renal disease. When provided by a registered dietitian or other nutrition professional, payment for MNT services is based on 80 percent of the actual charge, or 80 percent of 85 percent of the physician fee schedule amount, whichever is less. Registered dietitians and nutrition professionals must accept assignment.

G0275

G0275 Renal angiography, nonselective, one or both kidneys, performed at the same time as cardiac catheterization and/or coronary angiography, includes positioning or placement of any catheter in the abdominal aorta at or near the origins (ostia) of the renal arteries, injection of dye, flush aortogram, production of permanent images, and radiologic supervision and interpretation (List separately in addition to primary procedure)

Lay Description

The renal artery for one or both kidneys is radiologically examined using contrast material at the same time as cardiac catheterization. The catheter that has been threaded over the guidewire from the access site is positioned non-selectively in the abdominal aorta or near the origins of the renal arteries. Contrast medium is injected and a series of permanent images are taken to visualize the vessels and evaluate any abnormalities. A flush aortogram is included. The catheter is directed to the aorta and dye is injected as x-rays are taken to look for plaque build-up. The catheter is removed and pressure applied to the site. Radiological supervision and interpretation is included. List this separately in addition to the code for the main cardiac catheterization procedure.

G0278

G0278 Iliac and/or femoral artery angiography, nonselective, bilateral or ipsilateral to catheter insertion, performed at the same time as cardiac catheterization and/or coronary angiography, includes positioning or placement of the catheter in the distal aorta or ipsilateral femoral or iliac artery, injection of dye, production of permanent images, and radiologic supervision and interpretation (List separately in addition to primary procedure)

Lay Description

An iliac artery is radiologically examined using contrast material at the same time as cardiac catheterization. The catheter that has been threaded over the guidewire from the access site is positioned non-selectively in the distal aorta or iliac artery. Contrast medium is injected and a series of permanent images are taken to visualize the vessels and evaluate any abnormalities. The catheter is removed and pressure applied to the site. Radiological supervision and interpretation is included. List this code separately in addition to the code for the main cardiac catheterization procedure.

G0281-G0282

G0281 Electrical stimulation, (unattended), to one or more areas, for chronic Stage III and Stage IV pressure ulcers, arterial ulcers, diabetic ulcers, and venous stasis ulcers not demonstrating measurable signs of healing after 30 days of conventional care, as part of a therapy plan of care

G0282 Electrical stimulation, (unattended), to one or more areas, for wound care other than described in G0281

Lay Description

Electrical stimulation is the use of electric current that mimics the body's own natural bioelectric system's current when injured and will jump start or accelerate the wound healing process by attracting the body's repair cells, changing cell membrane permeability and hence cellular secretion, and orientating cell structures. A current is generated between the skin and inner tissues when there is a break in the skin. The current is kept flowing until the open skin defect is repaired. There may be different types of electricity used, controlled by different electrical sources. A moist wound environment is required for capacitatively coupled electrical stimulation, which involves using a surface electrode pad in wet contact (capacitatively coupled) with the external skin surface and/or wound bed. Two electrodes are required to complete the electric circuit and are usually placed over a wet conductive medium in the wound bed and on the skin away from the wound. One of the most safe and effective wavelengths used is monophasic twin peaked high voltage pulsed current (HVPC), allowing for selection of polarity, variation in pulse rates, and very short pulse duration. Significant changes in tissue pH and temperature are avoided, which is good for healing. Use G0281 for electrical stimulation to one or more areas for chronic stage III and IV pressure ulcers, arterial ulcers, diabetic ulcers, and venous stasis ulcers that do not demonstrate measurable signs of healing after 30 days of conventional care and G0282 for wounds other than stated in G0281.

Documentation Standards

Each claim must be submitted with ICD-9-CM diagnosis codes that reflect the condition of the patient and indicate the reason for which the service was performed. Claims submitted without ICD-9-CN diagnosis codes will be returned.

All providers performing CT scans on a mobile unit must maintain a record of the attending physician's order.

The medical records supporting the necessity for performing CT's, as well as the CT scan report, must be made available to the carrier upon request.

When a CT scan and MRI are performed on the same day for the same anatomical area, the medical record must clearly reflect the medical necessity for performing both tests.

Medicare Information

Electrical stimulation for the treatment of chronic stage III or IV pressure ulcers, arterial ulcers, diabetic ulcers, and venous stasis ulcers will be covered effective April 1, 2003. However, this modality will not be covered for the initial treatment of any other type of wound.

Coverage for electrical stimulation is provided only when an appropriate standard of wound care has been attempted for at least 30 days with no signs of healing. When electrical stimulation is being used, the physician must evaluate the wound at least every 30 days. Treatment is not covered if the wound fails to respond to electrical stimulation treatment within a 30–day period or when a 100 percent epithelialized wound bed is established.

G0283

G0283 Electrical stimulation (unattended), to one or more areas for indication(s) other than wound care, as part of a therapy plan of care

Lay Description

Electrical stimulation is the application of low doses of electrical current used or studied for many different applications. The electrical current may be direct current (DC), alternating current (AC), pulsed current (PC), pulsed electromagnetic induction, and spinal cord stimulation. The electrodes, leads, or devices are attached to the patient and the treatment started, but the therapist does not have to be present. This code should be used only when wound care is not the intended result. The electrical stimulation must be part of a plan of treatment for the patient.

Documentation Standards

The medical record must identify the physician responsible for the general medical care.

The services must be furnished according to a written treatment plan determined by the physician or by the therapist who will provide the treatment after an appropriate assessment of the condition (illness or injury). All providers rendering therapy must document the appropriate history, examination, diagnosis, functional assessment, type of treatment, the body areas to be treated, the date that therapy was initiated, and expected frequency and number of treatments.

Documentation should indicate the prognosis for potential restoration of function in a reasonable and generally predictable period of time or the need to establish a safe and effective maintenance program.

When both a modality/procedure and an evaluation service are billed, the evaluation may be reimbursed if the medical necessity for the evaluation is clearly documented. Standard medical practice may be one or two visits in addition to physical therapy treatments. Reimbursement beyond this standard utilization requires documentation supporting the medical necessity for the office visit.

Patients receiving services from independent physical or occupational therapists require reviews (dated and signed) of the treatment plan by the attending physician at least every 30 days.

Documentation supporting the medical necessity should be legible, maintained in the patient's medical record, and must be made available to Medicare upon request.

Medicare Information

Electrical stimulation for the treatment of chronic stage III or IV pressure ulcers, arterial ulcers, diabetic ulcers, and venous stasis ulcers will be covered effective April 1, 2003. However, this modality will not be covered for the initial treatment of any other type of wound.

Coverage for electrical stimulation is provided only when an appropriate standard of wound care has been attempted for at least 30 days with no signs of healing. When electrical stimulation is being used, the physician must evaluate the wound at least every 30 days. Treatment is not covered if the wound fails to respond to electrical stimulation treatment within a 30–day period or when a 100 percent epithelialized wound bed is established.

G0288

G0288 Reconstruction, computed tomographic angiography of aorta for surgical planning for vascular surgery

Lay Description

Report this code for the computer reconstruction of computerized tomography (CT) generated angiographic images of the aorta for the purpose of planning vascular surgery.

G0289

G0289 Arthroscopy, knee, surgical, for removal of loose body, foreign body, debridement/shaving of articular cartilage (chondroplasty) at the time of other surgical knee arthroscopy in a different compartment of the same knee

Lay Description

A surgical knee arthroscopy is done with removal of loose or foreign bodies and debridement of articular cartilage at the same surgical session as other arthroscopy done in a separate compartment of the knee. The physician makes 1.0 cm long portal incisions on either side of the patellar tendon for arthroscopic access into the knee joint. Any loose bodies (fragments of cartilage or bone) encountered are removed through the portal incisions. Small loose bodies are suctioned or irrigated from the joint. Larger loose or foreign bodies are grasped by a clamp and removed. A chondroplasty is done to debride or shave the partially fragmented or unstable articular cartilage with a motorized suction cutter. This smoothes the roughened or damaged cartilage and promotes bleeding and regeneration of cartilage. The joint is thoroughly flushed. A temporary drain may be applied and incisions are closed with sutures.

G0290-G0291

G0290 Transcatheter placement of a drug eluting intracoronary stent(s), percutaneous, with or without other therapeutic intervention, any method; single vessel

G0291 Transcatheter placement of a drug eluting intracoronary stent(s), percutaneous, with or without other therapeutic intervention, any method; each additional vessel

Lay Description

A drug-eluting intracoronary stent is placed percutaneously. A needle is inserted through the skin into the access blood vessel and a guidewire is threaded through the needle into the target coronary blood vessel. The needle is removed. A catheter with a stent-transporting tip is threaded over the guidewire into the vessel area requiring additional support through stent placement. The wire is then extracted and the compressed stent is passed from the catheter into the vessel, where it expands to support the vessel walls. The stent itself contains a drug that releases over time within the blood vessel and deters the build-up of plaque within the artery and/or helps prevent the formation of scar tissue and changes in the arterial wall. The catheter is then removed and pressure is applied over the puncture site to stop bleeding. Code G0290 is used for transcatheter placement of a drug-eluting agent into a single vessel and G0291 is reported in addition to G0290 once for every additional vessel.

G0293-G0294

G0293 Noncovered surgical procedure(s) using conscious sedation, regional, general, or spinal anesthesia in a Medicare qualifying clinical trial, per day

G0294 Noncovered procedure(s) using either no anesthesia or local anesthesia only, in a Medicare qualifying clinical trial, per day

Lay Description

Clinical trials are tests of a new procedure or drug using human patients to determine its effectiveness, side effects, and optimal dosage levels. Report G0293 for the use of the facility, staff time, and related supplies and drugs associated with an experimental procedure performed under regional, general, or spinal anesthesia. Report G0294 for the use of the facility, staff time, and related supplies and drugs associated with an experimental procedure performed without any type of anesthesia or under a local spinal anesthesia. These are daily charges and should not be reported more than once per calendar day.

Medicare Information
Effective January 1, 2003, Medicare began to cover the procedures associated with a qualified clinical trial.

G0295
G0295   Electromagnetic therapy, to one or more areas, for wound care other than described in G0329 or for other uses

Lay Description
Electromagnetic therapy is the application of low doses of electromagnetic current into the body. It is a form of electrical stimulation that is used for many different applications, including helping to heal wounds that have not been responding to conventional care. This code covers electromagnetic therapy applied for would care that is not any type of chronic stage III or IV ulcer.

Medicare Information
Medicare will cover electrical stimulation for the treatment of wounds only for chronic Stage III or Stage IV pressure ulcers, arterial ulcers, diabetic ulcers, and venous stasis ulcers. All other uses of electrical stimulation for the treatment of wounds are not covered by Medicare. Electrical stimulation will not be covered as an initial treatment modality.

The use of electrical stimulation will only be covered after appropriate standard wound care has been tried for at least 30 days and there are no measurable signs of healing. If electrical stimulation is being used, wounds must be evaluated periodically by the treating physician, but no less than every 30 days by a physician. Continued treatment with electrical stimulation is not covered if measurable signs of healing have not been demonstrated within any 30–day period of treatment. Additionally, electrical stimulation must be discontinued when the wound demonstrates a 100 percent epithelialized wound bed.

G0302-G0305
G0302   Preoperative pulmonary surgery services for preparation for LVRS, complete course of services, to include a minimum of 16 days of services

G0303   Preoperative pulmonary surgery services for preparation for LVRS, 10 to 15 days of services

G0304   Preoperative pulmonary surgery services for preparation for LVRS, 1 to 9 days of services

G0305   Postdischarge pulmonary surgery services after LVRS, minimum of 6 days of services

Lay Description
Lung volume reduction surgery (LVRS) is an invasive procedure to reduce the volume of a hyperinflated lung, allowing the underlying lung to expand to improve respiratory function. LRVS may also be called reduction pneumoplasty, lung shaving, or lung contouring. The procedure may be performed on patients with severe upper lobe predominant emphysema, or those with severe non-upper lobe emphysema with low exercise capacity. Report G0302 for preoperative services of 16 days or more; G0303 for preoperative services of 10-15 days; G0304 for preoperative services of one to nine days. Code G0305 reports post-operative services, which must be performed for a minimum of six days.

Medicare Information
Medicare coverage of this procedure began January 1, 2004 as a result of findings of the National Emphysema Treatment Trial (NETT). Medicare-covered LVRS approaches are limited to bilateral excision of a damaged lung with stapling performed via median sternotomy or video-assisted thoracoscopic surgery. Strict coverage criteria governs this procedure. The surgery must be performed at facilities identified by the National Heart, Lung, and Blood Institute to meet participation thresholds for NETT, and at sites that have been approved by Medicare as lung transplant facilities. The surgery must be preceded and followed by a program of diagnostic and therapeutic services consistent with those provided in the NETT. These services are designed to maximize the patient's potential to successfully undergo and recover from surgery. The program must include a six to ten-week series of at least 16, and no more than 20, preoperative sessions, each lasting a minimum of two hours. It must also include at least six, and no more than ten, postoperative sessions, each lasting a minimum of two hours, within eight to nine weeks of the LVRS.

G0306-G0307

G0306 Complete CBC, automated (HgB, HCT, RBC, WBC, without platelet count) and automated WBC differential count

G0307 Complete (CBC), automated (HgB, Hct, RBC, WBC; without platelet count)

Lay Description

A complete blood count (CBC) is a series of tests of peripheral blood that measure the hematocrit, hemoglobulin, red blood cell count (RBC), white blood cell count (WBC), and the proportion of different white cells as they appear on a blood smear. The CBC may or may not include an enumeration of platelets within the specimen. A WBC differential count is an enumeration, expressed as a percentage, of the different types of white blood cells, (e.g., leukocytes) which are present in a specific blood specimen. Both assays may be performed manually or automated. Report G0306 when the tests performed on a specific blood sample are an automated CBC that does not contain a platelet count, and an automated WBC differential. Report G0307 when the tests performed are an automated CBC that does not contain a platelet count, and when no WBC differential is performed.

Consolidated Billing

When the automated CBC with an automated WBC differential does include a platelet count, use CPT code 85025. An automated CBC with a platelet count and without a WBC differential is reported using CPT code 85027.

G0328

G0328 Colorectal cancer screening; fecal occult blood test, immunoassay, 1-3 simultaneous determinations

Lay Description

Colorectal cancer screening is a preventive measure to detect precancerous signs in the colon and rectum. A fecal-occult blood test is an examination that detects the presence of blood in the stool that cannot be seen with the naked eye. An immunoassay detects the presence of antigen or antibodies. Several methods of screening may be performed, including colonoscopy, barium enema, and fecal-occult blood tests. This code includes the use of a spatula or special brush to collect the appropriate number of samples.

Medicare Information

Effective for services furnished on or after January 1, 2004, Medicare payment may be made for fecal-occult blood immunoassays of one to three simultaneous determinations. The immunoassays must be performed in place of guaiac (reagent)-based test (G0107). Patients must be fifty years of age or older. Coverage is limited to one test every twelve months. The test requires a written order from the patient's attending physician.

G0329

G0329 Electromagnetic therapy, to one or more areas for chronic Stage III and Stage IV pressure ulcers, arterial ulcers, diabetic ulcers and venous stasis ulcers not demonstrating measurable signs of healing after 30 days of conventional care as part of a therapy plan of care

Lay Description

Electromagnetic therapy is a distinct form of treatment using application of electromagnetic fields rather than direct electrical current. Electromagnetic therapy is used for wound treatment for Stage III and/or Stage IV pressure ulcers, arterial ulcers, diabetic ulcers, and venous stasis ulcers. Electromagnetic therapy is only considered appropriate after standard wound therapy has been tried for a minimum of 30 days with documentation showing no measurable signs of healing.

G0333

G0333 Pharmacy dispensing fee for inhalation drug(s); initial 30-day supply as a beneficiary

Lay Description

Medicare will pay an initial dispensing fee to a pharmacy for the first 30-day period of inhalation drugs furnished through DME, regardless of the number of shipments or drugs dispensed during that time and regardless of the number of pharmacies used by a beneficiary during that time. This initial 30-day dispensing fee is a one-time fee applicable only to those who are using inhalation drugs for the first time as Medicare beneficiaries. Report G0333 for this Medicare-covered dispensing fee.

G0337

G0337 Hospice evaluation and counseling services, preelection

Lay Description

This code reports an evaluation of a terminally ill, Medicare beneficiary by a physician who is either the medical director or an employee of the hospice. This hospice consultation service is available to those who have not made a hospice election, nor received a previous hospice consultation. It includes an assessment of the patient's need for pain and symptom management, counseling regarding hospice and other care options, and may include advice regarding advanced care planning. The beneficiary or his or her physician must request this evaluation.

G0339-G0340

G0339   Image guided robotic linear accelerator-based stereotactic radiosurgery, complete course of therapy in one session or first session of fractionated treatment

G0340   Image guided robotic linear accelerator-based stereotactic radiosurgery, delivery including collimator changes and custom plugging, fractionated treatment, all lesions, per session, second through fifth sessions, maximum 5 sessions per course of treatment

Lay Description

Image-guided robotic linear accelerator-based stereotactic radiosurgery is treatment using a robotic device of a precisely defined area (stereotactic) with radiation generated by a linear accelerator. A linear accelerator is a device that increases the motion of ions to high energy or frequency levels. Electrodes are lined up with very small spaces between them creating very excited molecules that possess high levels of energy. The robotic device is guided by images taken during the course of treatment. This code includes collimator changes and custom plugging. This code represents all lesions treated in one treatment plan. Report G0339 when the complete course of treatment is given at one time, or for the first session of treatment that is broken or fractionated into different sessions; G0340 for each session for the second through fifth fractionated treatments. The maximum number of fractionated treatments allowed is five.

G0341-G0343

G0341   Percutaneous islet cell transplant, includes portal vein catheterization and infusion

G0342   Laparoscopy for islet cell transplant, includes portal vein catheterization and infusion

G0343   Laparotomy for islet cell transplant, includes portal vein catheterization and infusion

Lay Description

Islets cells are found in clusters throughout the pancreas and can be taken from an organ donor and transferred into the pancreas of the patient. Once transplanted, the cells can take over the task of destroyed cells. For example, diabetic Type I patients have a pancreas that no longer makes insulin and the patient must take insulin daily. Once implanted, the islet cells, which contain beta cells, begin to make insulin. Percutaneous islet cell transplant (G0341), laparoscopy islet transplant (G0342), and laparotomy for islet cell transplant (G0343) require access to the portal vein and are commonly accessed via a transhepatic approach.

G0364

G0364   Bone marrow aspiration performed with bone marrow biopsy through the same incision on the same date of service

Lay Description

The physician performs a bone marrow aspiration with a bone marrow biopsy through the same incision at the same surgical session. Bone marrow samples are usually taken from the pelvic bone or sternum. The skin over the bone is first cleaned with an antiseptic solution. A local anesthetic is injected. To obtain bone marrow aspirate, the physician inserts a needle beneath the skin and rotates it until the needle penetrates the cortex. At least half a teaspoon of marrow is sucked out of the bone by a syringe attached to the needle. If more marrow is needed, the needle is repositioned slightly, a new syringe is attached, and a second sample is taken. The samples are transferred from the syringes to slides and sent to a laboratory for analysis. To obtain a bone marrow biopsy, the physician inserts the needle, rotates the needle to the right and the left, withdraws the needle, and reinserts the needle at a slightly different angle. The procedure is repeated until a small chip is separated from the bone marrow. The needle is again removed and a piece of fine wire threaded through the tip transfers the specimen onto sterile gauze. The chip contains bone marrow that has not had the structure disturbed or destroyed. The bone marrow biopsy tissue must be decalcified overnight before it can be stained and examined.

Medicare Information

This code is specific to Medicare billing, but may be accepted by other payers. Report G0364 in addition to 38221 *Bone marrow biopsy* when the bone marrow aspiration is performed with bone marrow biopsy through the same skin incision on the same date of service.

G0365

G0365   Vessel mapping of vessels for hemodialysis access (services for preoperative vessel mapping prior to creation of hemodialysis access using an autogenous hemodialysis conduit, including arterial inflow and venous outflow)

Lay Description

The physician performs preoperative vessel mapping prior to creation of an autogenous hemodialysis conduit to assess suitability of the vessels for creation of the conduit. Both arterial inflow and venous outflow are evaluated. The forearm vessels are evaluated first. Creation of an arteriovenous fistula (AVF) requires an arterial diameter of at least 2 mm and a venous diameter of at least 2.5 mm. The arm is comfortably positioned at a 45-degree angle from the body. Antegrade radial arterial flow is evaluated at the wrist level, and the radial arterial diameter is determined. If the radial arterial diameter is less than 2 mm, the ulnar artery is evaluated. If either artery measures at least 2 mm, the physician places a tourniquet at the middle forearm and the distal forearm is percussed to promote vein distension. Special attention is paid to the cephalic and dorsal forearm veins. The cephalic vein is measured. If the cephalic vein is at least 2.5 mm in diameter, the cephalic vein is followed to the elbow and the cephalic vein branches assessed. The tourniquet is moved to the antecubital area and then to the upper arm and the veins assessed in the upper arm to the point of insertion of the cephalic vein into the subclavian vein. If the cephalic vein is occluded or measures less than 2.5 mm it may still be possible to create an AVF using the cephalic vein if the cephalic vein branches are of sufficient size. If it is determined that the cephalic vein is not suitable for an AVF, the physician evaluates veins in the dorsal and volar aspects to determine if another suitable vein exists. If blood vessels in the forearm are not suitable, the physician evaluates vessels in the upper arm. The brachial artery and the cephalic, basilic, and brachial veins are evaluated. Veins measuring 2.5 mm in diameter are followed to the insertion into the subclavian vein. Outflow in all draining veins is then assessed to identify any occlusion or stenosis. Adequate vein diameter is confirmed into the deep veins and deep vein drainage evaluated.

Medicare Information
This code is specific to Medicare billing, but may be accepted by other payers. Report G0365 in place of the imaging CPT codes when the imaging is used for the specific purpose of planning the creation of hemodialysis access.

G0372

G0372   Physician service required to establish and document the need for a power mobility device

Lay Description
A physician or treating nonphysician practitioner (a physician assistant, nurse practitioner, or clinical nurse specialist) must conduct a face-to-face examination of the patient and write a written order for a power mobility device (PMD). The written order must include the patient's name, the date of the face-to-face examination, the diagnoses and conditions that the PMD is expected to modify, a description of the item, the length of need, the physician or treating nonphysician practitioner's signature, and the date the order is written. The PMD supplier cannot deliver a Medicare-covered PMD unless the supplier has a written order for the PMD and the report of the face-to-face examination. Code G0372 represents a physician visit for the purpose of establishing and documenting the patient's need for a PMD.

G0378

G0378   Hospital observation service, per hour

Lay Description
Observation in a hospital setting is the monitoring, testing, short term treatment, and assessment of a patient, to determine if the patient will require further treatment as a hospital inpatient or can be discharged from the hospital. Observation status is commonly assigned to patients who present to the emergency department and who then require a significant period of treatment or monitoring in order to make a decision concerning their admission or discharge. Code G0378 represents one hour of observation care.

G0379

G0379   Direct admission of patient for hospital observation care

Lay Description
Observation is commonly assigned to patients who present to the emergency department and who then require a significant period of treatment or monitoring in order to make a decision concerning their admission or discharge. The decision to admit a patient for observation care may sometimes be made in the physician office or other community setting. Report G0379 when a patient is admitted to observation directly from the community without being seen in the hospital's clinic or emergency department.

G0380-G0384

G0380   Level 1 hospital emergency department visit provided in a type B emergency department; (the ED must meet at least one of the following requirements: (1) it is licensed by the state in which it is located under applicable state law as an emergency room or emergency department; (2) it is held out to the public (by name, posted signs, advertising, or other means) as a place that provides care for emergency medical conditions on an urgent basis without requiring a previously scheduled appointment; or (3) during the calendar

HCPCS Lay Descriptions

year immediately preceding the calendar year in which a determination under 42 CFR 489.24 is being made, based on a representative sample of patient visits that occurred during that calendar year, it provides at least one-third of all of its outpatient visits for the treatment of emergency medical conditions on an urgent basis without requiring a previously scheduled appointment)

G0381 Level 2 hospital emergency department visit provided in a type B emergency department; (the ED must meet at least one of the following requirements: (1) it is licensed by the state in which it is located under applicable state law as an emergency room or emergency department; (2) it is held out to the public (by name, posted signs, advertising, or other means) as a place that provides care for emergency medical conditions on an urgent basis without requiring a previously scheduled appointment; or (3) during the calendar year immediately preceding the calendar year in which a determination under 42 CFR 489.24 is being made, based on a representative sample of patient visits that occurred during that calendar year, it provides at least one-third of all of its outpatient visits for the treatment of emergency medical conditions on an urgent basis without requiring a previously scheduled appointment)

G0382 Level 3 hospital emergency department visit provided in a type B emergency department; (the ED must meet at least one of the following requirements: (1) it is licensed by the state in which it is located under applicable state law as an emergency room or emergency department; (2) it is held out to the public (by name, posted signs, advertising, or other means) as a place that provides care for emergency medical conditions on an urgent basis without requiring a previously scheduled appointment; or (3) during the calendar year immediately preceding the calendar year in which a determination under 42 CFR 489.24 is being made, based on a representative sample of patient visits that occurred during that calendar year, it provides at least one-third of all of its outpatient visits for the treatment of emergency medical conditions on an urgent basis without requiring a previously scheduled appointment)

G0383 Level 4 hospital emergency department visit provided in a type B emergency department; (the ED must meet at least one of the following requirements: (1) it is licensed by the state in which it is located under applicable state law as an emergency room or emergency department; (2) it is held out to the public (by name, posted signs, advertising, or other means) as a place that provides care for emergency medical conditions on an urgent basis without requiring a previously scheduled appointment; or (3) during the calendar year immediately preceding the calendar year in which a determination under 42 CFR 489.24 is being made, based on a representative sample of patient visits that occurred during that calendar year, it provides at least one-third of all of its outpatient visits for the treatment of emergency medical conditions on an urgent basis without requiring a previously scheduled appointment)

G0384 Level 5 hospital emergency department visit provided in a type B emergency department; (the ED must meet at least one of the following requirements: (1) it is licensed by the state in which it is located under applicable state law as an emergency room or emergency department; (2) it is held out to the public (by name, posted signs, advertising, or other means) as a place that provides care for emergency medical conditions on an urgent basis without requiring a previously scheduled appointment; or (3) during the calendar year immediately preceding the calendar year in which a determination under 42 CFR 489.24 is being made, based on a representative sample of patient visits that occurred during that calendar year, it provides at least one-third of all of its outpatient visits for the treatment of emergency medical conditions on an urgent basis without requiring a previously scheduled appointment)

Lay Description

Type B emergency departments (EDs) are areas within a hospital that provide emergency and urgent care to patients. Type B EDs meet the EMTALA definition of a dedicated ED, but do not meet the CPT definition of an ED. Hospitals that meet the CPT definition are labeled Type A EDs. Type B EDs most likely are not available 24 hours a day, 7 days a week as required for the Type A designation. A Type B ED must be licensed by the state in which it is located under applicable state law as an ED; or be held out to the public (by name, posted signs, advertising, or other means) as a place that provides care for emergency medical conditions on an urgent basis without requiring a previously scheduled appointment; or provide one third of all its outpatient visits for the treatment of emergency medical conditions on an urgent basis without requiring a previously scheduled appointment.

Hospitals may make their own determination as to the assignment of the various levels of care. Determination should be documented and consistently applied. Report G0380 for a level 1 Type B ED visit, G0381 for a level 2 visit, G0382 for a level 3 visit, G0383 for a level 4 visit, and G0384 for a level 5 visit.

G0389

G0389 Ultrasound B-scan and/or real time with image documentation; for abdominal aortic aneurysm (AAA) screening

Lay Description

Medicare will pay for one screening ultrasound for an abdominal aortic aneurysm (AAA) in the patient's lifetime. Coverage is limited to patients who receive a referral for this test as a result of the initial preventive physical examination, who have never previously had this test, and who are in a risk category. Risk categories are family history of AAA, male age 65-75 years who has smoked at least 100 cigarettes in his lifetime, othr risk factors as specified in the National Coverage Determination. The AAA screening must be performed by a provider or supplier authorized to provide covered diagnostic services.

G0390

G0390 Trauma response team associated with hospital critical care service

Lay Description

Trauma response teams are specialized teams of key hospital personnel who respond to triage information from prehospital caregivers in advance of the patient's arrival. The trauma team designation may only be used by trauma center/hospitals as licensed or designated by the state or local government authority entitled to do so, or as verified by the American College of Surgeons. Revenue code 068X is used for patients for whom a trauma activation occurred. Patients can only be billed the trauma activation fee charge if there has been prehospital notification for them; they meet either local, state, or American College of Surgeons field triage criteria; or they are delivered by inter-hospital transfers; and if they are given the appropriate team response. If a trauma activation occurs that would permit reporting a charge under revenue code 68X, the hospital may bill one unit of code G0390, which represents trauma activation associated with hospital critical care services. Report G0390 with revenue code 068X. CMS maintains that trauma activation is a one-time occurrence in association with critical care services, and therefore CMS will only pay for one unit of G0390 per day.

G0396-G0397

G0396 Alcohol and/or substance (other than tobacco) abuse structured assessment (e.g., AUDIT, DAST), and brief intervention 15 to 30 minutes
G0397 Alcohol and/or substance (other than tobacco) abuse structured assessment (e.g., AUDIT, DAST), and intervention, greater than 30 minutes

Lay Description

Alcohol and substance abuse may be assessed by several different methods, including a drug abuse screening test (DAST) and an alcohol use disorder identification test (AUDIT). Medicare does not cover screening services unless specifically mandated by statute. Report G0396 and G0397 when a brief intervention and a structured assessment of alcohol or substance abuse is performed in the context of the diagnosis or treatment of an illness or injury. When the brief intervention is 15 to 30 minutes, report G0396. When the brief intervention is more than 30 minutes, report G0397.

G0398-G0400

G0398 Home sleep study test (HST) with type II portable monitor, unattended; minimum of 7 channels: EEG, EOG, EMG, ECG/heart rate, airflow, respiratory effort and oxygen saturation
G0399 Home sleep test (HST) with type III portable monitor, unattended; minimum of 4 channels: 2 respiratory movement/airflow, 1 ECG/heart rate and 1 oxygen saturation
G0400 Home sleep test (HST) with type IV portable monitor, unattended; minimum of 3 channels

Lay Description

Sleep apnea is a serious sleep disorder in which breathing repeatedly stops and starts. There are two main types of sleep apnea: obstructive sleep apnea is the more common form that occurs when throat muscles relax; and central sleep apnea occurs when your brain doesn't send proper signals to the muscles that control breathing. Some people may have a complex sleep apnea, which is a combination of both. Medicare covers continuous positive airway pressure (CPAP) as a treatment for obstructive sleep apnea. Prior to March 13, 2008, the sleep testing necessary to diagnose obstructive sleep apnea had to be performed in a facility for Medicare coverage. Since March 13, 2008, Medicare accepts a diagnosis of obstructive sleep apnea as determined with a home sleep study. Sleep studies, whether in a facility or performed at home, generally have the following components: electroencephalogram (EEG) to measure brain activity; electrooculogram (EOG) to monitor eye movements; electromyogram (EMG) to monitor muscle movements; electrocardiogram (EKG) to monitor heart rate and rhythm; blood oxygen saturation; breathing effort or respiratory disturbance index (RDI); and airflow monitors. Chest and abdomen movements are also sometimes monitored. Home sleep studies used to diagnose obstructive sleep apnea are reported with the following: G0398 for a type II portable monitor that monitors a minimum of seven channels (EEG, EOG, EMG, EKG, RDI, oxygen saturation levels, and airflow); G0399 for a type III portable monitor that monitors a minimum of four channels (EKG, RDI, oxygen saturation levels, and airflow); and G0400 for a type IV portable monitor that monitors a minimum of three channels.

G0402

G0402 Initial preventive physical examination; face-to-face visit, services limited to new beneficiary during the first 12 months of Medicare enrollment

Lay Description

An initial preventive physical examination is provided to a new beneficiary during the first 12 months of Medicare enrollment. It is also referred to as a "Welcome to Medicare" physical examination. The physician performs a thorough review of the patient's health. The physician takes a medical history on the patient and performs an exam that includes a blood pressure check, height and weight assessment, and a vision screen. Depending on the medical history information provided by the patient and the results of the physical examination, the physician orders or performs additional tests as medically necessary. The physician also provides preventive medicine education and counseling services based on the patient's medical history and examination results. The physician provides a written plan of care to the patient detailing any follow-up screening or preventive services that the patient should receive.

Medicare Information

This code is specific to the Medicare physical examination. The exam must be performed within twelve months of the patient's initial Part B coverage date. The exam is allowed only once in a patient's lifetime. Bill separately any additional screening or preventive services, such as diabetes laboratory screening tests, ECGs, glaucoma screening, or medical nutrition therapy. All screening and other preventive services are subject to their own detailed coverage criteria.

G0403-G0405

G0403 Electrocardiogram, routine ECG with 12 leads; performed as a screening for the initial preventive physical examination with interpretation and report

G0404 Electrocardiogram, routine ECG with 12 leads; tracing only, without interpretation and report, performed as a screening for the initial preventive physical examination

G0405 Electrocardiogram, routine ECG with 12 leads; interpretation and report only, performed as a screening for the initial preventive physical examination

Lay Description

Electrocardiogram (ECG) services are performed as a component of the initial preventive physical examination provided to a new beneficiary during the first 12 months of Medicare enrollment. Twelve electrodes are placed on a patient's chest to record electrical activity of the heart. A physician interprets the findings. Report G0403 when the physician provides the combined technical (tracing) and professional (interpretation and report) components of the ECG. Report G0404 for the technical component (tracing) only. Report G0405 when the physician provides the professional component (interpretation and report) only.

Medicare Information

These codes are specific to EKGs ordered and performed as a part of the Medicare physical examination. The exam must be performed within six months of the patient's initial Part B coverage date. These codes are reportable only once in a patient's lifetime. Facilities may report only the tracing, G0404, on a UB-04 claim.

G3001

G3001 Administration and supply of tositumomab, 450 mg

Lay Description

Tositumomab (trade name Bexxar) is a murine monoclonal antibody that is directed against the CD20 antigen, which is found on the surface of normal and malignant B lymphocytes. When linked to Iodine I-131, it is used as an anti-neoplastic treatment of patients with CD20 positive, follicular, non-Hodgkin's lymphoma, with and without transformation, whose disease is refractory to rituximab, and whose disease has recurred following chemotherapy. The tositumomab therapeutic regimen is not indicated for the initial treatment of patients with CD20 positive non-Hodgkin's lymphoma. Prior to the administration of the radioactive Iodine I-131 tositumomab, non-radioactive tositumomab is given to determine the proper treatment dose for the patient. This code represents the 450 mg of the non-radioactive tositumomab dose used for treatment planning. It includes the intravenous administration of the drug.

G9001-G9012

G9001   Coordinated care fee, initial rate
G9002   Coordinated care fee, maintenance rate
G9003   Coordinated care fee, risk adjusted high, initial
G9004   Coordinated care fee, risk adjusted low, initial
G9005   Coordinated care fee, risk adjusted maintenance
G9006   Coordinated care fee, home monitoring
G9007   Coordinated care fee, scheduled team conference
G9008   Coordinated care fee, physician coordinated care oversight services
G9009   Coordinated care fee, risk adjusted maintenance, Level 3
G9010   Coordinated care fee, risk adjusted maintenance, Level 4
G9011   Coordinated care fee, risk adjusted maintenance, Level 5
G9012   Other specified case management service not elsewhere classified

Lay Description

In an effort to improve care and to contain costs, Medicare is testing several coordinated care demonstration projects. There are fifteen sites that manage or coordinate all care delivered to Medicare beneficiaries with certain complex chronic illnesses, including asthma, diabetes, congestive heart failure and related cardiac conditions, hypertension, coronary artery disease, cardiovascular and cerebrovascular conditions, and chronic lung disease. CMS implemented this demonstration to test whether coordinated care programs can improve medical treatment plans, reduce avoidable hospital admissions, and promote other desirable outcomes for chronically ill beneficiaries, without increasing costs. The selected projects include both case and disease management models in urban and rural settings. These codes should be used only by the fifteen approved demonstration projects. The codes correspond to the rates proposed and included in each specific demonstration project.

G9016

G9016   Smoking cessation counseling, individual, in the absence of or in addition to any other evaluation and management service, per session (6-10 minutes) [demo project code only]

Lay Description

CMS had been conducting a demonstration project to test smoking cessation as a Medicare benefit. The project examined the "quit" rates of Medicare beneficiaries receiving three different types of treatment. The three types are counseling only, counseling and an FDA-approved prescription or nicotine replacement drug therapy, and a telephone counseling hotline and nicotine replacement therapy. This code was used to bill individual counseling services when that counseling is the only service provided. It is reported for each session that must total between six and ten minutes in length. Code G9016 is to be used only for services provided by providers and beneficiaries enrolled in the demonstration project. The project has concluded. Report G0375 and G0376 for the Medicare benefit.

G9017

G9017   Amantadine HCl, oral, per 100 mg (for use in a Medicare-approved demonstration project)

Lay Description

Amantadine hydrochloride is a chemical that has pharmacological actions as both an anti-Parkinson and an antiviral drug. Its mechanism of action for either use is unknown. Amantadine hydrochloride is indicated for the treatment of Parkinsonism and drug-induced extrapyramidal reactions, as well as signs and symptoms of infections caused by the influenza Type A virus. The drug is self-administered orally. Each capsule contains 100 mg of amantadine hydrochloride. When used in a Medicare approved demonstration project, report HCPCS Level II code G9017 for generic name drug.

G9018

G9018   Zanamivir, inhalation powder, administered through inhaler, per 10 mg (for use in a Medicare-approved demonstration project)

Lay Description

Zanamivir is an antiviral drug that has an effect against the influenza virus. It inhibits the enzyme that the virus uses to separate itself from other cells. Inhibition of this enzyme allows antibodies to attack and destroy the virus. Zanamivir is indicated for treatment of uncomplicated acute infections with influenza A and B virus in patients 7 years of age and older. The patient should be symptomatic for no more than two days. It is not recommended for patients with an underlying airway disease, such as asthma or COPD. The drug is self-administered in an inhaled powder form via a supplied disk inhaler. HCPCS Level II code G9081 represents 10 mg of zanamivir generic for use in a Medicare approved demonstration project.

G9019

G9019 Oseltamivir phosphate, oral, per 75 mg (for use in a Medicare-approved demonstration project)

Lay Description

Oseltamivir phosphate is an oral anti-viral drug for the treatment of uncomplicated influenza in patients one year and older whose flu symptoms have not lasted more than two days. Oseltamivir phosphate is approved to treat Type A and B influenza. It is available in a 75 mg capsule form, as well as in a powder form for oral suspension. The oral suspension is reconstituted with water to contain 12 mg/mL oseltamivir base. Oseltamivir phosphate is an ethyl ester prodrug requiring ester hydrolysis for conversion to the active form, oseltamivir carboxylate. The proposed mechanism of action of oseltamivir phosphate is inhibition of influenza virus neuraminidase with the possibility of alteration of virus particle aggregation and release. HCPCS Level II code G9019 represents 75 mg of oseltamivir phosphate oral generic.

G9020

G9020 Rimantadine HCl, oral, per 100 mg (for use in a Medicare-approved demonstration project)

Lay Description

Rimantadine hydrochloride is an oral anti-viral drug for the treatment of influenza type A. The drug affects only certain susceptible strains of the influenza type A virus. It is available in a 100 mg capsule form, as well as in a syrup form. The mechanism of action is not entirely understood, but Rimantadine hydrochloride appears to interfere with the activity of the virus's genetic material, blocking an essential step in the process of viral replication by possibly inhibiting the uncoating of the virus. HCPCS Level II code G9020 represents 100 mg of rimantadine HCl generic for use in a Medicare-approved demonstration project.

G9033

G9033 Amantadine HCl, oral brand, per 100 mg (for use in a Medicare-approved demonstration project)

Lay Description

Amantadine hydrochloride is a chemical that has pharmacological actions as both an anti-Parkinson and an antiviral drug. Its mechanism of action for either use is unknown. Amantadine hydrochloride is indicated for the treatment of Parkinsonism and drug-induced extrapyramidal reactions, as well as signs and symptoms of infections caused by the influenza Type A virus. The drug is self-administered orally. Each capsule contains 100 mg of amantadine hydrochloride. When used in a Medicare approved demonstration project, report HCPCS Level II code G9033 for 100 mg of the brand name drug.

G9034

G9034 Zanamivir, inhalation powder, administered through inhaler, brand, per 10 mg (for use in a Medicare-approved demonstration project)

Lay Description

Zanamivir is an antiviral drug that has an effect against the influenza virus. It inhibits the enzyme that the virus uses to separate itself from other cells. Inhibition of this enzyme allows antibodies to attack and destroy the virus. Zanamivir is indicated for treatment of uncomplicated acute infections with influenza A and B virus in patients 7 years of age and older. The patient should be symptomatic for no more than two days. It is not recommended for patients with an underlying airway disease, such as asthma or COPD. The drug is self-administered in an inhaled powder form via a supplied disk inhaler. HCPCS Level II code G9034 represents 10 mg of zanamivir brand name for use in a Medicare approved demonstration project.

G9035

G9035 Oseltamivir phosphate, oral, brand, per 75 mg (for use in a Medicare-approved demonstration project)

Lay Description

Oseltamivir phosphate is an oral anti-viral drug for the treatment of uncomplicated influenza in patients 1 year and older whose flu symptoms have not lasted more than two days. Oseltamivir phosphate is approved to treat Type A and B influenza. It is available in a 75 mg capsule form, as well as in a powder form for oral suspension. The oral suspension is reconstituted with water to contain 12 mg/mL oseltamivir base. Oseltamivir phosphate is an ethyl ester prodrug requiring ester hydrolysis for conversion to the active form, oseltamivir carboxylate. The proposed mechanism of action of oseltamivir phosphate is inhibition of influenza virus neuraminidase with the possibility of alteration of virus particle aggregation and release. HCPCS Level II code G9035 represents 75 mg of oseltamivir phosphate oral brand name for use in a Medicare approved demonstration project.

G9036

G9036 **Rimantadine HCl, oral, brand, per 100 mg (for use in a Medicare-approved demonstration project)**

Lay Description

Rimantadine hydrochloride is an oral anti-viral drug for the treatment of influenza type A. The drug affects only certain susceptible strains of the influenza type A virus. It is available in a 100 mg capsule form, as well as in a syrup form. The mechanism of action is not entirely understood, but Rimantadine hydrochloride appears to interfere with the activity of the virus's genetic material, blocking an essential step in the process of viral replication by possibly inhibiting the uncoating of the virus. HCPCS Level II code G9036 represents 100 mg of rimantadine HCl oral brand name for use in a Medicare-approved demonstration project.

G9041

G9041 **Rehabilitation services for low vision by qualified occupational therapist, direct one-on-one contact, each 15 minutes**

Lay Description

This code reports low vision rehabilitation services provided by an occupational therapist participating in a low vision demonstration project. The low vision demonstration project permits low vision rehabilitation specialists to provide services in the home, office, or clinic under the general supervision of a physician. Under the low vision demonstration project, Medicare covers low vision rehabilitation services to individuals with a diagnosis of moderate to severe vision impairment at selected demonstration sites. Services are provided under an individualized, written plan of care developed by a physician or qualified occupational therapist. Rehabilitation services must be conducted within a three-month period appropriate to the patient's needs and shall not exceed the equivalent of nine weekly one-hour visits. All services must be individual, face-to-face services. No group services are covered. Patients usually receive therapy one to two days a week during 30 to 60 minute sessions. Rehabilitation services are generally not provided less frequently than every two weeks. The plan of care must be reviewed by the physician at a minimum of every 30 days. Periodic follow-up evaluations are required by the supervising physician at least every 30 days. This code reports only the rehabilitation component of the low vision services.

G9042

G9042 **Rehabilitation services for low vision by certified orientation and mobility specialists, direct one-on-one contact, each 15 minutes**

Lay Description

This code reports low vision rehabilitation services provided by an orientation and mobility specialist participating in a low vision demonstration project. The low vision demonstration project permits low vision rehabilitation specialists to provide services in the home, office, or clinic under the general supervision of a physician. Under the low vision demonstration project, Medicare covers low vision rehabilitation services to individuals with a diagnosis of moderate to severe vision impairment at selected demonstration sites. Services are provided under an individualized, written plan of care developed by a physician or qualified occupational therapist. Rehabilitation services must be conducted within a three-month period appropriate to the patient's needs and shall not exceed the equivalent of nine weekly one-hour visits. All services must be individual, face-to-face services. No group services are covered. Patients usually receive therapy one to two days a week during 30 to 60 minute sessions. Rehabilitation services are generally not provided less frequently than every two weeks. The plan of care must be reviewed by the physician at a minimum of every 30 days. Periodic follow-up evaluations are required by the supervising physician at least every 30 days. This code reports only the rehabilitation component of the low vision services.

G9043

G9043 **Rehabilitation services for low vision by certified low vision rehabilitation therapist, direct one-on-one contact, each 15 minutes**

Lay Description

This code reports low vision rehabilitation services provided by a low vision therapist participating in a low vision demonstration project. The low vision demonstration project permits low vision rehabilitation specialists to provide services in the home, office, or clinic under the general supervision of a physician. Under the low vision demonstration project, Medicare covers low vision rehabilitation services to individuals with a diagnosis of moderate to severe vision impairment at selected demonstration sites. Services are provided under an individualized, written plan of care developed by a physician or qualified occupational therapist. Rehabilitation services must be conducted within a three-month period appropriate to the patient's needs and shall not exceed the equivalent of nine weekly one-hour visits. All services must be individual, face-to-face services. No group services are covered. Patients usually receive therapy one to two days a week during 30 to 60 minute sessions. Rehabilitation services are generally not provided less frequently than every two weeks. The plan of care must be reviewed by the physician at a minimum of every 30 days. Periodic follow-up evaluations are required by the supervising physician at least every 30 days. This code reports only the rehabilitation component of the low vision services.

G9044

G9044 **Rehabilitation services for low vision by certified low vision rehabilitation teacher, direct one-on-one contact, each 15 minutes**

Lay Description

This code reports low vision rehabilitation services provided by a rehabilitation teacher participating in a low vision demonstration project. The low vision demonstration project permits low vision rehabilitation specialists to provide services in the home, office, or clinic under the general supervision of a physician. Under the low vision demonstration project, Medicare covers low vision rehabilitation services to individuals with a diagnosis of moderate to severe vision impairment at selected demonstration sites. Services are provided under an individualized, written plan of care developed by a physician or qualified occupational therapist. Rehabilitation services must be conducted within a three-month period appropriate to the patient's needs and shall not exceed the equivalent of nine weekly one-hour visits. All services must be individual, face-to-face services. No group services are covered. Patients usually receive therapy one to two days a week during 30 to 60 minute sessions. Rehabilitation services are generally not provided less frequently than every two weeks. The plan of care must be reviewed by the physician at a minimum of every 30 days. Periodic follow-up evaluations are required by the supervising physician at least every 30 days. This code reports only the rehabilitation component of the low vision services.

G9141

G9141 **Influenza A (H1N1) immunization administration (includes the physician counseling the patient/family)**

Lay Description

Use this code to report the administration of an influenza A (H1N1) virus vaccine. Do not bill an office visit if the only reason for the visit was to receive a vaccination.

G9142

G9142 **Influenza A (H1N1) vaccine, any route of administration**

Lay Description

Use this code to report the H1N1 vaccine. The vaccine is monovalent and comprised of inactivated influenza virus. The virus is reproduced in an embryonic chicken egg. The virus is concentrated, purified, and put into an isotonic solution for intramuscular administration. Recommended dose for children six to 35 months is 0.25 ml given twice with at least one month in between injections. Children 36 months to nine years receive 0.50 ml twice with at least one month between injections. Patients age ten and older should receive one 0.50 ml injection. If the vaccine is provided at no cost to the provider, report only the code for administration and not for the vaccine.

H0001

H0001 **Alcohol and/or drug assessment**

Lay Description

This code reports provision of alcohol and/or drug assessment services. A psychiatrist, clinical psychologist, or other specialized health care professional or team of professionals generally provides drug and/or alcohol assessments. Protocols vary, but an assessment is systematic and thorough and addresses all aspects of a patient's encounters with alcohol and/or drugs. A detailed family, social, and legal history is usually solicited and components may be verified independent of the patient interview. Quantity and frequency of alcohol and/or drug use is documented. Physical manifestations associated with alcohol or drug use or abuse may be noted if present, such as depression, mania, anxiety, etc. A physical medical examination may be a component of the assessment. Questionnaires and tests may be used as components of the assessment. A report is generally issued that characterizes the patient's contact with alcohol and/or drugs as casual, dependent, abusive, addictive, etc. Should alcohol or drug use be determined to have caused adverse effects in the life of the patient or others, a report is issued documenting abuse. In addition to a diagnostic status, an assessment of abuse can have legal repercussions. This assessment should be used to devise a plan of care in treating the patient effectively.

H0002

H0002 Behavioral health screening to determine eligibility for admission to treatment program

Lay Description

Behavioral health screening is done to determine a patient's eligibility for admission to a treatment program. Patients are screened for mental health conditions as well as substance use disorders and are medically assessed to ensure appropriate treatment is given.

H0003

H0003 Alcohol and/or drug screening; laboratory analysis of specimens for presence of alcohol and/or drugs

Lay Description

Alcohol and/or drug screening is performed through laboratory analysis of urine, blood, or hair specimens to determine the presence of alcohol and/or drugs in the patient's system.

H0004

H0004 Behavioral health counseling and therapy, per 15 minutes

Lay Description

This code reports provision of behavioral health counseling and therapy services. Behavioral health counseling and therapy provides individual counseling by a clinician for a patient in a private setting and is billed in 15-minute increments.

H0005

H0005 Alcohol and/or drug services; group counseling by a clinician

Lay Description

Alcohol and/or drug group counseling by a clinician provides the patient support in a group setting (two or more individuals) in abstaining from substance abuse and assisting the patient with sobriety maintenance. Group counseling focuses on cognitive or behavioral approaches that typically address triggers and relapse prevention, self evaluation, the process of recovery, and issues pertaining to changes in lifestyle. Group sizes and treatment plans may vary according to the needs of the individual.

H0006

H0006 Alcohol and/or drug services; case management

Lay Description

Case management for patients needing services relating to alcohol or drug abuse provides assistance and care coordination based on the needs of the individual. The case manager assesses the needs of the patient, assists in developing plans to benefit the patient, as well as implementation of the plans, and reviews and evaluates the patient's status.

H0007

H0007 Alcohol and/or drug services; crisis intervention (outpatient)

Lay Description

Crisis intervention for alcohol and/or drug services is an emergency response by a clinician to provide immediate face-to-face support for an individual.

H0008-H0009

H0008 Alcohol and/or drug services; subacute detoxification (hospital inpatient)

H0009 Alcohol and/or drug services; acute detoxification (hospital inpatient)

Lay Description

Code H0008 is for sub-acute detoxification services in which the patient is monitored on an inpatient hospitalization basis for the long-term symptoms associated with the withdrawal from alcohol and/or drugs. Sub-acute detoxification deals with severe symptoms such as alcohol and drug cravings. Code H0009 is for acute detoxification services in which the patient is medically managed and stabilized on an inpatient hospitalization basis for severe withdrawal syndrome associated with the withdrawal from alcohol/drugs. Acute withdrawal begins within hours and includes severe physical and psychological symptoms that may require medical management with medications such as methadone.

H0010-H0011

H0010 Alcohol and/or drug services; subacute detoxification (residential addiction program inpatient)
H0011 Alcohol and/or drug services; acute detoxification (residential addiction program inpatient)

Lay Description

Code H0010 reports subacute detoxification services in which the patient is monitored in an inpatient residential addiction program for long-term symptoms associated with the withdrawal from alcohol and/or drugs. Subacute detoxification deals with severe symptoms such as alcohol and drug cravings. Code H0011 reports acute detoxification services in which the patient is medically managed and stabilized in an inpatient residential addiction program for severe withdrawal syndrome associated with the withdrawal from alcohol/drugs. Acute withdrawal begins within hours and includes severe physical and psychological symptoms that may require medical management with medications such as methadone. During this treatment, the patient lives in a controlled and supportive environment having access to care during a 24-hour period.

H0012-H0013

H0012 Alcohol and/or drug services; subacute detoxification (residential addiction program outpatient)
H0013 Alcohol and/or drug services; acute detoxification (residential addiction program outpatient)

Lay Description

Code H0012 is for sub-acute detoxification service in which the patient is monitored as an outpatient coming to a residential addiction program for the treatment of long-term symptoms associated with the withdrawal from alcohol and/or drugs. Sub-acute detoxification deals with severe symptoms such as alcohol and drug cravings. Code H0013 is for acute detoxification services in which the patient is medically managed and stabilized as an outpatient coming to a residential addiction program for the treatment of severe withdrawal syndrome associated with the withdrawal from alcohol/drugs. Acute withdrawal begins within hours and includes severe physical and psychological symptoms that may require medical management with medications such as methadone.

H0014

H0014 Alcohol and/or drug services; ambulatory detoxification

Lay Description

Code H0014 is for ambulatory detoxification service for mild to moderate withdrawal from alcohol and/or drug abuse.

H0015

H0015 Alcohol and/or drug services; intensive outpatient (treatment program that operates at least 3 hours/day and at least 3 days/week and is based on an individualized treatment plan), including assessment, counseling; crisis intervention, and activity therapies or education

Lay Description

This code reports alcohol and drug related services within an intensive outpatient treatment program requiring the patient to participate at least 3 hours per day for at least 3 days per week. The patient is assessed medically and psychologically, provided counseling, intervention, and activity therapy or education, according to the needs of the patient and the individual's treatment plan.

H0016

H0016 Alcohol and/or drug services; medical/somatic (medical intervention in ambulatory setting)

Lay Description

This service includes the supervision of medication, physical examinations, or other medical needs required to maintain the physical health of the patient receiving medical intervention treatment for alcohol and drug related problems in an ambulatory setting.

H0017

H0017 Behavioral health; residential (hospital residential treatment program), without room and board, per diem

Lay Description

Residential treatment on a per diem basis for behavior health issues in a hospital residential treatment program is designed to provide a 24-hour group living situation in which the patient receives treatment under the care of a physician. This code does not include daily room and board.

H0018

H0018 Behavioral health; short-term residential (nonhospital residential treatment program), without room and board, per diem

Lay Description

Short-term residential treatment is typically less than 30 days. This code applies to a residential treatment program for behavior health issues that is not part of a hospital but provides a 24-hour group living situation in which the patient receives treatment and does not include daily room and board.

H0019

H0019 Behavioral health; long-term residential (nonmedical, nonacute care in a residential treatment program where stay is typically longer than 30 days), without room and board, per diem

Lay Description

Long-term residential treatment is typically more than 30 days. This code applies to a residential treatment program for behavioral health issues that is neither medical, nor acute in nature. This code is per diem, not including daily room and board.

H0020

H0020 Alcohol and/or drug services; methadone administration and/or service (provision of the drug by a licensed program)

Lay Description

Methadone administration and/or service programs provide opioid replacement treatment (ORT) or opioid maintenance treatment (OMT), including the administration of methadone to an individual for detoxification from opioids and/or maintenance treatment. Overall treatment must be delivered, which should include counseling/therapy, case review, and medication monitoring. ORT/OMT is delivered by providers functioning under a defined set of policies and procedures, including admission, discharge, and continued service criteria stipulated by state law and regulations, Substance Abuse and Mental Health Services Administration (SAMHSA) regulations, and Drug Enforcement Agency (DEA) regulations. The ORT must be licensed by the Drug Enforcement Agency. The ORT should also have accreditation from the Joint Commission on the Accreditation of Healthcare Organizations (JCAHO), Committee for Accreditation (COA), and/or the Commission on the Accreditation of Rehabilitation Facilities (CARF). The ORT/OMT must meet the requirements of the Substance Abuse and Mental Health Administration.

H0021

H0021 Alcohol and/or drug training service (for staff and personnel not employed by providers)

Lay Description

Code H0021 is used to report developing alcohol and/or drug service skills of staff and personnel that are not employed by an agency, such as training a counselor/clinician on proper techniques and approaches or sessions for clinicians on the effects of various types of drugs.

H0022

H0022 Alcohol and/or drug intervention service (planned facilitation)

Lay Description

Alcohol and drug intervention services provide treatment services and activities that assist the professionally trained interventionalist to pursue and detect alcohol and or drug addictions and to intercede to halt the progress of the addictions. These services also include early interventions.

H0023

H0023 Behavioral health outreach service (planned approach to reach a targeted population)

Lay Description

Behavioral health outreach is a service targeting specific, at-risk individuals in a given population who are in need of assistance with mental health issues. This may include mobile teams that contact at-risk individuals in the home, centers in which individuals can drop-in and obtain information regarding mental heath treatment or social services, or other various methods of contact that are not represented by a more specific code.

H0024-H0025

H0024 Behavioral health prevention information dissemination service (one-way direct or nondirect contact with service audiences to affect knowledge and attitude)

H0025 Behavioral health prevention education service (delivery of services with target population to affect knowledge, attitude and/or behavior)

Lay Description

Code H0024, behavioral health prevention information dissemination service, is used to provide facts to individuals in the community or in at-risk populations on issues of mental health. This service includes any form of direct or non-direct contact with the targeted audience to increase their awareness and knowledge of the issues and to affect their attitude. Code H0025, behavioral health prevention education service, is used to delivery services to individuals of a target population on issues of mental health education, to affect their knowledge, attitude, and behavior. It may include screenings to assist individuals in obtaining appropriate treatment. Causes and symptoms of disorders are discussed so as to encourage early intervention and reduce severity of mental illness.

H0026

H0026 Alcohol and/or drug prevention process service, community-based (delivery of services to develop skills of impactors)

Lay Description

Community-based, alcohol and/or drug prevention process services enhance the ability of a community to provide violence, alcohol, and/or drug abuse prevention services. The activities include planning, interagency collaboration, coalition building, and networking. Examples include multi-agency coordination and collaboration, community and volunteer training, and systemic planning.

H0027

H0027 Alcohol and/or drug prevention environmental service (broad range of external activities geared toward modifying systems in order to mainstream prevention through policy and law)

Lay Description

Alcohol and/or drug prevention environmental services (broad range of external activities geared toward modifying systems in order to mainstream prevention through policy and law) establish or change written and unwritten community standards and postures that influence the incidence and prevalence of violence and/or the abuse of alcohol and/or drugs used in the general population.

H0028

H0028 Alcohol and/or drug prevention problem identification and referral service (e.g., student assistance and employee assistance programs), does not include assessment

Lay Description

This code reports alcohol and/or drug prevention problem identification and referral services (e.g., student assistance and employee assistance programs). Prevention strategies aim to identify individuals who have engaged in illegal and age-inappropriate use of tobacco, alcohol, and/or drugs. Services may include employee assistance programs (EAP), student assistance programs, and driving under the influence (DUI) education programs. Append modifier HA to H0028 for 12 hours of education program within a community-based setting for youth younger than age 18 who are first-time offenders of alcohol or other drugs. Append modifier HB to H0028 for 10 hours of education/diversion program within the circuit court districts for 19 to 20 year olds who have been referred to the program due to an alcohol-related offense. Append modifier HK to H0028 for 30 hours of IPP within a community based setting for adolescents who have multiple offenses of alcohol or other drug use.

H0029

H0029 Alcohol and/or drug prevention alternatives service (services for populations that exclude alcohol and other drug use e.g., alcohol free social events)

Lay Description

This code reports alcohol and/or drug prevention alternative services (services for populations that exclude alcohol and other drug use e.g., alcohol free social events). Service strategies provide for the participation of specific inhabitants of a community in activities free from violence and/or alcohol/drug use. This strategy is to create attractive, healthy, and safe activities that increase an individual's commitment to abstain from violence and/or alcohol and drugs. These activities provide opportunities for low-risk choices when it comes to alcohol use and/or violent behavior. Examples include leadership camps, chemical free events, social activities, recreational activities, cultural activities, and behavioral activities at local community centers and other like places.

H0030

H0030 Behavioral health hotline service

Lay Description

Behavioral health hotline is a telephone service that provides crisis intervention and emergency management such as mental health referrals, treatment information, and other verbal assistance.

H0031

H0031 Mental health assessment, by nonphysician

Lay Description

Mental health assessment is provided by someone other than a physician who is a trained staff member. The assessment identifies factors of mental illness, functional capacity, and gathers additional information used for the treatment of mental illness.

H0032

H0032 Mental health service plan development by nonphysician

Lay Description

A mental health service plan is developed for treating a patient, including modifying goals, assessing progress, planning transitions, and addressing other needs. This service is provided by someone other than a physician, who is a clinical, professional, or other specialist.

H0033

H0033 Oral medication administration, direct observation

Lay Description

Patients are assisted or observed by professional medical staff during the administration of oral medication. This is often used in the administration of drugs such as methadone when it must be established that the patient has received the medication.

H0034

H0034 Medication training and support, per 15 minutes

Lay Description

Medication training and support is an educational service to assist the patient, family, or other caretaker in the proper management of prescribed medication regimens, drug interactions, and side effects. This code is reported per 15 minutes.

H0035

H0035 Mental health partial hospitalization, treatment, less than 24 hours

Lay Description

Partial hospitalization for mental health services is a treatment period of less than 24 hours care in which the patient is assisted with issues related to the individual's reintegration into society. This code is not considered an inpatient service.

H0041-H0042

H0041 Foster care, child, nontherapeutic, per diem
H0042 Foster care, child, nontherapeutic, per month

Lay Description

Foster care is a service in which custodial care of a child under the age of 18 is assumed by someone outside the individual's family. The child is cared for and nurtured within a family context, nontherapeutically, per diem in H0041 and per month in H0042.

H0043-H0044

H0043 Supported housing, per diem
H0044 Supported housing, per month

Lay Description

Supported housing service provides individuals with assistance for the responsibilities of obtaining and maintaining independent living. Once housing is established, the clients are monitored through periodic visits to confirm the continued appropriateness of the living situation including affordability, and ensure that issues of independent living are addressed. This service does not include therapeutic aspects. Report H0043 for services performed per diem and code H0044 for services per month.

H0045

H0045 Respite care services, not in the home, per diem

Lay Description

Respite care services provided outside the home give assistance to clients in place of primary care givers on a temporary per diem basis so the patient may be maintained at the current level of care required when the primary care givers are temporarily absent.

H0048

H0048 Alcohol and/or other drug testing: collection and handling only, specimens other than blood

Lay Description

Collection of specimens for alcohol/drug analysis is dependent on the type of biological sample obtained. Samples typically include urine or hair. This code represents the collection and handling of specimens other than blood samples. The handling of specimens requires a chain of custody from the point of collection throughout the analysis process to ensure the integrity of the specimen.

H0049

H0049 Alcohol and/or drug screening

Lay Description

Drug and alcohol screening is performed on patients in a drug and alcohol treatment program to detect the presence or absence of drugs or alcohol in the urine, blood, or breath. Screening tests are used to determine if an individual has recently ingested drugs or alcohol. A screening test does not quantify the amount of a drug in the urine, blood, or breath; it identifies only the presence or absence of these substances. If the individual tests positive, the individual may be tested with a more specific drug test to rule out any false positive results and to identify the specific substance ingested and the amount of the substance ingested.

H0050

H0050 Alcohol and/or drug services, brief intervention, per 15 minutes

Lay Description

A brief intervention for a patient in a drug and/or alcohol treatment program is performed. Professionally trained interventionists who are experts in chemical dependency meet briefly with the patient and/or family members to discuss a current treatment issue. The service may be initiated by the patient or the interventionist in response to a specific issue. The purpose of the intervention is to provide support and feedback related to chemical dependency issues that are currently affecting the patient and/or family members. This code is reported per 15 minute time increment spent in the intervention service.

H1000

H1000 Prenatal care, at-risk assessment

Lay Description

Prenatal at risk assessment is used to identify factors contributing to an increase risk for morbidity or mortality during pregnancy of the mother or fetus. Factors observed in risk assessment include obstetrical history, complicating health conditions or comorbidities, drug or alcohol use, prenatal care compliance, or other psychosocial circumstances that may jeopardize or complicate maternal or fetal health.

H2000

H2000 Comprehensive multidisciplinary evaluation

Lay Description

A comprehensive multidisciplinary evaluation consists of a thorough investigation in several areas to provide an accurate representation of the individual's needs and strengths. This evaluates areas such as psychiatric, physical, psychosocial, family, recreational, and occupational therapy.

H2011

H2011 Crisis intervention service, per 15 minutes

Lay Description

Mental health crisis intervention provides immediate support for an individual in personal crisis with outpatient status. The aim of this service is to stabilize the individual during a psychiatric emergency and is billed in 15-minute increments.

H2012

H2012 Behavioral health day treatment, per hour

Lay Description

Day treatment for behavior health focuses on maintaining and improving functional abilities for the individual. Clients may participate in activities in a therapeutic and social environment several times per week for several hours per day to improve personal skills. This code is reported per hour of daytime behavioral health treatment.

H2013

H2013 Psychiatric health facility service, per diem

Lay Description

A psychiatric health facility is specifically licensed as such and is differentiated from a hospital with an inpatient psychiatric ward, psychiatric hospital, or crisis residential services. This facility provides services in an acute non-hospital inpatient setting, and includes appropriate care in psychiatry, clinical psychology, social work, rehabilitation, drug administration, and other basic needs, per diem.

Medicare Information

This service is all-inclusive except for the day of admission and case management services. No other mental health procedures can be billed while the patient is in the facility.

H2014

H2014 Skills training and development, per 15 minutes

Lay Description

Skills training and development provides the patient with necessary abilities that will enable the individual to live independently and manage his/her illness and treatment. Training focuses on skills for daily living and community integration for patients with functional limitations due to psychiatric disorders, per 15 minutes.

H2019-H2020

H2019 Therapeutic behavioral services, per 15 minutes
H2020 Therapeutic behavioral services, per diem

Lay Description

Therapeutic behavioral services are provided for a short period of time for serious emotionally disturbed youth. This service is mandated when an individual is at risk for placement in a restrictive treatment facility, or when transitioning from a group home of rate classification level (RCL) 12 through 14 to a higher level. This service targets disruptive behaviors that jeopardize continued placement in the current setting. This service requires a staff member be available for one-to-one therapeutic assistance and intervention. The individual must be receiving other specialty mental health services, as well as being at risk of placement at a higher level of residential care. Report H2019 when billing in 15-minute increments and H2020 when billing services per diem.

H2021-H2022

H2021 Community-based wrap-around services, per 15 minutes
H2022 Community-based wrap-around services, per diem

Lay Description

Wrap-around community services are provided for a short period of time for seriously emotionally disabled youth. These services are provided for children/adolescents with a rate classification level (RCL) placement higher than 12. These codes include support and training for family members as an integral part of services provided. Code H2021 is per 15-minute increments and H2022 is for services per diem.

H2023-H2024

H2023 Supported employment, per 15 minutes
H2024 Supported employment, per diem

Lay Description

Supported employment services are available to individuals with serious mental illness. Employment specialists assist in obtaining and maintaining employment in the community and in continuing treatment for the client to ensure rehabilitation and productive employment. Report H2023 for 15-minute increments and H2024 for services per diem.

H2025-H2026

H2025 Ongoing support to maintain employment, per 15 minutes
H2026 Ongoing support to maintain employment, per diem

Lay Description

Ongoing support to maintain employment services are available to individuals with serious mental illness. Employment specialists provide supportive counseling and interventions within the work environment when needed to ensure the continued employment and self-sufficiency of the client. Report H2025 for 15-minute increments and H2026 for services per diem.

H2028-H2029

H2028 Sexual offender treatment service, per 15 minutes
H2029 Sexual offender treatment service, per diem

Lay Description

Sexual offender treatment services provide rehabilitation services that vary depending on the type of treatment facility, security level, and staffing ratios available. Code H2028 is for services per 15 minutes. Code H2029 is for services per diem.

H2030-H2031

H2030 Mental health clubhouse services, per 15 minutes
H2031 Mental health clubhouse services, per diem

Lay Description

Mental health clubhouse is a community service provided for people with mental illness and promotes a structured environment in which individuals can improve interpersonal skills, and develop personal goals that will assist with success in the community. Participants are required to take part in the operations of the clubhouse. Code H2030 is for services per 15 minutes. Code H2031 is for services per diem.

H2032

H2032 Activity therapy, per 15 minutes

Lay Description

Activity therapy such as music, dance, creative art, or any type of play, not for recreation, but related to the care and treatment of the patient's disabling mental health problems is reported for services per 15 minutes.

H2033

H2033 Multisystemic therapy for juveniles, per 15 minutes

Lay Description

Multisystemic therapy uses the strengths found in key environmental settings of juveniles to promote and maintain positive behavioral changes. These services focus on individual, family, and extrafamilial (such as peer, school, and neighborhood) influences, reported in 15 minute increments.

H2034-H2036

H2034 Alcohol and/or drug abuse halfway house services, per diem
H2035 Alcohol and/or other drug treatment program, per hour
H2036 Alcohol and/or other drug treatment program, per diem

Lay Description

Halfway house services for alcohol and chemical dependency provide a transitional living environment. These services are structured to promote sobriety and independent living, and assist with continued treatment. Patients are free to work or attend classes during the day, and return to the facility at night. Code H2034 is for services per diem. Code H2035 is for alcohol and/or other drug treatment program services, not specifically in a half-hay house setting, per hour and H2036 per diem.

H2037

H2037 Developmental delay prevention activities, dependent child of client, per 15 minutes

Lay Description

Developmental delay prevention activities are designed to reduce the occurrence of problems stemming from inhibited or suppressed development in children that can have effects carrying over into later years. The developmental activities promote the physical and mental well being of dependent children of patients in treatment for alcohol/drug abuse. These services focus on overall healthy development of the child, reported in 15-minute blocks.

J0120

J0120 Injection, tetracycline, up to 250 mg

Lay Description

Tetracycline is a broad-spectrum antibiotic prepared from cultures of certain species of streptomyces bacteria. It is thought to inhibit protein synthesis in bacteria creating cell death. Many microorganisms have developed a resistance to tetracycline and related antibiotics. Susceptibility studies should be performed prior to administration. Tetracycline can be effective against gram-negative and gram-positive organisms. Susceptible organisms include Rickettsiae, Mycoplasma pneumoniae, Borrelia recurrentis, Haemophilus ducreyi, Pasteurella pestis, Pasteurella tularensis, Bartonella bacilliformis, Bacteroides species, Vibrio comma, Vibrio fetus, Brucella species (in conjunction with streptomycin), Escherichia coli, Enterobacter aerogenes, Shigella species, Mima species, Herellea species, Haemophilus influenzae, and Klebsiella species. HCPCS Level II code J0120 represents 250 mg of injectable tetracycline.

J0129

J0129 Injection, abatacept, 10 mg

Lay Description

Abatacept is a protein combination of human cytotoxic T-lymphocyte-associated antigen 4 (CTLA-4) linked to a modified portion of human immunoglobulin G1 (IgG1). It is produced by recombinant DNA technology. Abatacept binds to specific receptor sites of T lymphocyte cells and inhibits their activation. Activated T lymphocytes are found in joint fluid of patients with rheumatoid arthritis. Abatacept is indicated for reducing signs and symptoms, slowing the progression of structural damage, and improving physical function of adult patients with moderately to severely active rheumatoid arthritis who have had an inadequate response to other drugs. The drug can be used singularly or in combination with other disease-modifying, anti-rheumatic drugs. The drug is administered by intravenous infusion over a 30-minute period. Dosage varies from 500 mg to 1 g depending on body weight. HCPCS Level II code J0129 represents 10 mg of abatacept.

J0130

J0130 Injection abciximab, 10 mg

Lay Description

Abciximab is a murine monoclonal antibody. It blocks certain glycoprotein receptors on platelets and prevents them from aggregating or sticking together. Abciximab also blocks receptors on vessel walls and smooth muscle cells preventing the platelets from aggregating in those sites. It is used as an adjunct with percutaneous transluminal coronary angioplasty (PTCA). Abciximab may be used to treat unstable angina when the patient is not responding to conventional therapy and PTCA is planned within 24 hours. The recommended dosage is 0.25 mg per kg of body weight. The drug is administered as an intravenous bolus 10 to 60 minutes prior to the PTCA, followed by continuous intravenous infusion for 12 hours. When given to unstable angina patients for whom PTCA is planned, a 0.25 mg bolus is administered followed by an 18 to 24 hour intravenous infusion. HCPCS Level II code J0130 represents 10 mg of abciximab.

J0132

J0132 Injection, acetylcysteine, 100 mg

Lay Description

Acetylcysteine is a derivative of the naturally occurring amino acid L-cysteine. It is used as an antidote for acetaminophen overdose to prevent life-threatening liver damage. Acetylcysteine reacts with the acetaminophen rendering some of the acetaminophen harmless. As an antidote for acetaminophen poisoning, acetylcysteine should be administered as soon as possible but within 24 hours after the overdose. Acetylcysteine is administered by intravenous infusion over 60 minutes. HCPCS Level II code J0132 represents 100 mg of acetylcysteine.

J0133

J0133 Injection, acyclovir, 5 mg

Lay Description

Acyclovir injection is used to treat herpes infections, including herpes zoster and varicella (chickenpox). It does not cure the infection but does reduce pain and may promote faster healing. Acyclovir is given intravenously over at least an hour. This code reports a 5 mg injection.

Medicare Information

See chapter titled "Medicare Guidelines," under "Drugs, Biologicals, and Radiopharmaceuticals," for Medicare billing and documentation information.

J0135

J0135 Injection, adalimumab, 20 mg

Lay Description

Adalimumab is a human IgG1 monoclonal antibody that is specific for human tumor necrosis factor (TNF). It is produced by recombinant DNA technology. Adalimumab binds specifically to TNF-alpha and blocks its interaction with cell surface TNF receptors and lyses surface TNF expressing cells. Adalimumab also modulates biological responses that are induced or regulated by TNF, including changes in the levels of adhesion molecules responsible for leukocyte migration. Adalimumab is indicated for reducing signs and symptoms and inhibiting the progression of structural damage in adult patients with moderately to severely active rheumatoid arthritis who have had an inadequate response to one or more disease modifying antirheumatic drugs and patients with active arthritis with psoriatic arthritis. Adalimumab can be used alone or in combination with methotrexate or other disease modifying antirheumatic drugs. Adalimumab is administered by subcutaneous injection and can be self-administered. HCPCS Level II code J0135 represents 20 mg of adalimumab.

Medicare Information

See the chapter titled "Medicare Guidelines," under "Drugs, Biologicals, and Radiopharmaceuticals," for Medicare information.

J0150-J0152

J0150 Injection, adenosine for therapeutic use, 6 mg (not to be used to report any adenosine phosphate compounds, instead use A9270)

J0152 Injection, adenosine for diagnostic use, 30 mg (not to be used to report any adenosine phosphate compounds; instead use A9270)

Lay Description

Adenosine is a nucleoside that is a component of RNA. Its nucleotides play major roles in the reactions and regulation of metabolism. Preparations of adenosine act as cardiac depressants, antiarrhythmics, and vasodilators. Adenosine is administered to convert paroxysmal supraventricular tachycardia (PSVT) to normal sinus rhythm. Diagnostic adenosine is administered to patients as an adjunct to a thallium myocardial perfusion scan for patients who are unable to adequately exercise. Recommended dose for therapeutic use is an initial 6 mg followed by 12 mg if the arrhythmia continues. Adenosine is administered via intravenous push injection. HCPCS Level II code J0150 represents 6 mg of adenosine for therapeutic use and J0152 represents 30 mg for diagnostic use.

Medicare Information

See the chapter titled "Medicare Guidelines," under "Drugs, Biologicals, and Radiopharmaceuticals," for Medicare information.

J0171

J0171 Injection, Adrenalin, epinephrine, 0.1 mg

Lay Description

Epinephrine hydrochloride (HCl), also known as adrenalin, is a synthetic version of a hormone secreted by the adrenal gland. Epinephrine is a potent stimulator of the sympathetic nervous system that increases blood pressure, stimulates the heart, and increases metabolic functions. Exogenous epinephrine is used as a cardiac stimulant, to increase blood pressure, and to relax bronchial smooth muscles. The injectable version of epinephrine HCl is administered subcutaneously or intramuscularly and is used to treat serious hypersenstivity (allergic) reactions and anaphylaxis, and to restore cardiac rhythym in cardiac arrest.

J0180

J0180   Injection, agalsidase beta, 1 mg

Lay Description

Agalsidase beta is a recombinant human a-galactosidase An enzyme with the same amino acid sequence as the naturally occurring enzyme. It is produced by recombinant DNA technology in a Chinese hamster ovary. Agalsidase beta is an orphan drug specifically targeted to Fabry disease. Fabry disease is an X-linked genetic disorder of glycosphingolipid metabolism. A deficiency of enzyme a-galactosidase A leads to progressive accumulation of glycosphingolipids, predominantly GL-3, in many body tissues, occurring over a period of years or decades. Clinical manifestations of Fabry disease include renal failure, cardiomyopathy, and cerebrovascular accidents. Recommended dose is 1.0 mg per kg of body weight. Agalsidase beta is administered by intravenous infusion. HCPCS Level II code J0180 represents 1 mg of agalsidase beta.

Medicare Information

See the chapter titled "Medicare Guidelines," under "Drugs, Biologicals, and Radiopharmaceuticals," for Medicare information.

J0190

J0190   Injection, biperiden lactate, per 5 mg

Lay Description

The injectable form of biperiden lactate has been discontinued.

J0200

J0200   Injection, alatrofloxacin mesylate, 100 mg

Lay Description

HCPCS Level II code J0200 represents alatrofloxacin mesylate. Per the FDA, this drug is no longer available in the United States.

J0205

J0205   Injection, alglucerase, per 10 units

Lay Description

Alglucerase is a modified form of beta-glucocerebrosidase prepared from pooled human placental tissue. It is an orphan drug used to treat Gaucher's disease caused by the lack of the enzyme glucocerebrosidase, which is crucial to the metabolism of fats. Alglucerase normalizes the pathway for membrane lipids. Dose is based on disease severity and individual patient response to treatment. Initial dosage may be as little as 2.5 units per kg of body weight three times a week up to as much as 60 units per kg administered as often as once a week or as infrequently as every four weeks. Alglucerase is administered by intravenous infusion over one to two hours. HCPCS Level II code J0205 represents 10 units of alglucerase.

J0207

J0207   Injection, amifostine, 500 mg

Lay Description

Amifostine is dephosphorylated in living tissue by an alkaline phosphate enzyme to become a biologically active form of free thiol in the body. Free thiol will bind to and detoxify the reactive metabolites of cisplatin, scavenges free radicals from tissues exposed to cisplatin. Amifostine is used to reduce the cumulative nephrotoxicity in patients who have received repeated doses of cisplatin because of advanced ovarian cancer, bladder cancer, testicular cancer, or non-small cell lung cancer. It is also newly used to reduce xerostomia in patients with head and neck cancer receiving postoperative radiation treatment. For patients on chemotherapy, it is injected over a 15-minute period one half hour before chemotherapy. For patients receiving radiation treatment, it is injected over a three minute period 15 to 30 minutes prior to radiation. HCPCS Level II code J0207 represents 500 mg of amifostine.

J0210

J0210   Injection, methyldopate HCl, up to 250 mg

Lay Description

Methyldopate hydrochloride is an aromatic-amino-acid decarboxylase inhibitor used primarily to treat hypertension or during a hypertensive crisis. It decreases the sympathetic outflow to the heart, kidneys, and peripheral vasculature. Decreased blood pressure may occur four to six hours after the administration of methyldopate hydrochloride and last 10 to 16 hours. The usual dose is 250 to 500 mg intravenously at six-hour intervals as required. The maximum recommended intravenous dose is 1 gram every six hours. Methyldopate hydrochloride is administered via intravenous infusion over 30 to 60 minutes. HCPCS Level II code J0210 represents up to 250 mg of methyldopate hydrochloride.

J0215

J0215 Injection, alefacept, 0.5 mg

Lay Description

Alefacept is an injectable drug that suppresses the immune system and is used for the treatment of moderate to severe chronic plaque psoriasis. It interferes with lymphocyte activation by binding to the lymphocyte antigen and interfering with the human leukocyte function antigen-3 and the CD2 binding interaction. It is produced by recombinant DNA technology in a Chinese hamster ovary (CHO) mammalian cell expression system. The recommended dose is 7.5 mg given once weekly as an intravenous injection or 15 mg given once weekly as an intramuscular injection. The recommended regimen is a course of 12 weekly injections. HCPCS Level II code J0215 represents up to 0.5 mg of alefacept.

J0220

J0220 Injection, alglucosidase alfa, 10 mg

Lay Description

Alglucosidase alfa is an exogenous source of the human enzyme alpha-glucosidase made from recombinant DNA technology using Chinese hamstrer ovaries. It is an orphan drug used to treat glycogen storage disease, type II (Pompe disease, GSD II or acid maltase deficiency). GSD II is caused by the lack of the enzyme alpha-glucosidase, which is crucial to the metabolism of glycogen. GSD II leads to a build up of intralysomal glycigen resulting in progressive muscle weakness. In infantile onset, GSD II may also lead to cardiomyopathy and impairment of respiratory function. The recommended dosage is 20 mg per kg of patient body weight. Alglucosidase alfa is administered by intravenous infusion, using an infusion pump, over four hours, every two weeks.

J0256

J0256 Injection, alpha 1-proteinase inhibitor — human, 10 mg

Lay Description

Alpha 1-proteinase inhibitor, human is a plasma product prepared from pooled human plasma of normal donors that contains high levels of purified human alpha 1-proteinase inhibitor (alpha1-PI) also known as alpha 1-antitrypsin. This is used to treat patients with alpha 1 antitrypsin deficiency (A1AD), a genetic protein deficiency that results in advanced emphysema showing up in young patients as an inherited disease, not related to smoking or environmental factors. It mimics COPD, asthma, and acquired emphysema and is therefore difficult to diagnose and rated as rare. Replacing the protein helps prevent the continued lung destruction caused by this deficiency. Recommended dose is 60 mg per kg of body weight once a week. Alpha 1-proteinase inhibitor is administered via intravenous infusion over 15 to 30 minutes. HCPCS Level II code J0256 represents 10 mg of alpha 1-proteinase inhibitor, human.

J0270-J0275

J0270 Injection, alprostadil, 1.25 mcg (code may be used for Medicare when drug administered under the direct supervision of a physician, not for use when drug is self-administered)

J0275 Alprostadil urethral suppository (code may be used for Medicare when drug administered under the direct supervision of a physician, not for use when drug is self-administered)

Lay Description

Alprostadil is a naturally occurring form of prostaglandin. It is a vasodilator that increases blood flow by expanding blood vessels. It is used for patients in need of palliative therapy for the temporary maintenance of patency of ductus arteriosus who have congenital heart defects and who depend upon the patent ductus for survival. Studies have shown that alprostadil reopens a closing ductus arteriosus. It is also indicated in the treatment of erectile dysfunction. Alprostadil increases cavernous arterial blood flow and inhibits platelet aggregation. It induces erection by relaxing the trabecular smooth muscle and dilating the cavernosal arteries. This leads to expansion of lacunar spaces and entrapment of blood by compressing the venules against the tunica. This is also known as the corporal veno-occlusive mechanism. It also lowers the blood pressure and increases cardiac output. Alprostadil can be administered into a large vein or umbilical artery for infants with congenital heart defects. It is administered via injection into the corpora cavernosa or as a urethral suppository for erectile dysfunction. Both of the methods for treatment of erectile dysfunction can be self-administered. HCPCS Level II code J0270 represents 1.25 mcg of alprostadil injection and J0275 represents an alprostadil urethral suppository.

J0278

J0278 Injection, amikacin sulfate, 100 mg

Lay Description

Amikacin sulfate is an antibiotic used to treat susceptible strains of Gram-negative bacteria. It binds to the RNA and will not allow the bacteria to synthesize protein that is essential to its growth. It is effective against Pseudomonas species, E. coli, Proteus species, Klebsiella-Enterobacter-Serratia species, Providencia species, Salmonella species, Citrobacter species, and S. aureus. Amikacin sulfate may be used to treat bacteremia, septicemia (including neonatal sepsis), osteomyelitis, septic arthritis, respiratory tract, urinary tract, intra-abdominal (including peritonitis) infections, and soft tissue abscesses. This medication is administered via intramuscular injection or intravenous infusion. HCPCS Level II code J0278 represents 100 mg of amikacin sulfate.

J0280

J0280   Injection, aminophyllin, up to 250 mg

Lay Description

Aminophylline is a bronchodilator that is used to treat breathing problems such as asthma, emphysema, and chronic bronchitis. It relaxes the smooth muscle in the bronchial airways and pulmonary blood vessels by interfering with phosphodiesterase, which is the enzyme that corrupts adenosine 3', 5'-cyclic monophosphate (cAMP). HCPCS Level II code J0280 represents up to 250 mg of aminophylline.

Medicare Information

See the chapter titled "Medicare Guidelines," under "Drugs, Biologicals, and Radiopharmaceuticals," for Medicare information.

J0282

J0282   Injection, amiodarone HCl, 30 mg

Lay Description

Amiodarone hydrochloride is an antiarrhythmic used in the treatment of ventricular fibrillation and hemodynamically unstable atrial fibrillation that do not respond to other treatment. It blocks the calcium channels and potassium channels and lengthens the cardiac action potential and slows the conduction and prolongation of refractoriness. It decreases the workload of the heart and the amount of oxygen it requires. Amiodarone hydrochloride can be administered orally or by intravenous push followed by intravenous infusion that may be continuous for several days. HCPCS Level II code J0282 represents 30 mg of amiodarone hydrochloride.

Medicare Information

See the chapter titled "Medicare Guidelines," under "Drugs, Biologicals, and Radiopharmaceuticals," for Medicare information.

J0285-J0289

J0285   Injection, amphotericin B, 50 mg
J0287   Injection, amphotericin B lipid complex, 10 mg
J0288   Injection, amphotericin B cholesteryl sulfate complex, 10 mg
J0289   Injection, amphotericin B liposome, 10 mg

Lay Description

Amphotericin B is an antibiotic derived from a strain of Streptomyces nodosus that has antifungal properties. The drug is effective against a wide variety of fungi and some species of Leishmania. It binds to the fungus cell membrane and changes the permeability causing the cell contents to leak out, which causes cell death. Amphotericin B may be administered by intravenous infusion or intracavitary instillation over two to six hours. A topical version is used to treat superficial candidiasis. The cholesteryl complex version is administered by intravenous infusion to treat disseminated aspergillosis in patients refractory to or intolerant of conventional amphotericin B. The lipid complex is administered by intravenous infusion to treat invasive fungal infections in patients refractory to or intolerant of conventional amphotericin B. The liposome complex is administered by intravenous infusion to treat sever fungal infections and visceral leishmaniasis in patients refractory to or intolerant of conventional amphotericin B. HCPCS Level II code J0285 represents 50 mg of amphotericin B; J0287 represents 10 mg of amphotericin B lipid complex; J0288 represents 10 mg of amphotericin B cholesteryl sulfate complex; and J0289 represents 10 mg of amphotericin B liposome.

Medicare Information

See the chapter titled "Medicare Guidelines," under "Drugs, Biologicals, and Radiopharmaceuticals," for Medicare information.

J0290

J0290   Injection, ampicillin sodium, 500 mg

Lay Description

Ampicillin is a form of penicillin used to treat respiratory or skin infections, urinary tract infections, bacterial meningitis, septicemia, and as a prophylaxis in dental procedures. It inhibits the formation of a cell wall during replication. It is effective against E. coli, P. mirabilis, enterococci, Shigella, S. typhosa and other Salmonella, non-penicillinase-producing N. gononhoeae, non-penicillinase-producing H. influenzae and staphylococci, and streptococci including streptococcus pneumoniae, Shigella, S. typhosa and other Salmonella, E. coli, P. mirabilis, and enterococci, and O. Meningitides. This drug may decrease the efficacy of oral contraceptives. HCPCS Level II code J0290 represents 500 mg of ampicillin sodium.

Medicare Information
See the chapter titled "Medicare Guidelines," under "Drugs, Biologicals, and Radiopharmaceuticals," for Medicare information.

J0295

J0295   Injection, ampicillin sodium/sulbactam sodium, per 1.5 g

Lay Description
Ampicillin sodium and sulbactam sodium are used to treat gynecologic, intra-abdominal, and skin infections. Ampicillin inhibits the formation of a cell wall during replication and sulbactam inactivates the enzyme produced by the bacteria to make them resistant to the ampicillin. It is effective against Staphylococcus aureus, Staphylococcus epidermidis, Staphylococcus saprophyticus, Streptococcus faecalis, Streptococcus pneumoniae, Streptococcus pyogenes, Streptococcus viridans, Haemophilus influenzae, Moraxella (Branhamella) catarrhalis, Escherichia coli, Klebsiella species, Proteus mirabilis, Proteus vulgaris, Providencia rettgeri, Providencia stuartii, Morganella morganii, Neisseria gonorrhoeae, Clostridium species, Peptococcus species, Peptostreptococcus species, and Bacteroides species, including B. fragilis. Ampicillin sodium and sulbactam sodium are administered via intramuscular injection, which is given only to adults, and intravenous injection, which is given by slow infusion over 10 to 15 minutes. HCPCS Level II code J0295 represents 1.5 grams of ampicillin sodium/sulbactam sodium.

J0300

J0300   Injection, amobarbital, up to 125 mg

Lay Description
Amobarbital is a barbiturate derivative that activates one of the major inhibitory neurotransmitters in the body, which reduces input resistance, depresses the electrical discharge along the cell and increases the conduction at the chloride channels, and increases the amplitude and decay time of inhibitory postsynaptic currents. It is also known as truth serum. Amobarbital is indicated as a treatment for convulsions, anxiety, epilepsy, and as a short-term treatment of insomnia. The drug is also used for preoperative sedation. It is a schedule II drug with the suppository being a schedule III drug. This medication is administered orally, rectally, via intramuscular injection, and via intravenous push injection. HCPCS Level II code J0300 represents up to 125 mg of amobarbital.

J0330

J0330   Injection, succinylcholine chloride, up to 20 mg

Lay Description
Succinylcholine chloride is skeletal muscle relaxant. It is used in combination with anesthesia to relax skeletal muscles for surgery, intubation, seizure control, and orthopedic manipulations. It reacts with cholinergic receptors of the motor end plates to create depolarization. Flaccid paralysis begins within one minute after administration and lasts approximately four to six minutes. HCPCS Level II code J0330 represents up to 20 mg of succinylcholine chloride.

Medicare Information
See the chapter titled "Medicare Guidelines," under "Drugs, Biologicals, and Radiopharmaceuticals," for Medicare information.

J0348

J0348   Injection, anidulafungin, 1 mg

Lay Description
Anidulafungin is a semisynthetic lipopeptide derived from the fungus *Aspergillus nidulans* It is used as an anitfungal drug. Anidulafungin disrupts the synthesis of a component of the fungal cell membrane. This component is not present in mammalian cells. Anidulafungin is indicated for the treatment of candidemia,intra-abdmoinal, peritoneal and esophageal *Candida* infections. The drug may cause allergic reactions. Anidulafungin must be administered by intravenous infusion. Recommended doasge for esophageal candidiasis is an initial dose of 100 mg followed by 50 mg daily. The duration of treatment depends upon the patient's response, but should be for a minimum of 14 days or for at least seven days following resolution of symptoms. Recommended dosage for candidemia, intra-abdominal and peritoneal *Candida* infections is am initial dose of 200 mg followed by 100 mg daily. The duration of treatment depends upon the patient's response, but should continue for least 14 days after the last positive culture.HCPCS Level II code J0348 represents 1 mg of anidulafungin.

J0350

J0350   Injection, anistreplase, per 30 units

Lay Description
Anistreplase is a complex composed of streptokinase and lys-plasminogen. It is also known as anisoylated plasminogen-streptokinase activator complex (APSAC). It is a thrombolytic agent used to dissolve blood clots that have formed in certain blood vessels. It binds to fibrin, converts plasminogen into

plasmin, and breaks down the thrombus into smaller components. Anistreplase is used primarily in the management of an acute myocardial infarction and should be administered as soon as possible after the onset of the heart attack symptoms. Anistreplase is administered via intravenous infusion. HCPCS Level II code J0350 represents 30 units of anistreplase.

J0360

J0360   Injection, hydralazine HCl, up to 20 mg

Lay Description

Hydralazine hydrochloride falls into a category of drugs known as antihypertensives. It works by exerting a vasodilating effect on vascular smooth muscle. It is used in combination with other drugs in treating a hypertensive crisis and eclampsia. Hydralazine hydrochloride can be administered by intramuscular injection, intravenous injection, or intravenous infusion. HCPCS Level II code J0360 represents up to 20 mg of hydralazine hydrochloride.

J0364

J0364   Injection, apomorphine HCl, 1 mg

Lay Description

Apomorphine hydrochloride is a non-ergoline dopamine agonist. It is used for the acute, intermittent treatment of hypomobility, "off" episodes ("end-of-dose wearing off" and unpredictable "on/off" episodes) associated with advanced Parkinson's disease. pomorphine should not be started without use of an associated antiemetic. Trimethobenzamide should be started three days prior to the initial dose of apomorphine and continued at least during the first two months of therapy. Ondansetron, granisetron, dolasetron, palonosetron, and alosetron should not be used as antiemetics due to reports of hypotension and loss of consciousness when given with apomorphine. The maximum recommended dose is 6 mg. Apomorphine is administered via subcutaneous injection. HCPCS Level II code J0364 represents 1 mg of apomorphine hydrochloride.

J0365

J0365   Injection, aprotinin, 10,000 kiu

Lay Description

Aprotonin is broad-spectrum protease inhibitor obtained from a bovine lung that diminishes the inflammatory response in cardiopulmonary bypass surgery. It preserves glycoprotein in platelets. This reduces bleeding and decreases the need for allogenic blood transfusions. Patients receive a 1 milliliter test dose, for allergic reaction, intravenously at least 10 minutes prior to the loading dose. The loading dose is administered via intravenous infusion over 20 to 30 minutes after induction of anesthesia but prior to sternotomy. A dose is also added to the cardiopulmonary bypass circuit and a constant infusion is maintained until the end of surgery. HCPCS Level II code J0365 represents 10,000 kiu of aprotonin.

J0380

J0380   Injection, metaraminol bitartrate, per 10 mg

Lay Description

Metaraminol bitartrate is classified as an adrenergic agent, direct-acting vasopressor. It releases norepinephrine from storage sites and stimulates alpha-receptors, which causes an increase in blood pressure, venous tone, and pulmonary pressure. Metaraminol bitartrate is used in treating surgery related hypotension, trauma, adverse drug reactions, and spinal anesthesia. Metaraminol bitartrate can be administered via subcutaneous injection, intramuscular injection, intravenous push, or intravenous infusion. HCPCS Level II code J0380 represents 10 mg of metaraminol bitartrate.

J0390

J0390   Injection, chloroquine HCl, up to 250 mg

Lay Description

Chloroquine is an anti-infective used primarily in treating malaria and extraintestinal amebiasis. The mechanism of action is not fully understood but the drug does interfere with certain enzymes. It is effective against Plasmodium vivax, Plasmodium malariae, P. ovale, and susceptible strains of Plasmodium falciparum (but not the gametocytes of P. falciparum). It is not effective against exoerythrocytic forms of the parasite. Chloroquine is administered orally. The injectable form has been discontinued.

J0395

J0395   Injection, arbutamine HCl, 1 mg

Lay Description

HCPCS Level II code J0395 represents arbutamine hydrochloride. Per the FDA, this drug is no longer available in the United States.

J0400

J0400   Injection, aripiprazole, intramuscular, 0.25 mg

Lay Description

Aripiprazole is an antipsychotic medication used to treat schizophrenia and bipolar disorder. The precise mechanism of action of aripiprazole is not known. The drug has a strong attraction to dopamine and serotonin receptor sites and acts as an agonist to various dopamine and serotonin subtypes. Aripiprazole is indicated for: treatment of schizophrenia in patients age 13 years or older; acute and maintenance treatment of manic and mixed episodes of bipolar I disorder with or without psychotic features; adjunctive treatment of major depressive disorders; and treatment of agitation associated with schizophrenia or bipolar disorder, manic, or mixed. Aripiprazole is available in oral and injectable forms. The recommended oral dosage is 10 to 15 mg a day for schizophrenia, and 30 mg a day to treat bipolar disorder. When administered with an antidepressant, dosages may be as low as 2 mg a day. When aripiprazole is used to treat agitation associated with schizophrenia or bipolar mania, the dosage is usually 9.75 mg administered by intramuscular injection. The maximum daily dose is 30 mg/day. Code J0400 represents 0.25 mg of injectable aripiprazole given intramuscularly.

J0456

J0456 Injection, azithromycin, 500 mg

Lay Description

Azithromycin is an antibiotic used in treating a wide range of bacterial infections including community acquired pneumonia, urethritis, and tonsillitis. It binds to the ribosomal subunit and disrupts microbial protein synthesis. It is effective against Staphylococcus aureus, Streptococcus pneumoniae, Haemophilus influenzae, Moraxella catarrhalis, Neisseria gonorrhoeae, Chlamydia pneumoniae, Chlamydia trachomatis, Legionella pneumophila, Mycoplasma hominis, Mycoplasma pneumoniae, Streptococcus agalactiae, Streptococcus pyogenes, and Haemophilus ducreyi. Recommended intravenous dose is 500 mg once a day for one or two days followed by an oral regimen. Azithromycin is administered orally or via intravenous infusion over one to three hours. HCPCS Level II code J0456 represents 500 mg of injectable azithromycin.

J0461

J0461 Injection, atropine sulfate, 0.01 mg

Lay Description

Atropine is an extract of an alkaloid from the plants belladonna, hyoscyamus, or stramonium. It is also made synthetically. Atropine sulfate is a highly toxic compound of atropine and sulfuric acid that has the same uses and effects as atropine. It blocks the neurotransmitter acetylcholine in muscarinic receptors of the parasympathetic system. Muscarinic receptors occur throughout the nervous system including in the heart, smooth muscles of the blood vessels, lungs, salivary glands, gastrointestinal tract, and eye. Atropine sulfate in clinical doses counteracts the peripheral vessel dilatation and abrupt decrease in blood pressure produced by other drugs or biologicals. Systemic doses slightly raise systolic and lower diastolic pressures, slightly increase cardiac output, and decrease central venous pressure. Atropine is used as an antispasmodic to relax smooth muscles, to reduce secretions in the respiratory tract, and to temporarily increase heart rate or decrease AV-block until definitive treatment can take place, and as an antidote for cholinergic drugs toxins, poisoning from organophosphorus insecticides or certain toxic mushrooms. Since it counteracts the side effects of neuromuscular blockers and gases used in anesthesia, it may also be administered as a preanesthesia medication. HCPCS Level II code J0461 represents 0.01 mg of the injectable version of atropine sulfate.

J0470

J0470 Injection, dimercaprol, per 100 mg

Lay Description

Dimercaprol, also known as BAL in oil, is a chemical compound dispersed in peanut oil used as a chelating agent. Certain heavy metals, especially arsenic, gold, lead, and mercury, bind with some of the pyruvate-oxidase enzymes and inhibit their normal functioning. Dimercaprol has a stronger attraction to the metal than the protein. It binds to the metal in a stable complex and carries it out of the body. It is indicated as a treatment for arsenic, gold, and mercury (soluble inorganic compounds) poisoning following ingestion, inhalation, or absorption through the skin of these metals or their salts, or following overdose of therapeutic agents containing these metals. Dimercaprol, in conjunction with edetate calcium disodium (calcium EDTA), is also used as a treatment for lead poisoning. Treatment should begin immediately after exposure. It is administered by intramuscular injection only and the drug needs to be administered repeatedly for several days. Dosages vary from 2.5 to 5 mg/kg of body weight every four to six hours depending on the metal that caused the poisoning. Pediatric dosages for lead poisoning vary from 50 to 75 mg per square meter of body surface area every four hours followed by calcium EDTA. HCPCS Level II code J0470 represents 100 mg of dimercaprol.

Medicare Information

See the chapter titled "Medicare Guidelines," under "Drugs, Biologicals, and Radiopharmaceuticals," for Medicare information.

J0475-J0476

J0475 Injection, baclofen, 10 mg
J0476 Injection, baclofen, 50 mcg for intrathecal trial

Lay Description

Baclofen is a chemical analogue of y-aminobutyric acid, an amino acid also known as GABA that is used as a muscle relaxant and antispastic. GABA is the principal inhibitory neurotransmitter in the brain, but is also found in several extraneural tissues, including kidney and pancreatic islet cells. GABA modulates membrane chloride permeability and inhibits postsynaptic cell firing. Although baclofen is an analogue of GABA, its exact mechanism of action is not fully understood. It inhibits both monosynaptic and polysynaptic reflexes at the spinal level, possibly by decreasing excitatory neurotransmitter release. Baclofen is available in an oral self-administered version and in an intrathecal version. It is used intrathecally to treat spasticity of cerebral origin, including trauma to the brain or cerebral palsy. The intrathecal administration is a long-term infusion delivered by an implantable pump. Prior to the pump implantation, patients usually receive a test or trial dose of 50 mcg administered via an intrathecal injection. HCPCS Level II code J0475 represents 10 mg of baclofen and J0476 represents 50 mcg of intrathecal baclofen.

Medicare Information

See the chapter titled "Medicare Guidelines," under "Drugs, Biologicals, and Radiopharmaceuticals," for Medicare information.

J0480

J0480 Injection, basiliximab, 20 mg

Lay Description

Basiliximab is a chimeric (murine/human) monoclonal antibody produced by recombinant DNA technology that is an immunosuppressive agent. Basiliximab binds to certain interleukin-2, also as CD25 antigen, receptor sites on activated T lymphocytes. By blocking these receptor sites, it prevents the interleukin-2 from activating the immune response, preventing rejection of allogenic transplants. Basiliximab in combination with cyclosporine and corticosteroids is indicated for the prophylaxis of acute organ rejection in patients receiving renal transplants. It is administered by intravenous bolus or by infusion over a 20-30 minute period. The dosage varies from 10 -20 mg. Basiliximab should only be administered once prior to the transplant when it has been determined that the patient will have the transplant with the concomitant immunosuppression. HCPCS Level II code J0480 represents 20 mg of basiliximab.

Medicare Information

See the chapter titled "Medicare Guidelines," under "Drugs, Biologicals, and Radiopharmaceuticals," for Medicare information.

J0500

J0500 Injection, dicyclomine HCl, up to 20 mg

Lay Description

Dicyclomine is a chemical compound that is an antispasmodic and anticholinergic (antimuscarinic) agent. It relieves smooth muscle spasms of the gastrointestinal tract. Dicyclomine appears to achieve this effect by inhibiting acetylcholine and by a direct effect on the smooth muscles. It is indicated for the treatment of irritable bowel syndrome. The injectable form is administered by intramuscular injection. Dosages are individualized to the patient depending upon response. HCPCS Level II code J0500 represents up to 20 mg of injectable dicyclomine hydrochloride.

J0515

J0515 Injection, benztropine mesylate, per 1 mg

Lay Description

Benztropine mesylate is a chemical compound containing atropine and diphenhydramine. The drug has anticholinergic and antihistamine effects. Benztropine mesylate is indicated as an adjunct treatment of Parkinson's disease and as a treatment for extrapyramidal disorders except tardive dyskinesia due to neuroleptic drugs. The drug is available in injectable and oral forms. The injectable form is recommended when a rapid response is desired and is useful for psychotic patients with acute dystonic reactions or other reactions that make oral medication difficult or impossible. The injectable form is administered by intramuscular on intravenous injection. Dosages vary from 0.5 to 6 mg depending upon response. HCPCS Level II code J0515 represents 1 mg of injectable benztropine mesylate.

J0520

J0520 Injection, bethanechol chloride, Myotonachol or Urecholine, up to 5 mg

Lay Description

Bethanechol chloride is a chemical compound that selectively stimulates the parasympathetic nervous system to release acetylcholine, a neurotransmitter. It stimulates the bladder muscles to contract and the motility of the gastric system. Bethanechol chloride is indicated for the treatment of acute postoperative and postpartum nonobstructive urinary retention and for neurogenic bladders with urinary retention. It is administered by subcutaneous injection.

Dosages vary depending upon type and severity of the condition. HCPCS Level II code J0520 represents up to 5 mg of injectable bethanechol chloride.

J0558

J0558 Injection, penicillin G benzathine and penicillin G procaine, 100,000 units

Lay Description

Penicillin G benzathine and penicillin G procaine is a suspension of equal amounts of each penicillin formulation. See the separate entries for penicillin G benzathine and penicillin G procaine for additional information. Penicillin G benzathine and penicillin G procaine is administered by deep intramuscular injection to the buttocks or thigh. The drug is slowly absorbed, released from the injection site. Once in the body, penicillin G benzathine and penicillin G procaine is hydrolyzed to penicillin G. The hydrolysis and slow absorption provide sustained, but lower blood levels of penicillin. Antibiotic action can be present for two to four weeks after a single injection. Susceptibility studies should be performed prior to the administration of this drug. Indications include severe upper respiratory tract infections of susceptible streptococci, scarlet fever, erysipelas, skin and soft tissue infections of susceptible streptococci, and severe pneumonia and otitis media due to susceptible pneumococci.

J0561

J0561 Injection, penicillin G benzathine, 100,000 units

Lay Description

Penicillin G benzathine, also known as benzathine benzylpenicillin, is a version of penicillin that contains dibenzylethylene diamine. Penicillins block the actions of transpeptidase, an enzyme needed to create the cell wall. This weakens the bacterial cell wall causing cellular death. This formulation is administered by deep intramuscular injection to the buttocks or thigh. The drug is slowly absorbed released from the injection site. Once in the body, penicillin G benzathine is hydrolyzed to penicillin G. The hydrolysis and slow absorption provide sustained, but lower blood levels of penicillin. Antibiotic action can be present for two to four weeks after a single injection. Susceptibility studies should be performed prior to the administration of penicillin G benzathine. Indications include mild to moderate upper respiratory tract infections of susceptible streptococci, syphilis, yaws, pinta, as a prophylaxis for rheumatic fever and chorea, and as a prophylactic follow-up for rheumatic heart disease and acute glomerulonephritis. Dosages vary from 300,000 units to 2,400,000 units depending upon the age of the patient and the disease being treated.

J0583

J0583 Injection, bivalirudin, 1 mg

Lay Description

Bivalirudin is a synthetic, 20 amino acid peptide that is a specific and reversible direct thrombin inhibitor. It binds to both circulating and clot-bound thrombin, which in turn prevents the thrombin from activating the coagulant cycle. Bivalirudin is indicated for use in conjunction with aspirin therapy as an anticoagulant in patients with unstable angina undergoing percutaneous transluminal coronary angioplasty (PTCA). The use of bivalirudin in conjunction with glycoprotein IIb/IIIa inhibitor is currently in clinical trials. Bivalirudin is also indicated for patients with or at risk for heparin-induced thrombocytopenia or heparin-induced thrombocytopenia with thrombosis syndrome who are undergoing percutaneous coronary interventions (PCI). Bivalirudin is not recommended for patients with acute coronary syndromes who are not undergoing PTCA or PCI. The drug is administered by intravenous injection and infusion. The recommended initial dosage is an intravenous bolus of 0.75 mg per kg of body weight. This is followed by an infusion of 1.75 mg per kg of body weight per hour for the duration of the procedure. Continued infusion of the drug after the procedure is left to the discretion of the treating physician. HCPCS Level II code J0583 represents 1 mg of bivalirudin.

J0585

J0585 Injection, onabotulinumtoxinA, 1 unit

Lay Description

Toxins are poisons, usually proteins produced by some higher plants, certain animals, and pathogenic bacteria, that are highly toxic for other living organisms. OnabotulinumtoxinA is a potent neurotoxin produced by the bacterium *Clostridium botulinum* type A. The toxin binds to sites on motor and sympathetic nerves and inhibits the release of acetylcholine. Injection of onabotulinumtoxinA produces partial chemical denervation at the injection site resulting in a localized reduction in muscular activity. OnabotulinumtoxinA is indicated as a cosmetic agent to provide temporary improvement in the appearance of moderate to severe glabellar lines associated with corrugator and/or procerus muscle activity. It may also be used as treatment for cervical dystonia in adults to decrease the severity of an abnormal head position and neck pain, severe primary axillary hyperhidrosis that is inadequately managed with topical agents, and strabismus and blepharospasm associated with dystonia in patients 12 years of age or older. OnabotulinumtoxinA is injected intramuscularly.

HCPCS Level II code J0585 represents 1 unit of onabotulinumtoxinA.

J0586

J0586 Injection, abobotulinumtoxinA, 5 units

Lay Description

AbobotulinumtoxinA is an acetylcholine release inhibitor and a neuromuscular blocker. It is used to treat adult cervical dystonia and the temporary treatment of glabellar lines in adults age 65 and over. It is a purified form of the Clostridium botulinum type A bacteria. The medication is injected into the affected muscles.

The recommended dose is 500 units for patients who have not been treated before. They should be divided between the muscles being treated. The injections may be done with EMG guidance. In clinical studies, it appears that the peak affect is about two to four weeks. If any retreatments are need, there should be a span of at least twelve weeks. Retreatment dosage is between 250 and 1,000 units.

The recommended dose for patients with glabellar lines is 50 units divided equally into the five areas. Retreatment should not be any more frequently than every three months.

J0587

J0587 Injection, rimabotulinumtoxinB, 100 units

Lay Description

Botulinum toxin type B is a purified form of the neurotoxin produced from fermentation of Colstridium botulinum type B. It inhibits acetylochine release at the nerve and is used as a neuromuscular blocking agent. Botulinum toxin type B is indicated for the treatment of cervical dystonia to reduce the severity of abnormal head position and associated neck pain caused by cervical dystonia. Botulinum toxin type B is administered by injection directly into the muscles that are affected. The average dose of botulinum toxin type B in adults for the treatment of cervical dystonia and associated abnormal head position and neck pain is one or more injections up to a total of 2,500 to 5,000 units. HCPCS Level II code J0587 represents 100 units of botulinum toxin type B.

J0592

J0592 Injection, buprenorphine HCl, 0.1 mg

Lay Description

Buprenorphine hydrochloride is a schedule V controlled substance. It is indicated for moderate to severe pain including postoperative pain and chronic pain of patients with terminal diseases. It is also used adjunctively with anesthesia as a means of providing postoperative pain relief. Although the action of the drug is not known, it binds with opiate receptors in the central nervous system and alters not only the perception of pain, but the emotional response as well. Buprenorphine hydrochloride is an injectable solution. It is administered by intramuscular, intravenous, or epidural injection. It may be administered by continuous intravenous infusion. HCPCS Level II code J0592 represents 0.1 mg of buprenorphine hydrochloride.

J0594

J0594 Injection, busulfan, 1 mg

Lay Description

Busulfan is a chemotherapeutic drug classified as a bifunctional alkylating agent that suppresses bone marrow function. Busulfan is used in combination with cyclophosphamide as a conditioning regiment prior to allogenic bone marrow or stem cell transplantation for chronic myelogenous leukemia. Injectable busulfan is administered as an intravenous infusion over two hours via a central venous catheter. The drug should be administered every six hours for four consecutive days for a total of 16 doses. The recommended dose is 0.8 mg per kg of adjusted ideal body weight. HCPCS Level II code J0594 represents 1 mg of injectable busulfan.

J0595

J0595 Injection, butorphanol tartrate, 1 mg

Lay Description

Butorphanol tartrate is a schedule IV controlled substance. It is indicated for moderate to severe pain, including postoperative pain and labor. It is also used prior to the administration of anesthesia and adjunctively with anesthesia. Although the action of the drug is not known, it binds with opiate receptors in the central nervous system and alters not only the perception of pain, but the emotional response as well.. Butorphanol tartrate is administered by intramuscular and intravenous push injection. HCPCS Level II code J0595 represents 1 mg of butorphanol tartrate.

J0598

J0598 Injection, C-1 esterase inhibitor (human), Cinryze, 10 units

Lay Description

C1 esterase inhibitor is a protein found in the blood that regulates the complement system. The complement system is a group of proteins found in the blood. There are nine complements. These complements work with the immune system. Low C1 estrace could be the result of hereditary angioedema which is a rare condition passed down in families. The recommended dose varies. C1 esterase inhibitor is administered by IV infusion.

J0600

J0600   Injection, edetate calcium disodium, up to 1,000 mg

Lay Description

Edetate calcium disodium is a chelating drug that is used as an antidote for lead poisoning and lead encephalopathy in adults and children. The mode of action of the drug is to form a stable chelate with any metal that has the ability to displace calcium, particularly lead. Edetate calcium disodium is used alone for patients with very high blood lead levels (≥70 mcg/dl). When lead poisoning is present, the drug should be used in combination with dimercaprol. Therapy is administered over a five-day period, followed by an interruption of two to four days (to allow for redistribution of the lead, as well as to prevent depletion of other essential metals such as zinc), and then another treatment course is administered. Most often two courses of therapy are administered. Edetate calcium disodium is provided in injectable form only. The drug may be administered intramuscularly (preferred route for pediatric patients), as well as for all patients with lead encephalopathy. Intravenously, the drug is administered as a slow infusion over a period of eight to 12 hours. HCPCS Level II code J0600 represents up to 1,000 mg of edetate calcium disodium.

J0610

J0610   Injection, calcium gluconate, per 10 ml

Lay Description

Calcium is a metallic element that is the most abundant element in the human body. It is found in almost all organized tissues. Calcium, in combination with phosphorus, forms calcium phosphate, the dense, hard material of the teeth and bones. It is an essential dietary element, an electrolyte essential for the maintenance of normal heartbeat and functioning of nerves and muscles. Calcium also plays a role in multiple phases of blood coagulation and in many enzymatic processes. Calcium gluconate is a form of calcium used to replace and maintain adequate levels of calcium. It is indicated as a nutritional supplement, for the prophylaxis and treatment of hypocalcemia related to hypoparathyroidism, rickets, osteomalacia, lead poisoning, and magnesium sulfate overdose. It is also indicated as treatment of hyperkalemia and as an adjunct treatment for cardiac arrest. HCPCS Level II code J0610 represents 10 ml of injectable calcium gluconate.

J0620

J0620   Injection, calcium glycerophosphate and calcium lactate, per 10 ml

Lay Description

Calcium is a metallic element that is the most abundant element in the human body. It is found in almost all organized tissues. Calcium, in combination with phosphorus, forms calcium phosphate, the dense, hard material of the teeth and bones. It is an essential dietary element, an electrolyte essential for the maintenance of normal heartbeat and functioning of nerves and muscles. Calcium also plays a role in multiple phases of blood coagulation and in many enzymatic processes. Calcium glycerophosphate and calcium lactate are electrolytes used to replace and maintain adequate levels of calcium. They are indicated for the prophylaxis and treatment of hypocalcemia. Calcium glycerophosphate and calcium lactate are administered by intramuscular or intravenous injection. HCPCS Level II code J0620 represents 10 ml of injectable calcium glycerophosphate and calcium lactate.

J0630

J0630   Injection, calcitonin salmon, up to 400 units

Lay Description

Calcitonin-salmon is a synthetic version of the hormone calcitonin originally obtained from salmon, but now produced by recombinant DNA technology. The salmon version has a slightly different amino acid sequence than the human form, but it produces the same effects. Calcitonin lowers plasma calcium and phosphate levels, inhibits bone resorption, and acts as an antagonist to the parathyroid hormone. Calcitonin-salmon is indicated for the treatment of symptomatic Paget"s disease of bone, hypercalcemia, and postmenopausal osteoporosis. The drug is provided in injection solution for subcutaneous or intramuscular injection. HCPCS Level II code J0630 represents up to 400 units of calcitonin-salmon.

J0636

J0636   Injection, calcitriol, 0.1 mcg

Lay Description

Calcitrol is a form of cholecalciferol that is a parathyroid-like hormone. It increases the ability of the body to absorb vitamin D and to distribute calcium throughout the body. It is indicated for the treatment of hypocalcemia, hypophosphatemia, rickets, osteodystrophy associated with long-term dialysis, and such disorders as hypoparathyroidism and pseudo-hypoparathyroidism. It is available in oral and injectable forms. The injectable form is administered by intravenous injection. Dosages vary from 0.25 to 3 mcg depending upon the form and indication. HCPCS Level II code J0636 represents 0.1 mcg of injectable calcitriol.

J0637

J0637   Injection, caspofungin acetate, 5 mg

Lay Description

Caspofungin acetate is an antifungal with the ability to inhibit one of the integral components of the cell wall of the fungus. It is indicated for treatment of presumed fungal infections in patients that are febrile and neutropenic, esophageal candidiasis, intra-abdominal candidiasis, pleural space candida infection, candida peritonitis, and for the treatment of invasive aspergillosis in patients who are intolerant of or refractory to other therapies. Caspofungin acetate is administered by slow intravenous infusion over one hour. It should not be mixed or infused with another drug. For the majority of indications, a 70 mg initial loading dose is administered on the first day, followed by 50 mg daily. HCPCS Level II code J0637 represents 5 mg of caspofungin acetate.

J0640

J0640   Injection, leucovorin calcium, per 50 mg

Lay Description

Leucovorin calcium (folinic acid, citrovorum factor) is a form of folic acid. When used with the chemotherapy drug 5-fluorouraci (Adrucil, 5-FU), it increases the ability of that drug to reduce or stop cell growth in advanced colorectal cancer. Leucovorin calcium is also indicated as a treatment for or to prevent toxicities associated with folic acid antagonists including methotrexate (MTX, Rheumatrex), trimetrexate (Neutrexin), trimethoprim (Proloprim, Trimpex), trimethoprim/sulfamethoxazole (Bactrim, Septra), pyrimethamine (Daraprim), and pyrimethamine/sulfadoxine (Fansidar). Leucovorin calcium is also used for the treatment of folate-deficient megaloblastic anemias. Leucovorin calcium is available in injectable and oral forms. Doses and route of administration vary with regards to the condition being treated.

J0641

J0641   Injection, levoleucovorin calcium, 0.5 mg

Lay Description

Levoleucovorin is similar to folate and used to reduce the toxicity in high-dose methotrexate therapy in osteosarcoma. Methotrexate is a folic acid antagonist. Folate is one of the B vitamins necessary for the production of DNA and RNA. Recommended dose is 7.5 mg administered as an IV infusion. It should not be mixed with other agents in the same mixture. HCPCS Level II code J0641 represents 0.5 mg of levoleucovorin calcium.

J0670

J0670   Injection, mepivacaine HCl, per 10 ml

Lay Description

Mepivacaine hydrochloride is a local anesthetic available in concentrations of 1%, 1.5%, and 2% for injection. As a local anesthetic, mepivacaine hydrochloride blocks the generation and conduction of nerve impulses. It may be administered by local infiltration, as a peripheral nerve block, or for caudal and lumbar epidural blocks. Dosages and concentrations of the drug vary with regards to how it is being administered. HCPCS Level II code J0670 represents 10 ml of mepivacaine hydrochloride.

J0690

J0690   Injection, cefazolin sodium, 500 mg

Lay Description

Cefazolin sodium is a semi-synthetic cephalosporin that inhibits synthesis of the cell wall used to prevent and treat a wide range of bacterial infections. Susceptibility studies should be performed prior to the administration of cefazolin sodium. Susceptible bacteria include S. pneumoniae, Klebsiella species, H. influenzae, S. aureus, group A beta-hemolytic streptococci, E. coli, P. mirabilis, S. aureus, and some strains of Enterobacter and enterococci. Cefazolin sodium is available in an injectable form for intravenous and intramuscular injection or intravenous infusion. Dosages vary from 25 mg to 1 g depending on the indication and for children, their body weight. HCPCS Level II code J0690 represents 500 mg of cefazolin sodium.

J0692

J0692   Injection, cefepime HCl, 500 mg

Lay Description

Cefepime hydrochloride is a semi-synthetic, broad spectrum, fourth generation cephalosporin antibiotic. It works by inhibiting synthesis of the cell wall and is used to treat a wide range of bacterial infections, as well as for empiric treatment for febrile neutropenia. Susceptibility studies should be performed prior to the administration of cefazolin sodium. Susceptible bacteria include Streptococcus pneumoniae, Pseudomonas aeruginosa, Klebsiella pneumoniae, Enterobacter species, Escherichia coli, Proteus mirabilis, Staphylococcus aureus, Streptococcus pyogenes, Bacteroides fragilis, and some strains of Enterobacter and streptococci. Intramuscular administration is used only for infections caused by E. coli. Otherwise, the intravenous route is used and the drug is administered by infusion over a period of 30 minutes. Dosages vary from 0.5 to 2 g depending on the indication and for children, their body weight. HCPCS Level II code J0692 represents 500 mg of cefepime hydrochloride.

J0694

J0694 Injection, cefoxitin sodium, 1 g

Lay Description

Cefoxitin sodium is a broad spectrum, third generation cephalosporin antibiotic. It works by inhibiting synthesis of the cell wall and is used to treat a wide range of bacterial infections. Cefoxitin sodium is administered by intravenous or intramuscular injection. Dosages vary from 80 mg to 2 g depending on the type and severity of the infection being treated and for children, their body weight. HCPCS Level II code J0694 represents 1 g of cefoxitin sodium.

J0696

J0696 Injection, ceftriaxone sodium, per 250 mg

Lay Description

Ceftriaxone sodium is a semisynthetic, third generation, broad-spectrum cephalosporin antibiotic for intravenous or intramuscular administration. It works by inhibiting synthesis of the cell wall and is used to treat a wide range of bacterial infections, as well as preoperative prevention. For IV use, it is mixed with 50 to 100 ml of compatible solution for infusion over a period of 30 minutes. Dosages depend on the type of infection being treated, as well as the patient's age and the weight of children. For adults, the dosage ranges from 1 to 2 g IV daily. For children age 12 or younger, 50 to 100 mg/kg IM or IV every 12 hours. HCPCS Level II code J0696 represents 250 mg of ceftriaxone sodium.

J0697

J0697 Injection, sterile cefuroxime sodium, per 750 mg

Lay Description

Cefuroxime sodium is a semisynthetic, second generation, broad-spectrum cephalosporin antibiotic for intravenous or intramuscular administration. It works by inhibiting synthesis of the cell wall and is used to treat a wide range of bacterial infections, as well as preoperative prevention. For IV use, it may be infused over a period of 15 to 60 minutes or injected directly over a period of three to five minutes. Dosages and the form of administration depend on the type and severity of the infection being treated, as well as the patient's age and the weight of children. There is also an oral form, cefuroxime axetil, that is available in a suspension as well as tablets. HCPCS

Level II code J0697 represents 750 mg of cefuroxime sodium.

J0698

J0698 Injection, cefotaxime sodium, per g

Lay Description

Cefotaxime sodium is a semisynthetic, third generation, broad-spectrum cephalosporin antibiotic for intravenous or intramuscular administration. It works by inhibiting synthesis of the cell wall and is used to treat a wide range of bacterial infections, as well as preoperative prevention. For IV use, it may be infused over a period of 20 to 30 minutes or injected directly over a period of three to five minutes. Dosages and the form of administration depend on the type and severity of the infection being treated, as well as the patient's age and the weight of children. HCPCS Level II code J0698 represents 1 g of cefotaxime sodium.

J0702

J0702 Injection, betamethasone acetate 3 mg and betamethasone sodium phosphate 3 mg

Lay Description

Betamethasone acetate and betamethazone sodium phosphate are injectable corticosteroid suspensions with anti-inflammatory and immunosuppressive abilities. The injectable corticosteroid suspensions are used to treat a wide variety of medical problems, including endocrine disorders, rheumatic disorders, collagen diseases, allergic states, ophthalmic diseases, gastrointestinal diseases, respiratory diseases, dermatologic diseases, hematologic disorders, neoplastic disorders, edematous states, nervous system disorders, tuberculous meningitis, and trichinosis with neurologic or myocardial involvement. The route of administration depends on the condition being treated. For most conditions, betamethasone acetate and betamethazone sodium phosphate are administered by intramuscular injection. For conditions such as bursitis, tenosynovitis, peritendonitis, ganglion cysts, or bone cysts, the injection is administered directly into the bursa, tendon sheath, or cystic lesions. For rheumatoid arthritis and osteoarthritis, administration is by intra-articular injection. .

J0706

J0706 Injection, caffeine citrate, 5 mg

Lay Description

Caffeine is a methylxanthine that is a central nervous system stimulant, bronchial smooth muscle relaxant, cardiac stimulant, and a diuretic. Caffeine citrate is a compound of caffeine and citric acid. It is indicated for adjunct treatment of apnea in premature neonates between 28 to 33 weeks gestational age. The exact action of caffeine citrate is not known, but it is thought to stimulate the respiratory center; increase minute ventilate; diminish diaphragm fatigue; increase metabolic rate skeletal tone, and oxygen consumption response; and decrease the threshold to and increase the response to hypercapnia. A loading dose of 1 mg per kg of body weight is administered by intravenous infusion over a period of 30 minutes using an infusion pump followed by a maintenance dose of 5 mg per kg of body weight over a 10-minute period every 24 hours. HCPCS Level II code J0706 represents 5 mg of caffeine citrate.

J0710
J0710 Injection, cephapirin sodium, up to 1 g

Lay Description
HCPCS Level II code J0710 represents cephapirin sodium. Per the FDA, this drug is no longer available in the United States.

J0713
J0713 Injection, ceftazidime, per 500 mg

Lay Description
Ceftazidime is a cephalosporin, a bactericidal agent that prevents cell wall production, causing osmotic imbalance in cellular pressure, and leading to cell death. This drug is used to treat serious infections of the lower respiratory and genitourinary tract, the central nervous system, and skin. It is also used in cases of bacteremia and septicemia from susceptible Streptococci, Staphylococcus aureus, E. coli, Klebsiella, Enterobacter, and Pseudomonas. Side effects include phlebitis, thrombophlebitis, rashes, urticaria, sterile abscesses of the skin, vaginitis, candidiasis, cramps, vomiting, diarrhea, hypersensitivity reactions, and other hematologic conditions. Concomitant use with aminoglycosides produces an additive effect against some microorganisms and may increase nephrotoxicity. Chloramphenicol is antagonistic to the action of ceftazidime. This anti-infective is administered by IV or IM injection with sodium carbonate, arginine, or as a premix infusion solution. This code is for a 500 mg injection.

J0715
J0715 Injection, ceftizoxime sodium, per 500 mg

Lay Description
Ceftizoxime sodium is a semisynthetic, third generation, broad-spectrum, beta-lactamase resistant cephalosporin antibiotic. It works by inhibiting synthesis of the cell wall and is used to treat a wide range of bacterial infections. Susceptibility studies should be performed prior to the administration of ceftizoxime sodium. Susceptible bacteria include Klebsiella, Serratia, Enterobacter, Pseudomonas, Peptococcus, Peptostreptococcus, Bacteroides species, Proteus mirabilis, Escherichia coli, Haemophilus influenzae, Staphylococcus aureus, P. vulgaris, Providencia rettgeri, Morganella morganii, Neisseria gonorrhoeae, Streptococcus agalactiae, Staphylococcus epidermidis, and Streptococcus species excluding enterococci. Ceftizoxime sodium is administered by intravenous or intramuscular injection. Dosages vary from 200 mg to 2 g depending on the type and severity of the infection and for children, their body weight. HCPCS Level II code J0715 represents 500 mg of ceftizoxime sodium.

J0718
J0718 Injection, certolizumab pegol, 1 mg

Lay Description
Certolizumab pegol is a tumor necrosis factor (TNF) blocker used to treat rheumatoid arthritis and the symptoms of Crohn's disease in patients who have not responded to conventional treatment. It is a recombinant humanized antibody Fab fragment that is manufactured in E. coli. For rheumatoid arthritis, the initial recommended dose is 400 mg (given as two subcutaneous injections of 200 mg). The same dose is given at weeks two and four. It is then reduced to 200 mg every other week. For maintenance, 200 mg may be given every four weeks. For Crohn's disease, the recommended initial adult dose is 400 mg (given as two subcutaneous injections of 200 mg). The same dose is given at weeks two and four. In patients who obtain a clinical response, the recommended maintenance regimen is 400 mg every four weeks. Certolizumab pegol is given as a subcutaneous injection.

J0720
J0720 Injection, chloramphenicol sodium succinate, up to 1 g

Lay Description
Chloramphenicol sodium is a potent antibiotic that is useful for, and should be reserved for, serious infections caused by organisms susceptible to its antimicrobial effects when other therapeutic agents that are potentially less hazardous are ineffective or contraindicated. The drug is able to inhibit bacterial protein synthesis and exert a bacteriostatic effect. Chloramphenicol is injected intravenously over a period of three to five minutes. Dosages depend on the type and severity of the infection being treated, as well as the patient's age, weight, and the presence of hepatic or renal function impairment. It should be used very cautiously in children and newborns with immature metabolic function. The adult dose is 50 to

100 mg/kg IV daily, divided into doses every six hours. For children, the dose is 50 mg/kg per day divided into four doses at six hour intervals. When cerebrospinal fluid concentrations of the drug are required, such as for meningitis, a dosage of up to 100 mg/kg a day can be administered. In newborns that are less than 2 weeks of age, a total of 25 mg/kg per day is administered in four equal doses at intervals of six hours. HCPCS Level II code J0720 represents up to 1 g of chloramphenicol sodium succinate.

J0725

J0725 Injection, chorionic gonadotropin, per 1,000 USP units

Lay Description

Chorionic gonadotropin is a hormone with actions nearly the same as luteinizing hormone (LH), which is produced by the pituitary gland and is the same as the hormone produced by the placenta during pregnancy. Indications for the use of chorionic gonadotropin vary with males and females. Used in many in-vitro fertilization programs, chorionic gonadotropin is used to aid conception and is usually administered in combination with other drugs including menotropins and urofollitropin. In male patients, LH and chorionic gonadotropin stimulate the testes to produce male hormones such as testosterone for the treatment of cryptorchidism, male infertility, and hypogonadism. Although chorionic gonadotropin may be prescribed as a weight loss drug, it should not be used for this indication. It is available in an injectable form only. The dose and the frequency with which it is administered are determined based on the indication for its use. For the treatment of male patients with low male hormone levels, 1,000 to 4,000 units are provided intramuscularly (IM) two or three times weekly. Treatment may range from several weeks to several months. For women undergoing fertility treatment, 5,000 to 10,000 units are administered IM per the physician's instructions. Children being treated for cryptorchidism will receive 1,000 to 5,000 units IM two or three times weekly for up to a total of 10 doses. HCPCS Level II code J0725 represents 1,000 USP units of chorionic gonadotropin.

J0735

J0735 Injection, clonidine HCl, 1 mg

Lay Description

Clonidine hydrochloride is used in addition to opiates to treat severe pain caused by cancer. Although the action of the drug is not known, it is thought to stimulate alpha2-adrenergic receptors and inhibit central vasomotor centers, which lowers sympathetic outflow to the kidneys, heart, and peripheral vascular system lowering vascular resistance, blood pressure, and heart rate. HCPCS Level II code J0735 represents 1 mg of injectable clonidine hydrochloride.

J0740

J0740 Injection, cidofovir, 375 mg

Lay Description

Cidofovir is an injectable antiviral that is indicated for the treatment of cytomegalovirus (CMV) retinitis in patients with AIDS. By selective inhibition of viral DNA synthesis, Cidofovir is able to suppress the replication of CMV. Dosage is based on the weight of the patient and is 5 mg/kg. It is infused intravenously over a period of one hour every two weeks. HCPCS Level II code J0740 represents 375 mg of cidofovir.

J0743

J0743 Injection, cilastatin sodium; imipenem, per 250 mg

Lay Description

Cilastatin sodium imipenem is a potent, broad-spectrum antibiotic for intravenous (IV) and intramuscular (IM) administration. Its action is to inhibit bacterial cell-wall synthesis. Because of breakdown in the kidneys, it is able to provide adequate levels of drug in the urine. Dosage and the route and frequency of administration are determined by the type of infection and the body area affected, the weight of the patient, and the age of the patient (e.g., adult, child 3 months of age and older, infants, and neonates). HCPCS Level II code J0743 represents 250 mg of cilastatin sodium imipenem.

J0744

J0744 Injection, ciprofloxacin for intravenous infusion, 200 mg

Lay Description

Ciprofloxacin is a fluoroquinolone antibiotic that inhibits the synthesis of bacterial DNA. The broad-spectrum action of the drug makes it useful against a wide range of infections and organisms. Dosage, route, and frequency of administration depend on the type of infection, the age of patient (adult or child), and the weight of children. HCPCS Level II code J0744 represents 200 mg of ciprofloxacin for intravenous infusion.

J0745

J0745 Injection, codeine phosphate, per 30 mg

Lay Description

Codeine phosphate is an opioid analgesic indicated for the treatment of mild to moderate pain. Although the action is unknown, it is known to bind with opiate receptors in the central nervous system and alter the perception of and response to pain. It is provided in an injectable form for subcutaneous (SC), intramuscular (IM), and intravenous (IV) use. The dosage, route of, and frequency of administration are determined by the degree of pain (e.g., mild to moderate), as well as the age of the patient. When administered by IV, it is injected slowly into a large vein. HCPCS Level II code J0745 represents 30 mg of injectable codeine phosphate.

J0760

J0760   Injection, colchicine, per 1 mg

Lay Description

Colchicine is an antigout drug. Although the action is not known, it is thought to decrease WBC motility, phagocytosis, and the production of lactic acid, which in turn reduces the deposits of urate crystals and inflammation. The drug may be administered intravenously (IV) by slow IV push over a period of two to five minutes. It is also provided orally as tablets. The dosage and route of administration depend on whether it is being used to prevent acute attacks of gout, including preoperatively, or for the treatment of an acute attack. For prophylactic and maintenance therapy, oral doses of 0.5 to 0.6 mg are administered three to four times weekly. Patients who have more than one attack of gout a year should take the medication daily. As much as 1 to 1.8 mg may be administered daily in severe cases. For preoperative prophylaxis, patients are given 0.5 to 0.6 mg three times daily for the three days prior to and after surgery. For acute attacks, patients receive an initial oral dose of 0.5 to 1.2 mg, repeated every one or two hours until the pain is relieved, gastrointestinal symptoms appear, or the maximum dose of 8 mg is attained. Intravenously, the patient is given 2 mg IV to start with, then 0.5 mg every six hours as needed up to a maximum of 4 mg. As an alternative, 3 mg IV may be administered. HCPCS Level II code J0760 represents 1 mg of colchicine.

J0770

J0770   Injection, colistimethate sodium, up to 150 mg

Lay Description

Colistimethate sodium is an antibiotic that disrupts the bacterial cell membrane causing its death. It is effective against Enterobacter aerogenes, Escherichia coli, Klebsiella pneumoniae, and Pseudomonas aeruginosa. Recommended dose is 2.5 mg/kg based on ideal body weight divided into two to four doses a day. Medication can be administered by intravenous infusion over three to five minutes every 12 hours or one half of the dose by intravenous infusion over three to five minutes and the rest by continuous intravenous infusion. HCPCS Level II code J0770 represents up to 150 mg of colistimethate sodium.

J0775

J0775   Injection, collagenase, clostridium histolyticum, 0.01 mg

Lay Description

Collagenase clostridium histolyticum is a purified form of the exotoxin collagenase produced by the bacteria *Clostridium histolyticum*. Collagenases are enzymes that break down collagen. This drug is indicated as a treatment for Dupuytren's contracture, which causes a build up of collagen in tendon sheathes in the hands. This drug is administered as an injection directly into the collagen cord of the hand.

J0780

J0780   Injection, prochlorperazine, up to 10 mg

Lay Description

Prochlorperazine/prochlorperazine maleate is an antiemetic used for severe nausea and vomiting, such as that associated with the administration of chemotherapy and prior to induction of anesthesia to control nausea and vomiting during and after surgery. The drug inhibits nausea and vomiting by acting on the chemoreceptor trigger zone and partially depresses the vomiting center. Prochlorperazine is also indicated for treating adult psychiatric illnesses including schizophrenia, non-psychotic anxiety, and mild psychotic disorders. Prochlorperazine is available in injection form for intramuscular (IM) and intravenous (IV) use, in tablets, extended release capsules and syrup for oral administration, and in suppository form. The dosage, route of administration, and frequency of administration depends on the patient's diagnosis, the severity of symptoms, and, in the injectable form, by the patient's weight. Parenteral adult doses range from 2.5 to 10 mg at no more than 5 mg/minute IV for adults or 5 to 20 mg IM. The maximum parenteral adult dose is 40 mg a day. The drug should be injected or infused slowly. For children, 0.132 mg/kg may be administered IM. Oral doses range from 5 to 10 mg three or four times a day for tablets, or for extended-release capsules, 15 mg daily or 10 mg every 12 hours. HCPCS Level II code J0780 represents up to 10 mg of injectable prochlorperazine.

J0795

J0795   Injection, corticorelin ovine triflutate, 1 mcg

Lay Description

Corticorelin ovine triflutate is used to differentiate pituitary and ectopic production of adrenocorticotropic hormone (ACTH) in Cushing's syndrome. After the hypercortisolism is determined to be caused from Cushing's syndrome and autonomous adrenal hyperfunction is eliminated as the cause, the corticorelin test is used to determine the source of the excessive ACTH. Blood samples are drawn 15 minutes before and immediately before the medication is administered. A baseline is determined by averaging the two samples. The corticorelin is administered by intravenous infusion over 30 to 60 second intervals at a dose of 1 mcg/kg body weight. Additional blood samples are drawn 15, 30, and 60 minutes after the patient receives the medication. HCPCS Level II code J0795 represents 1 mcg of corticorelin ovine triflutate.

J0800

J0800   Injection, corticotropin, up to 40 units

Lay Description

Corticotropin is a pituitary hormone released in response to corticotrophin-releasing hormone (CRH), which is released by the hypothalamus. Corticotropin is administered as a diagnostic indicator or adrenocortical function, as well as an anti-inflammatory or immunosuppressant for conditions such as multiple sclerosis. Corticotropin replaces the body's own hormones and stimulates the adrenal cortex to secrete hormones. Corticotropin may be administered intravenously (IV), intramuscularly (IM), or subcutaneously (SC). Intravenously it is administered over a period of eight hours. Dosages, frequency, and method of administration vary according to the indication for the drug, as well as the age of the patient (adult or child). IV doses range from 10 to 25 units every 12 hours for one or two days. IM and SC doses range from 20 to 120 units every 24 to 72 hours. HCPCS Level II code J0800 represents up to 40 units of corticotropin.

J0833-J0834

J0833   Injection, cosyntropin, not otherwise specified, 0.25 mg
J0834   Injection, cosyntropin (Cortrosyn), 0.25 mg

Lay Description

Cosyntropin is a synthetic version of adrenocorticotrophic hormone (ACTH). It is a polypeptide that comprises the first 24 of the 39 amino acids of natural ACTH and has the same effect as natural ACTH. Cosyntropin is used as a diagnostic agent to screen patients with presumed adrenocortical insufficiency. Since it exerts a rapid effect on the adrenal cortex, it may be used to perform a 30-minute test of adrenal function (plasma cortisol response) as an office or outpatient procedure. Cosyntropin may be administered by intramuscular or intravenous injection for a rapid screening test of adrenal function. It may also be administered as an intravenous infusion over four to eight hours for greater stimulus to the adrenal glands. One of the rapid screening tests of adrenal function involves the collection of a control blood sample followed by an intramuscular injection of cosyntropin. A dose of 0.25 mg is provided to adults; for children 2 years of age or younger, a dose of 0.125 mg is adequate. A second blood sample is collected exactly 30 minutes after injection. When administered as an infusion, 0.25 mg is given over a six-hour period.

J0850

J0850   Injection, cytomegalovirus immune globulin intravenous (human), per vial

Lay Description

Immune globulins are glycoproteins in the blood that function as antibodies. Immune globulins specific to a certain disease are antibodies with specific amino acid sequences that interact only with the antigen that stimulated its creation or with antigens that are closely related to the stimulating antigen. Immune globulins are usually derived from the pooled plasma of human donors who have antibodies to the specific disease. The antibodies from the exogenous immune globulin help the body to fight off a disease. Cytomegalovirus (CMV) is a virus of the subfamily Betaherpesvirinae that produces unique large cells with intranuclear inclusions. The majority of CMV infections are very mild. Depending on the age and immune status of the person, CMV infections can cause several serious diseases. CMV infections can include mononucleosis, encephalitis, retinitis, and pneumonia. In immunocompromised patients, CMV can cause a disseminated and sometimes fatal illness. In severely infected infants, CMV may cause hepatosplenomegaly, jaundice, retinitis, purpura, microcephaly, cerebral calcifications, blindness, deafness, quadriplegia, and mental retardation. CMV can be transmitted by respiratory droplets or from the mother to infant during birth or breast-feeding. CMV immune globulin is administered intravenously for the treatment and prophylaxis of CMV disease in transplant recipients and other immunocompromised patients. HCPCS Level II code J0850 represents one vial of CMV immune globulin.

J0878

J0878   Injection, daptomycin, 1 mg

Lay Description

Daptomycin is an antibiotic of the class cyclic lipopeptide. It binds to the bacterial membrane causing a rapid depolarization that leads to bacterial cell death. Daptomycin is indicated for the treatment of complicated skin and skin-structure infections caused by susceptible gram-positive bacteria. Susceptible bacteria include Staphylococcus aureus, including methicillin-resistant strains (MRSA); Streptococcus pyogenes; Streptococcus agalactiae; Streptococcus dysgalactiae subspecies equisimilis; and vancomycin-susceptible strains of Enterococcus faecalis. Daptomycin may be given in combination with other antibiotics. It is administered by intravenous infusion over a 30-minute period once every 24 hours for seven to 14 days. Dosage is based upon body weight with a recommended dose of 4 mg per kg. HCPCS Level II code J0878 represents 1 mg of daptomycin.

J0881-J0882

J0881 Injection, darbepoetin alfa, 1 mcg (non-ESRD use)
J0882 Injection, darbepoetin alfa, 1 mcg (for ESRD on dialysis)

Lay Description

Darbepoetin alfa is a drug used to stimulate red blood cell production. It is produced by recombinant DNA technology in Chinese hamster ovaries. Darbepoetin alfa contains more carbohydrate chains and sialic acid residues than epoetin alfa. This reduces the rate of clearance, extends the half-life, and allows for less frequent administration. It acts in the body similar to erythropoietin, which is produced by the kidneys. Erythropoietin is a hormone that is released into the blood system by the kidneys to prompt the production of red blood cells when low levels of oxygen are detected in the blood. Patients with chronic renal failure will not be able to produce adequate levels of erythropoietin in the kidneys. Darbepoetin alfa is used to treat patients with anemia due to chronic renal failure or due to chemotherapy for patients with nonmyeloid cancer. Dose is based on patient condition and indication. Darbepoetin alfa can be administered by subcutaneous or intravenous injection. HCPCS Level II code J0881 represents 1 mcg of darbepoetin alfa for patients who do not have chronic kidney disease and those patients who have chronic kidney disease but are not on maintenance dialysis. HCPCS Level II code J0882 represents 1 mcg of darbepoetin alfa for patients who are on maintenance dialysis.

J0885-J0886

J0885 Injection, epoetin alfa, (for non-ESRD use), 1000 units
J0886 Injection, epoetin alfa, 1000 units (for ESRD on dialysis)

Lay Description

Epoetin alfa is used to stimulate red blood cell production. It is produced by recombinant DNA technology in mammalian cells. It acts in the body similar to erythropoietin, which is produced by the kidneys. Erythropoietin is a hormone that is released into the blood system by the kidneys to prompt the production of red blood cells when low levels of oxygen are detected in the blood. Patients with chronic renal failure will not be able to produce adequate levels of erythropoietin in the kidneys. Epoetin alfa is used to treat patients with anemia due to chronic renal failure, due to chemotherapy for patients with non-myeloid cancer, or anemia for HIV patients being treated with zidovudine. Epoetin alfa is also indicated in the preoperative treatment of anemic patients scheduled to undergo surgery with significant, anticipated blood loss who cannot donate autologous blood. Dose is based on patient condition and indication. Epoetin alfa can be administered by subcutaneous or intravenous injection. HCPCS Level II code J0885 represents 1,000 units of epoetin alfa for patients who do not have chronic kidney disease and those patients who have chronic kidney disease but are not on maintenance dialysis. HCPCS Level II code J0886 represents 1,000 units of epoetin alfa for patients who are on maintenance dialysis.

J0894

J0894 Injection, decitabine, 1 mg

Lay Description

Decitabine is an antineoplastic drug that is an analogue of the nucleoside 2-deoxycytidine. It incorporates itself into cellular DNA suppressing methylation. It is thought that suppression of the methylation of DNA may restore normal function to genes. Decitabine is indicated as a treatment for patients with myelodysplastic syndromes (MDS) , both previsouly treated and untreated. The drug may used for newly diagnosed and secondary MDS. The recommended dosage is 15 mg per m^2 of body surface. Decitabine is administered by intravenous infusion over three hours repeated every eight hours for three days. This cycle is repeated every six weeks for a recommended four cycles. Patient responce may take longer than four cycles and treatments may be continued as long as the patient benefits. HCPCS Level II code J0894 represents 1 mg of decitabine.

J0895

J0895 Injection, deferoxamine mesylate, 500 mg

Lay Description

Deferoxamine mesylate is an iron-chelating agent that forms a stable complex with the iron and prevents it from being broken down any further in the body. It is indicated for the treatment of both acute iron intoxication and for chronic iron overload due to transfusion-dependent anemias. In acute iron intoxication, deferoxamine mesylate is administered along with standard measures for the treatment of acute iron intoxication. In patients with chronic iron overload secondary to multiple transfusions, deferoxamine mesylate can promote the excretion of iron. With long-term use, the drug can slow the accumulation of hepatic iron and slow or stop the progression of hepatic fibrosis. The action of the drug has been found to be poor in patients younger than 3 years of age without significant iron overload and should not be used unless the mobilization of 1 mg (or more) of iron per day can be demonstrated. This drug is not indicated for treating primary hemochromatosis. The drug is provided for intramuscular, subcutaneous, and intravenous administration. HCPCS Level II code J0895 represents 500 mg of deferoxamine mesylate.

Medicare Information

See chapter titled "Medicare Guidelines," under "Infusion Pumps, External; Equipment and Supplies," for Medicare billing and documentation information.

J0900

J0900   Injection, testosterone enanthate and estradiol valerate, up to 1 cc

Lay Description

Testosterone enanthate is an androgen. Estradiol valerate is an estrogen. Please see the separate entries for each drug for additional information. This combination is indicated for the treatment of menopausal symptoms including hot flashes, unusual sweating, dizziness, and chills. It is administered by intramuscular injection. HCPCS Level II code J0900 represents up to 1 cc of testosterone enanthate and estradiol valerate.

J0945

J0945   Injection, brompheniramine maleate, per 10 mg

Lay Description

Brompheniramine maleate is an antihistamine that blocks the effects of histamine in the body and provides relief of allergy symptoms including hives, rashes, itching, watery eyes, runny nose, and sneezing. It is also indicated for the treatment of motion sickness, anxiety or tension, and sleeplessness. Brompheniramine maleate is available in oral and injectable forms. The injectable form is administered by intramuscular injection. HCPCS Level II code J0945 represents 10 mg of injectable brompheniramine maleate.

J1000

J1000   Injection, depo-estradiol cypionate, up to 5 mg

Lay Description

Depo-estradiol cypionate is a long-acting estrogen in a sterile oil solution for intramuscular use. Depo-estradiol cypionate increases the synthesis of RNA, DNA and protein in tissues and inhibits the release of follicle stimulating and luteinizing hormones from the pituitary gland. Depo-estradiol cypionate is indicated for the treatment of atrophic vaginitis, the palliative treatment of inoperable breast and prostate cancer, severe vasomotor symptoms associated with menopause, and hypoestrogenism due to hypogonadism, castration, or primary ovarian failure. Dosage is based on the condition being treated as well as the patient's response to treatment and ranges from 10 mg every four weeks to 30 mg every week. HCPCS Level II code J1000 represents up to 5 mg of depo-estradiol cypionate.

J1020-J1040

J1020   Injection, methylprednisolone acetate, 20 mg
J1030   Injection, methylprednisolone acetate, 40 mg
J1040   Injection, methylprednisolone acetate, 80 mg

Lay Description

Methylprednisolone is a corticosteroid used to treat a variety of conditions. Indications include allergic disorders, arthritis, blood diseases, breathing problems, certain cancers, eye diseases, intestinal disorders, and collagen and skin diseases. Methylprednisolone may also be used with other medications as a replacement for certain hormones. Methylprednisolone works by decreasing the body's immune response to these diseases and reducing symptoms such as swelling and redness. Methylprednisolone may be administered orally, by intramuscular injection in the form of methylprednisolone acetate, or by intravenous infusion in the form of methylprednisolone sodium succinate. HCPCS Level II codes J1020, J1030, and J1040 represent 20 mg, 40 mg, and 80 mg of methylprednisolone acetate injections respectively.

J1051

J1051   Injection, medroxyprogesterone acetate, 50 mg

Lay Description

Medroxyprogesterone acetate is a progestin used in a variety of disorders and as a long-term injectable contraceptive. Medroxyprogesterone acetate suppresses ovulation by inhibiting the secretion of pituitary gonadotropin, which prevents maturation of follicles and causes thinning of the endometrial lining. It is indicated as antineoplastic treatment in endometrial, breast, and renal carcinoma. medroxyprogesteron acetate is administered by subcutaneous or intramuscular injection. HCPCS Level II code J1051 represents 50 mg of medroxyprogesterone acetate.

J1055

J1055 Injection, medroxyprogesterone acetate for contraceptive use, 150 mg

Lay Description

Medroxyprogesterone acetate is a as a long-term injectable contraceptive. Medroxyprogesterone acetate suppresses ovulation by inhibiting the secretion of pituitary gonadotropin, which prevents maturation of follicles and causes thinning of the endometrial lining. It is administered by subcutaneous or intramuscular injection. HCPCS Level II code J1055 represents 150 mg of medroxyprogesterone acetate for contraceptive use.

J1056

J1056 Injection, medroxyprogesterone acetate/estradiol cypionate, 5 mg/25 mg

Lay Description

Medroxyprogesterone acetate and estradiol cypionate is a monthly injectable contraceptive. The drug inhibits the secretion of gonadotropin, which prevents ovulation and the maturation of follicles. It also thins the endometrium and causes a reduction and thickening of the cervical mucus. The drug, indicated for women age 16 and older, is administered intramuscularly. HCPCS Level II code J1056 represents a combination of 5 mg of medroxyprogesterone acetate and 25 mg of estradiol cypionate.

J1060

J1060 Injection, testosterone cypionate and estradiol cypionate, up to 1 ml

Lay Description

Testosterone cypionate is an androgen. Estradiol cypionate is an estrogen. Please see the separate entries for each drug for additional information. This combination is indicated for the treatment of menopausal symptoms including hot flashes, unusual sweating, dizziness, and chills. It is administered by intramuscular injection. HCPCS Level II code J1060 represents up to 1 ml of testosterone cypionate and estradiol cypionate.

J1070-J1080

J1070 Injection, testosterone cypionate, up to 100 mg
J1080 Injection, testosterone cypionate, 1 cc, 200 mg

Lay Description

Testosterone cypionate is an anabolic steroid that stimulates the normal development of target tissues in men with androgen deficiency. It also has antiestrogen qualities that make it useful to treat estrogen dependent breast cancers. Administered intramuscularly (IM) or subcutaneously (SC), the dosages of testosterone cypionate and the frequency with which it is administered vary with regards to the condition being treated. For the treatment of male hypogonadism, the dose is 50 to 400 mg of testosterone cypionate IM every two to four weeks. For the treatment of metastatic breast cancer in women after menopause, 200 to 400 mg is administered IM every two to four weeks. In combination with estradiol cypionate, it is also indicated for the treatment of menopausal symptoms including hot flashes, unusual sweating, dizziness, and chills. HCPCS Level II code J1070 represents up to 100 mg of testosterone cypionate and J1080 represents 200 mg of testosterone cypionate.

J1094-J1100

J1094 Injection, dexamethasone acetate, 1 mg
J1100 Injection, dexamethasone sodium phosphate, 1 mg

Lay Description

Dexamethasone is a synthetic corticosteroid that is similar to a natural hormone produced by the adrenal gland. It is 25 times as potent as cortisol. Dexamethasone has anti-inflammatory, antiemetic and immunosuppressant properties. It is used to treat a wide variety of disorders. It is also used as a diagnostic aid in the detection of Cushing's syndrome in dexame-thasone suppression testing. HCPCS Level II code J1094 represents 1 mg of dexamethasone acetate; J1100 represents 1 mg of dexamethasone sodium phosphate.

J1110

J1110 Injection, dihydroergotamine mesylate, per 1 mg

Lay Description

Dihydroergotamine mesylate is indicated for acute treatment of migraine and cluster headaches. By stimulating alpha receptors, it causes peripheral vasoconstriction and may abort vascular headaches by direct vasoconstriction of the dilated carotid artery bed. It may be administered parenterallyÑintravenously (IV), intramuscularly (IM), and subcutaneously (SC) with a dose of 1 mg that may be repeated every hour or two up to a maximum of 2 mg IV or 3 mg IM and SC in a 24-hour period. When administered IV, it is given by a slow injection over three minutes. The weekly maximum is 6 mg. HCPCS Level II code J1110 represents 1 mg of dihydroergotamine mesylate.

J1120

J1120 Injection, acetazolamide sodium, up to 500 mg

Lay Description

Acetazolamide sodium is a carbonic anhydrase inhibitor indicated as adjunctive treatment of edema caused by congestive heart failure or drugs, and for rapid relief of ocular tension. Acetazolamide sodium is a nonbacteriostatic sulfonamide that acts to inhibit secretion of aqueous humor, reduce abnormal discharges from central nervous system neurons, and increase diuresis in the kidneys. The drug is administered by venous injection of a reconstituted powder that has been mixed with sterile water. HCPCS Level II code J1120 represents up to 500 mg of acetazolamide sodium.

J1160

J1160 Injection, digoxin, up to 0.5 mg

Lay Description

Digoxin is a cardiac glycoside extracted from the leaf of the digitalis (foxglove) plant. Digoxin acts directly on cardiac muscle and indirectly on the cardiovascular system and autonomic nervous system to both strengthen heart contractions and slow the heart rate. It is a therapy for congestive heart failure, paroxysmal supraventricular tachycardia, and atrial fibrillation. HCPCS Level II code J1160 represents 0.5 mg of digoxin.

J1162

J1162 Injection, digoxin immune fab (ovine), per vial

Lay Description

Digoxin immune Fab (ovine) is an antigen binding fragment (Fab) substance raised in sheep. Sheep are immunized with human antibodies specific to digoxin to produce antibodies specific for the antigenic determinants of the digoxin molecule. The antibody is then papin digested and the digoxin specific Fab fragments of the antibody are isolated and purified by affinity chromatography. Digoxin immune Fab is used to treat life-threatening toxicity due to digoxin or digitoxin overdose. Life-threatening manifestations include severe ventricular arrhythmias, progressive bradyarrhythmias, or second- or third-degree heart block. The drug can be administered by intravenous injection if cardiac arrest seems eminent, or by intravenous infusion over 30 minutes. Improvement ordinarily is seen within a half hour after administration. HCPCS Level II code J1162 represents per vial of digoxin immune Fab.

J1165

J1165 Injection, phenytoin sodium, per 50 mg

Lay Description

Phenytoin sodium is an anticonvulsant medication for the control of tonic-clonic and temporal lobe seizures. It can be taken daily as an oral medication for prophylactic treatment of seizures or be administered intravenously for treatment of acute episodes. Phenytoin sodium is somewhat related to barbiturates in chemical structure and acts upon the motor cortex to inhibit seizure activity. Therapeutic levels vary greatly among patients. HCPCS Level II code J1165 represents an injection of up to 50 mg of phenytoin sodium.

J1170

J1170 Injection, hydromorphone, up to 4 mg

Lay Description

Hydromorphone is a narcotic and opioid analgesic classified as a schedule II controlled substance. This drug binds to opiate nerve center receptors and alters the human pain response, as well as suppressing the cough reflex. It is available in oral and injectable forms. The injectable form can be administered by intramuscular, subcutaneous, and intravenous injection, or by intravenous infusion. Hydromorphone hydrochloride is indicated for the relief of moderate to severe pain. HCPCS Level II code J1170 represents up to 4 mg of hydromorphone.

J1180

J1180 Injection, dyphylline, up to 500 mg

Lay Description

Dyphylline is a derivative of theophylline. Theophylline is a xanthine compound that naturally occurs in tea leaves and can be made synthetically. Dyphylline acts directly on the bronchial smooth muscles as a bronchodilator. It is indicated to treat and prevent the symptoms of bronchial asthma, chronic bronchitis, and emphysema by relaxing the bronchial airways and improving the air flow through the lungs. The injectable form is administered by intramuscular injection for acute conditions. Dosage varies based on the severity of the condition and response. HCPCS Level II code J1180 represents an injection of up to 500 mg of dyphylline.

J1190

J1190 Injection, dexrazoxane HCl, per 250 mg

Lay Description

Dexrazoxane hydrochloride is an intracellular chelating agent derived from ethylenediaminetetraacetic acid (EDTA). Dexrazoxane hydrochloride acts as a cardioprotective agent when used in conjunction with chemotherapeutic agents classified as anthracyclines. Anthracyclines, such as doxorubicin and daunorubicin, are known for their high rate of cardiotoxicity. The method of action is not entirely understood. However, in laboratory studies, dexrazoxane hydrochloride is converted intracellularly to a chelating agent that interferes with iron-mediated free radical generation thought to be responsible, in part, for anthracycline-induced cardiomyopathy. Dexrazoxane hydrochloride is supplied in 250 mg or 500 mg single use vials and is administered by intravenous infusion. HCPCS Level II code J1190 represents 250 mg of dexrazoxane hydrochloride.

J1200

J1200 Injection, diphenhydramine HCl, up to 50 mg

Lay Description

Diphenhydramine hydrochloride is an antihistamine, a histamine receptor antagonist that has anticholinergic, antitussive, antiemetic, antivertigo, antipruritic, antidyskinetic, and sedative effects. It blocks the effects of histamine on the smooth muscle of the bronchial tubes, GI tract, uterus, and blood vessels. It also acts as a local anesthetic by preventing transmission of nerve impulses. Diphenhydramine hydrochloride is indicated for the treatment of anaphylaxis, Parkinsonism when the patient cannot tolerate other medications, drug-induced extrapyramidal disorders, motion sickness, allergies, vertigo, insomnia, and to suppress nausea and prevent vomiting. Its antiemetic effects allow it to be prescribed to treat nausea and vomiting associated with chemotherapy. Diphenhydramine hydrochloride is available in self-administrable oral forms and in an injectable form. The injectable form is administered by intramuscular or intravenous injection. HCPCS Level II code J1200 represents up to 50 mg of injectable diphenhydramine hydrochloride.

J1205

J1205 Injection, chlorothiazide sodium, per 500 mg

Lay Description

Chlorothiazide sodium is a thiazide diuretic. The mechanism of action of thiazides is unknown. They affect the distal renal tubular process of electrolyte reabsorption, increasing the excretion of sodium and chloride and, to a lesser extent, potassium and bicarbonate. Chlorothiazide sodium does not usually affect normal blood pressure. It is indicated, solely or in combination, for the treatment of edema associated with congestive heart failure, hepatic cirrhosis, diabetes insipidus, and renal dysfunction. It is administered by intravenous injection or infusion. Dosages are dependent upon response and are individualized to the patient. HCPCS Level II code J1205 represents up to 500 mg of chlorothiazide sodium.

J1212

J1212 Injection, DMSO, dimethyl sulfoxide, 50%, 50 ml

Lay Description

Dimethyl sulfoxide, also known as DMSO, is an industrial solvent produced as a chemical byproduct of wood pulp in the production of paper. DMSO is FDA approved only as a preservative for transplant organs and for treating interstitial cystitis. It is also used as a preservative for stem cells collected from newborn umbilical cords, and has many off-label uses for medication delivery and pain control. DMSO has the ability to pass through membranes, including the skin barrier, carrying other drugs with it across those membranes. For interstitial cystitis, a 50 percent solution of DMSO is instilled in the bladder via catheter or syringe. The DMSO remains in the bladder for 15 minutes, when the patient is instructed to void. HCPCS Level II code J1212 represents 50 ml of 50 percent dimethyl sulfoxide.

J1230

J1230 Injection, methadone HCl, up to 10 mg

Lay Description

Methadone hydrochloride is a synthetic opioid analgesic that has effects similar to those of morphine and heroin. It is a schedule II controlled substance. Methadone hydrochloride is indicated for the treatment of severe pain and also as a substitute drug in the detoxification of heroin dependence. It is available in injectable and self-administrable oral forms. The injectable form can be administered by intrathecal, intravenous, subcutaneous, or intramuscular injection. Generally speaking, injections and tablets are administered as pain treatment and the oral solution or dissolved tablets administered as part of a detoxification program. The usual dosage for detoxification is 15 to 20 mg. Dosages for pain management vary dependent upon the severity of the pain and the response. HCPCS Level II code J1230 represents up to 10 mg of methadone hydrochloride injection.

J1240
J1240 Injection, dimenhydrinate, up to 50 mg

Lay Description

Dimenhydrinate is a histamine receptor antagonist that has anticholinergic, antiemetic, antivertigo, and sedative effects. It is used as an antiemetic in the treatment and prevention of motion sickness or in cases of nausea and dizziness due to inner ear disturbances. It is thought that antihistamines may affect neural pathways that originate in the labyrinth, which inhibits nausea and vomiting. HCPCS Level II code J1240 represents up to 50 mg of dimenhydrinate.

J1245
J1245 Injection, dipyridamole, per 10 mg

Lay Description

Dipyridamole inhibits platelet aggregation and is a coronary vasodilator. It is indicated as a prophylaxis to prevent thromboembolisms in patients with prosthetic heart valves, and to prevent additional events in patients who have had transient ischemic attacks or an ischemic stroke due to thrombosis. An infusion of dipyridamole may also be administered during diagnostic thallium myocardial perfusion imaging as an alternative to exercise. It is available in oral and injectable forms. The injectable form is administered by intravenous injection. The recommended dosage for prophylactic use is 75 to 100 mg. The recommended dosage for diagnostic testing is 0.142 mg/kg of body weight. HCPCS Level II code J1245 represents up to 10 mg of dipyridamole.

J1250
J1250 Injection, Dobutamine HCl, per 250 mg

Lay Description

Dobutamine hydrochloride is a synthetic catecholamine that acts primarily on beta1 adrenergic receptors. It directly stimulates the heart muscle to increase its contractions and blood flow. Dobutamine hydrochloride is indicated for the treatment of cardiac decompensation in congestive heart failure or following cardiac surgery. It is administered by intravenous infusion through a central line or large peripheral vein. Dosage varies depending upon body weight and response. HCPCS Level II code J1250 represents up to 250 mg of dobutamine hydrochloride.

J1260
J1260 Injection, dolasetron mesylate, 10 mg

Lay Description

Dolasetron mesylate is an antiemetic drug with a chemical compound that is a selective blocker of serotonin 5-HT3 receptors. Serotonin 5-HT3 receptors are present on the vagal nerve and at sensory nerve endings. Cytotoxic chemotherapy appears to trigger the release of serotonin in the small intestine, which may trigger the 5-HT3 receptors and initiate the vomiting reflex. It is indicated to prevent and treat nausea and vomiting associated with chemotherapy or surgery. HCPCS Level II code J1260 represents up to 10 mg of injectable dolasetron mesylate.

J1265
J1265 Injection, dopamine HCl, 40 mg

Lay Description

Dopamine hydrochloride (HCl) is a sympathomimetic amine vasopressor. This drug causes a release of norepinephrine and acts on the nerves in the central nervous system. It is a chemical naturally produced in the brain that increases heart rate and blood pressure. It is used to treat hemodynamic imbalances caused by myocardial infarction, trauma, endotoxic septicemia, open-heart surgery, renal failure, and chronic cardiac decompensation as in heart failure. Dopamine is administered via intravenous infusion. HCPCS Level II code J1265 represents 40 mg of dopamine hydrochloride.

J1267
J1267 Injection, doripenem, 10 mg

Lay Description

Doripenem is a synthetic, broad-spectrum carbapenem antibiotic structurally related to beta-lactam antibiotics. It inhibits bacterial cell wall synthesis by binding to penicillin binding proteins. It is used to treat complicated intraabdominal and urinary tract infections. The normal dose for doripenem is 500 mg administered by IV infusion over one hour. HCPCS Level II code J1267 represents 10 mg of doripenem.

J1270
J1270 Injection, doxercalciferol, 1 mcg

Lay Description

Doxercalciferol is a synthetic analogue of vitamin D that acts directly upon the parathyroid glands to suppress parathyroid hormone synthesis and secretion in order to control the levels of calcium and phosphate in the blood and bones. It is indicated in the treatment of secondary hyperparathyroidism in dialysis patients with chronic renal failure. HCPCS Level II code J1270 represents up to 1 mcg of doxercalciferol.

J1290

J1290   Injection, ecallantide, 1 mg

Lay Description
Ecallantide is a chemical compound that is a selective reversible inhibitor of plasma kallikrein. Kallikreins are enzymes that break peptide bonds in proteins. Ecallantide binds to the plasma kallikrein preventing the creation of bradykinin. Bradykinin is a vasodilator thought to be responsible for edema, inflammations, and pain. This medication is used to treat acute attacks of hereditary angioedema for patients who are 16 years of age or older. The recommended dosage is 30 mg administered subcutaneously in three injections.

J1300

J1300   Injection, eculizumab, 10 mg

Lay Description
Eculizumab is a monoclonal antibody produced from murine myeloma cell cultures. The antibody in the drug binds specifically to the complement protein C5, preventing the generation of a terminal complement complex that hemolyzes red blood cells. Eculizumab is indicated as a treatment for patients with paroxysmal nocturnal hemoglobinuria (PNH) to reduce hemolysis. PNH is a chronic acquired blood cell dysplasia with proliferation of a clone of stem cells producing erythrocytes, platelets, and granulocytes that are abnormally susceptible to lysis by complement. PHN patients have episodes of intravascular hemolysis causing hemolytic anemia, and venous thromboses, especially of the hepatic veins. Eculizumab is administered via intravenous infusion over 35 minutes. It should not be administered as a push or bolus. If an adverse reaction occurs during the administration, the infusion may be slowed, but total infusion time should not exceed two hours. The recommended dosage is 600 mg every 7 days for the first 4 weeks, followed by 900 mg for the fifth dose 7 days later, then 900 mg every 14 days thereafter. Since the use of this drug increases a patient's susceptibility to serious meningococcal infections (septicemia and/or meningitis), all patients without a history of prior meningococcal vaccination must receive the vaccine at least 2 weeks prior to receiving the first dose of eculizumab and be revaccinated according to current medical guidelines. Code J1300 represents 10 mg of eculizumab.

J1320

J1320   Injection, amitriptyline HCl, up to 20 mg

Lay Description
Amitriptyline is a tricyclic antidepressant, a dibenzocycloheptadiene derivative with additional sedative effects. It inhibits the membrane pump mechanism responsible for uptake of norepinephrine and serotonin. It is indicated for the treatment of depression, enuresis, and bulimia nervosa. The recommended dosage is 20 to 30 mg four times a day. HCPCS Level II code J1320 represents up to 20 mg of amitriptyline hydrochloride.

J1324

J1324   Injection, enfuvirtide, 1 mg

Lay Description
Enfuvirtide is a synthetic peptide that inhibits the fusion of human immunodeficiency virus, serotype 1 (HIV-1) into CD4+ cells. HIV-1 causes the majority of infections worldwide. Enfuvirtide, in combination with other antiretroviral agents, is indicated as a second-line therapy for the treatment of HIV-1 infections in patients who have evidence of continued HIV-1 replication despite ongoing antiretroviral therapy. The drug is administered by subcutaneous injection into the upper arm, anterior thigh or abdomen. Recommended dosage is 90 mg twice a day. Enfuvirtide may be self-administered. HCPCS Level II code J1324 represents 1 mg of enfuvirtide.

J1325

J1325   Injection, epoprostenol, 0.5 mg

Lay Description
Epoprostenol is a prostaglandin that acts as a direct vasodilator of pulmonary and systemic arteries and an inhibitor of platelet aggregation. It is usually administered parenterally through a permanent indwelling central venous catheter as a long-term medication to treat primary pulmonary hypertension and pulmonary hypertension secondary to scleroderma in NYHA Class III and IV patients. Initial administration may be through a peripheral intravenous infusion until a central venous catheter is established. It is manufactured as a powder that must be reconstituted with sterile diluent specific to the epoprostenol. Dosages vary dependent upon body weight and response. Once a regimen of epoprostenol has been established, it should never be stopped suddenly. HCPCS Level II code J1325 represents up to 0.5 mg of epoprostenol.

J1327

J1327 Injection, eptifibatide, 5 mg

Lay Description

Eptifibatide is an intravenous cyclical heptapeptide that prevents platelet aggregation and has a short half-life of 2.5 hours. It prevents the binding of fibrinogen, von Willebrand factor, and other ligands to glycoprotein IIb/IIIa stopping the platelets from joining. Eptifibatide is indicated as a treatment for acute coronary syndrome and to prevent thrombosis in patients undergoing percutaneous coronary interventions. Eptifibatide is administered by continuous intravenous infusion. Patients generally receive an infusion of eptifibatide for up to 96 hours following surgery or during medical hospitalization. Dosage is based on body weight. HCPCS Level II code J1327 represents up to 5 mg of eptifibatide.

J1330

J1330 Injection, ergonovine maleate, up to 0.2 mg

Lay Description

Ergonovine maleate is a natural or synthetic version of an ergot alkaloid. It is an oxytocic medication that acts to stimulate uterine and vascular smooth muscle contractions to reduce postpartum or post-abortion bleeding. It also is used to induce coronary artery spasms in diagnostic testing. Ergonovine maleate is available in oral and injectable forms. The injectable form is administered by intravenous or intramuscular injection. HCPCS Level II code J1330 represents up to 0.2 mg of ergonovine maleate.

J1335

J1335 Injection, ertapenem sodium, 500 mg

Lay Description

Ertapenem sodium is a synthetic parenteral antibiotic that is structurally related to penicillin and cephalosporin. It works by prohibiting the creation of bacterial cells walls, causing cellular death. Susceptibility studies should be performed prior to the administration of ertapenem sodium. Susceptible bacteria includes E. coli, Clostridium clostridiiforme, Eubacterium lentum, Peptostreptococcus species, Bacteroides fragilis, Bacteroids distasonis, Bacteroids ovatus, Bacteroids thetaiotaomicron, Bacteroids uniformis, Staphylococcus aureus, Streptococcus agalactiae, Streptococcus pyogenes, Klebsiella pneumoniae, Proteus mirabilis, Porphyromonas asaccharolytica, Prevotella bivia, Streptococcus pneumoniae, Haemophilus influenzae, and Moraxella catarrhalis. Ertapenem sodium is administered as a daily 30-minute intravenous infusion. The recommended dosage for a patient age 13 years or older is 1 g daily. HCPCS Level II code J1335 represents up to 500 mg of ertapenem sodium.

J1364

J1364 Injection, erythromycin lactobionate, per 500 mg

Lay Description

Erythromycin lactobionate is a macrolide antibiotic produced by the bacterium Streptomyces erythreus. It inhibits protein synthesis causing cellular death. Susceptibility studies should be performed prior to the administration of erythromycin lactobionate. Susceptible bacteria include Streptococcus pyogenes, Streptococcus pneumoniae, Haemophilus influenzae, Listeria monocytogenes, Bordetella pertussis, Mycoplasma pneumoniae, Staphylococcus aureus, Corynebacterium diphtheriae, Corynebacterium minutissimum, Treponema pallidum, Neisseria gonorrhoeae, Chlamydia trachomatis, Ureaplasma urealyticum, and Legionella pneumophila. Erythromycin lactobionate is administered by intravenous injection or infusion. Dosage varies depending on the indication and the extent of the infection. HCPCS Level II code J1364 represents up to 500 mg of erythromycin lactobionate.

J1380

J1380 Injection, estradiol valerate, up to 10 mg

Lay Description

Estradiol valerate is an exogenous form of the natural hormone estrogen produced semisynthetically. Estradiol is produced naturally by the ovaries and placenta. It increases synthesis of DNA, RNA, and protein in responsive tissues and reduces the release of FSH from the pituitary gland. Estradiol valerate is a long-acting estrogen suspended in oil. It is indicated as a hormone replacement therapy for female hypogonadism, primary ovarian failure, absence of ovaries, postmenopausal osteoporosis, vasomotor menopausal symptoms, atrophic vaginitis, atrophic urethritis, and vulvar squamous metaplasia. It may also be used to treat advanced prostate cancer. Estradiol valerate is administered by deep intramuscular injection.

J1410

J1410 Injection, estrogen conjugated, per 25 mg

Lay Description

Estrogen conjugates are an exogenous form of the natural hormone estrogen. They may be derived from the urine of pregnant mares or produced synthetically. It increases synthesis of RNA, DNA, and protein in responsive tissue and inhibit release of FSH and luteinizing hormones from the pituitary gland. Estrogen conjugates are indicated as a hormone replacement therapy for female hypogonadism, primary ovarian failure, absence of ovaries, dysfunctional uterine bleeding, postmenopausal osteoporosis, vasomotor menopausal symptoms, atrophic vaginitis, atrophic urethritis, and vulvar squamous metaplasia. It may also be used to treat advanced prostate cancer. HCPCS Level II code J1410 represents up to 25 mg of estrogen conjugated.

J1430

J1430   Injection, ethanolamine oleate, 100 mg

Lay Description

Ethanolamine oleate is a mild sclerosing agent consisting of ethanolamine combined with oleic acid in an aqueous solution. When injected intravenously for local use, it irritates the venous endothelium and produces an inflammatory response that results in fibrosis and potential occlusion of the vein. It is indicated as a treatment for varicose veins and esophageal varices. HCPCS code J1430 represents up to 100 mg of ethanolamine oleate.

Medicare Information

See chapter titled "Medicare Guidelines," under "Drugs, Biologicals, and Radiopharmaceuticals," for Medicare billing and documentation information.

J1435

J1435   Injection, estrone, per 1 mg

Lay Description

Estrone is the oxidation product of estradiol, a long-acting exogenous form of the natural hormone. Estrone may be produced synthetically or derived from human or animal urine, human ovarian fluid or placenta, or from palm kernel oil. It is produced naturally by the ovaries and placenta. It is less potent than estradiol but more so than estriol and is metabolically convertible to estradiol. Estrone increases synthesis of DNA, RNA, and protein in responsive tissues and reduces the release of FSH from the pituitary gland. It is a long-acting estrogen and given as an intramuscular injection. Estrone is indicated as a hormone replacement therapy for female hypogonadism, primary ovarian failure, absence of ovaries, dysfunctional uterine bleeding, postmenopausal osteoporosis, vasomotor menopausal symptoms, atrophic vaginitis, atrophic urethritis, and vulvar squamous metaplasia. It may also be used to treat advanced prostate cancer. HCPCS Level II code J1435 represents up to 1 mg of estrone.

J1436

J1436   Injection, etidronate disodium, per 300 mg

Lay Description

Etidronate disodium is a diphosphate compound, also known as EHDP, that regulates bone metabolism. It inhibits formation and growth of hydroxyapatite crystals to calcium surfaces, and in so doing, slows resorption and accretion in abnormal bone turnover. Etidronate disodium is indicated as a treatment for osteitis deformans, heterotopic ossification, and hypercalcemia of malignancy. The drug is available in oral and injectable forms. The injectable form is administered by intravenous infusion over a two-hour period. HCPCS Level II code J1436 represents up to 300 mg of etidronate disodium.

J1438

J1438   Injection, etanercept, 25 mg (code may be used for Medicare when drug administered under the direct supervision of a physician, not for use when drug is self-administered)

Lay Description

Etanercept is an antirheumatic agent that binds to tumor necrosis factor, blocking its action and thereby causing a decrease in inflammation and autoimmune response. It is indicated for the treatment of juvenile rheumatoid arthritis, rheumatoid arthritis, psoriatic arthritis, ankylosing spondylitis, and chronic plaque psoriasis. Etanercept is administered by subcutaneous injection, typically the thigh, abdomen, or upper arm, once or twice weekly. The recommended adult dosage is 50 mg per week. The recommended dosage for patients 4 to 17 years of age is 0.8 mg/kg of body weight. The drug may be self-administered by the patient. HCPCS Level II code J1438 represents up to 25 mg of etanercept administered under the direct supervision of a physician.

J1440-J1441

J1440   Injection, filgrastim (G-CSF), 300 mcg
J1441   Injection, filgrastim (G-CSF), 480 mcg

Lay Description

Filgrastim is a synthetic, human granulocyte colony-stimulating factor (G-CSF). It is produced by recombinant DNA technology using E. coli bacteria. The drug binds to surface receptors on hematopoietic and stimulates neutrophil production, differentiation, maturation, and function. It is indicated as a treatment for neutropenia in patient receiving myelosuppressive therapy for nonmyeloid malignancies. Filgrastim is also used to mobilize hematopoietic progenitor cells for leukapheresis to be used for bone marrow transplants. The drug is administered by subcutaneous or intravenous injection and intravenous infusion. Recommended dosage varies from 5 to 10 mcg/kg of body weight per day depending on the indication. HCPCS Level II code J1440 represents up to 300 mcg of filgrastim and J1441 represents up to 480 mcg.

J1450

J1450   Injection, fluconazole, 200 mg

Lay Description

Fluconazole is a synthetic triazole antifungal agent. It is indicated as a treatment for vaginal, oropharyngeal, and esophageal candidiasis and cryptococcal meningitis. Fluconazole is also used as a prophylaxis for candidiasis in patients undergoing bone marrow transplantation, radiation therapy, or cytotoxic chemotherapy. It is available in oral and injectable forms. The injectable form is administered by intravenous infusion. Recommended dosage varies from 3 to 12 mg/kg of body weight depending on the indication. HCPCS Level II code J1450 represents 200 mg of injectable fluconazole.

J1451

J1451   Injection, fomepizole, 15 mg

Lay Description

Fomepizole is a competitive inhibitor of alcohol dehydrogenase, the enzyme that catalyzes the initial steps in the metabolism of ethylene glycol and methanol and prevents these two substances from forming the toxic metabolites that cause metabolic acidosis and renal damage. Fomepizole is indicated for use as an antidote in confirmed or suspected ethylene glycol (antifreeze) poisoning and methanol poisoning. It may be used alone or with hemodialysis. Fomepizole is administered by intravenous infusion. The usual initial dose is 15 mg/kg of body weight administered over 30 minutes. Subsequent doses are usually reduced to 10 mg/kg of body weight given every 12 hours over 30 minutes until ethylene glycol or methanol concentration decreases to less than 20 mg per dl. HCPCS Level II code J1451 represents up to 15 mg of fomepizole.

Medicare Information

See chapter titled "Medicare Guidelines," under "Drugs, Biologicals, and Radiopharmaceuticals," for Medicare billing and documentation information.

J1452

J1452   Injection, fomivirsen sodium, intraocular, 1.65 mg

Lay Description

Fomivirsen sodium intravitreal injection is indicated for the local treatment of cytomegalovirus (CMV) retinitis in patients with acquired immunodeficiency syndrome (AIDS). Fomivirsen intravitreal injection is a local treatment that does not affect CMV infections of other sites. Treatment of bilateral CMV retinal infections requires injections in both eyes. Fomivirsen inhibits human cytomegalovirus (HCMV) replication by binding to the target mRNA and inhibiting IE2 protein synthesis, which prevents virus replication. Initial intravitreal injection for treatment of CMV retinitis is 330 mcg into the affected eye every other week for two doses. After the two initial doses, maintenance doses of 330 mcg are administered every four weeks. HCPCS Level II code J1452 represents up to 1.65 mg of fomivirsen sodium for intraocular injection.

Medicare Information

See chapter titled "Medicare Guidelines," under "Drugs, Biologicals, and Radiopharmaceuticals," for Medicare billing and documentation information.

J1453

J1453   Injection, fosaprepitant, 1 mg

Lay Description

Fosaprepitant is a lyophilized prodrug of aprepitant. When fosaprepitant is administered intravenously, it is quickly converted to aprepitant. It is administered before chemotherapy to eliminate or reduce acute nausea and vomiting. Fosaprepitant is administered 30 minutes prior to chemotherapy by IV infusion over 15 minutes. The recommended dose is 115 mg. HCPCS Level II code J1453 represents 1 mg of fosaprepitant.

J1455

J1455   Injection, foscarnet sodium, per 1,000 mg

Lay Description

Foscarnet sodium is an antiviral indicated for treatment of cytomegalovirus (CMV) retinitis in patients with acquired immune deficiency syndrome. It is also indicated for treatment of herpes simplex virus types 1 and 2 (HPV-1, HPV-2) mucocutaneous infections in immunocompromised patients. It works by inhibiting in vitro viral replication by binding to the pyrophosphate binding site on virus-specific DNA polymerases. Foscarnet sodium is administered by intravenous infusion over one to two hours. Dose is dependent on specific viral infection being treated, as well as body weight of the patient. HCPCS Level II code J1455 represents up to 1,000 mg of foscarnet sodium.

Medicare Information

See chapter titled "Medicare Guidelines," under "Infusion Pumps, External; Equipment and Supplies," for Medicare billing and documentation information.

J1457

J1457   Injection, gallium nitrate, 1 mg

Lay Description

Gallium is a rare metal that is liquid at room temperature. Gallium nitrate is a hydrated nitrate salt of gallium used in the treatment of symptomatic cancer-related hypercalcemia that has not responded to hydration therapy. Generally, patients should have serum calcium (corrected for albumin) equal to or greater than 12 mg/dl. The recommended usage for gallium nitrate is 200 mg per m2 of body surface daily infused over 24 hours for five consecutive days. HCPCS Level II code J1457 represents 1 mg of gallium nitrate.

J1458

J1458   Injection, galsulfase, 1 mg

Lay Description

Galsulfase is a human enzyme produced by recombinant DNA technology in a Chinese hamster ovary. Galsulfase is an orphan drug used to treat the inherited metabolic disorder mucopolysaccharidosis VI (MPS VI or Maroteaux-Lamy Syndrome). Mucopolysaccharidosis VI is caused by a lack of the enzyme arylsulfatase B that normally breaks down certain carbohydrates known as glycosaminoglycans. While intelligence is not affected, MPS VI causes widespread cumulative organ and tissue damage. The drug is administered via a four-hour infusion every week. HCPCS Level II code J1458 represents 1 mg of galsulfase.

J1459

J1459   Injection, immune globulin (Privigen), intravenous, nonlyophilized (e.g., liquid), 500 mg

Lay Description

Immune globulins are glycoproteins in the blood that function as antibodies. Immune globulins specific to a certain disease are antibodies with specific amino acid sequences that interact only with the antigen that stimulated its creation or with antigens that are closely related to the stimulating antigen. Immune globulins are usually derived from the pooled plasma of human donors who have antibodies to the specific disease. The antibodies from the exogenous immune globulin help the body to fight off a disease. The term intravenous immune globulin, IVIg, used with a qualifier generally refers to the full range of immunoglobulins contained within the blood. Immunoglobulins are divided into five classes, IgM, IgG, IgA, IgD, and IgE, on the basis of structure and biologic activity. IVIg is administered by intravenous injection or infusion. IVIg is indicated as a treatment for primary immune deficiency disorders, idiopathic thrombocytopenia purpura, autoimmune diseases, and as an adjunct treatment of Kawasaki disease. It is also indicated as a prophylaxis of infectious diseases associated with chronic lymphocytic leukemia, pediatric HIV infection, and bone marrow transplants. IVIg is available as a solution or in a lyophilized or freeze-dried form.

J1460, J1560

J1460   Injection, gamma globulin, intramuscular, 1 cc
J1560   Injection, gamma globulin, intramuscular, over 10 cc

Lay Description

Gamma globulins are serum globulins having the least rapid electrophoretic migration. Since the gamma globulin fractions are composed almost entirely of immune globulin, gamma globulin has come to be used as a synonym of immune globulin or immunoglobulin. Immune globulins are glycoproteins in the blood that function as antibodies. Immune globulins specific to a certain disease are antibodies with specific amino acid sequences that interact only with the antigen that stimulated its creation or with antigens that are closely related to the stimulating antigen. Immune globulins are usually derived from the pooled plasma of human donors who have antibodies to the specific disease. The antibodies from the exogenous immune globulin help the body to fight off a disease. The term immune globulin used with a qualifier generally refers to the full range of immunoglobulins contained within the blood. Immunoglobulins are divided into five classes, IgM, IgG, IgA, IgD, and IgE, on the basis of structure and biologic activity. Gamma globulins are administered by intramuscular injection. They are indicated as a treatment for primary immune deficiency disorders or as a prophylaxis after exposure to hepatitis A, measles, rubella, and varicella.

J1561, J1566-J1569, J1572-J1573

J1561 Injection, immune globulin, (Gamunex), intravenous, nonlyophilized (e.g., liquid), 500 mg
J1566 Injection, immune globulin, intravenous, lyophilized (e.g., powder), not otherwise specified, 500 mg
J1568 Injection, immune globulin, (Octagam), intravenous, nonlyophilized (e.g., liquid), 500 mg
J1569 Injection, immune globulin, (Gammagard liquid), intravenous, nonlyophilized, (e.g., liquid), 500 mg
J1572 Injection, immune globulin, (Flebogamma/Flebogamma Dif), intravenous, nonlyophilized (e.g., liquid), 500 mg
J1573 Injection, hepatitis B immune globulin (Hepagam B), intravenous, 0.5 ml

Lay Description

Immune globulins are glycoproteins in the blood that function as antibodies. Immune globulins specific to a certain disease are antibodies with specific amino acid sequences that interact only with the antigen that stimulated its creation or with antigens that are closely related to the stimulating antigen. Immune globulins are usually derived from the pooled plasma of human donors who have antibodies to the specific disease. The antibodies from the exogenous immune globulin help the body to fight off a disease. The term intravenous immune globulin, IVIg, used with a qualifier generally refers to the full range of immunoglobulins contained within the blood. Immunoglobulins are divided into five classes, IgM, IgG, IgA, IgD, and IgE, on the basis of structure and biologic activity. IVIg is administered by intravenous injection or infusion. IVIg is indicated as a treatment for primary immune deficiency disorders, idiopathic thrombocytopenia purpura, autoimmune diseases, and as an adjunct treatment of Kawasaki disease. It is also indicated as a prophylaxis of infectious diseases associated with chronic lymphocytic leukemia, pediatric HIV infection, and bone marrow transplants. IVIg is available as a solution or in a lyophilized or freeze-dried form.

J1562

J1562 Injection, immune globulin (Vivaglobin), 100 mg

Lay Description

Immune globulins are glycoproteins in the blood that function as antibodies. Immune globulins specific to a certain disease are antibodies with specific amino acid sequences that interact only with the antigen that stimulated its creation or with antigens that are closely related to the stimulating antigen. Immune globulins are usually derived from the pooled plasma of human donors who have antibodies to the specific disease. The antibodies from the exogenous immune globulin help the body to fight off a disease. The term immune globulin, used without a qualifier, generally refers to the full range of immunoglobulins contained within the blood. Immunoglobulins are divided into five classes, IgM, IgG, IgA, IgD, and IgE, on the basis of structure and biologic activity. Subcutaneous immune globulin is indicated as a treatment for primary immune deficiency disease. Recommended total weekly dosage for the subcutaneous version is 100 to 200 mg per kg of patient body weight. The subcutaneous version may be self-administered. HCPCS Level II code J1562 represents 100 mg of immune globulin administered subcutaneously.

J1566-J1569

J1566 Injection, immune globulin, intravenous, lyophilized (e.g., powder), not otherwise specified, 500 mg
J1568 Injection, immune globulin, (Octagam), intravenous, nonlyophilized (e.g., liquid), 500 mg
J1569 Injection, immune globulin, (Gammagard liquid), intravenous, nonlyophilized, (e.g., liquid), 500 mg

Lay Description

Please refer to code J1561 for the description, coding, and billing information.

J1570

J1570 Injection, ganciclovir sodium, 500 mg

Lay Description

Ganciclovir sodium is a synthetic guanine derivative active against cytomegalovirus (CMV). It is indicated for treatment and prevention of CMV in patients with acquired immune deficiency syndrome (AIDS). It is also indicated for prevention of CMV in organ transplant patients. It works by inhibiting the replication of the virus. Ganciclovir is available as sterile lyophilized powder in 500 mg vials for intravenous administration. It is also available in 250 mg and 500 mg capsules for oral administration. For AIDS patients with CMV infection, initial treatment is by intravenous injection infused over one hour every 12 hours for 14 to 21 days. Dose is dependent on body weight. Following the intravenous course of treatment, maintenance therapy is administered by intravenous infusion once per day five to seven days per week or in oral capsule form. Maintenance intravenous therapy dose is dependent on body weight. Usual oral dose is 1,000 mg tid. Organ transplant patients typically receive initial intravenous therapy for up to 21 days, followed by maintenance doses by intravenous infusion or orally.

HCPCS Level II code J1570 represents up to 500 mg of ganciclovir sodium.

Medicare Information

See chapter titled "Medicare Guidelines," under "Infusion Pumps, External; Equipment and Supplies," for Medicare billing and documentation information.

J1571

J1571 Injection, hepatitis B immune globulin (Hepagam B), intramuscular, 0.5 ml

Lay Description

Immune globulins are glycoproteins in the blood that function as antibodies. Immune globulins specific to a certain disease are antibodies with specific amino acid sequences that interact only with the antigen that stimulated its creation or with antigens that are closely related to the stimulating antigen. Immune globulins are usually derived from the pooled plasma of human donors who have antibodies to the specific disease. The antibodies from the exogenous immune globulin help the body to fight off a disease. Hepatitis B is a viral infection of the liver. The virus is shed in all body fluids from infected individuals. While it is possible to become infected via oral transmission, it is more commonly transmitted by parenteral routes, such as blood transfusion, contaminated needles, and sexual contact. Hepatitis B has an incubation period of about 90 days with a range of 40 to 180 days. It can cause fever, malaise, anorexia, nausea and vomiting, jaundice, urticaria, angioedema, arthritis, and, rarely, glomerulonephritis or a serum sickness-like syndrome. Hepatitis B can cause massive liver necrosis. It is thought that the disease may be a cause of cirrhosis and primary liver cancer. Most patients recover completely. Some may remain chronic carriers or develop chronic active or persistent hepatitis. The disease is endemic worldwide. Hepatitis B immune globulin is derived from persons with high titers of antibodies against the hepatitis B surface antigen. It is administered by intramuscular injection for the prophylaxis of persons exposed to the virus or infants of mothers who test positive for the antigen.

J1572-J1573

J1572 Injection, immune globulin, (Flebogamma/Flebogamma Dif), intravenous, nonlyophilized (e.g., liquid), 500 mg
J1573 Injection, hepatitis B immune globulin (Hepagam B), intravenous, 0.5 ml

Lay Description

Please refer to code J1561 for the description, coding, and billing information.

J1580

J1580 Injection, garamycin, gentamicin, up to 80 mg

Lay Description

Garamycin/gentamycin is an antibiotic used to treat a wide variety of bacterial infections. It is indicated for use in the treatment of primary and secondary infections caused by sensitive strains of Group A beta-hemolytic, alpha-hemolytic streptococci, S. aureus, P. aeruginosa, A. aerogenes, E. coli, P. vulgaris, and K. pneumoniae. HCPCS Level II code J1580 represents up to 80 mg of garamycin or gentamycin.

J1590

J1590 Injection, gatifloxacin, 10 mg

Lay Description

Gatifloxacin falls into the category of drugs known as fluoroquinolones. It is used in treating chronic bronchitis, acute sinusitus, and community-acquired pneumonia caused by streptococcus pneumoniae as well as skin infections caused by streptococcus aureus. Gatifloxacin acts by inhibiting bacterial replication. Some adverse reactions may include headache, palpitations, hematuria, dyspnea, and/or back pain. It is contraindicated in patients with untreated hypokalemia. This code reports a 10 mg injection.

J1595

J1595 Injection, glatiramer acetate, 20 mg

Lay Description

Glatiramer acetate is used in the treatment of relapsing-remitting multiple sclerosis (MS) and is indicated to reduce the frequency of relapses. The mechanism by which glatiramer acetate exerts its effects in patients with MS is not fully understood; however, it is thought that it has an effect on immune processes that are believed to be responsible for the origin and development of MS. Glatiramer acetate is available in 20 mg single dose, prefilled vials and is administered by subcutaneous injection. The recommended dose is 20 mg per day. Glatiramer acetate may be self-administered. HCPCS Level II code J1595 represents up to 20 mg of glatiramer acetate.

J1600

J1600 Injection, gold sodium thiomalate, up to 50 mg

Lay Description

Gold sodium thiomalate is a gold salt indicated for the treatment of adult and juvenile rheumatoid arthritis. The mechanism of action in gold salts is not well understood. However, in patients with inflammatory arthritis, such as adult and juvenile rheumatoid arthritis, gold salts decrease the inflammation of the joint lining, preventing destruction of bone and cartilage. Gold salts, such as gold sodium thiomalate, are second-line drugs prescribed when anti-inflammatory drugs, such as nonsteroidal anti-inflammatory drugs (NSAID) and corticosteroids, are ineffective in preventing the progression of inflammatory arthritis. Gold sodium thiomalate is available as a 50 mg/ml injectable suspension to be administered by intramuscular injection. HCPCS Level II code J1600 represents up to 50 mg of gold sodium thiomalate.

J1610

J1610 Injection, glucagon HCl, per 1 mg

Lay Description

Glucagon hydrochloride is a synthetic polypeptide identical to human glucagon. It is produced by recombinant DNA technology using E. coli bacteria. An injection of glucagon stimulates the liver to release stored glycogen and convert it to glucose in order to raise blood glucose levels. It also relaxes smooth muscles of the gastrointestinal tract. Its principal use is in an emergency setting, as a treatment for severe insulin reaction in which the patient is unconscious or otherwise unable to eat or drink. An emergency glucagon kit containing a vial of powdered glucagon and a syringe of sterile water is usually maintained in the homes of insulin-dependent diabetics. Glucagon is also useful as a diagnostic aid in radiological examination of the stomach and lower gastrointestinal tract when diminished motility would be advantageous, because glucagon acts as a smooth muscle relaxant. The diagnostic kit also contains a vial of powdered glucagon and a syringe of sterile water. Glucagon can be administered by subcutaneous, intravenous, or intramuscular injection. It can be administered in a non-medical setting by non-medical personnel. HCPCS Level II code J1610 represents 1 mg of glucagon hydrochloride administered by medical personnel.

J1620

J1620 Injection, gonadorelin HCl, per 100 mcg

Lay Description

Gonadorelin HCl is used primarily as a diagnostic agent for evaluating the functional capacity and response of the anterior pituitary gonadotropins. Side effects may include headache, abdominal discomfort, flushing, bronchospasm, and/or local swelling at the injection site. The use of gonadorelin is contraindicated in patients who are hypersensitive to gonadorelin hydrochloride or any of its components. This code reports a 100 mcg injection. HCPCS Level II code J1620 represents up to 100 mcg of gonadorelin hydrochloride.

J1626

J1626 Injection, granisetron HCl, 100 mcg

Lay Description

Granisetron HCl is an antiemetic used to prevent postoperative and chemotherapy or radiation related nausea and vomiting. It is a selective antagonist of serotonin receptors located in the vagus nerve and in the central nervous system's chemoreceptor trigger zone. Granisetron hydrochloride may be administered orally in solution or tablets or by intravenous injection. It is usually given 30 minutes to one hour before chemotherapy, with a second oral dose often following 12 hours later. HCPCS Level II code J1626 represents up to 100 mcg of granisetron hydrochloride for injection.

J1630-J1631

J1630 Injection, haloperidol, up to 5 mg
J1631 Injection, haloperidol decanoate, per 50 mg

Lay Description

Haloperidol and haloperidol decanoate are antipsychotics that are used in treating chronic psychosis due to schizophrenia, Tourette''s syndrome, and other psychotic disorders. These drugs block the postsynaptic dopamine receptors in the brain. The injectable form is available in 5 mg/ml doses and may be administered by intravenous or intramuscular injection. The Haloperidol decanoate is a long-acting form of haloperidol and is administered by intramuscular injection only. Haloperidol decanoate is available in 50 mg/ml and 100 mg/ml doses. Dosing is dependent on individual patient requirements and response to treatment. HCPCS Level II code J1630 represents up to 5 mg of haloperidol and J1631 represents up to 50 mg of haloperidol deconoate.

J1640

J1640 Injection, hemin, 1 mg

Lay Description

Hemin is an iron containing metaalloporphyrin. It is an enzyme inhibitor derived from prodesses red blood cells and acts to limit the hepatic and marrow synthesis of porphyrn. Hemin is an orphan drug indicated for the treatment of acute intermittent porphyria, porphyria variegata, and hereditary coproporphyria. Hemin therapy must be administered under close supervision of a physician, and it is not curative. The drug is administered by an intravenous infusion of 10 to 15 minutes. Recommended dosage is 1 to 4 mg/kg of body weight daily. The infusions are given for three to 14 days depending on the clinical signs. HCPCS Level II code J1640 represents up to 1 mg of hemin.

Medicare Information
See chapter titled "Medicare Guidelines," under "Drugs, Biologicals, and Radiopharmaceuticals," for Medicare billing and documentation information.

J1642-J1644

J1642   Injection, heparin sodium, (heparin lock flush), per 10 units
J1644   Injection, Heparin sodium, per 1000 units

Lay Description
Heparin is an anticoagulant indicated for the treatment and prevention of blood clots, including pulmonary embolism and deep vein thrombosis. It is also used to ensure patency of indwelling intravenous catheters. Heparin inhibits reactions that lead to the clotting of blood and the formation of fibrin clots. It works by acting as an accelerant in forming antithrombin III-thrombin complex, which deactivates thrombin. This prevents the conversion of fibrinogen to fibrin. Heparin sodium is derived from bovine or porcine pulmonary or intestinal tissue and standardized for anticoagulant activity. It is administered by subcutaneous or intravenous injection. Heparin sodium is available in doses of 1,000, 5,000, and 10,000 units/ml. Heparin lock flush is available in 10 and 100 units/ml syringes or vials. HCPCS Level II code J1642 represents up to 10 units of heparin sodium for use as a heparin lock flush and J1644 represents up to 1,000 units of heparin sodium.

J1645

J1645   Injection, dalteparin sodium, per 2500 IU

Lay Description
Dalteparin sodium is a low molecular weight heparin that is produced through controlled nitrous acid depolymerization of sodium heparin from porcine intestinal mucosa followed by a chromatographic purification process. It acts by enhancing the inhibition of Factor Xa and thrombin by antithrombin. Dalteparin sodium is an injected drug that is used for the prophylaxis of ischemic complications in unstable angina and non-Q-wave myocardial infarction when administered in conjunction with aspirin therapy. This drug is also indicated for the prophylaxis of deep vein thrombosis (DVT), which may lead to pulmonary embolism (PE) for patients who are undergoing hip replacement surgery or abdominal surgery and are at risk for thromboembolic complications or a patient who is at risk for thromboembolic complications due to severely restricted mobility during acute illness. The dosage recommended for patients with unstable angina or non-Q-wave myocardial infarction is 120 IU per kg of body weight (but not more than 10,000 IU) subcutaneously every 12 hours with concurrent oral aspirin therapy for a duration of five to eight days. Dosage for hip replacement therapy varies as to the regime, but the first dose of 2,500 or 5,000 IU is administered prior to surgery and follow-up administration of 2,500 to 5,000 IU is administered postoperatively. In patients undergoing abdominal surgery with a risk of thromboembolic complications, the recommended dosage is 2,500 IU once daily beginning one to two hours prior to surgery and then once daily for five to 10 days. If the patient is at high risk of thromboembolic complications, dosage is increased to 5,000 IU. Dosage for patients with severely restricted mobility is 5,000 IU administered once daily. Dalteparin sodium is administered by subcutaneous injection. HCPCS Level II code J1645 represents 2,500 IU of dalteparin sodium.

J1650

J1650   Injection, enoxaparin sodium, 10 mg

Lay Description
Enoxaparin sodium is a low molecular weight heparin that has antithrombotic properties. When given at a dose of 1.5 mg/kg, enoxaparin has a higher ratio of anti-Factor Xa to anti-Factor IIa activity when compared to the ratios observed for heparin. Enoxaparin sodium is used for the prophylaxis of ischemic complications in unstable angina and non-Q-wave myocardial infarction when administered in conjunction with aspirin therapy and for the prophylaxis of deep vein thrombosis (DVT), which may lead to pulmonary embolism (PE) for patients who are undergoing hip or knee replacement surgery or abdominal surgery and are at risk for thromboembolic complications. It is also prescribed to patients who are at risk for thromboembolic complications due to severely restricted mobility during acute illness. This drug is administered via subcutaneous injection. Dosage varies depending upon the clinical indication. When administered to patients undergoing abdominal surgery, the usual dosage is 40 mg once per day beginning two hours prior to surgery for a seven to 10 day duration. When administered to patients undergoing hip or knee replacement surgery, 30 to 40 mg is injected subcutaneously 12 to 24 hours prior to surgery and then once daily for seven to 10 days. When administered to patients who are at risk for thromboembolic complications due to severely restricted mobility during an acute illness, the recommended dosage is 40 mg per day for six to 11 days. Injections of 1 mg/kg of enoxaparin sodium subcutaneously every 12 hours in conjunction with aspirin therapy is administered for treatment of

unstable angina. HCPCS Level II code J1650 represents 10 mg of enoxaparin sodium.

J1652

J1652   Injection, fondaparinux sodium, 0.5 mg

Lay Description

Fondaparinux sodium is a synthetic inhibitor of activated factor X (Xa). It has no known effect on platelet function because it does not affect thrombin (activated factor II). Fibrinolytic activity or bleeding times are not affected. Fondaparinux sodium is a low molecular weight heparin that has antithrombotic properties. Fondaparinux sodium is indicated for the prophylaxis of deep vein thrombosis, which may lead to pulmonary embolism in patients undergoing hip fracture surgery, including extended prophylaxis, hip replacement surgery, knee replacement surgery, and abdominal surgery for patients who are at risk for thromboembolic complications. Fondaparinux sodium is also indicated for the treatment of acute deep vein thrombosis when administered in conjunction with warfarin sodium, and the treatment of acute pulmonary embolism when administered in conjunction with warfarin sodium when initial therapy is administered in the hospital. Dosage is dependent upon the condition being treated and body weight. HCPCS Level II code J1652 represents 0.5 mg of fondaparinux sodium.

J1655

J1655   Injection, tinzaparin sodium, 1000 IU

Lay Description

Tinzaparin sodium is a low weight heparin that is used to treat the deep vein thrombosis with or without pulmonary embolism. Tinzaparin interfers with the body"s natural blood clotting mechanism by inactivating thrombin. Thrombin is an important constituent in blood clot formation. Tinzaparin is available in multiple use 2 ml vials. Each ml contains 20,000 IU of tinzaparin for a total of 40,000 IU per vial. Tinzaparin is administered by subcutaneous injection. The recommended dosage for the treatment of deep vein thrombosis is 175 IU/kg of body weight once daily for at least six days. HCPCS Level II code J1655 represents 1,000 IU of tinzaparin sodium.

J1670

J1670   Injection, tetanus immune globulin, human, up to 250 units

Lay Description

Immune globulins are glycoproteins in the blood that function as antibodies. Immune globulins specific to a certain disease are antibodies with specific amino acid sequences that interact only with the antigen that stimulated its creation or with antigens that are closely related to the stimulating antigen. Immune globulins are usually derived from the pooled plasma of human donors who have antibodies to the specific disease. The antibodies from the exogenous immune globulin help the body to fight off a disease. Tetanus is an acute, often fatal, infectious disease caused by the bacterium Clostridium tetani. This bacterium produces a neurotoxin called tetanospasmin. Generalized tetanus is characterized by muscular contractions and hyperreflexia, resulting in trismus (lockjaw), glottal spasm, generalized muscle spasm, opisthotonos, respiratory spasm, seizures, and paralysis. Localized tetanus may be mild, with localized muscular twitching and spasm of muscle groups near the site of injury. Localized tetanus may progress to the generalized form. Tetanus usually enters the body through a puncture wound, such as a splinter or bite. It may also enter through a burn, surgical wound, skin ulcer, injection site of drug abusers, the umbilical stump, or postpartum uterus. Tetanus immune globulin is administered by intramuscular injection. It is administered for the prophylaxis or treatment of tetanus. HCPCS Level II code J1670 represents up to 250 units of human tetanus immune globulin.

J1675

J1675   Injection, histrelin acetate, 10 mcg

Lay Description

Histrelin acetate is the acetate salt of a synthetic nonapeptide that corresponds to a component of naturally occurring human growth hormone. Initially the drug stimulates release of human growth hormone-releasing hormone. However, chronic use desensitizes responsiveness of the pituitary gonadotropin, causing a reduction in ovarian and testicular steroidogenesis. Decreases in LH, FSH, and sex steroid levels are observed within three months of initiation of therapy. It is an orphan drug indicated for the treatment of children with central precocious puberty (idiopathic or neurogenic) occurring before 8 years of age in girls or 9.5 years of age in boys. Report J1675 for an injection of 10 mcg of histrelin acetate.

Medicare Information

See chapter titled "Medicare Guidelines," under "Drugs, Biologicals, and Radiopharmaceuticals," for Medicare billing and documentation information. Note that OPPS facilities are not allowed to report J1675.

J1680

J1680 Injection, human fibrinogen concentrate, 100 mg

Lay Description

Fibrinogen (factor I) is a component in the blood that helps with clotting and it used to treat patients with congenital fibrinogen deficiency including afibrinogenemia and hypofibrinogenemia. It is a physiological substrate of three enzymes: thrombin, factor XIIIa, and plasmin and is manufactured from pooled human plasma that has been purified and concentrated. During the coagulation process, its molecules are used by the thrombin, factor XIIIa, and plasmin to produce a fibrin monomer. This monomer along with calcium ions and factor XIII makes the clot stronger and more elastic. The dose is dependent on the patient's body weight, condition, and blood levels. The solution is administered by intravenous injection.

J1700-J1720

J1700 Injection, hydrocortisone acetate, up to 25 mg
J1710 Injection, hydrocortisone sodium phosphate, up to 50 mg
J1720 Injection, hydrocortisone sodium succinate, up to 100 mg

Lay Description

Hydrocortisone is a steroid hormone produced by the adrenal cortex. A preparation of this hormone may be obtained from natural sources or produced synthetically. It is a corticosteroid that decreases inflammation and suppresses the immune system. Hydrocortisone acetate, sodium phosphate, and sodium succinate are used to treat severe inflammation, shock reactions, adrenal insufficiency, ulcerative colitis, and other inflammatory processes. HCPCS Level II code J1700 represents up to 25 mg of injectable hydrocortisone acetate; J1710 represents up to 50 mg of injectable hydrocortisone sodium phosphate; and J1720 represents up to 100 mg of injectable hydrocortisone sodium succinate.

J1730

J1730 Injection, diazoxide, up to 300 mg

Lay Description

Diazoxide is a vasodilator when administered intra-venously and a drug used to treat hypoglycemia when administered orally. Intravenous administration is indicated in the emergency reduction of blood pressure in severe nonmalignant and malignant hypertension. It is also used to reduce extremely high blood pressure caused by kidney disease where other medicines have not been effective. Diazoxide works by causing the muscle in the walls of the blood vessels to relax. This allows the arteries to widen rapidly and reduces blood pressure. Intravenous dose is dependent on body weight. HCPCS Level II code J1730 represents up to 300 mg of diazoxide.

J1740

J1740 Injection, ibandronate sodium, 1 mg

Lay Description

Ibandronate sodium is a chemical compound that inhibits bone resorption. It binds to hydroxyapatite, which is part of the mineral matrix of bone. Ibandronate inhibits osteoclast activity reducing bone resorption and turnover. The drug is indicated for the prophylaxis and treatment of osteoporosis in postmenopausal women where it reduces the elevated rate of bone turnover, leading to a net gain in bone mass density. HCPCS Level II code J1740 represents 1 mg of injectable ibandronate sodium.

J1742

J1742 Injection, ibutilide fumarate, 1 mg

Lay Description

Ibutilide fumarate is an antiarrhythmic drug. Ibutilide fumarate is indicated for the rapid conversion of atrial fibrillation or atrial flutter of recent onset. It prolongs action potential duration in isolated adult cardiac myocytes and increases both atrial and ventricular refractoriness. This allows prolongation of atrial and ventricular action potential duration and refractoriness, aiding in a normal cardiac rhythm. It is supplied in single dose 10 ml vials containing 1 mg of ibutilide fumarate for intravenous injection. Usual adult dose is 1 mg administered by intravenous push over a 10-minute period. HCPCS Level II code J1742 represents up to 1 mg of ibutilide fumarate.

J1743

J1743 Injection, idursulfase, 1 mg

Lay Description

Idursulafse is an exogenous, purified form of a human enzyme produced by recombinant DNA technology in a human cell line. Idursulfase is an orphan drug used to treat the inherited metabolic disorder mucopolysaccharidosis II (MPS II or Hunter's Syndrome). MPS II is caused by a lack of the enzyme iduraonate-2-sulfase that normally breaks down certain carbohydrates known as glycosaminoglycans. MPS II causes widespread cumulative organ and tissue damage. The recommended dosage is 0.5 mg per kg of body weight. The drug is administered as an intravenous infusion every week. The infusion may be administered over one to three hours.

J1745

J1745 Injection infliximab, 10 mg

Lay Description

Infliximab is an injectable antibody that blocks the effects of tumor necrosis factor alpha (TNF alpha), a substance made by cells of the body that has an important role in promoting inflammation. Specifically, infliximab is used for treating the inflammation of Crohn's disease, rheumatoid arthritis, and psoriatic arthritis. Infliximab is administered by intravenous infusion, and dosage varies depending on the condition being treated. Dosage may range from 3 mg/kg of body weight (rheumatoid arthritis) to 5 mg/kg of body weight for moderate to severe Crohn's disease. HCPCS Level II code J1745 represents 10 mg of infliximab.

J1750

J1750 Injection, iron dextran, 50 mg

Lay Description

Iron dextran is used to treat iron deficiency anemia. It is a complex of ferric hydroxide and dextran. It is absorbed from the injection site into the capillaries and the lymphatic system. The iron is bound to the protein and forms iron. This iron is used to resupply the body with iron. Recommended dose of iron dextran varies based on the patient's hemoglobin level. It is administered by IV or intramuscular injection.

J1756

J1756 Injection, iron sucrose, 1 mg

Lay Description

Iron sucrose is a form of iron that is safe for the treatment of iron deficiency anemias in patients with kidney disease. It is used primarily in patients receiving ongoing hemodialysis and patients who are taking the hormone erythropoietin to help balance the iron deficiency caused by hemodialysis. Iron sucrose provides elemental iron, which is essential in the formation of hemoglobin. Iron sucrose is administered by intravenous injection over a 15-minute period. The dosage varies dependent on the degree of iron deficiency and type of renal disease the patient suffers. HCPCS Level II code J1756 represents 1 mg of iron sucrose.

Medicare Information

Medicare covers iron sucrose injection as a first line treatment of iron deficiency anemia when furnished intravenously to patients undergoing chronic hemodialysis who are receiving supplemental erythropoietin therapy.

J1786

J1786 Injection, imiglucerase, 10 units

Lay Description

Imiglucerase is an enzyme used to treat and alleviate the symptoms of Gaucher's disease, a lysosomal storage disorder caused by a genetic lack of the enzyme glucocerebrosidase. Gaucher cells accumulate in the liver, spleen, and bone marrow, resulting in severe abdominal swelling, causing the spleen to break down red blood cells more rapidly than they are produced. Imiglucerase is a synthetic form of protein beta-glucocerebrosidase that works by catalyzing the hydrolysis of glucocerebrosidase to glucose and ceramide. Imiglucerase is used for the treatment of Type 1 Gaucher's disease that results in one or more of the following: anemia, thrombocytopenia, bone disease, hepatomegaly, or splenomegaly. Dosage is determined by body weight. The usual dose is 15 to 60 units/kg of body weight administered by intravenous injection over one to two hours.

J1790

J1790 Injection, droperidol, up to 5 mg

Lay Description

Droperidol is used as an adjunct to general or regional anesthesia or as a general anesthetic in diagnostic procedures. It also has an antiemetic effect and may be used prior to surgery or postoperatively to prevent nausea and vomiting. It is administered by intramuscular or intravenous injection. Dosage is dependent upon patient's age and weight. HCPCS Level II code J1790 represents up to 5 mg of droperidol.

J1800

J1800 Injection, propranolol HCl, up to 1 mg

Lay Description

Propranolol is a nonselective beta-blocker used to treat tremors, angina, heart rhythm disorders, hypertension, and other cardiac conditions. It has also been found to prevent myocardial infarction and lessen the severity of migraine headaches. It works by blocking catecholamine-induced increases in heart rate, blood pressure, and force of myocardial contraction, thereby reducing cardiac oxygen demand. It also depresses renin secretion and prevents vasodilation of the cerebral arteries. It may be administered orally by capsule, tablet, or oral suspension, or by intravenous injection or infusion. Intravenous administration is only used in life-threatening arrhythmias or those occurring under anesthesia. The usual dose ranges from 1 to 3 mg. HCPCS Level II code J1800 represents up to 1 mg of propranolol hydrochloride.

J1810

J1810 Injection, droperidol and fentanyl citrate, up to 2 ml ampule

Lay Description

HCPCS Level II code J1810 represents a combination of droperidol and fentanyl citrate. Per the FDA, this drug is no longer available in the United States.

J1815-J1817

J1815 Injection, insulin, per 5 units
J1817 Insulin for administration through DME (i.e., insulin pump) per 50 units

Lay Description

Insulin is a hormone secreted by the beta cells of the pancreas that controls the metabolism and cellular uptake of sugars, proteins, and fats. As a drug, it is used principally to control Type I diabetes mellitus. Different forms of insulin may also be used to control blood sugar levels in patients with gestational diabetes to prevent fetal complications caused by maternal hyperglycemia. The use of insulin in Type II diabetes mellitus is typically only for patients who have failed to control their blood sugars with diet, exercise, and oral drugs. In the past, insulin for injection was obtained from beef or porcine pancreas. Most insulin now in use is made by recombinant DNA technology and is equivalent to human insulin from an immunological perspective. Dosage varies by the level of control of blood sugar needed. Insulin is administered by subcutaneous injection or by insulin pump. HCPCS Level II code J1815 represents 5 units of insulin. HCPCS Level II code J1817 represents 50 units of insulin administered by DME through an insulin pump.

J1830

J1830 Injection interferon beta-1b, 0.25 mg (code may be used for Medicare when drug administered under the direct supervision of a physician, not for use when drug is self-administered)

Lay Description

Interferon beta-1b is a biologic response modifier possessing both antiviral and immunoregulatory activities. Interferon beta-1b is indicated for the treatment of relapsing-remitting multiple sclerosis in ambulatory patients. The mechanisms by which interferon beta-1b exerts its actions in multiple sclerosis are not clearly understood. However, the biologic response-modifying properties are known to be mediated through its interactions with specific cell receptors found on the cell membrane, which cause cellular changes, including increased protein synthesis of human cells. The usual dosage is 0.25 mg self-injected subcutaneously every other day. HCPCS Level II code J1830 represents 0.25 mg interferon beta-1b when administered under the supervision of a physician.

J1835

J1835 Injection, itraconazole, 50 mg

Lay Description

Itraconazole is an antifungal used for the treatment of patients with aspergillosis, blastomycosis, histoplasmosis, esophageal and oropharyngeal candidiasis, and onychomycosis. It is also used to prevent fungal infections in patients with human immunodeficiency virus (HIV) or acquired immunodeficiency syndrome (AIDS). Itraconazole is in a class of antifungals called triazoles. It works by slowing the growth of fungi that cause infection. It may be administered orally as a capsule or oral solution or by intravenous infusion. Itraconazole administered by intravenous infusion is used primarily for immunocompromised patients with severe lung or systemic fungal infections. Usual intravenous dosage is 200 mg infused over one hour. HCPCS Level II code J1835 represents 50 mg of itraconazole.

J1840-J1850

J1840 Injection, kanamycin sulfate, up to 500 mg
J1850 Injection, kanamycin sulfate, up to 75 mg

Lay Description

Kanamycin sulfate is a bacterial antibiotic used to treat E. coli, Proteus species (both indole-positive and indole-negative), Enterobacter aerogenes, Kiebsiella pneumoniae, Serratia marcescens, and Acinetobacter species. It inhibits the synthesis of protein in susceptible microorganisms. The recommended dose is 15 mg per kg per day divided equally for intramuscular injection and should not exceed 15 mg per kg per day for intravenous infusion. Kanamycin can be administered intramuscularly or intravenously over 30 to 60 minutes. HCPCS Level II code J1840 represents a dose of up to 500 mg of kanamycin sulfate and J1850 represents a dose up to 75 mg of kanamycin sulfate.

J1885

J1885 Injection, ketorolac tromethamine, per 15 mg

Lay Description

Ketorolac tromethamine is a nonsteroidal anti-inflammatory drug (NSAID) that is indicated for short-term (up to five days in adults) management of moderately severe acute pain that requires analgesia at the opioid level. Ketorolac tromethamine is available for intravenous (IV) or intramuscular (IM) administration as 15 mg in 1 mL (1.5%) and 30 mg in 1 mL (3%) in sterile solution; 60 mg in 2 mL (3%) of ketorolac tromethamine in sterile solution is available for IM administration only. HCPCS Level II code J1885 represents up to 15 mg of ketorolac tromethamine.

J1890

J1890 Injection, cephalothin sodium, up to 1 g

Lay Description

Cephalosporins are used in the treatment of infections caused by bacteria. They work by killing bacteria or preventing their growth. Cephalosporins are used to treat infections in many different parts of the body. They are sometimes given with other antibiotics. Some cephalosporins given by injection are also used to prevent infections before, during, and after surgery. Cephalothin will not work against infections caused by viruses such as colds or the flu. HCPCS Level II code J1890 represents up to 1 gram of cephalothin sodium. HCPCS Level II code J1890 represents cephalothin sodium. Per the FDA, this drug is no longer available for human use in the United States.

J1930

J1930 Injection, lanreotide, 1 mg

Lay Description

Lanreotide is an orphan drug used to treat acromegaly, often due to a benign pituitary gland tumor. It is a rare and potentially life-threatening disease in which abnormal growth hormone is secreted by the pituitary gland. This abnormal growth hormone can cause enlargement of the hands, feet, facial bones, and internal organs such as the heart and liver. Patients who are untreated may have a shortened life span from heart and respiratory diseases, diabetes mellitus, and colon cancer. Lanreotide is used to treat patients who are not able to undergo surgery or radiotherapy. The recommended dose is 90 milligrams. This medication is administered by deep subcutaneous injection every four weeks for three months. HCPCS Level II code J1930 represents a 1 milligram dose.

J1931

J1931 Injection, laronidase, 0.1 mg

Lay Description

Laronidase is a polymorphic variant of the human enzyme L-iduronidase that is produced by recombinant DNA technology in a Chinese hamster ovary cell line. It is used to treat Hurler and Hurler-Scheie forms of mucopolysaccharidosis in patients who have moderate to severe symptoms. Laronidase has been shown to improve pulmonary function and walking capacity. Laronidase has not been evaluated for effects on the central nervous system manifestations of the disorder. The recommended dosage is 0.58 mg/kg of body weight administered once weekly as an intravenous infusion. HCPCS Level II code J1931 represents 0.1 mg of laronidase.

Medicare Information

See the chapter titled "Medicare Guidelines," under "Drugs, Biologicals, and Radiopharmaceuticals," for Medicare information.

J1940

J1940 Injection, furosemide, up to 20 mg

Lay Description

Furosemide is a diuretic that is an anthranilic acid derivative. It is used to treat edema, hypertension, and pulmonary edema. Dosage recommendations vary by the type of condition being treated, route of administration (oral, IV, or IM), and age and size of patient. HCPCS Level II code J1940 represents up to 20 mg of furosemide.

J1945

J1945 Injection, lepirudin, 50 mg

Lay Description

Lepirudin is a bivalent direct thrombin inhibitor derived from yeast cells that reduces the risk of serious consequences of heparin-induced thrombocytopenia (HIT). It is indicated for anticoagulation in patients with HIT and associated thromboembolic diseases. The usual dosage is 0.4 mg/kg body weight (up to 110 kg) administered slowly intravenously (e.g., over 15 to 20 seconds) as a bolus dose, followed by 0.15 mg/kg body weight (up to 110kg/hour) as a continuous intravenous infusion for two to 10 days or longer if clinically needed. HCPCS Level II code J1945 represents up to 50 mg of lepirudin.

Medicare Information

See chapter titled "Medicare Guidelines," under "Drugs, Biologicals, and Radiopharmaceuticals," for Medicare billing and documentation information.

J1950

J1950 Injection, leuprolide acetate (for depot suspension), per 3.75 mg

Lay Description

Leuprolide acetate is a synthetic analogue of the luteinizing hormone-releasing hormone (LHRH) that is used as an antineoplastic drug and a treatment for central precocious puberty, endometriosis, and uterine fibroids. It first stimulates and then suppresses follicle stimulating and luteinizing hormone release, resulting in suppression of testosterone and estrogen. A depot suspension is a drug that remains in the body long-term in storage and is slowly released into the blood. The leuprolide acetate depot suspension in dosages of 3.75 mg monthly and the 12.25 mg every three months are injected intramuscularly to treat endometriosis and uterine fibroids. When used to treat central precocious puberty, the dosage is individualized to the child and can range from 7.5 to 15 mg. Leuprolide acetate in doses of 7.5 mg and greater is injected subcutaneously and is used as a palliative treatment for advanced prostate cancer. HCPCS Level II code J1950 represents 3.75 mg of leuprolide acetate in depot suspension.

J1953

J1953   Injection, levetiracetam, 10 mg

Lay Description

Levetiracetam is an anticonvulsant indicated as an adjunctive therapy to help control partial onset seizures or myoclonic seizures in adults with juvenile myoclonic epilepsy. This injection is used when oral administration is not feasible. The precise mechanism by which levetiracetam controls seizure activity is unknown. The recommended dose is 500 milligrams twice a day. The dose can be increased every two weeks up to 3,000 milligrams. Levetiracetam is administered by IV injection over 15 minutes. HCPCS Level II code J1953 represents 10 milligrams.

J1955

J1955   Injection, levocarnitine, per 1 g

Lay Description

Levocarnitine is a naturally occurring substance required for energy metabolism. It has been shown to facilitate long-chain, fatty acid entry into cellular mitochondria, therefore delivering substrate for oxidation and subsequent energy production. With the exception of the brain, all tissues use fatty acids as an energy substrate and serve as a major fuel source in skeletal tissue and cardiac muscle. Levocarnitine is prescribed for the treatment of patients with an inherent error of metabolism that results in secondary carnitine deficiency. It is also used to prevent and treat carnitine deficiency in patients with end-stage renal disease who are on hemodialysis. The recommended dosage is a loading dose of 50 mg/kg given as a bolus injection over two to three minutes followed by 50 mg/kg daily by intravenous infusion. HCPCS Level II code J1955 represents 1 g of levocarnitine.

J1956

J1956   Injection, levofloxacin, 250 mg

Lay Description

Levofloxacin is a quinolone antibiotic. It inhibits DNA synthesis causing cell death. Susceptibility studies should be performed prior to the administration of levofloxacin. Susceptible bacteria include Streptococcus pneumoniae, Haemophilus influenzae, Moraxella catarrhalis, Staphylococcus aureus, Haemophilus parainfluenzae, Pseudomonas aeruginosa, Serratia marcescens, E. coli, Klebsiella pneumoniae, Chlamydia pneumoniae, Legionella pneumophila, Mycoplasma pneumoniae, Enterococcus faecalis, Streptococcus pyogenes, Proteus mirabilis, Staphylococcus epidermidis, Enterobacter cloacae, Staphylococcus saprophyticus, and Bacillus anthracis. HCPCS Level II code J1956 represents 250 mg of injectable levofloxacin.

J1960

J1960   Injection, levorphanol tartrate, up to 2 mg

Lay Description

Levorphanol tartrate is a potent synthetic opioid analgesic used to manage moderate to severe pain or as a pre- or postoperative medication where an opioid analgesic is appropriate. It may be administered by injection, intravenous infusion, or orally. The usual recommended starting dose for intravenous administration is up to 1 mg, given in divided doses, by slow push technique. This may be repeated every three to six hours as needed. The usual recommended starting dose administration by injection is 1 to 2 mg subcutaneously or intramuscularly repeated every six to eight hours as needed. HCPCS Level II code J1960 represents up to 2 mg of levorphanol tartrate.

J1980

J1980   Injection, hyoscyamine sulfate, up to 0.25 mg

Lay Description

Hyoscyamine sulfate is a component of belladonna alkaloid and is used as an anticholinergic and antispasmodic. Hyoscyamine sulfate inhibits gastrointestinal propulsive motility and decreases gastric acid secretion. This drug also decreases pharyngeal, tracheal, and bronchial secretions. Hyoscyamine sulfate is used as an adjunct therapy for the treatment of peptic ulcer disease, to control gastric secretion or excessive saliva production, and to decrease visceral spasm and hypermotility in such conditions as spastic colitis, spastic bladder, cystitis, and pylorospasm. It may also be used to prevent drug induced bradycardia during surgery. Hyoscyamine sulfate may be administered by several forms including sublingual, oral, injection, or intravenously. Dosage varies depending upon the condition being treated, patient age, and the size and weight of the patient. It can range from 0.25 mg to 0.5 mg for adults. HCPCS Level II code J1980 represents up to 0.25 mg of hyoscyamine sulfate.

J1990

J1990   Injection, chlordiazepoxide HCl, up to 100 mg

Lay Description

Chlordiazepoxide is a member of the benzodiazepine class of drugs. It acts on the gamma amino butyric acid (GABA) receptors in the brain resulting in the release of GABA and reducing the function of certain areas of the brain. GABA is a major inhibitory chemical in the brain that assists with inducing sleepiness and helps to control anxiety. Chlordiazepoxide is most commonly used to treat insomnia; however, it can also be used to relieve anxiety, particularly preoperative anxiety, and help alleviate alcohol withdrawal symptoms. It can be habit forming and is only used on a short-term basis. Dosage is dependent upon the condition being treated and the response of the individual patient. HCPCS Level II code J1990 represents up to 100 mg of chlordiazepoxide hydrochloride.

J2001

J2001   Injection, lidocaine HCl for intravenous infusion, 10 mg

Lay Description

Lidocaine hydrochloride stabilizes the neuronal membrane by inhibiting the conduction of pain impulses, thereby providing local anesthesia. It also stabilizes heart rhythms when administered intravenously. Lidocaine hydrochloride is indicated for local or regional anesthesia by infiltration techniques, such as percutaneous injection and intravenous regional peripheral nerve block techniques, and for treatment of cardiac arrhythmias. The drug is available in topical and injectable forms. The injectable form can be administered by intravenous infusion, caudal, epidural, retrobulbar, peripheral nerve block, and sympathetic nerve block. HCPCS Level II code J2001 represents up to 10 mg of lidocaine hydrochloride administered by intravenous infusion.

J2010

J2010   Injection, lincomycin HCl, up to 300 mg

Lay Description

Lincomycin hydrochloride (HCl) is an antibiotic used to treat serious, susceptible strains of streptococci, pneumococci, and staphylococci infections. It is specifically effective against the following organisms: Streptococcus pyogenes, Viridans group streptococci, Corynebacterium diphtheriae, Propionibacterium acnes, Clostridium tetani, and Clostridium perfringens.It is used for patients who are allergic to penicillin or for whom penicillin treatment is inappropriate. Recommended dose is 600 mg intramuscularly every 24 hours and 600 mg to 1 gram via intravenous infusion every eight to 12 hours. Intravenous lincomycin should be infused over one hour or more. HCPCS Level II code J2010 represents up to 300 mg of lincomycin HCl.

J2020

J2020   Injection, linezolid, 200 mg

Lay Description

Linezolid is a synthetic antibacterial of the oxazolidinone class. This drug inhibits bacterial protein synthesis by binding to a specific site on RNA and preventing the translation process. This method of action is different from other antibacterials; cross-resistance between linezolid and other antibiotics is unlikely. Susceptibility studies should be performed prior to the administration of cefazolin sodium. Susceptible bacteria include vancomycin-resistant Enterococcus faecium, methicillin-susceptible and resistant Staphylococcus aureus, Streptococcus pneumoniae, Streptococcus pyogenes, and Streptococcus agalactiae. Linezolid is available in injectable and oral forms. The injectable form is administered by intravenous infusion over a period of 30 to 120 minutes. Dosage varies by the route of administration, and by type and severity of the infection. HCPCS Level II code J2020 represents 200 mg of linezolid.

J2060

J2060   Injection, lorazepam, 2 mg

Lay Description

Lorazepam is a psychotropic drug with potent hypnotic and sedative effects. Lorazepam injection may be prescribed as a preanesthetic medication. Lorazepam is also indicated for the management of anxiety disorders or for the short-term relief of symptoms of anxiety or anxiety associated with depressive symptoms. When administered by intramuscular injection, usual dosage is 0.05 mg/kg of body weight up to a maximum of 4 mg. For intravenous injection for the purposes of sedation or relief of anxiety, the usual dose is 0.02 mg/kg of body weight to a maximum of 2 mg. HCPCS Level II code J2060 represents 2 mg of lorazepam.

J2150

J2150   Injection, mannitol, 25% in 50 ml

Lay Description

Mannitol is an osmotic diuretic that is readily diffused through the kidney. It is used to induce diuresis in the treatment and/or prevention of the oliguric phase of acute renal failure before irreversible damage is established. Mannitol is also used to reduce intracranial pressure and cerebral edema by reducing brain mass, to reduce elevated intraocular pressure, and to promote urinary excretion of toxic substances. Mannitol is administered by intravenous infusion. Dosage is dependent upon the condition being treated, with usual adult dosage ranging from 20 to 100 g in a 24-hour period.

J2170

J2170   Injection, mecasermin, 1 mg

Lay Description

Mecasermin is a synthesized version of human insulin-like growth factor-1 (IGF-1). It is produced by recombinant DNA technology using strains of *E. coli* bacteria. IGF-1 (formerly called somatomedin C) is a serum peptide formed within the liver and other tissues. IGF-1 in the human body is stimulated by human growth hormone and in turn stimulates cell growth and replication by increasing the metabolic uptake of glucose, fatty acids, and amino acids. Mecasermin is indicated for the long-term treatment of growth failure in children with severe primary IGF-1 deficiency or with genetic growth gene deletion who has developed neutralizing antibodies to growth hormone. The drug is not indicated for treatment of secondary forms of IGF-1 deficiency. Mecasermin should not be used in patients with closed epiphyses. Dosage is individualized to each patient and varies from an initial dose of 0.5 mg to 2 mg per kg of patient body weight. Mecasermin is administered subcutaneously and can be self-administered. HCPCS Level II code J2170 represents 1 mg of mecasermin.

J2175

J2175   Injection, meperidine HCl, per 100 mg

Lay Description

Meperidine hydrochloride is a narcotic analgesic with similar effects as morphine. Meperidine hydrochloride is used for analgesia and sedation. It is primarily used to treat moderate to severe pain, as a preoperative medicate, and as a form of anesthesia. HCPCS Level II code J2175 represents 100 mg of meperidine hydrochloride.

Medicare Information

See chapter titled "Medicare Guidelines," under "Infusion Pumps, External; Equipment and Supplies," for Medicare billing and documentation information.

J2180

J2180   Injection, meperidine and promethazine HCl, up to 50 mg

Lay Description

Meperidine and promethazine hydrochloride is a compound of a narcotic analgesic with similar effects as morphine (meperidine hydrochloride) and a phenothiazine derivative that provides antiemetic, sedative, and antihistaminic actions. It is primarily used to treat moderate to severe pain, as a preoperative medicate, and as a form of anesthesia. This drug is usually administered intramuscularly but the intravenous route may be employed. When used intravenously, it is preferable to use a push technique. Usual adult dosage is 50 mg every three to four hours; children's dosage is 0.5 mg/kg. HCPCS Level II code J2180 represents up to 50 mg of meperidine and promethazine hydrochloride.

J2185

J2185   Injection, meropenem, 100 mg

Lay Description

Meropenem is a broad spectrum carbapenem antibiotic for intravenous administration. It is indicated for the treatment of infections of the skin, intra-abdominal infections such as peritonitis, and bacterial meningitis when caused by susceptible bacterial agents. Dosage varies depending upon the severity of the condition and the age and weight of the patient. In adults, the recommended dosage is 500 mg every eight hours for skin infections and 1 g given every eight hours for intra-abdominal infections. Pediatric patients receive doses of 10, 20, or 40 mg/kg every eight hours depending on the type of infection. The usual technique is intravenous infusion over 15 to 30 minutes; however, a bolus dose over three to five minutes may be prescribed. HCPCS Level II code J2185 represents 100 mg of meropenem.

J2210

J2210   Injection, methylergonovine maleate, up to 0.2 mg

Lay Description

Methylergonovine maleate is a blood-vessel constrictor that is used to prevent or control postpartum hemorrhage caused by subinvolution or uterine atony. It works by causing the uterine muscles to contract, thereby reducing blood loss.

Methylergonovine maleate is available in tablet and injectable forms. The injectable form can be administered by intramuscular or intravenous injection; however, intravenous injection is administered only for life-threatening postpartum hemorrhage. HCPCS Level II code J2210 represents 0.2 mg of methylergonovine maleate.

J2248

J2248   Injection, micafungin sodium, 1 mg

Lay Description

Micafungin sodium is a semisynthetic lipopeptide produced from Coleophoma empetri, a plant fungus. It is used as an antifungal drug. Micafungin sodium disrupts the synthesis of a component of the fungal cellular membrane. This component is not present in mammalian cells. Micafungin sodium is indicated for the treatment of esophageal candidiasis and as a prophylactic therapy to prevent candida infections in patients undergoing hematopoietic stem cell transplants. The drug may cause allergic reactions including anaphylaxis. Micafungin sodium must be administered via an intravenous infusion over one hour. It should not be mixed with or infused with any other medication. HCPCS Level II code J2248 represents 1 mg of micafungin sodium.

J2250

J2250   Injection, midazolam HCl, per 1 mg

Lay Description

Midazolam hydrochloride is a benzodiazepine, a group of chemically similar psychotropic drugs. Because midazolam hydrochloride is associated with a high incidence of partial or complete recall impairment, it is used as preoperative sedation, sedation during diagnostic or therapeutic procedures, or for induction of general anesthesia. Dosage varies depending on the reason for administration and the age and weight of the patient. HCPCS Level II code J2250 represents 1 mg of midazolam hydrochloride.

J2260

J2260   Injection, milrinone lactate, 5 mg

Lay Description

Milrinone lactate is a member of a class of bipyridine inotropic/vasodilator agents with phosphodiesterase inhibitor activity that is distinct from digitalis or catecholamines. Milrinone lactate is indicated for the short-term intravenous treatment of acute heart failure. It is administered intravenously with a loading dose of 50 mcg/kg followed by a maintenance dose of no more than 1.13 mg/kg/day. HCPCS Level II code J2260 represents 5 mg of milrinone lactate.

J2270-J2275

J2270   Injection, morphine sulfate, up to 10 mg
J2271   Injection, morphine sulfate, 100 mg
J2275   Injection, morphine sulfate (preservative-free sterile solution), per 10 mg

Lay Description

Morphine sulfate is an opioid analgesic that principally affects the central nervous system and gastrointestinal tract. The drug increases the patient's tolerance for pain and decreases patient discomfort. The patient, however, may still recognize the presence of pain. Sedation also occurs. Dosage varies by route of administration, patient's age, weight, severity of illness, and comorbidities. HCPCS Level II code J2270 represents up to 10 mg of morphine sulfate; J2271 represents 100 mg of morphine sulfate; and J2275 represents 10 mg of preservative free morphine sulfate.

Medicare Information

See chapter titled "Medicare Guidelines," under "Infusion Pumps, External; Equipment and Supplies," for Medicare billing and documentation information.

J2278

J2278   Injection, ziconotide, 1 mcg

Lay Description

Ziconotide is a synthetic equivalent conopeptide produced from piscivorous marine snails. It binds to N-type calcium channels in the afferent nerves of the dorsal horn in the spinal column preventing the transmission of pain sensation. This drug must be administered intrathecally via an implanted variable-rate microinfusion device or an external microinfusion device and catheter. Ziconotide is indicated for the management of severe chronic pain in patients who are intolerant or refractory to other treatments. The effective dose of ziconotide is variable and the dose should be adjusted according to the patient's severity of pain, response to therapy, and the occurrence of adverse events. HCPCS Level II code J2278 represents 1 mcg of ziconitide.

J2280

J2280   Injection, moxifloxacin, 100 mg

Lay Description

Moxifloxacin hydrochloride is a synthetic, broad spectrum antibacterial agent. It is used to treat adult patient with acute bacterial sinusitis, acute bacterial exacerbation of chronic bronchitis, community acquired pneumonia, skin infections, and complicated intra-abdominal infections when caused by susceptible bacterial organism such as Streptococcus pneumoniae, Haemophilus influenzae,

Haemophilus parainfluenzae, Klebsiella pneumoniae, methicillin-susceptible Staphylococcus aureus, or Moraxella catarrhalis. The usual dosage is 400 mg daily. HCPCS Level II code J2280 represents 100 mg of moxifloxacin.

J2300

J2300   Injection, nalbuphine HCl, per 10 mg

Lay Description
Nalbuphine hydrochloride is a synthetic opioid analgesic that is chemically related to naloxone and oxymorphone. Nalbuphine hydrochloride is prescribed for the relief of moderate to severe pain or as a supplement to balanced anesthesia. It is also used for pre- and postoperative pain relief or obstetrical analgesia during labor and delivery. It may be administered by subcutaneous, intramuscular, or intravenous injection. The usual adult dose is 10 mg for every 70 kg every three to six hours as needed, adjusted according to the pain severity, condition of the patient, and other medications. HCPCS Level II code J2300 represents 10 mg of nalbuphine hydrochloride.

J2310

J2310   Injection, naloxone HCl, per 1 mg

Lay Description
Naloxone hydrochloride injection is indicated for the complete or partial reversal of narcotic depression induced by opioids, including natural and synthetic narcotics. Naloxone hydrochloride injection is also indicated for the diagnosis of suspected acute opioid overdosage. It may be administered intravenously, intramuscularly, or subcutaneously. The most rapid onset of action is achieved by intravenous administration, and this route is recommended in emergency situations. The usual intravenous dosage is 2 mg of naloxone hydrochloride in 500 mL of IV solution. Intramuscular or subcutaneous injection dosage varies depending upon patient's response. HCPCS Level II code J2310 represents 1 mg of naloxone hydrochloride.

J2315

J2315   Injection, naltrexone, depot form, 1 mg

Lay Description
Naltrexone depot is an opioid antagonist. The drug binds to specific opioid receptors blocking the effects stimulated by alcohol ingestion. A depot suspension is a drug that remains in the body long term in storage and is slowly released into the blood. The depot form is indicated as a treatment of alcohol dependence in patients who are unable to abstain from alcohol consumption during outpatient therapy treatments. The drug should be a part of a comprehensive treatment management program.

Patients should not be actively consuming alcohol during the time of initiation of naltrexone depot treatment. Naltrexone depot is administered by intramuscular injection into the gluteus once a month. Recommended dosage is 380 mg once a month. The depot form is not self-administrable. HCPCS Level II code J2315 represents 1 mg of naltrexone depot.

J2320

J2320   Injection, nandrolone decanoate, up to 50 mg

Lay Description
Nandrolone decanoate is a long-acting synthetic version of testosterone that has strong anabolic properties and weak androgenic or masculinizing properties. Anabolic properties are any constructive metabolic process by which organisms convert substances into other components of the organism"s chemical architecture. Nandrolone decanoate stimulates erythropoiesis, promotes tissue growth and building processes, and reverses tissue destruction. It is indicated as a treatment for chronic wasting diseases and anemia associated with renal insufficiency. Nandrolone decanoate is administered by intramuscular injection.

J2323

J2323   Injection, natalizumab, 1 mg

Lay Description
Natalizumab is a monoclonal antibody produced with recombinant DNA technology in murine myeloma cells. Natalizumab binds to the surface of leukocyte cells (except neutrophils) preventing their migration to the site of inflamed tissue. It is indicated as a monotherapy for the treatment of relapsing forms of multiple sclerosis in patients who cannot tolerate or have not adequately responded to other treatments. The recommended dose is 300 mg administered via intravenous infusion every four weeks. Note that this drug can only be prescribed, distributed and infused by providers, infusion centers and pharmacies registered with the manufacturer's TOUCH program. Patients must also be enrolled with the program.

J2325

J2325   Injection, nesiritide, 0.1 mg

Lay Description
Nesiritide is a human, B-type natriuretic peptide produced by recombinant DNA technology from E. coli. It has the same amino acid sequence as the endogenous peptide produced by the ventricular myocardium. Nesiritide binds to receptors of vascular smooth muscle and endothelial cells and increases intracellular concentrations of guanosine

cyclic monophosphate (cGMP), which creates smooth muscle cell relaxation. Use of this drug should be strictly limited to patients with acutely decompensated heart failure with a clinical presentation severe enough to warrant hospitalization. It should be administered in a clinical setting where blood pressure can be closely monitored. Nesiritide is currently in a clinical trial to asses its use in intermittent and scheduled infusions to treat severely ill congestive heart failure patients in an outpatient setting. However, this setting and indication is not recommended and has not yet been approved. Nesiritide is not intended for use as a diuretic. The drug is administered by intravenous infusion. The recommended dose is an initial intravenous bolus of 2 mcg/kg of body weight followed by a continuous infusion of 0.01 mcg/kg of body weight per minute. HCPCS Level II code J2325 represents 0.1 mg of nesiritide.

Medicare Information

See chapter titled "Medicare Guidelines," under "Drugs, Biologicals, and Radiopharmaceuticals," for Medicare billing and documentation information.

J2353-J2354

J2353 Injection, octreotide, depot form for intramuscular injection, 1 mg

J2354 Injection, octreotide, nondepot form for subcutaneous or intravenous injection, 25 mcg

Lay Description

Octreotide is a synthetic analogue of the natural hormone somatostatin. It causes the same effects as somatostatin, but has a prolonged duration. Somatostatin is a peptide produced by the hypothalamus gland and by pancreatic islet cells that inhibit the release of growth hormone, thyrotropin, corticotropin, insulin, glucagon, gastrin, renin, and secretin. The depot version is octreotide encased in biodegradable microspheres. The microspheres control the rate of drug release and allow it to be dispensed over longer periods of time. Both depot and non-depot formulations of octreotide are indicated as a treatment for acromegaly, as a symptomatic treatment for diarrhea, and flushing associated with metastatic carcinoid and vasoactive intestinal peptide tumors. Non-depot octreotide is administered by subcutaneous or intravenous injection. Dosages for the non-depot version vary from 50 to 600 mcg depending on the disease and response to treatment. Octreotide depot is administered by deep intramuscular injection into the buttocks every four weeks. Dosage for the depot version is usually 20 mg for patients who have been receiving the non-depot version. HCPCS Level II code J2353 represents 1 mg of octreotide depot and J2354 represents 25 mcg of the non-depot octreotide.

J2355

J2355 Injection, oprelvekin, 5 mg

Lay Description

Oprelvekin is a synthetic interleukin-11 produced by recombinant DNA technology using E. coli bacteria. Interleukin-11 is a growth factor produced by bone marrow stromal cells that stimulates the production of hematopoietic stem cells and megakaryocyte progenitor cells and B cell differentiation. Oprelvekin is indicated for prevention of thrombocytopenia following myelosuppressive chemotherapy in patients with non-myeloid malignancies. It is administered by subcutaneous injection. The recommended dosage is 50 mg/kg of body weight. HCPCS Level II code J2355 represents 5 mg of oprelvekin.

J2357

J2357 Injection, omalizumab, 5 mg

Lay Description

Omalizumab is a monoclonal antibody produced by recombinant DNA technology using Chinese hamster ovaries. It binds specifically to human immunoglobulin E (IgE) and inhibits the binding of IgE to mast cells and basophils. The reduction in IgE binding limits the allergic response. Omalizumab is indicated for patients age 12 years or older with moderate to severe persistent asthma who are reactive to air-borne allergens and whose symptoms are not adequately controlled by inhaled corticosteroids. It is administered by subcutaneous injection. Dosages vary from 150 to 375 mg every two to four weeks. Dosage depends on the patient's body weight and the serum level of IgE. HCPCS Level II code J2357 represents 5 mg of omalizumab.

Medicare Information

See the chapter titled "Medicare Guidelines," under "Drugs, Biologicals, and Radiopharmaceuticals," for Medicare information.

J2360

J2360 Injection, orphenadrine citrate, up to 60 mg

Lay Description

Orphenadrine citrate is a synthetic analogue of diphenhydramine having analgesic, antihistaminic, anti-cholinergic, and antispasmodic properties. The drug acts on the brain stem selectively blocking facilitatory functions of the reticular formation. This produces a blocking of the pain transmission signals. Its therapeutic effects are not completely understood, but appear to be related to its analgesic properties. Orphenadrine is indicated for symptomatic relief of pain associated with acute musculoskeletal disorders. It can be used as an adjunct to rest, physical therapy, and other analgesic measures. Orphenadrine is available in an oral, self-administrable form and in an injectable form. The oral form is usually combined with aspirin and caffeine. Dosages of the oral form vary from 25 to 200 mg per day. Recommended dosage of the injectable form is 60 mg twice a day. The Injectable form is administered by intravenous or intramuscular injection. HCPCS Level II code J2360 represents up to 60 mg of injectable orphenadrine citrate.

J2370

J2370   Injection, phenylephrine HCl, up to 1 ml

Lay Description

Phenylephrine hydrochloride is an amine that is related to epinephrine and ephedrine. The drug is longer-acting than epinephrine or ephedrine. It affects the sympathetic nervous system by stimulating alpha adrenergic receptors. It functions predominately as a vasoconstrictor. Injectable phenylephrine hydrochloride is indicated for the treatment of hypotension, vascular failure in shock, and paroxysmal supraventricular tachycardia. The drug is also used to maintain adequate blood pressure during inhalation and spinal anesthesia and as a vasoconstrictor in regional analgesia. Injectable phenylephrine hydrochloride may be administered by intramuscular, subcutaneous, or intravenous injection and by intravenous infusion. HCPCS Level II code J2370 represents an injection of up to 1 ml of phenylephrine hydrochloride.

J2400

J2400   Injection, chloroprocaine HCl, per 30 ml

Lay Description

Chloroprocaine hydrochloride (HCl) is a local anesthetic that blocks the feeling of pain by inhibiting the conduction of nerve impulses. The order of loss of nerve function is pain, temperature, touch, proprioception, and skeletal muscle tone. It is often used for dental procedures and during labor and delivery. Chloroprocaine can be administered by infiltration, caudal, epidural, or peripheral block. HCPCS Level II code J2400 represents 30 ml of chloroprocaine HCl.

J2405

J2405   Injection, ondansetron HCl, per 1 mg

Lay Description

Ondansetron hydrochloride is a chemical compound that is a selective blocker of serotonin 5-HT3 receptors. It is an antiemetic drug available in oral and injectable forms. Serotonin 5-HT3 receptors are present on the vagal nerve and at sensory nerve endings. Cytotoxic chemotherapy appears to trigger the release of serotonin in the small intestine, which may trigger the 5-HT3 receptors and initiate the vomiting reflex. Ondansetron hydrochloride is indicated for the prevention of nausea and vomiting associated with surgery and antineoplastic drugs. The oral version is also indicated for the prevention of nausea and vomiting associated with radiation therapy. The drug is available in oral and injectable versions. The injectable version is administered by intravenous injection. When administered in conjunction with antineoplastic drugs, ondansetron hydrochloride should be diluted. The recommended dosage for this indication is a single 32 mg or three doses at 0.15 mg/kg of body weight infused over 15 minutes. Subsequent dosages may be infused at four and eight hours after the initial dose. When used to suppress postoperative vomiting, the drug does not need to be diluted. The recommended dose is 4 mg or 0.1 mg/kg of body weight administered by intravenous or intramuscular injection. Dosages for the oral version vary from 8 to 24 mg depending on the indication and patient. HCPCS Level II code J2405 represents 1 mg of injectable ondansetron hydrochloride.

J2410

J2410   Injection, oxymorphone HCl, up to 1 mg

Lay Description

Oxymorphone hydrochloride is a semi-synthetic opioid substitute for morphine that is a potent analgesic and sedative. Oxymorphone hydrochloride exerts its effect on the central nervous system (CNS) and gastrointestinal tract. It binds to specific opiate receptors in the CNS providing an analgesic effect. The exact mechanism of action for its analgesic effect is unknown. Oxymorphone hydrochloride also produces respiratory depression; decreases gastric, biliary, and pancreatic secretions; and increases smooth muscle tone in the urinary tract. It is a schedule II controlled substance. Oxymorphone hydrochloride is indicated for the relief of moderate to severe pain, as an anesthetic premedication, and for the relief of anxiety related to dyspnea associated with pulmonary edema in patients with acute left ventricular dysfunction. HCPCS Level II code J2410 represents up to 1 mg of injectable oxymorphone hydrochloride

J2425

J2425   Injection, palifermin, 50 mcg

Lay Description

Palifermin is a human keratinocyte growth factor (KGF) produced by recombinant DNA technology in Escherichia coli (E. coli). It is different from endogenous human growth factor (EGF) in that the first 23 N-terminal amino acids have been deleted to improve protein stability. It stimulates the epithelial cells that line and protect the oral mucosa. It is used to treat severe oral mucositis that is often found as a side effect of high dose chemotherapy and/or radiation therapy in patients with hematologic malignancies. The recommended dose of palifermin is 60 mcg per kg per day. The medication is administered for three consecutive days prior to the myelotoxic therapy and three consecutive days after. Palifermin is administered by intravenous bolus injection. HCPCS Level II code J2425 represents 50 mcg of palifermin.

J2426

J2426 Injection, paliperidone palmitate extended release, 1 mg

Lay Description

Paliperidone palmitate is a psychotropic agent used to treat schizophrenia in adults. The recommended dose is 234 mg on the first day of treatment and 156 mg one week later administered as an IM injection into the deltoid muscle. The recommended maintenance dose is 117 mg monthly administered as in IM injection in the deltoid or gluteal muscle. The maintenance dose may vary based on individual response to the treatment.

J2430

J2430 Injection, pamidronate disodium, per 30 mg

Lay Description

Pamidronate disodium is used to treat hypercalcemia from cancer, Paget's disease, osteolytic bone metastases of breast cancer, and osteolytic bone lesions of multiple myeloma. Pamidronate disodium acts as an antihypercalcemic, inhibiting the resorption of bone and blocking the formation of mature osteoclasts. Cardiovascular side effects of atrial fibrillation and tachycardia may occur, with hypertension a common side-effect as well as fatigue, abdominal pain, nausea, constipation, anorexia, and anemia. This code reports a 30 mg intravenous injection.

J2440

J2440 Injection, papaverine HCl, up to 60 mg

Lay Description

Papaverine hydrochloride is an alkaloid extracted from opium or synthetically produced. The drug relaxes smooth muscles, especially when is has been contracted in spasm. The drug directly relaxes the cardiac and vascular systems, bronchial muscles, and gastrointestinal, biliary, and urinary tracts. Its effect on the vascular system includes coronary, cerebral, peripheral, and pulmonary arteries. It has minimal effect on the central nervous system, though large doses can cause some sedation. Papaverine hydrochloride is indicated in erectile dysfunction and various conditions where spasms occur, such as vascular spasm associated with acute myocardial infarction, angina pectoris, peripheral embolism, pulmonary embolism, and visceral spasms such as gastrointestinal colic and ureteral or biliary spasms. It may also be useful in peripheral vascular disease with vasospastic elements and certain cerebral angiospasms. HCPCS Level II code J2440 represents up to 60 mg of papaverine hydrochloride.

J2460

J2460 Injection, oxytetracycline HCl, up to 50 mg

Lay Description

Oxytetracycline hydrochloride is a broad-spectrum antibiotic of the tetracycline group produced by the bacterium Streptomyces rimosus. Its mechanism of action is not known, but it is thought to inhibit protein synthesis. Oxytetracycline is effective against a wide range of both gram-positive and gram-negative organisms. Susceptibility studies should be performed prior to the administration of this drug. Cross resistance among drugs in the tetracycline family is common. Susceptible organisms include rickettsiae, Mycoplasma pneumoniae, Borrelia recurrentis, Escherichia coli, Enterobacter aerogenes, Pseudomonas aeruginosa, Haemophilus aegyptius, Shigella species, Mima species, Herellea species, Haemophilus influenzae, Klebsiella species, Diplococcus pneumoniae, Staphylococcus aureus, Neisseria gonorrhoeae, Treponema pallidum, Treponema pertenue, Listeria monocytogenes, Clostridium species, Bacillus anthracis, Fusobacterium fusiforme, and Actinomyces species. It may also be used in combination with amebicides to treat acute intestinal amebiasis. HCPCS Level II code J2460 represents up to 50 mg of oxytetracycline hydrochloride.

J2469

J2469 Injection, palonosetron HCl, 25 mcg

Lay Description

Palonosetron hydrochloride is a chemical compound that is a selective blocker of serotonin 5-HT3 receptors. Serotonin 5-HT3 receptors are present on the vagal nerve and at sensory nerve endings. Cytotoxic chemotherapy appears to trigger the release of serotonin in the small intestine, which may trigger the 5-HT3 receptors and initiate the vomiting reflex. It is indicated to prevent and treat nausea and vomiting associated with chemotherapy. Palonosetron hydrochloride is administered by intravenous injection. The recommended dosage of the injectable form is 25 mcg. HCPCS Level II code

J2469 represents 25 mcg of palonosetron hydrochloride.

Medicare Information
See the chapter titled "Medicare Guidelines," under "Drugs, Biologicals, and Radiopharmaceuticals," for Medicare information.

J2501
J2501   Injection, paricalcitol, 1 mcg

Lay Description
Paricalcitol is a synthetic analogue of calcitriol, vitamin D. Vitamins are organic compounds that are necessary for the metabolic functioning of the body. Vitamin D is a fat-soluble vitamin that is a group of related compounds commonly called calciferol. Two common forms are cholecalciferol and ergocalciferol. Vitamin D is a steroid hormone precursor and helps to maintain calcium and phosphorus levels throughout the body. Human skin can produce vitamin D when exposed to sunlight, specifically UVB. Secondary hyperparathyroidism is characterized by an increase in parathyroid hormone to compensate for inadequate levels of active vitamin D hormone. Paricalcitol is indicated for the prevention and treatment of hyperparathyroidism secondary to chronic renal failure. The injectable form is administered by intravenous injection and is primarily used when the patient has stage 5 chronic renal disease. HCPCS Level II code J2501 represents up to 1 mcg of paricalcitol.

J2503
J2503   Injection, pegaptanib sodium, 0.3 mg

Lay Description
Pegaptanib sodium is a pegylated oligonucleotide for intravitreous injection. Pegylating is the addition of a polyethylene glycol (PEG) molecule, which allows a slow release of the carried substance. Pegaptanib sodium is a selective vascular endothelial growth factor antagonist that inhibits the growth of additional blood vessels. Pegaptanib sodium is indicated for the treatment of neovascular or wet age-related macular degeneration. The recommended dose is 0.3 mg administered by intravitreous injection to the affected eye once every six weeks. HCPCS Level II code J2503 represents 0.3 mg of pegaptanib sodium.

J2504
J2504   Injection, pegademase bovine, 25 IU

Lay Description
Pegademase bovine is an orphan drug that provides an exogenous source for the enzyme adenosine deaminase. It is derived from bovine intestines. A deficiency of adenosine deaminase allows adenosine and some of its derivatives to accumulate in cells. This accumulation is toxic to lymphocytes, which are a main component of the immune system. Pegademase is indicated as a replacement enzyme in patients with severe combined immunodeficiency disease in whom the disease is due to the lack of adenosine deaminase. Pegademase is administered by intramuscular injection. Dosage needs to be individualized to the patient and varies from 10 to 30 IU/kg of body weight. HCPCS Level II code J2504 represents 25 IU of pegademase.

Medicare Information
See chapter titled "Medicare Guidelines," under "Drugs, Biologicals, and Radiopharmaceuticals," for Medicare billing and documentation information.

J2505
J2505   Injection, pegfilgrastim, 6 mg

Lay Description
Pegfilgrastim is a pegylated form of filgrastim. Pegylated means that polyethylene glycol, a dispensing agent, has been added to the drug. Filgrastim is a synthetic human granulocyte colony-stimulating factor (G-CSF). Pegfilgrastim is produced by recombinant DNA technology using E. coli bacteria. The drug binds to surface receptors on hematopoietic and stimulates neutrophil production, differentiation, maturation, and function. Pegfilgrastim is longer acting than filgrastim. It is indicated as a treatment for neutropenia in patients receiving myelosuppressive therapy for nonmyeloid malignancies. The drug is administered by subcutaneous injection. Recommended dosage is 6 mg once each chemotherapy cycle. HCPCS Level II code J2505 represents 6 mg of pegfilgrastim.

J2510
J2510   Injection, penicillin G procaine, aqueous, up to 600,000 units

Lay Description
Penicillin G procaine is a version of penicillin that contains procaine, a local anesthesic agent. Penicillins block the actions of transpeptidase, an enzyme needed to create the cell wall. This weakens the bacterial cell wall causing cellular death. The procaine provides a local anesthetic action and contributes to a slower release of the penicillin G from the injection site. Penicillin G procaine is not as long acting as penicillin G benzathine. Once in the body, penicillin G procaine is hydrolyzed to penicillin G. The hydrolysis and slow absorption provide sustained, but lower blood levels of penicillin. Susceptibility studies should be performed prior to the administration of penicillin G procaine. This formulation is administered by deep intramuscular injection. Dosage depends upon the

bacterial infection being treated. HCPCS Level II code J2510 represents up to 600,000 units of penicillin G procaine.

J2513

J2513 Injection, pentastarch, 10% solution, 100 ml

Lay Description

Pentastarch is a derivative of starch composed of 90 percent amylopectin. It is used in plasma volume expander. Intravenous infusion of pentastarch results in expansion of the plasma volume in excess of the volume infused. This expansion persists for approximately 18 to 24 hours and is expected to improve the hemodynamic status for 12 to 18 hours. It is indicated for plasma volume expansion when needed to manage shock due to hemorrhage, surgery, sepsis, burns, or other trauma. It is not a substitute for red blood cells or coagulation factors in plasma. Pentastarch is administered by intravenous infusion only. Total dosage and rate of infusion depend upon the amount of blood or plasma lost. HCPCS Level II code J2513 represents up to 100 ml of pentastarch 10% solution.

Medicare Information

See chapter titled "Medicare Guidelines," under "Drugs, Biologicals, and Radiopharmaceuticals," for Medicare billing and documentation information.

J2515

J2515 Injection, pentobarbital sodium, per 50 mg

Lay Description

Pentobarbital sodium is a short- to intermediate-acting barbiturate. Barbiturates are derivatives of barbituric acid that act as central nervous system depressants producing a wide variety of effects, from mild sedation to anesthesia. They enhance the neurotransmitter gamma aminobutyric acid (GABA), which inhibits the excitation of nerves. Pentobarbital sodium is indicated as a sedative, presurgical adjunct to anesthesia, as a short-term treatment for insomnia, and as an anticonvulsant. HCPCS Level II code J2515 represents up to 50 mg of pentobarbital sodium.

J2540

J2540 Injection, penicillin G potassium, up to 600,000 units

Lay Description

Penicillin G potassium is a version of penicillin that contains potassium. Penicillins block the actions of transpeptidase, an enzyme needed to create the cell wall. This weakens the bacterial cell wall causing cellular death. Susceptibility studies should be performed prior to the administration of penicillin G potassium. The drug is available in oral and injectable forms. The injectable form can be administered by intramuscular, subcutaneous, intracavity, and intrathecal injection or continuous intravenous infusion. Dosage depends upon the bacterial infection being treated, as well as the form of the penicillin. HCPCS Level II code J2540 represents up to 600,000 units of penicillin G potassium.

J2543

J2543 Injection, piperacillin sodium/tazobactam sodium, 1 g/0.125 g (1.125 g)

Lay Description

Piperacillin is a semisynthetic broad-spectrum penicillin. Penicillins block the actions of transpeptidase, an enzyme needed to create the cell wall. This weakens the bacterial cell wall causing cellular death. Many bacteria have developed a resistance to penicillin. Resistant bacteria produce an enzyme, penicillinase or beta-lactamase, that protects it from the effects of penicillin. Tazobactam inhibits the penicillinase so the piperacillin is effective against a greater number of bacteria. Susceptibility studies should be performed prior to the administration of piperacillin. Susceptible bacteria include E. coli, Pseudomonas aeruginosa, enterococci, Clostridium spp., Bacteroides spp., Klebsiella spp., Proteus spp., Neisseria gonorrhoeae, Enterobacter spp., Serratia spp., Streptococcus pneumoniae, Haemophilus influenzae, Acinetobacter spp., Morganella morganii, and Providencia rettgeri. Piperacillin/tazobactam is administered by intramuscular injection or intravenous injection and infusion. Dosage varies from 2 to 6 g depending on the organism and extent of the infection. HCPCS Level II code J2543 represents 1 g of piperacillin with 0.125 g of tazobactam.

J2545

J2545 Pentamidine isethionate, inhalation solution, FDA-approved final product, noncompounded, administered through DME, unit dose form, per 300 mg

Lay Description

Pentamidine isethionate is an aromatic diamidine that is an anti-protozoal. Its mechanism of action is not completely known. It is thought the drug interferes with the synthesis of DNA, RNA, and protein causing cell death. Pentamidine isethionate is indicated as a treatment for Pneumocystis carinii, trypanosomiasis, and leishmaniasis. The drug may be administered by intramuscular injection, inhalation, or intravenous infusion over one hour.

HCPCS Lay Descriptions

Dosage is usually 300 mg. HCPCS Level II code J2545 represents 300 mg of the inhaled form of pentamidine isethionate administered through DME by a nebulizer.

J2550

J2550 Injection, promethazine HCl, up to 50 mg

Lay Description
Promethazine hydrochloride is a phenothiazine derivative with antihistamine, sedative, antiemetic, and anticholinergic properties. The drug binds to histamine receptors preventing the histamine from dilating capillaries, constricting the bronchial smooth muscles, and increasing gastric secretions. Promethazine hydrochloride is indicated as an antiemetic, a sedative in anesthesia, as a treatment for motion sickness, and for allergic reactions, including rhinitis and pruritic skin reactions. The drug may be combined with other drugs in cough and cold preparations. Promethazine hydrochloride is available in injectable, oral, and rectal suppository forms. The injectable form is administered by intramuscular or intravenous injection although the preferred method is by IM injection. Dosage varies from 25 to 50 mg.

J2560

J2560 Injection, phenobarbital sodium, up to 120 mg

Lay Description
Phenobarbital sodium is a long-acting barbiturate. Barbiturates are derivatives of barbituric acid that act as central nervous system depressants that produce a wide variety of effects, from mild sedation to anesthesia. They enhance the neurotransmitter gamma aminobutyric acid (GABA), which inhibits the excitation of nerves. Phenobarbital sodium is indicated as a sedative, presurgical adjunct to anesthesia, as a short-term treatment for insomnia, and as an anticonvulsant. It is a schedule IV narcotic. HCPCS Level II code J2560 represents up to 120 mg of phenobarbital sodium.

J2562

J2562 Injection, plerixafor, 1 mg

Lay Description
Plerixafor is a hematopoietic stem cell mobilizer that helps move hematopoietic stem cells to the peripheral blood for collection prior to autologous transplant in patients with non-Hodgkin's lymphoma and multiple myeloma (MM). It inhibits the CXCR4 chemokine receptor and blocks binding the stromal cell-derived factors. Those factors direct the hematopoietic stem cells to the bone marrow. Once the stem cells are circulating in the peripheral blood, they can be extracted and prepared for transplant. The recommended dose is 0.24 mg/kg body weight about 11 hours before starting the apheresis for up to four consecutive days. Plerixafor is given by subcutaneous injection.

J2590

J2590 Injection, oxytocin, up to 10 units

Lay Description
Oxytocin is an animal-derived or synthetic form of the hormone secreted by the hypothalamus and stored in the pituitary gland. Oxytocin promotes uterine contractions and stimulates milk secretion. It is indicated to induce labor, to promote uterine contractions after delivery of the placenta or abortion, and to control postpartum hemorrhage. Dosage depends upon uterine response. HCPCS Level II code J2590 represents up to 10 units of oxytocin.

J2597

J2597 Injection, desmopressin acetate, per 1 mcg

Lay Description
Desmopressin acetate, also known as DDAVP, is a potent synthetic analogue of the natural hormone vasopressin. Vasopressin is a hormone produced by the posterior pituitary gland. Vasopressin has an antidiuretic effect causing the renal tubules to reabsorb water. Desmopressin acetate is indicated for the treatment of diabetes insipidus, primary nocturnal enuresis, treatment of temporary polyuria and polydipsia secondary to trauma to or surgery in the pituitary region, and to increase coagulation factor VIII activity before surgical procedures in patients with hemophilia A and von Willebrand's disease. HCPCS Level II code J2597 represents up to 1 mcg of desmopressin acetate.

J2650

J2650 Injection, prednisolone acetate, up to 1 ml

Lay Description
Prednisolone is a synthetic adrenal corticosteroid. Corticosteroids are natural substances produced by the adrenal glands located adjacent to the kidneys. Corticosteroids are widely used to treat allergies, inflammation, and many disease processes. Prednisolone is used to treat a wide variety of conditions. Oral and injectable prednisolone is used to suppress inflammation in many inflammatory and allergic conditions. Examples include rheumatoid arthritis, systemic lupus, acute gouty arthritis, psoriatic arthritis, ulcerative colitis, and Crohn's disease. Severe allergic conditions that fail conventional treatment may also be treated with

© 2010 Ingenix

prednisolone. Examples include bronchial asthma, allergic rhinitis, drug-induced dermatitis, and contact and atopic dermatitis. Prednisolone is also used in the treatment of leukemia and lymphomas, idiopathic thrombocytopenia purpura, and autoimmune hemolytic anemia. Other miscellaneous conditions treated with this medication include thyroiditis and sarcoidosis. Prednisolone is used as a hormone replacement in patients whose adrenal glands are unable to produce sufficient amounts of corticosteroids. Prednisolone injection or sterile suspension can be injected into a muscle, joint, lesion, or soft tissue. When used as an intra-articular injection, prednisolone is indicated as a treatment for joint pain and inflammation, epicondylitis, bursitis, and synovitis. HCPCS Level II code J2650 represents up to 1 ml of prednisolone acetate injection.

J2670

J2670   Injection, tolazoline HCl, up to 25 mg

Lay Description

Tolazoline hydrochloride is a chemical compound that is an adrenergic blocking agent and peripheral vasodilator. Per the FDA, this drug is no longer available in the United States for human use. It is still available for veterinary use.

J2675

J2675   Injection, progesterone, per 50 mg

Lay Description

Progesterone is an animal-derived or synthetic form of the natural human hormone produced by the adrenal cortex, ovaries, and placenta. The hormone prepares the uterus for the reception and development of the fertilized ovum and maintains an optimal intrauterine environment for pregnancy. Exogenous progesterone is used as a treatment for dysfunctional uterine bleeding, secondary amenorrhea, infertility, and as part of postmenopausal hormone replacement therapy. HCPCS Level II code J2675 represents 50 mg of injectable progesterone.

J2680

J2680   Injection, fluphenazine decanoate, up to 25 mg

Lay Description

Fluphenazine decanoate is a phenothiazine derivative that blocks dopamine receptors in hypothalamus and pituitary glands. Fluphenazine decanoate has a slower release from the injection site than the fluphenazine hydrochloride, which results in a prolonged duration of action. The precise mechanism of action is not known, but it is believed to depress the reticular activating system. Fluphenazine decanoate is indicated in the management of manifestations of schizophrenia. Adult dosage varies from 1 to 10 mg daily depending on the severity and duration of symptoms. Fluphenazine decanoate is administered by intramuscular or subcutaneous injection. HCPCS Level II code J2680 represents up to 25 mg of fluphenazine decanoate.

J2690

J2690   Injection, procainamide HCl, up to 1 g

Lay Description

Procainamide hydrochloride is a benzoic acid derivative that depresses heart function. The drug increases the refractory period of the cardiac atria and ventricles. Procainamide hydrochloride is indicated as a treatment for documented life-threatening ventricular arrhythmias, such as sustained ventricular tachycardia. The drug is available in injectable and oral forms. The injectable form is administered by intramuscular or intravenous injection or intravenous infusion. Dosage varies from 100 to 1,000 mg depending upon response. HCPCS Level II code J2690 represents up to 1 g of injectable procainamide hydrochloride.

J2700

J2700   Injection, oxacillin sodium, up to 250 mg

Lay Description

Oxacillin sodium is a semi-synthetic penicillin that is penicillinase resistant. Penicillins block the actions of transpeptidase, an enzyme needed to create the cell wall. This weakens the bacterial cell wall causing cellular death. Many bacteria have developed a resistance to penicillin. Resistant bacteria produce an enzyme, penicillinase or beta-lactamase, that protects it from the effects of penicillin. Susceptibility studies should be performed prior to the administration of oxacillin sodium. Oxacillin sodium is indicated in the treatment of infections caused by penicillinase-producing staphylococci. HCPCS Level II code J2700 represents up to 250 mg of oxacillin sodium.

J2710

J2710   Injection, neostigmine methylsulfate, up to 0.5 mg

Lay Description

Neostigmine methylsulfate is a chemical that blocks the passage of nerve signals in the parasympathetic system. It competes with acetylcholine by attaching itself to the same receptors on a cell. Neostigmine methylsulfate is indicated for treatment of myasthenia gravis, prevention and postoperative treatment of distention and urinary retention, and reversal of the effects of nondepolarizing neuromuscular blocking agents, such as tubocuranne, metocurine, gallamine, or pancuronium following surgery. The recommended dose is dependent on the condition being treated. For myasthenia gravis, the recommended dose is 1:2000 solution (0.5 mg) administered by subcutaneous or intramuscular injection. For prevention and postoperative treatment of distention and urinary retention, the recommended dose is 1:4000 solution (0.25 mg) administered by subcutaneous or intramuscular injection. For reversal of the effects of nondepolarizing neuromuscular blocking agents, the recommended dose is 1:2000 solution (0.5 mg) administered by subcutaneous or intramuscular injection. HCPCS Level II code J2710 represents up to 0.5 mg of neostigmine methylsulfate.

J2720

J2720   Injection, protamine sulfate, per 10 mg

Lay Description
Protamine sulfate is a simple protein with a low molecular weight. It occurs naturally in the sperm of salmon and certain other species of fish. When given alone, it has a weak anticoagulant effect. However, when given in the presence of heparin, a stable salt is formed and both drugs lose their anticoagulant effect. Protamine sulfate is indicated for the treatment of heparin overdose. Protamine sulfate is administered intravenously and has a rapid onset of action. Neutralization of heparin occurs within five minutes following intravenous administration. Each mg of protamine will neutralize approximately 90 USP units of heparin activity derived from beef lung tissue or about 115 USP units of heparin activity derived from porcine intestinal mucosa. Protamine sulfate is given by very slow intravenous injection in doses 50 mg or less over a 10-minute period. HCPCS Level II code J2720 represents 10 mg of protamine sulfate.

J2724

J2724   Injection, protein C concentrate, intravenous, human, 10 IU

Lay Description
Protein C concentrate is used to replace congenitally deficient protein C. Protein C is a vitamin K-dependent plasma protein. When activated by thrombin, protein C inhibits the clotting mechanism by enzymatically breaking up the activated forms of clotting factors V and VIII. It also enhances fibrinolysis. Protein C concentrate is derived from pooled human plasma and uses a column of mouse monoclonal antibodies. It is indicated for the treatment of severe congenital protein C deficiency for the prevention and treatment of venous thrombosis and purpura fulminans. Protein C concentrate may be used for an acute episode, short-term prophylaxis, and long-term prophylaxis. The dosage, frequency, and duration of treatment depends on the severity of the patient's deficiency and the patient's age, clinical condition, and the plasma levels of protein C. Protein C concentrate is administered by intravenous infusion. Code J2724 represents 10 IU of Protein C concentrate.

J2725

J2725   Injection, protirelin, per 250 mcg

Lay Description
Protirelin is a synthetic peptide similar to the endogenous thyrotropin releasing hormone produced by the hypothalamus. Thyrotropin releasing hormone stimulates the anterior pituitary gland to release thyroid stimulating hormone (TSH). Protirelin is indicated for diagnosis of mild hyperthyroidism, Graves' disease, and for differentiating between primary, secondary, and tertiary hypothyroidism. The drug is administered via an intravenous bolus with a recommended dosage of 500 mcg. TSH serum levels are then measured at different intervals. HCPCS Level II code J2725 represents 250 mcg of protirelin.

J2730

J2730   Injection, pralidoxime chloride, up to 1 g

Lay Description
Pralidoxime chloride, also known as p2-PAM chloride, is a chemical that reactivates the parasympathetic nervous system. Pralidoxime chloride is indicated as an antidote in the treatment of poisoning due to pesticides and chemicals of the organophosphate class that block nerve signal transmission in the parasympathetic nervous system. Pralidoxime chloride is also indicated in the control of overdosage by some drugs used in the treatment of myasthenia gravis. The principal indications for the use of pralidoxime chloride are muscle weakness and respiratory depression. The principal action of pralidoxime chloride is to reactivate cholinesterase that has been inactivated by an organophosphate pesticide or related compound. This facilitates destruction of accumulated acetylcholine, which allows nerve signals to function normally. The most critical effect of pralidoxime chloride is in relieving paralysis of the respiratory muscles. Because pralidoxime chloride is less effective in relieving depression of the respiratory center, atropine is always administered concomitantly to block the effect of accumulated acetylcholine of the respiratory center. Pralidoxime chloride is administered by intravenous, intramuscular, or subcutaneous injection or infusion. HCPCS Level II code J2730 represents up to 1 gm of pralidoxime chloride.

J2760

J2760 Injection, phentolamine mesylate, up to 5 mg

Lay Description

Phentolamine mesylate is a chemical compound that produces a short-term block of the adrenal hormones epinephrine and norepinephrine. It is indicated for the diagnosis of pheochromocytoma, the prophylaxis and treatment of hypertensive episodes in patients with pheochromocytoma, and the prophylaxis and treatment of dermal necrosis following intravenous administration or extravasation of norepinephrine. Pheochromocytoma is a neoplasm, usually benign, of the adrenal medulla or sympathetic paraganglia that results in increased secretion of epinephrine and norepinephrine. The drug is administered by intramuscular or intravenous injection. Dosage ranges from 5 to 10 mg. HCPCS Level II code J2760 represents up to 5 mg of phentolamine mesylate.

J2765

J2765 Injection, metoclopramide HCl, up to 10 mg

Lay Description

Metoclopramide hydrochloride is a chemical compound that acts as a dopamine receptor antagonist. Dopamine produces nausea and vomiting by stimulating the chemoreceptor trigger zones. Metoclopramide hydrochloride blocks the stimulation of these zones. It stimulates upper gastrointestinal tract motility without stimulating the gastric, biliary, or pancreatic secretions. Metoclopramide hydrochloride is indicated for use as an antiemetic and in the treatment of gastroesophageal reflux and gastroparesis. HCPCS Level II code J2765 represents up to 10 mg of metoclopramide hydrochloride.

J2770

J2770 Injection, quinupristin/dalfopristin, 500 mg (150/350)

Lay Description

Quinupristin-dalfopristin is an antibiotic in the class known as streptogramins. The streptogramins are macromolecular antibiotics produced by Streptomyces pristinaepiralis. Quinupristin-dalfopristin is indicated for treatment of susceptible bacterial infections caused by antibiotic-resistant, gram-positive organisms, including severe infections caused by vancomycin-resistant E. faecium, nosocomial pneumonia, infections due to the use of intravenous catheters, and complicated skin and skin structure infections caused by methicillin-susceptible Staphylococcus aureus and Streptococcus pyogenes (group A streptococcus). The mechanism of action of quinupristin-dalfopristin is primarily inhibition of protein synthesis. Dalfopristin acts to block an early step in protein synthesis forming a bond with a ribosome and preventing elongation of the peptide chain. Quinupristin acts to block a later step preventing the extension of peptide chains and causing incomplete chains to be released. Quinupristin-dalfopristin is administered by intravenous injection or infusion. HCPCS Level II code J2770 represents 500 mg of quinupristin-dalfopristin (150/350).

J2778

J2778 Injection, ranibizumab, 0.1 mg

Lay Description

Ranibizumab is a monoclonal antibody produced by recombinant DNA technology using a strain of E.coli bacteria. The drug binds to receptor sites of human vascular endothelial growth factor A (VEGF-A) and inhibits its activity. VEGF-A has been shown to cause new vascularization and leakage of blood vessels in the eye and contributes to the progression of age-related macular degeneration. Ranibizumab is indicated as a treatment for neovascular or wet, age-related macular degeneration. The drug is administered by intravitreal injection only. Recommended doage is 0.5 mg once a month.

J2780

J2780 Injection, ranitidine HCl, 25 mg

Lay Description

Ranitidine hydrochloride is a chemical compound that binds to histamine receptors preventing the histamine from increasing gastric acid secretions. Ranitidine hydrochloride, singularly or in combination, is indicated as a treatment and as maintenance therapy for gastric ulcers, duodenal ulcers, gastroesophageal reflex disease, pathological gastric hypersecretory conditions, and erosive esophagitis. Oral forms of ranitidine hydrochloride are available in smaller dosages over-the-counter. Larger dosages are prescription only and available in oral and injectable forms. The injectable form is administered by intramuscular or intravenous injection. HCPCS Level II code J2780 represents 25 mg of injectable ranitidine hydrochloride.

J2783

J2783 Injection, rasburicase, 0.5 mg

Lay Description

Rasburicase is a synthetic enzyme produced by recombinant DNA technology in Saccharomyces cerevisiae yeast. It catalyzes the oxidation of uric acid into an inactive and soluble metabolite. Rasburicase is indicated for the initial management of plasma uric acid levels in pediatric patients with leukemia, lymphoma, and solid tumor malignancies who are receiving antineoplastic therapy expected to result in tumor lysis and subsequent elevation of plasma uric acid. The drug is administered by intravenous infusion over 30 minutes. Recommended dosage is 0.15 or 0.20 mg/kg of body weight daily for five days. HCPCS Level II code J2783 represents 0.5 mg of rasburicase.

J2785

J2785   Injection, regadenoson, 0.1 mg

Lay Description

Regadenoson is a vasodialator medication used as a cardiac stressing agent prior to myocardial perfusion imaging. This is an alternate to exercise stress when the patient is not a candidate for exercise stress. It is administered as a rapid IV push. The recommended dose is 0.4 mg of regadenoson. HCPCS level II code J2785 represents 0.1 mg of regadenoson.

J2788-J2792

J2788   Injection, Rho D immune globulin, human, minidose, 50 mcg (250 i.u.)
J2790   Injection, Rho D immune globulin, human, full dose, 300 mcg (1500 i.u.)
J2791   Injection, Rho(D) immune globulin (human), (Rhophylac), intramuscular or intravenous, 100 IU
J2792   Injection, Rho D immune globulin, intravenous, human, solvent detergent, 100 IU

Lay Description

Rh factors are a group of antigens present on the membrane of erythrocytes. When a person who is Rh-negative receives an Rh-positive transfusion or becomes pregnant with an Rh-positive fetus, the person develops antibodies against Rh-positive blood. These antibodies will in future exposures, attack and kill any Rh-positive erythrocytes. Rho (D) immune globulin suppresses the immune response of the Rh-negative person preventing antibody formation against the Rh-positive blood. Recommendations for administration during a pregnancy include a full dose of 300 mcg antepartum at 28 weeks and another full dose within 72 hours of delivery when there is known incompatibility between the mother and fetus. In cases of abortion, spontaneous or induced, of a fetus of less than 12 weeks, a mini-dose of 50 mcg is recommended. The mini-dose should be administered within three hours of the event. Dosages administered when an Rh incompatible blood transfusion occurs depend upon the volume of incompatible blood transfused and should be administered within 72 hours of the transfusion. Rho (D) immune globulin may be treated in several different ways to ensure that the pooled donor plasma has no pathogens. The immune globulin may be ultrafiltered, solvent washed, or detergent washed. It can be administered by intramuscular or intravenous injection. HCPCS Level II code J2788 represents 50 mcg of Rho (D) immune globulin; J2790 represents 300 mcg of Rho (D) immune globulin; and J2792 represents 100 IU of Rho (D) immune globulin intravenous that has been solvent or detergent washed.

J2793

J2793   Injection, rilonacept, 1 mg

Lay Description

Rilonacept is an interleukin 1 blocker used in the treatment and prevention of genetic conditions; cryopyrin associated periodic syndromes (CAPS), including Muckle Wells Syndrome (MWS); and familial cold auto inflammatory syndrome (FCAS) in adults and children age 12 or older. Although, used to treat and prevent these conditions, Rilonacept cannot cure these inherited conditions. Rilonacept is expressed in recombinant Chinese hamster ovary cells and comes in a sterile single use glass vial containing lyophilized powder for reconstitution. Recommended dose for adults is a loading dose of 320 mg administered by two separate subcutaneous injections. A maintenance dose of 160 mg is administered once a week by subcutaneous injection. Patients 12 to 17 years of age should receive a loading dose of 4.4 mg/kg with a maximum of 320 mg administered as one or two subcutaneous injections. Following that, the patient should receive 2.2 mg/kg with a maximum of 160 mg, once a week.

J2794

J2794   Injection, risperidone, long acting, 0.5 mg

Lay Description

Risperidone is an antipsychotic drug of the class of benzisoxazole derivatives. The drug's mechanism of action is unknown. It is thought that the drug acts by mediating dopamine and serotonin levels. Long-acting risperidone is encased within microspheres so that the drug is slowly released over a two-week period. Risperidone is indicated for the treatment of schizophrenia. Long-acting risperidone is injected via deep muscular gluteal injection every two weeks with a recommended initial dosage of 25 mg. This drug should not be administered intravenously. If patients do not respond to the 25 mg injections, 37.5 mg or 50 mg injections may be administered every two weeks. Different strengths should not be combined within a single administration. HCPCS Level II code J2794 represents an injection of 0.5 mg of injectable, long-acting risperidone only.

J2795

J2795 Injection, ropivacaine HCl, 1 mg

Lay Description

Ropivacaine hydrochloride is a chemical compound that is an amino amide local anesthetic agent. It locally blocks the generation and conduction of nerve transmissions. Ropivacaine hydrochloride is used as a peripheral nerve block, for percutaneous infiltration anesthesia, and as an epidural block. It may also be administered by continuous epidural infusion for acute postoperative pain management. Dosage varies by indication and extent of the anesthesia required. HCPCS Level II code J2795 represents 1 mg of ropivacaine hydrochloride.

J2796

J2796 Injection, romiplostim, 10 mcg

Lay Description

Romiplostim increases platelet production and is used to treat patients with idiopathic thrombocytopenic purpura (ITP) for whom other treatments have not been successful. It should be used for patients who have bleeding problems and not only for normalizing a patient's platelet count. Romiplostim is derived using DNA segments in *Escherichia coli* (*E. coli*). Recommended dose is 1 mcg/kg based on the patient's weight. The dose is adjusted depending on the patient's platelet count. Romiplostim is administered by subcutaneous injection. HCPCS Level II code J2796 is reported for a 10 mcg dose.

J2800

J2800 Injection, methocarbamol, up to 10 ml

Lay Description

Methocarbamol is a skeletal muscle relaxant, indicated for the treatment of muscle spasms and muscle pain and stiffness. Methocarbamol acts on the central nervous system to produce its muscle relaxant effects. HCPCS Level II code J2800 represents up to 10 ml of methocarbamol.

J2805

J2805 Injection, sincalide, 5 mcg

Lay Description

Sincalide is a gastrointestinal hormone peptide injected intravenously. It is used to stimulate gallbladder contractions for assessment via a cholecystogram or ultrasound; to stimulate pancreatic secretin prior to the obtaining of a duodenal aspirate; or to accelerate the transit of barium through the small bowel for fluoroscopic or x-ray examination of the intestinal tract. HCPCS Level II code J2805 represents 5 mcg of sincalide.

J2810

J2810 Injection, theophylline, per 40 mg

Lay Description

Theophylline is a methylxanthine drug with structural and pharmacological similarity to caffeine. It is naturally found in black and green tea. Theophylline's exact mechanism of action is unknown. It is suggested that it is a nonspecific inhibitor of phosphodiesterase enzymes, which are enzymes that control the tissue concentration of various hormones and other enzymes. Inhibiting the phosphodiesterase enzymes would allow for increases in intracellular cyclic AMP. Cyclic AMP is a nucleotide involved in the activities of many hormones and cellular functions. Theophylline relaxes the smooth bronchial muscles and allows for easier breathing. It also increases the force of contraction of the diaphragmatic muscles. It is indicated for the prophylaxis and treatment of chronic asthma and COPD. Theophylline is also indicated as an emergency treatment in an acute severe asthma episode .Theophylline carries a high incidence of side effects when used at its upper therapeutic range. The drug is also affected by many other drugs including antibiotics, cimtedine, and phytoin among others. HCPCS Level II code J2810 represents 40 mg of injectable theophylline.

J2820

J2820 Injection, sargramostim (GM-CSF), 50 mcg

Lay Description

Sargramostim is a synthetic granulocyte-macrophage colony-stimulating factor (GM-CSF) produced by recombinant DNA technology in S. cerevisiae yeast. GM-CSF binds to receptor sites on stem cells and supports the survival, expansion, and differentiation of hematopoietic progenitor cells into granulocytes and macrophages. Sargramostim is indicated to stimulate hematopoiesis and decrease neutropenia as an adjunct to myelosuppressive cancer chemotherapy in patients with acute myelogenous leukemia and non-Hodgkin's lymphoma, to promote myeloid engraftment in bone marrow transplantation or hematopoietic stem cell transplantation, and to enhance peripheral progenitor cell yield in autologous hematopoietic stem cell transplantation. The drug is administered by intravenous infusion. Dosage varies from 250 mcg per m^2 of body surface per day. HCPCS Level II code J2820 represents 50 mcg of sargramostim.

J2850

J2850 Injection, secretin, synthetic, human, 1 mcg

Lay Description

Secretin is a synthetic version of the natural hormone secretin secreted by the mucosa of the duodenum and upper jejunum. Secretin stimulates the release of pancreatic juice by the pancreas and bile by the liver. Both bile and the pancreatic juices contain bicarbonate and change the pH of the duodenum from acid to alkaline which facilitates the action of intestinal digestive enzymes. Secretin is used in diagnostic tests for gastrinoma and pancreatic exocrine function, and to facilitate the identification of the ampulla of Vater and accessory papilla during endoscopic retrograde cholangiopancreatography (ERCP). Dosage is 0.2-0.4 mcg per kg of body weight depending on the indication. The drug is administered by intravenous injection. HCPCS Level II code J2850 represents 1 mcg of secretin.

J2910

J2910 Injection, aurothioglucose, up to 50 mg

Lay Description

Aurothioglucose is a gold salt used in treating inflammatory arthritis. The mechanism of action in gold salts is not well understood. However, in patients with inflammatory arthritis, such as adult and juvenile rheumatoid arthritis, gold salts decrease the inflammation of the joint lining, preventing destruction of bone and cartilage. Gold salts, such as aurothioglucose, are second-line drugs prescribed when anti-inflammatory drugs, such as nonsteroidal anti-inflammatory drugs (NSAID) and corticosteroids, are ineffective in preventing the progression of inflammatory arthritis. Aurothioglucose is available as a 50 mg/ml injectable suspension to be administered by intramuscular injection. HCPCS Level II code J2910 represents up to 50 mg of aurothioglucose.

J2916

J2916 Injection, sodium ferric gluconate complex in sucrose injection, 12.5 mg

Lay Description

Sodium ferric gluconate is an iron oxide hydrate directly bound to sucrose and chelated with gluconate. The drug replenishes iron, which is critical for normal hemoglubulin synthesis to maintain oxygen transport. Iron is also required for the metabolism and synthesis of DNA and various enzymes. Sodium ferric gluconate is indicated for the treatment of iron deficiency in ESRD patients undergoing hemodialysis who are also receiving erythropoietin therapy. It is administered by intravenous infusion over one hour. The recommended dosage is 125 mg. HCPCS Level II code J2916 represents 12.5 mg of sodium ferric gluconate.

J2920-J2930

J2920 Injection, methylprednisolone sodium succinate, up to 40 mg

J2930 Injection, methylprednisolone sodium succinate, up to 125 mg

Lay Description

Methylprednisolone is a corticosteroid used to treat a variety of conditions. Indications include allergic disorders, arthritis, blood diseases, breathing problems, certain cancers, eye diseases, intestinal disorders, and collagen and skin diseases. Methylprednisolone may also be used with other medications as a replacement for certain hormones. Methylprednisolone works by decreasing the body's immune response to these diseases and reducing symptoms such as swelling and redness. Methylprednisolone may be administered orally, by intramuscular injection in the form of methylprednisolone acetate, or by intravenous infusion in the form of methylprednisolone sodium succinate. HCPCS Level II codes J2920 and J2930 represent up to 40 mg and up to 125 mg of methylprednisolone sodium succinate injections respectively

Documentation Standards

A prescription (order) for the drug that has been signed and dated by the ordering physician must be kept on file by the supplier. A new prescription is required if there is a change in dose or frequency of administration.

Claims for the first month's supply of drugs must include a copy of the CMN form if filed hard copy.

If another immunosuppressive drug is added after the original CMN has been submitted, or if the code for a drug is changed (e.g., from a miscellaneous code to a specific J-code), another "initial" CMN form is required and must be submitted to the DME MAC. However, if there is a change in the dose or frequency of administration of an already approved drug, a revised CMN is not required, but the supplier must keep the new prescription on file. Providers must document this information in the patient's medical record.

Medicare Information

The national drug code (NDC) number identifies the manufacturer's product in terms of strength, quantity, and other details. Any entity billing drugs to a DME MAC must use the NDC number effective April 1, 2003.

Coverage of parenteral methylprednisolone (J2920, J2930) is limited to those situations in which the medication cannot be tolerated or absorbed if taken orally and if it is self-administered by the patient. There is no coverage under the immunosuppressive drug benefit for supplies used in conjunction with the administration of parenteral immunosuppressive drugs.

Note: See chapter titled "Medicare Guidelines," under "Drugs, Biologicals, and Radiopharmaceuticals," for additional Medicare billing and documentation information.

J2940

J2940   Injection, somatrem, 1 mg

Lay Description

Somatrem is a version of human growth hormone (HGH) produced by recombinant DNA technology from a strain of E. coli bacteria. It contains the identical sequence of the 191 amino acids that compromise endogenous HGH. HGH has a direct effect on the metabolism of protein, carbohydrates, and fat and controls skeletal and visceral growth. Somatrem is indicated for the treatment of idiopathic HGH deficiency in children with growth failure. Treatment with somatrem should be discontinued when the epiphyses are fused. The drug is administered subcutaneously or intramuscularly at a dosage of 0.30 mg per body weight and may be self-administered. HCPCS Level II code J2940 represents 1 mg of somatrem.

J2941

J2941   Injection, somatropin, 1 mg

Lay Description

Somatropin is another name for human growth hormone (HGH). Most versions are produced by recombinant DNA technology from a strain of E. coli bacteria. It contains the identical sequence of the 191 amino acids that compromise endogenous HGH. HGH has a direct effect on the metabolism of protein, carbohydrates, and fat and controls skeletal and visceral growth. Somatropin is indicated for the treatment of growth failure in children born small for their gestational age, children with growth failure due to HGH deficiency, chronic renal insufficiency, Turner's syndrome, or Prader-Willi syndrome. Another indication is the treatment of adult patients with HGH deficiency, either primary or secondary to pituitary or hypothalamic diseases, radiation therapy, surgery, or trauma. The drug is administered subcutaneously or intramuscularly at a dosage of 0.30 mg per body weight and may be self-administered. HCPCS Level II code J2941 represents 1 mg of somatropin.

J2950

J2950   Injection, promazine HCl, up to 25 mg

Lay Description

Promazine hydrochloride belongs to a group of medications known as the phenothiazine antipsychotics. Promazine hydrochloride is indicated for the treatment of agitation alone and agitation and restlessness in the elderly. The mechanism of action involves blocking a variety of receptors in the brain, particularly dopamine receptors. Dopamine is a chemical that aids in transmission of signals between brain cells. An excess of dopamine in the brain can cause over-stimulation of dopamine receptors. Because dopamine receptors normally act to modify behavior, over-stimulation can result in psychotic illness. Promazine hydrochloride prevents over-stimulation by blocking these receptors, which then helps to control psychotic illness. HCPCS Level II code J2950 represents up to 25 mg of promazine hydrochloride.

J2993

J2993   Injection, reteplase, 18.1 mg

Lay Description

Reteplase is a longer-acting derivative of alteplase, a synthetic tissue plasminogen activator. Reteplase is produced by recombinant DNA technology in E. coli bacteria. Tissue plasminogen activators are enzymes produced by endothelial cells that catalyze the breakdown of thrombi or blood clots. The drug is indicated as a treatment of acute myocardial infarction. Treatment should begin as soon as possible after the onset of symptoms. The drug is administered by two intravenous bolus injections. Each bolus should be 18.1 mg. HCPCS Level II code J2993 represents 18.1 mg of reteplase.

J2995

J2995   Injection, streptokinase, per 250,000 IU

Lay Description

Streptokinase is a protein produced by beta hemolytic streptococci bacteria that binds to plasminogen and breaks down thrombi or blood clots. Streptokinase is indicated as a treatment of acute myocardial infarction, acute pulmonary embolism, deep venous thrombosis, acute arterial thrombi or emboli, and occlusion of an arteriovenous shunt. Treatment of the acute myocardial infarction should begin within four hours of the onset of symptoms. Treatment of acute pulmonary embolism, deep venous thrombosis, and acute arterial thrombi or emboli should begin as soon as possible from onset of the event, preferably within seven days. The drug is administered by intravenous infusion. Recommended dosage varies from 1,000,000 to 1,500,000 units depending upon the indication. HCPCS Level II code J2995 represents 250,000 IUs of streptokinase.

J2997

J2997 Injection, alteplase recombinant, 1 mg

Lay Description
Alteplase is a synthetic tissue plasminogen activator produced by recombinant DNA technology in Chinese hamster ovaries. Tissue plasminogen activators are enzymes produced by endothelial cells that catalyze the breakdown of thrombi or blood clots. Alteplase is indicated as a treatment of acute myocardial infarction, acute ischemic stroke, acute massive pulmonary embolism, or to restore the function of a thrombosed central venous access device. Treatment of the acute myocardial infarction should begin as soon as possible after the onset of symptoms. Treatment of acute ischemic stroke should begin within three hours of the onset of symptoms and after it has been determined that no intracranial hemorrhage has occurred. Treatment of acute massive pulmonary embolism should begin after objective confirmation of the diagnosis has been obtained. The drug is administered by intravenous injection and infusion. Recommended total dosage is based upon body weight, but should not exceed 100 mg. HCPCS Level II code J2997 represents up to 1 mg of alteplase.

J3000

J3000 Injection, streptomycin, up to 1 g

Lay Description
Streptomycin was the first of the aminoglycoside antibiotics. Aminoglycoside antibiotics are those derived from various species of Streptomyces bacteria or produced synthetically. Aminoglycosides inhibit bacterial protein synthesis by binding with the 30S ribosomal subunit and are bactericidal. Streptomycin is derived from Streptomyces griseus. It inhibits protein synthesis causing cell death. Streptomycin is now in limited use due to the emergence of resistant bacterial strains. Susceptibility studies should be performed prior to the administration of streptomycin. It is indicated in the treatment of tuberculosis in combination with other drugs. Streptomycin is indicated in the treatment infections caused by gram-negative bacillary bacteria, Pasteurella pestis, Francisella tularensis, Brucella, Calymmatobacterium granulomatis, H. ducreyi, H. influenzae, K. pneumoniae, E. coli, Proteus, A. aerogenes, K. pneumoniae, Enterococcus faecalis, Streptococcus viridans, and Enterococcus faecalis. Streptomycin is available only in an injectable form. It is administered by intramuscular injection to the buttocks or thigh. Dosages vary from 15 to 40 mg/kg of body weight depending on the frequency of administration, patient age, and indication. HCPCS Level II code J3000 represents up to 1 g of streptomycin.

J3010

J3010 Injection, fentanyl citrate, 0.1 mg

Lay Description
Fentanyl is a schedule II, controlled substance pain medication in the narcotic and opioid analgesic class. Fentanyl is used as an adjunct to anesthesia, to manage chronic pain, and breakthrough persistent pain in cancer patients who have an increased physical tolerance to current opioid therapy. Fentanyl interacts primarily with the opioid mu-receptor. These mu-binding sites are distributed throughout the human brain, spinal cord, and other tissues. In clinical settings, fentanyl exerts its principal pharmacologic effects on the central nervous system. It is administered via intravenous push injection, intramuscular injection, transdermal patch, or transmucosal lozenges. HCPCS Level II code J3010 represents 0.1 mg of fentanyl citrate.

Medicare Information
See chapter titled "Medicare Guidelines," under "Infusion Pumps, External; Equipment and Supplies," for Medicare billing and documentation information.

J3030

J3030 Injection, sumatriptan succinate, 6 mg (code may be used for Medicare when drug administered under the direct supervision of a physician, not for use when drug is self-administered)

Lay Description
Sumatriptan succinate is given to treat migraines and acute treatment of cluster headaches. It is thought to act by stimulating the specific serotonin receptors of the cranial arteries and the dura mater to cause vasoconstriction of the cerebral arteries, without affecting systemic vessels or blood pressure. Recommended injection dose is 6 mg. It can be administered by subcutaneous injection, through tablets, or nasal inhalation. The injection can be self-administered. HCPCS Level II code J3030 represents 6 mg of sumatriptan succinate injection.

J3070

J3070 Injection, pentazocine, 30 mg

Lay Description
Pentazocine is an opioid analgesic used for moderate to severe pain and during labor. It is thought that pentazocine HCl binds with opiate receptors in the central nervous system (CNS), which then alters both the emotional response to and perception of

pain. HCPCS Level II code J3070 represents 30 mg of pentazocine injection.

J3095

J3095 Injection, telavancin, 10 mg

Lay Description

Telavancin is a lipoglycopeptide antibacterial that is a synthetic derivative of vancomycin. It is indicated for the treatment of adults with complicated skin and skin structure infections caused by susceptible gram-positive bacteria, including *Staphylococcus aureus, Streptococcus pyogenes, Streptococcus agalactiae,* the *Streptococcus anginosus* group, or vancomycin susceptible *Enterococcus faecalis*. Telavancin is supplied in single use vials that contain 250 mg or 750 mg of a sterile and lyophilized powder. It should be administered as an infusion over 60 minutes.

J3101

J3101 Injection, tenecteplase, 1 mg

Lay Description

Tenecteplase is a thrombolytic enzyme used in treating the effects of a myocardial infarction. It is a tissue plasminogen activator (TPA) produced by recombinant DNA technology using Chinese hamster ovary cells. It binds with fibrin and converts plasminogen to plasmin. Tenecteplase is used to treat acute myocardial infarction and should be administered as soon as possible after the onset of symptoms. This medication is administered intravenously. HCPCS Level II code J3101 represents 1 mg of tenecteplase.

J3105

J3105 Injection, terbutaline sulfate, up to 1 mg

Lay Description

Terbutaline sulfate is a bronchodilator that relaxes both bronchial and uterine smooth muscle by stimulating beta2 receptors and is used primarily to treat bronchospasm in patients with reversible obstructive airway disease. It is available as tablets, aerosol inhaler, or subcutaneous injection. Side effects may include nervousness, palpitations, tachycardia, and/or diaphoresis. This code reports an injection of up to 1 mg.

J3110

J3110 Injection, teriparatide, 10 mcg

Lay Description

Teriparatide is a recombinant human parathyroid hormone (1-34) that has an identical structure to the naturally occurring hormone. Teriparatide is manufactured from a strain of Escherichia coli, and modified by recombinant DNA technology. Teriparatide is indicated for the treatment of postmenopausal women with osteoporosis who are at high risk for fracture. This includes women with a history of osteoporotic fracture, who have multiple risk factors for fracture, or who have failed or are intolerant of previous osteoporosis therapy. Teriparatide is also indicated to increase bone mass in men with primary or hypogonadal osteoporosis who are at high risk for fracture. This includes men with a history of osteoporotic fracture, who have multiple risk factors for fracture, or who have failed or are intolerant to previous osteoporosis therapy. Recommended dose is 20 mcg of teriparatide each day for up to 28 days. Teriparatide should be administered as a subcutaneous injection into the thigh or abdominal wall and can be self-administered. HCPCS Level II code J3110 represents 10 mcg of teriparatide.

Medicare Information

Medicare does not cover self-administrable drugs.

J3120-J3130

J3120 Injection, testosterone enanthate, up to 100 mg
J3130 Injection, testosterone enanthate, up to 200 mg

Lay Description

Testosterone enanthate is a hormonal drug in the androgens grouping for injection. Testosterone is used in treating male hypogonadism and delayed puberty, as it stimulates the targeted gonadal tissue to develop normally. It is also used in treating some estrogen-dependent breast cancers as it has some counter-estrogenic action in women. Testosterone enanthate is absorbed more slowly so it can be given less often than free testosterone. Doses vary from 50 to 400 mg every two to four weeks. Testosterone enanthate is administered by intramuscular injection. HCPCS Level II code J3120 represents up to 100 mg of testosterone enanthate and J3130 represents up to 200 mg of testosterone enanthate.

J3140

J3140 Injection, testosterone suspension, up to 50 mg

Lay Description

Testosterone is an anabolic steroid used primarily to treat male hypogonadism. It stimulates targeted tissues to develop normally in androgen-deficient men. Testosterone may also have some anti-estrogen properties, making it useful in treating certain estrogen-dependent breast cancers. This drug is used to treat male hypogonadism, unusually late sexual maturity, myotonia congenita, inflammation and rotation of the testes, undescended testicle, absence of testicles, Klinefelter syndrome, anemia, and in the prevention of breast pain and engorgement in postpartum women. HCPCS Level II code J3140 represents up to 50 mg of testosterone suspension.

J3150

J3150 Injection, testosterone propionate, up to 100 mg

Lay Description

Testosterone propionate is a hormonal drug in the androgens grouping for injection. Testosterone is used in treating male hypogonadism and delayed puberty, as it stimulates the targeted gonadal tissue to develop normally. Testosterone propionate is absorbed more slowly so it can be given less often than free testosterone. Testosterone propionate is administered via intramuscular injection. HCPCS Level II code J3150 represents a dose up to 100 mg of testosterone propionate.

J3230

J3230 Injection, chlorpromazine HCl, up to 50 mg

Lay Description

Chlorpromazine hydrochloride (HCl) is used in the treatment of manic psychosis, preoperative sedation, acute intermittent porphyria, an adjunct treatment for tetanus, intractable hiccups, some behavior problems in children, and nausea and vomiting. The main pharmacological actions are psychotropic. The mechanism of action is not known. It has a sedative and antiemetic effect. HCPCS Level II code J3230 represents up to 50 mg of injectable chlorpromazine hydrochloride.

J3240

J3240 Injection, thyrotropin alpha, 0.9 mg, provided in 1.1 mg vial

Lay Description

Thyrotropin alpha is indicated for use as an adjunctive diagnostic tool for serum thyroglobulin (Tg) testing in the follow-up of patients with well-differentiated thyroid cancer. This may be done with or without radioiodine imaging. It contains a highly purified recombinant form of human thyroid stimulating hormone (TSH), a glycoprotein that is produced by recombinant DNA technology in Chinese hamster ovaries. A dose of 0.9 mg can be administered every day for three days. Thyrotropin alpha is administered via intramuscular injection. HCPCS Level II code J3240 represents a dose of 0.9 mg in 1.1 mg vial of thyrotropin alpha.

J3243

J3243 Injection, tigecycline, 1 mg

Lay Description

Tigecycline is an antibiotic of the class glycylcycline. The drug disrupts RNA protein synthesis in bacteria causing cellular death. Tigecycline has proven effective in drug-resistant strains of many anaerobic and aerobic, gram-negative, and positive microorganisms. It is indicated in the treatment of complicated skin and skin-structure infections, and complicated intra-abdominal infections caused by susceptible strains of bacteria in patients 18 years of age or older. Susceptible bacteria include Escherichia coli; Staphylococcus aureus, including methicillin-resistant strains (MRSA); Streptococcus pyogenes; Streptococcus agalactiae; the Streptococcus anginosis group; vancomycin-susceptible strains of Enterococcus faecalis; Bacteroides fragilis; Citrobacter freundii; Enterobacter cloacae; Klebsiella oxytoca; Klebsiella pneumoniae; Bacteroides thetaiotaomicron; Bacteroides uniformis; Bacteroides vulgatus; Clostridium perfringens; and Peptostreptococcus micros. Tigecycline should be administered via an intravenous infusion over 30 to 60 minutes every 12 hours. HCPCS Level II code J3248 represents 1 mg of tigecycline.

J3246

J3246 Injection, tirofiban HCl, 0.25 mg

Lay Description

Tirofiban hydrochloride is an antiplatelet drug used to treat or prevent blood clots. It is used to treat certain types of angina, such as acute coronary syndrome, and may also be used prophylactically prior to angiography and angioplasty procedures. Tirofiban hydrochloride is a reversible antagonist of fibrinogen binding to the GP IIb/IIIa receptor, the major platelet surface receptor involved in platelet aggregation, thereby inhibiting ex vivo platelet aggregation. Tirofiban hydrochloride is administered by intravenous infusion at a recommended infusion rate of 0.4 mcg/kg/min initially for 30 minutes and then continuing at 0.1 mcg/kg/min for the duration of the infusion. HCPCS Level II code J3246 represents 0.25 mg of tirofiban hydrochloride.

J3250

J3250 Injection, trimethobenzamide HCl, up to 200 mg

Lay Description

Trimethobenzamide hydrochloride (HCl) is an antiemetic used to alleviate nausea and vomiting. The mechanism of action is not known but it appears to act on the chemoreceptor trigger zone (CTZ) in the brain where vomiting impulses are transmitted.

It can be administered via intramuscular injection. Trimethobenzamide HCl also comes in capsule and suppository forms. HCPCS Level II code J3250 represents a dose of up to 200 mg of trimethobenzamide HCl injection.

J3260

J3260   Injection, tobramycin sulfate, up to 80 mg

Lay Description

Tobramycin is an aminoglycoside antibiotic. Aminoglycoside antibiotics are those derived from various species of Streptomyces bacteria or produced synthetically. Aminoglycosides inhibit bacterial protein synthesis by binding with the 30S ribosomal subunit and are bactericidal. Streptomycin is derived from *Streptomyces tenebrarius*. It inhibits protein synthesis causing cell death. Susceptibility studies should be performed prior to the administration of tobramycin. It is indicated in the treatment of infections caused by gram-negative bacillary bacteria including *Pseudomonas aeruginosa, Staphylococcus aureus, Escherichia coli, Klebsiella* species, *Enterobacter* species, *Serretia* species, *Proteus* species, *Providencia* species, and *Citrobacter* species. The injectable form is administered by intramuscular injection and intravenous infusion. Dosages vary depending on the form of administration, frequency of administration, and indication.

J3262

J3262   Injection, tocilizumab, 1 mg

Lay Description

Tocilizumab is a chemical compound that is an interleukin-6 receptor inhibitor. Interleukin-6 is a protein secreted by a variety of cells to stimulate immune response to trauma or other tissue damage leading to inflammation. Tocilizumab is indicated for adult patients with moderate to severe active rheumatoid arthritis who have had an inadequate response to one or more tumor necrosis factor inhibitors. This medication may be used as monotherapy or with methotrexate or other disease modifying antirheumatic drugs. The recommended dose is 4 mg to 8 mg per kg of patient weight. The drug is administered as a 60 minute IV infusion.

J3265

J3265   Injection, torsemide, 10 mg/ml

Lay Description

Torsemide is a diuretic that is used to treat patients with heart or liver failure, hypertension, or for those with hepatic cirrhosis. Torsemide acts on the loop of Henle by enhancing excretion of sodium, water, and chloride. HCPCS Level II code J3265 represents 10 mg/ml of torsemide.

J3280

J3280   Injection, thiethylperazine maleate, up to 10 mg

Lay Description

Thiethylperazine maleate is indicated for the relief of nausea and vomiting. The exact mechanism of action is not known. However, it appears to have an effect on the vomiting center and the chemoreceptor trigger zone (CTZ) of the brain. Recommended oral dose is 10 to 30 mg a day. Thiethylperazine maleate can be administered orally or by intramuscular injection. Recommended intramuscular injection dose is 10 mg one to three times a day. HCPCS Level II code J3280 represents a dose of up to 10 mg of thiethylperazine maleate injection.

J3285

J3285   Injection, treprostinil, 1 mg

Lay Description

Treprostinil is a prostacyclin, an analogue of prostaglandin, that is a vasodilator. The drug directly dilates pulmonary and systemic arterial beds and inhibits platelet aggregation. Treprostinil is indicated for the treatment of pulmonary arterial hypertension patients who have New York Heart Association Class II-IV symptoms. The drug may be administered via a continuous subcutaneous infusion. If the patient cannot tolerate subcutaneous infusion, the drug may be administered via continuous intravenous infusion by a central venous line. Treprostinil may be self-administered using an infusion pump. Dosage is dependent upon the patient's body weight and the relief of symptoms. HCPCS Level II code J3285 represents 1 mg of treprostinil.

J3300-J3303

J3300   Injection, triamcinolone acetonide, preservative free, 1 mg
J3301   Injection, triamcinolone acetonide, not otherwise specified, 10 mg
J3302   Injection, triamcinolone diacetate, per 5 mg
J3303   Injection, triamcinolone hexacetonide, per 5 mg

Lay Description

Triamcinolone is a synthetic corticosteroid, which is analogous to corticosteroids produced by the adrenal cortex. The drug is one to two times more potent than prednisone. Its mechanism of action is not clearly defined. Triamcinolone does decrease inflammation by stabilizing leukocytes, suppress the chemicals normally released in immune response, and stimulate bone marrow. Triamcinolone acetonide is a more potent derivative of triamcinolone, approximately eight times more potent than prednisone. Triamcinolone acetonide is the version most commonly used in preparations. Diacetate and hexacetonide are different formulations of triamcinolone with hexacetonide having the longest acting effect. The drug has a number of uses, including hormone replacement when the adrenal gland does not produce adequate supplies. The injectable version may be administered intramuscularly, intra-articularly, intravitreally, or intralesionally. The injectable version is indicated for the treatment of a large number of symptoms and diseases, which are far too numerous to list. HCPCS Level II code J3300 represents 1 mg of preservative free injectable triamcinolone acetonide; J3301 represents 10 mg of injectable triamcinolone acetonide; J3302 represents 5 mg of injectable triamcinolone diacetate; and J3303 represents 5 mg of injectable triamcinolone hexacetonide.

J3305

J3305   Injection, trimetrexate glucuronate, per 25 mg

Lay Description

Trimetrexate glucuronate is a nonclassical folate antagonist. It is a synthetic inhibitor of the enzyme dihydrofolate reductase (DHFR) and is used as an alternative therapy for the treatment of moderate-to-severe Pneumocystis carinii pneumonia (PCP) in immunocompromised patients. It interferes with the RNA, DNA, and protein synthesis, which results in cell death. Leucovorin calcium should be given with this medication to protect the patient from life-threatening toxicities. Trimetrexate glucoronate is administered by intravenous infusion over 60 minutes. HCPCS Level II code J3265 represents 25 mg of trimetrexate glucoronate.

J3310

J3310   Injection, perphenazine, up to 5 mg

Lay Description

Perphenazine is used in treating psychosis and severe nausea and vomiting. The mechanism of action is not known. However, it does have an effect on the entire central nervous system particularly the hypothalamus. Dose is based on the condition and response of the patient. Perphenazine is administered orally. Per the FDA, the injectable form is no longer available in the United States.

J3315

J3315   Injection, triptorelin pamoate, 3.75 mg

Lay Description

Triptorelin pamoate is a synthetic decapeptide agonist analog of luteinizing hormone releasing hormone (LHRH or GnRH) with greater potency than the naturally occurring LHRH. It is used in the palliative treatment of advanced prostate cancer. This medication prevents gonadotropin secretion when given continuously in therapeutic doses. After the first dose there is an increase in the luteinizing hormone (LH), follicle-stimulating hormone (FSH), testosterone, and estradiol levels. Following continuous administration, there is a persistent decrease in LH and FSH secretion. There is also a significant decrease of testicular and ovarian steroidogenesis. The reduction of serum testosterone is that usually found in surgically castrated men. Recommended dose is 3.75 mg monthly. Triptorelin pamoate is administered by intramuscular injection. HCPCS Level II code J3315 represents 3.75 mg of triptorelin pamoate.

J3320

J3320   Injection, spectinomycin dihydrochloride, up to 2 g

Lay Description

Spectinomycin dihydrochloride is an aminocyclitol antibiotic produced by the Streptomyces spectabilis species of soil microorganism. Spectinomycin dihydrochloride is indicated for treatment of susceptible, drug-resistant strains of acute N. gonorrhea. Spectinomycin dihydrochloride works by inhibiting protein synthesis in the bacterial cell. Spectinomycin dihydrochloride is administered by intramuscular injection. HCPCS Level II code J3320 represents up to 2 g of spectinomycin dihydrochloride.

J3350

J3350   Injection, urea, up to 40 g

Lay Description

Urea is an organic compound of carbon, nitrogen, oxygen, and hydrogen. It is the chief nitrogenous end-product from the metabolism of proteins. Intravenous infusions of urea are used as a diuretic and to lower intracranial pressure. Intravenous urea is indicated as a treatment for fluid accumulation in the brain, high intraocular pressure, or glaucoma. HCPCS Level II code J3350 represents up to 40 g of urea.

J3355

J3355 Injection, urofollitropin, 75 IU

Lay Description
Urofollitropin is a highly purified, follicle-stimulating hormone extracted from the urine of post-menopausal women. Follicle stimulating hormone is a gonadotropic hormone produced in the anterior pituitary gland. It stimulates the growth and maturation of follicles in the ovary. Urofollitropin is used to induce ovulation in polycystic ovary disease. It is administered by subcutaneous or intramuscular injection. HCPCS Level II code J3355 represents 75 IU of urofollitropin.

Medicare Information
See chapter titled "Medicare Guidelines," under "Drugs, Biologicals, and Radiopharmaceuticals," for Medicare billing and documentation information.

J3357

J3357 Injection, ustekinumab, 1 mg

Lay Description
Ustekinumab is a human monoclonal antibody used to treat patients diagnosed with moderate to severe plaque psoriasis. The recommended dose is based on the patient's body weight. After initial administration, the second dose is given four weeks later and then every 12 weeks thereafter. Ustekinumab is administered by subcutaneous administration.

J3360

J3360 Injection, diazepam, up to 5 mg

Lay Description
Diazepam is an antianxiety drug that acts on the central nervous system (CNS). This benzodiazepine produces anxiolytic effects by aiding the action of a specific inhibitory neurotransmitter in the brain, depressing the CNS in the limbic and subcortical areas, as well as seizure activity focused in the cortex and thalamus. Diazepam is used for anxiety, acute alcohol withdrawal, muscle spasm, and before endoscopic procedures. Dosages range from 2 to 20 mg based on patient condition. Diazepam can be administered via intramuscular injection or intravenous push. HCPCS Level II code J3360 represents up to 5 mg of diazepam.

J3364-J3365

J3364 Injection, urokinase, 5,000 IU vial
J3365 Injection, IV, urokinase, 250,000 IU vial

Lay Description
Urokinase is urokinase-type plasminogen activator (uPA) and is a serine protease. It is a thrombolytic agent obtained from human neonatal kidney cells grown in tissue culture. Urokinase is a thrombolytic enzyme used for treatment of acute pulmonary embolism, acute coronary arterial thrombosis, and to clear thrombi from intravenous catheters. Urokinase binds to fibrin, converts plasminogen into plasmin, and breaks down the thrombus into smaller components. Urokinase is administered via intravenous infusion. HCPCS Level II code J3364 represents a 5,000 IU vial of urokinase and J3365 represents a 250,000 IU vial of urokinase.

J3370

J3370 Injection, vancomycin HCl, 500 mg

Lay Description
Vancomycin is used to treat serious infections including septicemia, bone infections, endocarditis, lower respiratory tract infections, and skin and skin structure infections. It is effective against Diphtheroids, Enterococci (e.g., Enterococcus faecalis), Staphylococci including Staphylococcus aureus and Staphylococcus epidermidis (including heterogeneous methicillin-resistant strains), Streptococcus bovis, Viridans group streptococci, Listeria monocytogenes, Streptococcus pyogenes, Streptococcus pneumoniae (including penicillin-resistant strains), Streptococcus agalactiae, Actinomyces species, and Lactobacillus species. Oral vancomycin HCl is used in treating antibiotic-associated pseudomembranous colitis caused by C. difficile and staphylococcal enterocolitis. Vancomycin HCl is not effective by the oral route for other types of infections. Vancomycin interferes with RNA synthesis and damages the bacterial cell's plasma membrane, making it susceptible to the forces of osmotic pressure. HCPCS Level II code J3370 represents up to 500 mg of vancomycin HCl.

J3385

J3385 Injection, velaglucerase alfa, 100 units

Lay Description
Velaglucerase alfa is a hydrolytic lysosomal glucocerebroside specific enzyme used in the treatment of long-term enzyme replacement therapy (ERT) for adults or pediatric patients who are diagnosed with Type 1 Gaucher disease. Gaucher disease occurs in patients who do not produce an adequate amount of an enzyme called glucocerebrosidase, which can result in harmful

amounts of lipid buildup in the spleen, bones, liver, nervous system, and bone marrow and may also prevent organs and cells from functioning properly. Velaglucerase alfa is used as a replacement for another enzyme replacement therapy, imiglucerase. Velaglucerase alfa comes in the form of a lyophilized powder to be reconstituted with diluted water and is administered by intravenous infusion.

J3396

J3396 Injection, verteporfin, 0.1 mg

Lay Description

Verteporfin is a benzoporphyrin derivative that is a photosensitizer or light-activated drug. Verteporfin is used together with a nonthermal red laser light to treat abnormal blood vessel formation in a part of the eye that, if left untreated, can lead to a loss of eyesight. Treatment with verteporfin and laser light occurs in two steps. First, the verteporfin is injected into the body. Second, 15 minutes later, a laser light is directed at the affected eye. Photodynamic therapy with verteporfin is approved to treat age-related macular degeneration (AMD) with neovascular changes, known as choroidal neovascularization (CNV). CNV can be described as classic or occult, based on appearance on fluorescein angiography. CNV can also be described by its location: extrafoveal, juxtafoveal, and subfoveal. Verteporfin is indicated for patients with predominately classic subfoveal CNV due to AMD, pathologic myopia, or presumed ocular histoplasmosis. Laser light treatment must follow verteporfin injection 15 minutes after the start of the injection. Once activated, the drug probably creates free radical formation, which causes cellular damage and eventually results in thrombosis of the vessels and slowing of the progression of CNV. The drug is injected intravenously into the patient"s arm. HCPCS Level II code J3396 represents 0.1 mg of verteporfin.

Medicare Information

Verteporfin is only covered when used in conjunction with ocular photodynamic therapy (OPT) when furnished intravenously. OPT with verteporfin is covered for patients with a diagnosis of neovascular age-related macular degeneration (AMD) with:

- Predominately classic subfoveal choroidal neovascularization (CNV) lesions (where the area of classic CNV occupies 50 percent of the area of the entire lesion) at the initial visit as determined by a fluorescein angiogram. (CNV lesions are comprised of classic and/or occult components.) Subsequent follow-up visits require a fluorescein angiogram prior to treatment. There are no requirements regarding visual acuity, lesion size, and number of retreatments when treating predominantly classic lesions.
- Subfoveal occult with no classic associated with AMD.
- Subfoveal minimally classic CNV (where the area of classic CNV occupies less than 50 percent of the area of the entire lesion) associated with AMD.

Other uses of OPT with verteporfin to treat AMD will continue to be noncovered. This includes, but is not limited to, the following AMD indications: juxtafoveal or extrafoveal CNV lesions (lesions outside the fovea), inability to obtain a fluorescein angiogram, or atrophic or "dry" AMD.

Other ocular indications, such as pathologic myopia or presumed ocular histoplasmosis may be covered through a local coverage determination at the individual contractor's discretion.

J3400

J3400 Injection, triflupromazine HCl, up to 20 mg

Lay Description

HCPCS Level II code J3400 represents triflupromazine hydrochloride. Per the FDA, this drug is no longer available in the United States.

J3410

J3410 Injection, hydroxyzine HCl, up to 25 mg

Lay Description

Hydroxyzine is a piperazine derivative that has central nervous system depressant, antispasmodic, antihistamine, and antifibrillatory properties. It is used to treat a variety of conditions such as anxiety, pruritus from allergies, psychiatric and emotional emergencies, and nausea and vomiting. Hydroxyzine may be used as a complete therapeutic substitute for intravenous antiemetic therapy at the time of a chemotherapy treatment. It is often used as a preoperative medication. It tends to increase the effect of meperidine and barbiturates. It can be administered via intravenous push, intramuscular injection, or orally. Hydroxyzine hydrochloride is used to treat anxiety, manifestations of allergic dermatoses, as an antiemetic, and as a preoperative medication. It is administered by intramuscular injection or orally. Hydroxyzine pamoate has uses similar to the hydrochloride version. HCPCS Level II code J3410 represents up to 25 mg of hydroxyzine HCl.

J3411

J3411 Injection, thiamine HCl, 100 mg

Lay Description

Vitamins are organic compounds that are necessary for the metabolic functioning of the body. Thiamine, also known as vitamin B1, is a water-soluble vitamin that acts by binding with adenosine triphosphate to form a coenzyme needed for carbohydrate metabolism. It is found particularly in pork, organ meats, legumes, nuts, and whole grain or enriched cereals and breads. Thiamine hydrochloride is used to treat deficiency states including beriberi, alcoholic neuritis, and Wernicke-Korsakoff syndrome. It is available in injectable and oral forms. Oral forms are sold over-the-counter in singular or combined products and are self-administered. The injectable form can be administered by intramuscular or intravenous injection. HCPCS Level II code J3411 represents 100 mg of thiamine HCl.

J3415

J3415 Injection, pyridoxine HCl, 100 mg

Lay Description

Pyridoxine is one of the forms of vitamin B6. Vitamins are organic compounds that are necessary for the metabolic functioning of the body. Vitamin B6 is a water-soluble vitamin used by the body in the metabolism of amino acids, in the degradation of tryptophan, and in the breakdown of glycogen to glucose-1-phosphate. Pyridoxine hydrochloride is used for patients with vitamin B6 deficiency, to prevent seizures during cycloserine therapy, and as an antidote for isoniazid and cycloserine poisoning. HCPCS Level II code J3415 represents 100 mg of pyridoxine hydrochloride.

J3420

J3420 Injection, vitamin B-12 cyanocobalamin, up to 1,000 mcg

Lay Description

Vitamin B12 cyanocobalamin is a coenzyme that stimulates metabolic cell function. It is required for cell replication, hematopoiesis, and nucleoprotein and myelin production. This medication is indicated for treatment of pernicious anemia, vitamin B12 malabsorption, and/or methylmalonicaciduria. Malabsorption can be caused by many conditions including neoplasms, AIDS, Crohn's Disease, parasites, and tapeworms. HCPCS Level II code J3420 represents up to 1,000 mcg of vitamin B12 cyanocobalamin.

J3430

J3430 Injection, phytonadione (vitamin K), per 1 mg

Lay Description

Phytonadione (vitamin K injection) is given to prevent hemorrhagic conditions and promote liver formation of prothrombin. Hypoprothrombinemia occurs when the body lacks vitamin K, sometimes occurring secondary to malabsorption, oral anticoagulants, drug therapy, or too much vitamin A. Phytonadione is often used for pregnant women, those who are breast-feeding, and neonates who have hemorrhagic disease or vitamin K deficiency through breast milk. Phytonadione is administered by subcutaneous injection, intramuscular injection, intravenous infusion over two or three hours, or orally. HCPCS Level II code J3430 represents 1 mg of phytonadione (vitamin K).

J3465

J3465 Injection, voriconazole, 10 mg

Lay Description

Voriconazole is an antifungal used to treat infections of the skin, abdomen, bladder wall, kidney, and esophageal candidiasis. It inhibits an essential protein found in the mitochondria of the cell that is needed for biosynthesis. This medication is effective against species of Aspergillus other than A. fumigatus, Scedosporium apiospermum (asexual form of Pseudallescheria boy'dii), and Fusarium species, including Fusarium solani, in patients intolerant of, or refractory to, other therapy. Voriconazole is administered via intravenous infusion over one to two hours or orally. HCPCS Level II code J3465 represents 10 mg of voriconazole.

J3470

J3470 Injection, hyaluronidase, up to 150 units

Lay Description

Hyaluronidase is a protein enzyme produced from purified bovine testicular tissue. Hyaluronidase is a diffusing substance that modifies the permeability of connective tissue through the hydrolysis of hyaluronic acid, a polysaccharide. Hyaluronidase hydrolyzes hyaluronic acid by splitting the glucosaminidic bond between C1 of the glucosamine moiety and C4 of glucuronic acid. This temporarily decreases the viscosity of the cellular cement and promotes diffusion of injected fluids or of localized transudates or exudates facilitating their absorption. Hyaluronidase is indicated as an adjunct to increase the absorption and dispersion of other injected drugs, for hypodermoclysis, and as an adjunct in subcutaneous urography for improving resorption of radiopaque agents. This code represents up to a 150 unit injection.

Medicare Information
See the chapter titled "Medicare Guidelines," under "Drugs, Biologicals, and Radiopharmaceuticals," for Medicare information.

J3471-J3472

J3471 Injection, hyaluronidase, ovine, preservative free, per 1 USP unit (up to 999 USP units)
J3472 Injection, hyaluronidase, ovine, preservative free, per 1,000 USP units

Lay Description
Hyaluronidase is a protein enzyme. The ovine version is manufactured from purified testicular tissue and is preservative-free. Hyaluronidase is a diffusing substance that modifies the permeability of connective tissue through the hydrolysis of hyaluronic acid, a polysaccharide. Hyaluronidase hydrolyzes hyaluronic acid by splitting the glucosaminidase bond between C1 of the glucosamine moiety and C4 of glucuronic acid. This temporarily decreases the viscosity of the cellular cement and promotes diffusion of injected fluids or of localized transudates or exudates facilitating their absorption. Hyaluronidase is indicated as an adjunct to increase the absorption and dispersion of other injected drugs, for hypodermoclysis, and as an adjunct in subcutaneous urography for improving resorption of radiopaque agents. When the dose administered is less than 1,000 units, report HCPCS Level II code J3471 in one-unit increments. If the dose is 1,000 units, report HCPCS Level II code J3472 in 1,000 unit increments.

J3473

J3473 Injection, hyaluronidase, recombinant, 1 USP unit

Lay Description
Hyaluronidase is a protein enzyme. The ovine version is manufactured from purified testicular tissue and is preservative free. The recombinant version is a purified protein produced by recombinant DNA technology in Chinese hamster ovaries. Hyaluronidase is a diffusing substance that modifies the permeability of connective tissue through the hydrolysis of hyaluronic acid, a polysaccharide. Hyaluronidase hydrolyzes hyaluronic acid by splitting the glucosaminidase bond between C1 of the glucosamine moiety and C4 of glucuronic acid. This temporarily decreases the viscosity of the cellular cement and promotes diffusion of injected fluids or of localized transudates or exudates facilitating their absorption. Hyaluronidase is indicated as an adjunct to increase

the absorption and dispersion of other injected drugs, for hypodermoclysis, and as an adjunct in subcutaneous urography for improving resorption of radiopaque agents..

J3475

J3475 Injection, magnesium sulfate, per 500 mg

Lay Description
Magnesium sulfate is used to prevent or control seizures occurring in eclampsia or pre-eclampsia, for hypomagnesemia, acute nephritis in children, uterine tetany management of paroxysmal atrial tachycardia, and for constipation. Magnesium sulfate functions as an anticonvulsant and as a fluid and electrolyte replacement. Its anticonvulsant properties are thought to come by inhibiting the release of acetylcholine at the myoneural junction and thus reducing muscle contractions. HCPCS Level II code J3475 represents 500 mg of magnesium sulfate.

J3480

J3480 Injection, potassium chloride, per 2 mEq

Lay Description
Potassium chloride is an electrolyte that is used to prevent hypokalemia, digitalis intoxication, hypokalemic familial periodic paralysis, and to treat an acute myocardial infarction. Dose is based on age, weight, and clinical condition of the patient. Potassium ions are necessary for many essential physiological functions, including the maintenance of intracellular tonicity; the transmission of nerve impulses; the contraction of cardiac, skeletal, and smooth muscle; and the maintenance of normal renal function. HCPCS Level II code J3480 represents 2 mEq of potassium chloride injection.

J3485

J3485 Injection, zidovudine, 10 mg

Lay Description
Zidovudine is an antiviral used for treating human immunodeficiency virus (HIV) infection and to prevent maternal-fetal transmission of HIV. It prevents elongation of the DNA chain within the viral cells and stops the DNA growth. HCPCS Level II code J3485 represents 10 mg of zidovudine.

J3486

J3486 Injection, ziprasidone mesylate, 10 mg

Lay Description
Ziprasidone mesylate is used in the treatment of schizophrenia by inhibiting both the dopamine and serotonin-2 receptors, reducing schizophrenic symptoms. Some adverse reactions may include orthostatic hypotension, dry mouth, dysmenorrhea,

rash, flu-like syndrome, and/or dyspepsia. Ziprasidone is contraindicated in patients who have experienced a recent myocardial infarction (MI) or have a history of long QT (time between the beginning of the QRS [ventricular depolarization] complex and the end of the T-wave) syndrome. This code reports a 10 mg injection.

J3487

J3487 Injection, zoledronic acid (Zometa), 1 mg

Lay Description

Zoledronic is used for the treatment of hypercalcemia of malignancy. It is a bisphosphonates that appears to counteract the bone mineral density loss seen in patients with multiple myeloma and bone metastases from solid tumor cancers. Hypercalcemia is an abnormally high concentration of calcium in the bloodstream and results in malignancy cases from secretions by the cancer cells that promote the release of calcium stored in the bones into the blood stream. Hypercalcemia can be life threatening. Zoledronic acid is thought to act by inhibiting or killing osteoclasts, which activate the calcium release signals, or by binding to the bone and cartilage to block osteoclastic activity. Zoledronic is administered by intravenous infusion over no less than 15 minutes. HCPCS Level II code J3487 represents 1 mg of zoledronic acid.

J3488

J3488 Injection, zoledronic acid (Reclast), 1 mg

Lay Description

Zoledronic acid is used to treat high levels of calcium in the blood that may be caused by certain types of cancer. Zoledronic acid is also used along with cancer chemotherapy to treat bone damage caused by multiple myeloma or by cancer that began in another part of the body but has spread to the bones. Zoledronic acid is not cancer chemotherapy, and it will not slow or stop the spread of cancer. However, it can be used to treat bone disease in patients who have cancer. Zoledronic acid is in a class of medications called bisphosphonates. It works by slowing bone breakdown and decreasing the amount of calcium released from the bones into the blood. Zoledronic acid comes as a solution (liquid) to infuse (inject slowly) intravenously (into a vein) over at least 15 minutes. It is usually injected by a health care provider in a doctor's office, hospital, or clinic. When zoledronic acid is used to treat high blood levels of calcium caused by cancer it is usually given as a single dose. A second dose may be given at least 7 days after the first dose if blood calcium does not drop to normal levels or remain at normal levels. When zoledronic acid is used to treat bone damage caused by multiple myeloma or cancer that has spread to the bones, it is usually given once every 3-4 weeks.

J3490

J3490 Unclassified drugs

Lay Description

Use this code to represent a drug that has been administered and that does not have any other specified level I or level II HCPCS code to represent it.

J3520

J3520 Edetate disodium, per 150 mg

Lay Description

Edetate disodium is indicated for the treatment of severe acute hypercalcemia and digitalis toxicity. It forms chelates, which displace calcium from molecules. A stable chelate will form with any metal that has the ability to displace calcium from the molecule, a feature shared by lead, zinc, cadmium, manganese, iron, and mercury. Edetate disodium is not well absorbed in the gastrointestinal tract. It does not seem to penetrate cells and is found mainly in the extracellular fluid. Edetate disodium is administered by intravenous infusion over three or more hours. HCPCS Level II code J3520 represents 150 mg of edetate disodium.

J3530

J3530 Nasal vaccine inhalation

Lay Description

Use this code to represent a drug that has been administered, when the route of administration is nasal, and it does not have any other specified level I or level II HCPCS code to represent it.

J3535

J3535 Drug administered through a metered dose inhaler

Lay Description

Use this HCPCS code to represent a drug that has been administered through a meter does inhaler and the drug does not have any other specified level I or level II HCPCS code to represent it.

J3570

J3570 Laetrile, amygdalin, vitamin B-17

Lay Description

Laetrile is a compound that contains a chemical called amygdalin. Amygdalin is found in the pits of many fruits, raw nuts, and plants. It is believed that the active anticancer ingredient in laetrile is cyanide.

Laetrile has shown little anticancer effects in laboratory studies, animal studies, and human studies. The side effects of laetrile are like the symptoms of cyanide poisoning. Laetrile is not approved by the Food and Drug Administration (FDA). Laetrile is given by intravenous injection. HCPCS Level II code J3570 does not specify dose.

J3590

J3590   Unclassified biologics

Lay Description

Use this code to represent a biologic that as been administered and does not have any other specified level I or level II HCPCS code to represent it.

J7030-J7040, J7050

J7030   Infusion, normal saline solution, 1,000 cc
J7040   Infusion, normal saline solution, sterile (500 ml=1 unit)
J7050   Infusion, normal saline solution, 250 cc

Lay Description

The infusion of normal saline solution replaces electrolytes and fluid loss in hyponatremia and/or severe salt depletion. Oral tablet form is also available. Normal saline solution may cause edema or pulmonary edema if administered too rapidly. Lab values may show electrolyte imbalance. Code J7030 is for a 1000 cc infusion of normal saline solution and J7050 is for a 250 cc infusion of normal saline solution. Code J7040 is for the 500 ml infusion of normal, saline solution that is sterile.

J7042

J7042   5% dextrose/normal saline (500 ml = 1 unit)

Lay Description

Dextrose/normal saline is a water-soluble sugar that minimizes glyconeogenesis and promotes anabolism in patients whose oral caloric intake is limited. It is used to provide fluid replacement and caloric supplementation for patients with cirrhosis, hepatitis, high metabolic stress, and for nutritional support for patients with renal failure. Some side effects may include fever, nausea, glycosuria, weight gain, and/or osteoporosis. This code is for the intravenous infusion of 5 percent dextrose/normal saline.

J7050

J7050   Infusion, normal saline solution, 250 cc

Lay Description

Please refer to codes J7030-J7040 for the description, coding, and billing information.

J7060

J7060   5% dextrose/water (500 ml = 1 unit)

Lay Description

A 5 percent dextrose/water solution is used to replace fluid and calories in patients that are not able to maintain adequate oral intake or are restricted from doing so. Side effects may include fever, confusion, hypertension, and/or pulmonary edema. Dextrose/water is contraindicated in patients with a known allergy to corn or corn related products. This code reports 500 ml as one unit.

J7070

J7070   Infusion, D-5-W, 1,000 cc

Lay Description

D5W is 5 percent dextrose in water. A 5 percent dextrose/water solution is used to replace fluid and calories in patients that are not able to maintain adequate oral intake or are restricted from doing so. This is also known as glucose, which is the main source of energy for all cells. D5W is administered via intravenous infusion. HCPCS Level II code J7070 represents 1,000 cc of D5W.

J7100-J7110

J7100   Infusion, dextran 40, 500 ml
J7110   Infusion, dextran 75, 500 ml

Lay Description

Dextran is used as a hemodiluent in extracorporeal circulation, for plasma volume expansion, and in the prevention of venous thrombosis. It is made from glucose molecules and binds to platelets, red blood cells, and the lining of the vessel walls. This decreases their capability of binding together and forming clots. Dextran is administered by intravenous infusion. HCPCS Level II code J7100 represents 500 ml of dextran 40, J7110 represents 500 ml of dextran 75.

J7120

J7120   Ringers lactate infusion, up to 1,000 cc

Lay Description

Ringer's lactate solution, or infusion, is a replacement solution for treating fluid and electrolyte imbalance. It contains sodium, potassium, calcium, chloride, and lactate in amounts that approximate the levels found in blood plasma. Ringer's lactate is administered by intravenous infusion. HCPCS Level II code J7120 represents up to 1,000 cc of ringer's lactate.

J7130

J7130 Hypertonic saline solution, 50 or 100 mEq, 20 cc vial

Lay Description

Hypertonic saline solution is a high concentration of sodium chloride and is approximately eight times saltier than physiologic saline used in most hospital IVs.

J7184

J7184 Injection, von Willebrand factor complex (human), Wilate, per 100 IU VWF:RCo

Lay Description

Von Willebrand's factor complex is a concentrated blood-clotting factor extracted from human blood and pasteurized and used to treat hemophilia A. It contains highly concentrated levels of antihemophiliac/von Willebrand factors and ristocetin cofactor (VWF:RCo). It is indicated for use in adult and pediatric patients for treatment of spontaneous and trauma-induced bleeding episodes in severe von Willebrand's disease and in mild to moderate von Willebrand's disease where use of desmopressin is known or suspected to be inadequate. Other indications include the treatment of adult patients with hemophilia A (classic hemophilia). Von Willebrand's factor complex is administered by intravenous injection and can be self administered.

J7185

J7185 Injection, factor VIII (antihemophilic factor, recombinant) (XYNTHA), per IU

Lay Description

Antihemophilic factor recombinant is used as a preventive measure before a surgical procedure for patients with hemophilia A (congenital factor VIII deficiency). XYNTHA does not contain plasma or albumin. The antihemophilic factor is secreted by Chinese hamster ovary cells and is grown in a culture medium that contains recombinant insulin. It does not contain von Willebrand factor and is not appropriate for patients with von Willebrand's disease. It is used as a short-term, routine prophylaxis to reduce bleeding incidences during surgery. Dose and length of treatment is based on the patient's body weight, condition, the procedure being performed, and the extent of bleeding. Antihemophilic factor recombinant is administered by IV infusion. The medication can be self-administered.

J7186

J7186 Injection, antihemophilic factor VIII/von Willebrand factor complex (human), per factor VIII i.u.

Lay Description

Von Willebrand's factor complex is a concentrated blood-clotting factor extracted from human blood and pasteurized. It contains highly concentrated levels of antihemophiliac/von Willebrand factors. It is indicated for use in adult and pediatric patients for treatment of spontaneous and trauma-induced bleeding episodes in severe von Willebrand's disease and in mild to moderate von Willebrand's disease where use of desmopressin is known or suspected to be inadequate. Other indications include the treatment of adult patients with hemophilia A (classic hemophilia). Von Willebrand's factor complex is administered by intravenous injection and can be self-administered.

J7187

J7187 Injection, von Willebrand factor complex (Humate-P), per IU VWF:RCO

Lay Description

Von Willebrand's factor complex is a concentrated blood-clotting factor extracted from human blood and pasteurized used to treat hemophilia A and . It contains highly concentrated levels of antihemophiliac/von Willebrand factors and ristocetin cofactor (VWF:RCo). It is indicated for use in adult and pediatric patients for treatment of spontaneous and trauma-induced bleeding episodes in severe von Willebrand's disease and in mild to moderate von Willebrand's disease where use of desmopressin is known or suspected to be inadequate. Other indications include the treatment of adult patients with hemophilia A (classic hemophilia). Von Willebrand's factor complex is administered by intravenous injection and can be self-administered.

J7189

J7189 Factor VIIa (antihemophilic factor, recombinant), per 1 mcg

Lay Description

Factor VIIa recombinant is an antihemophilia drug that is a purified protein produced by recombinant DNA technology in baby hamster kidney cells. It is a vitamin K-dependent glycoprotein that is involved in the extrinsic pathway of blood coagulation. In conjunction with tissue factor, it activates coagulation Factor X and Factor IX to Factor IXa. These factors then assist in the conversion of prothrombin to thrombin and fibrinogen to fibrin inducing local hemostasis. Factor VIIa recombinant is indicated for the treatment of bleeding episodes in hemophilia A or B patients with inhibitors to Factor VIII or Factor IX. The drug is available only in an injectable form. It should be administered as an intravenous bolus only under the direct supervision of a physician experienced in the treatment of hemophilia. The recommended dosage for hemophilia A or B patients with inhibitors varies from 35 to 120 µg/kg of body weight every two hours until hemostasis is achieved, or until the treatment has been judged to be inadequate. Dosage and administration intervals are dependent upon the severity of the bleeding and patient response.

J7190-J7192

J7190 Factor VIII (antihemophilic factor, human) per IU
J7191 Factor VIII (antihemophilic factor (porcine)), per IU
J7192 Factor VIII (antihemophilic factor, recombinant) per IU, not otherwise specified

Lay Description

Factor VIII, antihemophilic factor is used to replace deficient clotting factor and treat bleeding in patients with hemophilia A or to prevent bleeding when surgery is needed. The desired level of factor VIII to be given is calculated from a formula multiplying body weight in kilograms by the level of desired factor VIII increase (or the percent of normal) by 0.5. The percent of normal used depends on the purpose of administration: to prevent spontaneous hemorrhage, 5 percent of normal is used; for moderate hemorrhage and minor surgery, 30 to 50 percent of normal is used. Severe hemorrhage requires 80 to 100 percent of normal antihemophilic factor. Factor VIII is administered by intravenous injection and can be self-administered. HCPCS Level II code J7190 represents 1 IU of human factor VIII; J7191 represents 1 IU of porcine factor VIII; and J7192 represents 1 IU of factor VIII recombinant not otherwise specified.

Documentation Standards

Medical record documentation maintained in the patient's file must document the condition for which the blood-clotting factor is being given. In addition, the name of the factor and the dosage required and/or given must be included in the records. This information is normally found in the office/progress notes, pharmacy forms, hospital records, and/or treatment notes.

Medicare Information

Medicare covers the costs of administering blood clotting factors to Medicare beneficiaries. Bill Factor VIII charges using one of these HCPCS codes. The units of blood clotting factor also must be reported. To determine the number of units to report on the claim, divide the number of international units (IU)

administered by 100 and round the answer to the nearest whole number. Payment is made for blood clotting factors only if one of the following hemophilia ICD-9-CM diagnosis codes is listed on the claim:

286.0
Coagulation defects, congenital factor VIII disorder

286.1
Coagulation defects, congenital factor IX disorder

286.2
Coagulation defects, congenital factor XI deficiency

286.3
Coagulation defects, congenital deficiency of other clotting factors

286.4
Coagulation defects, Von Willebrand's disease

286.5
Coagulation defects, hemorrhagic disorder due to circulating anticoagulants

The contractor's determination of the amount of clotting factors that may be covered is based on patterns of historical usage by the patient and the need to keep an emergency supply on hand at home.

J7193

J7193 Factor IX (antihemophilic factor, purified, nonrecombinant) per IU

Lay Description

Factor IX nonrecombinant is an antihemophilia drug. Factor IX nonrecombinant is a sterile, stable, lyophilized concentrate of factor IX prepared from pooled human plasma and is indicated for treatment of factor IX deficiency, also known as hemophilia B or Christmas disease. Factor IX is isolated from the source material by use of a murine monoclonal antibody and extraneous plasma-driven proteins, including factors II, VII, and X, are removed by use of immunoaffinity chromatography. Once factor IX has been isolated and other proteins removed, the factor IX is dissociated from the monoclonal antibody and further purified, resulting in a highly purified form of factor IX. Factor IX nonrecombinant is administered by intravenous infusion. Each vial of factor IX nonrecombinant contains the labeled amount of factor IX activity expressed in international units (IU). One IU represents the activity of factor IX present in 1 ml of normal, pooled plasma. HCPCS Level II code J7193 represents 1 IU of factor IX nonrecombinant.

Medicare Information

Medicare covers the costs of administering blood clotting factors to Medicare beneficiaries. Bill Factor

Coders' Desk Reference for HCPCS

IX charges using this HCPCS code. The units of blood clotting factor also must be reported. To determine the number of units to report on the claim, divide the number of international units (IU) administered by 100 and round the answer to the nearest whole number. Payment is made for blood clotting factors only if one of the following hemophilia ICD-9-CM diagnosis codes is listed on the claim:

286.0
Coagulation defects, congenital factor VIII disorder

286.1
Coagulation defects, congenital factor IX disorder

286.2
Coagulation defects, congenital factor XI deficiency

286.3
Coagulation defects, congenital deficiency of other clotting factors

286.4
Coagulation defects, Von Willebrand's disease

286.5
Coagulation defects, hemorrhagic disorder due to circulating anticoagulants

The contractor's determination of the amount of clotting factors that may be covered is based on patterns of historical usage by the patient and the need to keep an emergency supply on hand at home.

J7194

J7194   Factor IX complex, per IU

Lay Description

Factor IX complex is an antihemophilia drug. Factor IX complex is a sterile, dried, plasma fraction containing coagulation factors II, IX, X, and low levels of factor VII. Factors II, VII, IX, and X are the vitamin K dependent coagulation factors that are synthesized in the liver. Factor IX complex is indicated for treatment of factor IX deficiency, also known as hemophilia B or Christmas disease, in patients with current or impending bleeding episodes. It is also indicated for treatment of bleeding episodes in patients with hemophilia A (factor VIII deficiency) who have inhibitors to factor VIII. Factor IX complex is also used in emergency situations, usually as a secondary measure following the administration of fresh frozen plasma, to treat patients with coumadin-induced hemorrhage when prompt reversal is required. Factor IX complex administered for these indications raises the plasma level of factor IX and restores hemostasis in patients with the listed conditions. Factor IX complex is administered by intravenous infusion. Each vial of factor IX complex contains the labeled amount of factor IX activity expressed in international units (IU). One IU represents the activity of factor IX present in 1 ml of normal, pooled plasma. HCPCS Level II code J7194 represents 1 IU of factor IX complex.

J7195

J7195   Factor IX (antihemophilic factor, recombinant) per IU

Lay Description

Factor IX recombinant is an antihemophilia drug. Factor IX recombinant is a purified protein produced by recombinant DNA technology and indicated in the treatment of factor IX deficiency, also known as hemophilia B or Christmas disease. Indications also include control or prevention of bleeding during surgery in factor IX deficient individuals. Recombinant DNA technology involves the use of a genetically engineered animal cell line that secretes recombinant factor IX into a cell culture medium. The brand name drug BeneFIX® uses a genetically engineered Chinese hamster ovary (CHO) cell line shown to be free of infectious agents. The stored cell banks are also free of blood or plasma products. The CHO cell line secretes recombinant factor IX into a defined cell culture medium that does not contain any proteins derived from animal or human sources. The recombinant factor IX in BeneFIX® is then purified by a chromatography purification process without the use of a monoclonal antibody yielding a high-purity, active product. The potency is verified by use of in vitro clotting assay. Factor IX recombinant is administered by intravenous infusion. Each vial of factor IX recombinant contains the labeled amount of factor IX activity expressed in international units (IU). One IU represents the activity of factor IX present in 1 ml of normal, pooled plasma. HCPCS Level II code J7195 represents 1 IU of factor IX recombinant.

J7197

J7197   Antithrombin III (human), per IU

Lay Description

Antithrombin III is a sterile, nonpyrogenic, stable, lyophilized preparation of purified human antithrombin III. Antithrombin III is normally present in human plasma and is the major plasma inhibitor of thrombin. Antithrombin III is indicated for the treatment of patients with hereditary antithrombin III deficiency in connection with surgical or obstetrical procedures or when they suffer from thromboembolism. Antithrombin III is prepared from pooled units of human plasma from normal donors. Antithrombin III is administered by intravenous infusion. Each vial of antithrombin III contains the labeled amount of antithrombin III activity expressed in international units (IU).

HCPCS Level II code J7197 represents 1 IU of antithrombin III.

J7198

J7198   Antiinhibitor, per IU

Lay Description

Anti-inhibitor is a sterile product prepared from pooled human plasma. Anti-inhibitor contains, in concentrated form, variable amounts of activated and precursor vitamin K-dependent clotting factors. Factors of the kinin generating system are also present. The product is standardized by its ability to correct the clotting time of Factor VIII deficient plasma or Factor VIII deficient plasma that contains inhibitors to Factor VIII. Anti-inhibitor is indicated for use in patients with Factor VIII or Factor IX inhibitors who are bleeding or are to undergo surgery. Anti-inhibitor is intended to control bleeding episodes in such patients. Anti-inhibitor is administered by intravenous infusion. Anti-inhibitor is labeled with the number of Hyland Factor VIII Correctional Units that it contains. One Hyland Factor VIII Correctional Unit is that quantity of activated prothrombin complex that, upon addition to an equal volume of Factor VIII deficient or inhibitor plasma, will correct the clotting time to a normal time of 35 seconds. The recommended dosage depends on the severity of hemorrhage and ranges from 25 to 100 Hyland Factor VIII Correctional Units per kg of body weight. The dose may be repeated if no improvement is observed approximately six hours following the initial administration. HCPCS Level II code J7198 represents 1 IU of anti-inhibitor.

Documentation Standards

Medical record documentation maintained in the patient's file must document the condition for which the blood-clotting factor is being given. In addition, the name of the factor and the dosage required and/or given must be included in the records. This information is normally found in the office/progress notes, pharmacy forms, hospital records, and/or treatment notes.

Medicare Information

Medicare covers the costs of administering blood clotting factors to Medicare beneficiaries. Bill antiinhibitor charges using this HCPCS code. The units of blood clotting factor also must be reported. To determine the number of units to report on the claim, divide the number of international units (IU) administered by 100 and round the answer to the nearest whole number. Payment is made for blood clotting factors only if one of the following hemophilia ICD-9-CM diagnosis codes is listed on the claim:

286.0
Coagulation defects, congenital factor VIII disorder

286.1
Coagulation defects, congenital factor IX disorder

286.2
Coagulation defects, congenital factor XI deficiency

286.3
Coagulation defects, congenital deficiency of other clotting factors

286.4
Coagulation defects, Von Willebrand's disease

286.5
Coagulation defects, hemorrhagic disorder due to circulating anticoagulants

The contractor's determination of the amount of clotting factors that may be covered is based on patterns of historical usage by the patient and the need to keep an emergency supply on hand at home.

J7199

J7199   Hemophilia clotting factor, not otherwise classified

Lay Description

Use this code to represent a hemophilia clotting factor that has been administered and does not have any other specified level I or level II HCPCS code to represent it.

J7300

J7300   Intrauterine copper contraceptive

Lay Description

An intrauterine copper contraceptive, also called the copper IUD, is a long-term, reversible, method of birth control that is comparable to oral contraceptives and tubal ligation in efficacy. This is an alternative choice for women who do not use hormonal contraceptives due to smoking or other conditions that contraindicate their use. The contraceptive device is about the size of a quarter in a T-shape, made of soft, flexible plastic with copper, and is designed to fit in the uterus. The physician inserts in the device, which requires no further attention outside of monthly chain checks and may be left in for continuous use up to 10 years. The copper IUD may be removed at any time. Use of this device is contraindicating in women with pelvic inflammatory disease (PID) or any history of PID.

J7302

J7302 **Levonorgestrel-releasing intrauterine contraceptive system, 52 mg**

Lay Description

Levonorgestrel-releasing intrauterine contraceptive system (LNG-IUS) consists of a Nova T-device and a Silastic rod impregnated with 52 mg of levonorgestrel. The silastic rod is attached to the vertical arm of the device and is covered with a rate limiting silastic membrane that allows release of progestin levonorgestrel at a constant rate of 20 mcg per day directly to the lining of the uterus. The LNG-IUS is a combination hormonal and intrauterine method of birth control. The LNG-IUS appears to work by suppressing the production of human chorionic gonadotropin, thereby preventing fertilization. A physician must fit the LNG-IUS into the uterus. The LNG-IUS is an effective, long-acting, reversible contraceptive, with an effective life span of at least five years. After five years, it must be removed and replaced. HCPCS Level II code J7302 represents a 52 mg implant system.

J7303

J7303 **Contraceptive supply, hormone containing vaginal ring, each**

Lay Description

This code reports the contraceptive supply of a hormone containing vaginal ring. Unlike the daily contraceptive pill, hormone containing vaginal rings are used on a monthly basis. The ring is inserted once a month in the vaginal wall and stays in place for about three weeks depending on the product used. During this time the contraceptive medication releases a dose of hormones needed to prevent pregnancy. The patient usually takes a week break before inserting a new ring. The two hormones released include estrogen and progestin, which prevent the ovaries from producing mature eggs. The hormones are absorbed by the vaginal walls and distributed in the bloodstream. HCPCS Level II code J7303 represents each ring.

J7304

J7304 **Contraceptive supply, hormone containing patch, each**

Lay Description

A birth control patch is applied to the skin and releases hormones through the skin into the bloodstream to prevent pregnancy. The progesterone and estrogen prevents ovulation (mature eggs are not produced). The patch will also thicken the mucus produced in the cervix making it difficult for sperm to enter and reach an egg that may have been released. The hormones may also affect the lining of the uterus so that if an egg is fertilized it may have a hard time attaching itself to the wall of the uterus. The patch must be placed on the skin on the first day of the menstrual cycle (there may be differences with difference suppliers of birth control patches). The patch should only be applied to one of four areas: abdomen, buttocks, upper arm, or upper torso, except for the breasts. The patch is worn for three weeks and no patch for the fourth week. Follow all manufacturers' instructions. HCPCS Level II code J7304 is reported for each patch.

J7306

J7306 **Levonorgestrel (contraceptive) implant system, including implants and supplies**

Lay Description

Levonorgestrel is a synthetic hormone used as contraception in females. A long-term administration is available as an implant system. Typically, the contraceptive is available as a kit of soft plastic capsules, which are imbedded under the skin of the upper arm. Depending on the kit selected, one, two, or up to six rods may be inserted. A small subdermal incision is made and a trocar is used to deliver each matchstick-sized capsule. The six capsules are arranged in a fanlike manner to facilitate drug dispersion and later removal of the capsules. The drug diffuses gradually through the walls of the capsule into the bloodstream. Protection can last up to five years with the six-capsule system. Fertility is restored within weeks upon removal of the implants. Report J7306 for supply of each Levonorgestrel implant system.

J7307

J7307 **Etonogestrel (contraceptive) implant system, including implant and supplies**

Lay Description

An etonogestrel implant system is a progestin-only female contraceptive that is implanted under the skin. Once the rod is implanted under the skin, it slowly releases the hormone that can prevent pregnancy for a period of up to 3 years. This is a completely reversible method of contraception. The implant system works in three ways: first, it suppresses ovulation; second, the hormone increases the thickness of the cervical mucus in order to prevent the egg from implanting itself into the uterine wall; third, the hormone alters that inner lining of the uterus also in an effort to prevent the egg from implanting itself. Code J7307 represents the drug, the actual implant, and the supplies.

J7308

J7308　Aminolevulinic acid HCl for topical administration, 20%, single unit dosage form (354 mg)

Lay Description
Aminolevulinic acid hydrochloride is a topical solution that photosensitizes the skin to which it is applied. It is applied topically, directly on the individual lesions. Aminolevulinic acid hydrochloride is used in conjunction with blue light photodynamic therapy applied 14-18 hours later. This photodynamic therapy is indicated as a treatment for nonhyperkeratotic actinic keratoses of the face or scalp. This drug should not be applied to the eyes or mucous membranes. Actinic keratoses are pre-cancerous skin lesions, appearing as scaly red or brown patches of skin, which if left untreated may become malignant. HCPCS Level II code J7308 represents one singe unit dose applicator, which contains 354 mg of aminolevulinic acid hydrochloride.

J7310

J7310　Ganciclovir, 4.5 mg, long-acting implant

Lay Description
Ganciclovir implant is an antiviral indicated for the treatment of cytomegalovirus (CMV) retinitis in individuals with acquired immune deficiency syndrome (AIDS). The ganciclovir implant does not cure the CMV retinitis; however, it does keep the infection under control and can help to prevent the CMV retinitis from worsening. The implant is surgically inserted. The ganciclovir is released into the eye over a five to eight month period after which it is surgically removed. At the time of removal, another ganciclovir implant may be inserted to provide ongoing treatment for the CMV retinitis. The implants contain a minimum of 4.5 mg of ganciclovir. HCPCS Level II code J7310 represents one 4.5 mg ganciclovir implant.

J7311

J7311　Fluocinolone acetonide, intravitreal implant

Lay Description
The fluocinolone acetonide intravitreal implant is a tablet designed to slowly release the synthetic corticosteroid fluocinolone to the posterior segment of the eye. It must be placed via a surgical incision into the ciliary disk or pars plana. Each tablet contains 0.59 mg of fluocinolone acetonide. The implant is indicated for the treatment of chronic noninfectious uveitis affecting the posterior segment of the eye. It is contraindicated in most viral diseases, vaccina, varicella, mycobacterial and fungal eye infections. The fluocinolone acetonide implant has a life of approximately 30 months. If uveitis recurs, the implant may be replaced. HCPCS Level II code J7311 represents one intravitreal implant of fluocinolone acetonide.

J7312

J7312　Injection, dexamethasone, intravitreal implant, 0.1 mg

Lay Description
Dexamethasone intravitreal implant is a corticosteroid indicated for the treatment of macular edema following branch retinal vein occlusion or central retinal vein occlusion, and for the treatment of noninfectious uveitis affecting the posterior segment of the eye. Each intravitreal implant contains 0.7 mg of dexamethasone.

J7321-J7325

J7321　Hyaluronan or derivative, Hyalgan or Supartz, for intra-articular injection, per dose
J7323　Hyaluronan or derivative, Euflexxa, for intra-articular injection, per dose
J7324　Hyaluronan or derivative, Orthovisc, for intra-articular injection, per dose
J7325　Hyaluronan or derivative, Synvisc or Synvisc-One, for intra-articular injection, 1 mg

Lay Description
Hyaluronan is a substance that doctors inject directly into the knee joint to supplement the knee joint's natural synovial fluid, relieving pain and improving use of the knee. This treatment is also called visco supplementation. Treatment includes three or five shots into the knee joint over three to five weeks. After an injection, some people may experience pain or swelling. Hyaluronan (hyaluronic acid) is used to treat osteoarthritis of the knee that has not improved with other treatment, such as acetaminophen and physical therapy. Some study results have indicated improved symptoms of osteoarthritis and joint function, while other studies have been inconclusive about the effectiveness of hyaluronan injections. Hyaluronan is a high-molecular-mass polysaccharide found in the extracellular matrix, especially of soft connective tissues. It is synthesized in the plasma membrane of fibroblasts and other cells by addition of sugars to the reducing end of the polymer, whereas the nonreducing end protrudes into the pericellular space. The polysaccharide is catabolized locally or carried by lymph to lymph nodes or the general circulation, from where it is cleared by the endothelial cells of the liver sinusoids. The overall turnover rate is surprisingly rapid for a connective tissue matrix component (0.5 to a few days). Hyaluronan has been assigned various physiological functions in the intercellular matrix (e.g., in water

and plasma protein homeostasis). Hyaluronan production increases in proliferating cells and the polymer may play a role in mitosis. Extensive hyaluronidase-sensitive coats have been identified around mesenchymal cells. They are anchored firmly in the plasma membrane or bound via hyaluronan-specific binding proteins (receptors). Such receptors have now been identified on many different cells (e.g., the lymphocyte homing receptor CD 44). Interaction between a hyaluronan receptor and extracellular polysaccharide has been connected with locomotion and cell migration. Hyaluronan seems to play an important role during development and differentiation and has other cell regulatory activities. Hyaluronan has also been recognized in clinical medicine. A concentrated solution of hyaluronan (10 mg/ml) has, through its tissue protective and rheological properties, become a device in ophthalmic surgery. Analysis of serum hyaluronan is promising in the diagnosis of liver disease and various inflammatory conditions (e.g., rheumatoid arthritis). Interstitial edema caused by accumulation of hyaluronan may cause dysfunction in various organs.

J7330

J7330 Autologous cultured chondrocytes, implant

Lay Description

Autologous cultured chondrocytes, also known as Carticel, are a type of cartilage tissue graft indicated for the repair of cartilage defects of the knee, including meniscal knee injuries, osteochondritis dissecans, chondromalacia, and other disorders of cartilage of the knee. Autologous cultured chondrocytes are derived from healthy cartilage tissue cells that are harvested from the patient. The harvested cells are sent to a laboratory and grown in a tissue culture. The cultured chondrocytes are then implanted into the patient's knee at the site of the injury or defect by periosteal injection. The amount of autologous cultured chondrocytes needed to repair damaged knee cartilage varies and is dependent on the size of the damaged area. Most patients receive between 0.64 million and 3.3 million cells for each square centimeter of damaged area. HCPCS Level II code J7330 represents one implant of autologous cultured chondrocytes.

J7335

J7335 Capsaicin 8% patch, per 10 sq cm

Lay Description

A capsaicin patch is a localized dermal delivery system. It is a synthetic version of the natural occurring substance found in chili peppers. Capsaicin is an irritant that causes sensation of heat and pain. The capsaicin selectively binds to a protein known as TRPV1 (aka capsaicin receptor) that resides on pain and heat sensing neurons. When capsaicin binds to TRPV1, it overwhelms the neuron and depletes one of the neurotransmitters for pain and heat. Neurons that do not contain TRPV1 are unaffected. The capsaicin patch is indicated to relieve the pain of postherpetic neuralgia caused by shingles.

J7500-J7501

J7500 Azathioprine, oral, 50 mg
J7501 Azathioprine, parenteral, 100 mg

Lay Description

Azathioprine is an immunosuppressant used to prevent rejection of kidney transplants. It is also indicated to treat severe rheumatoid arthritis when other medications and treatments have not helped. Less frequently, azathioprine is used to treat ulcerative colitis. Azathioprine is available in oral and injectable forms. Its mechanism of action is not known. The drug suppresses hypersensitivities of the cell-mediated type and causes variable alterations in antibody production. HCPCS Level II code J7500 represents 50 mg of oral azathioprine. HCPCS Level II code J7501 represents 100 mg of parenteral azathioprine.

Documentation Standards

A prescription (order) for the drug that has been signed and dated by the ordering physician must be kept on file by the supplier. A new prescription is required if there is a change in dose or frequency of administration.

Claims for the first month's supply of drugs must include a copy of the CMN form if filed hard copy.

If another immunosuppressive drug is added after the original CMN has been submitted, or if the code for a drug is changed (e.g., from a miscellaneous code to a specific J-code), another "initial" CMN form is required and must be submitted to the DME MAC. However, if there is a change in the dose or frequency of administration of an already approved drug, a revised CMN is not required, but the supplier must keep the new prescription on file. Providers must document this information in the patient's medical record.

Medicare Information

Coverage of parenteral azathioprine (J7501) is limited to those situations in which the medication cannot be tolerated or absorbed if taken orally and if it is self-administered by the patient. There is no coverage under the immunosuppressive drug benefit for supplies used in conjunction with the administration of parenteral immunosuppressive drugs.

See chapter titled "Medicare Guidelines," under "Drugs, Biologicals, and Radiopharmaceuticals," for additional Medicare billing and documentation information.

J7502

J7502   Cyclosporine, oral, 100 mg

Lay Description

Cyclosporine is used to prevent rejection of skin, pancreas, kidney, liver, heart, small intestine, and bone marrow transplants. When a patient receives an allogenic tissue or organ transplant, lympho-cytes in the allograft recipient recognize the foreign tissue and attack the transplanted tissue or organ. Cyclosporine can also be used to treat rheumatoid arthritis that is not responding to methotrexate and severe psoriasis. The exact mechanism of action is not known. T-lymphocytes are preferentially inhibited. The 1-helper cell is the primary target, but the 1-suppressor cell may also be suppressed. Cyclosporine also inhibits lymphokine production and release including interleukin-2 or 1-cell growth factor (TCGF). It should be administered with adrenal corticosteroids but not with other immunosuppressive agents. HCPCS Level II code J7502 represents 100 mg of oral cyclosporine

Documentation Standards

A prescription (order) for the drug that has been signed and dated by the ordering physician must be kept on file by the supplier. A new prescription is required if there is a change in dose or frequency of administration.

Claims for the first month's supply of drugs must include a copy of the CMN form if filed hard copy.

If another immunosuppressive drug is added after the original CMN has been submitted, or if the code for a drug is changed (e.g., from a miscellaneous code to a specific J-code), another "initial" CMN form is required and must be submitted to the DME MAC. However, if there is a change in the dose or frequency of administration of an already approved drug, a revised CMN is not required, but the new prescription must be kept on file by the supplier. Providers must document this information in the patient's medical record.

Medicare Information

See chapter titled "Medicare Guidelines," under "Drugs, Biologicals, and Radiopharmaceuticals," for additional Medicare billing and documentation information.

J7504

J7504   Lymphocyte immune globulin, antithymocyte globulin, equine, parenteral, 250 mg

Lay Description

Lymphocyte immune globulin, antithymocyte globulin helps to prevent organ rejection in renal allograft transplant patients. It is given at the time of rejection or as an adjunct with other immunosuppressants to delay onset of the first rejection episode. It reduces the number of thymus-dependent lymphocytes. It changes the T lymphocyte immunity, which is partially responsible for cell-mediated immunity. Other medications may be prescribed to help prevent rejection of the transplanted kidney (e.g., corticosteroids, azathioprine) and/or prevent infection (e.g., antibiotics, antifungals, antivirals). It is also used for the treatment of moderate to severe aplastic anemia in patients who cannot undergo bone marrow transplantation. Lymphocyte immune globulin, antithymocyte globulin is administered via intravenous infusion over at least four hours. HCPCS Level II code J7504 represents 250 mg of lymphocyte immune globulin, antithymocyte globulin, equine.

Medicare Information

The national drug code (NDC) number identifies the manufacturer's product in terms of strength, quantity, and other details. Any entity billing drugs to a DME MAC must use the NDC number.

Lymphocyte immune globulin, anti-thymocyte globulin (equine) is covered under Medicare only when used in the management of allograft rejection episodes in renal transplantation. It is covered when used to supplement conventional immunosuppressive drugs or as alternatives to elevated or accelerated dosing with conventional immunosuppressive agents.

Anti-thymocyte globulins are not safely administered in the home setting and will be denied as not medically necessary in that setting.

See chapter titled "Medicare Guidelines," under "Drugs, Biologicals, and Radiopharmaceuticals," for additional Medicare billing and documentation information.

J7505

J7505   Muromonab-CD3, parenteral, 5 mg

Lay Description

Muromonab-CD3 is a murine monoclonal antibody specific to the CD3 antigen of human T cells. It inhibits the functioning of T cells, which play a major role in acute allograft rejection. It is an immunosuppressant. Muromonab is a monoclonal antibody used to prevent organ transplant rejection in patients who have received kidney, heart, and liver transplants. It blocks the function of the T cells, which play a major role in organ transplant rejection. Recommended adult dose is 5 mg per day in an intravenous injection. HCPCS Level II code J7505 represents 5 mg of muromonab-CD3.

Documentation Standards

A prescription (order) for the drug that has been signed and dated by the ordering physician must be kept on file by the supplier. A new prescription is required if there is a change in dose or frequency of administration.

Claims for the first month's supply of drugs must include a copy of the CMN form if filed hard copy.

If another immunosuppressive drug is added after the original CMN has been submitted, or if the code for a drug is changed (e.g., from a miscellaneous code to a specific J-code), another "initial" CMN form is required and must be submitted to the DME MAC. However, if there is a change in the dose or frequency of administration of an already approved drug, a revised CMN is not required, but the new prescription must be kept on file by the supplier. Providers must document this information in the patient's medical record.

Medicare Information

Monoclonal antibodies are not safely administered in the home setting and they will be denied as not medically necessary in that setting.

See chapter titled "Medicare Guidelines," under "Drugs, Biologicals, and Radiopharmaceuticals," for additional Medicare billing and documentation information.

J7506

J7506   Prednisone, oral, per 5 mg

Lay Description

Prednisone is a corticosteroid. Corticosteroids are widely used in medicine to control allergies, inflammation, and many disease processes. Prednisone is similar to a natural hormone produced by the adrenal glands. It is often used to replace this chemical when the body does not make enough. It relieves inflammation and is used to treat certain forms of arthritis; skin, blood, kidney, eye, thyroid, and intestinal disorders; severe allergies; and asthma. Prednisone also is used with other drugs to prevent rejection of transplanted organs and to treat certain types of cancer. HCPCS Level II code J7506 represents 5 mg of oral prednisone.

Documentation Standards

A prescription (order) for the drug that has been signed and dated by the ordering physician must be kept on file by the supplier. A new prescription is required if there is a change in dose or frequency of administration.

Claims for the first month's supply of drugs must include a copy of the CMN form if filed hard copy.

If another immunosuppressive drug is added after the original CMN has been submitted, or if the code for a drug is changed (e.g., from a miscellaneous code to a specific J-code), another "initial" CMN form is required and must be submitted to the DME MAC. However, if there is a change in the dose or frequency of administration of an already approved drug, a revised CMN is not required, but the supplier must keep the new prescription on file. Providers must document this information in the patient's medical record.

Medicare Information

See chapter titled "Medicare Guidelines," under "Drugs, Biologicals, and Radiopharmaceuticals," for additional Medicare billing and documentation information.

J7507

J7507   Tacrolimus, oral, per 1 mg

Lay Description

Tacrolimus is used to reduce the risk of rejection by the body of liver and kidney allogeneic transplants and of bone marrow transplants, usually used with corticosteroids. Recent trials show it to be effective in managing heart, pancreas, pancreatic island cell transplants, and small bowel disease patients. Tacrolimus prevents rejection by impeding T lymphocyte cells, cells that are in the immune system. A lower dose can be used than with cyclosporine because of its potency. Tacrolimus should not be used at the same time as cyclosporine. The current drug should be stopped at least 24 hours before beginning the other one. Tacrolimus can be administered orally, topically, or via intravenous infusion. HCPCS Level II code J7507 represents 1 mg of oral tacrolimus.

Documentation Standards

A prescription (order) for the drug that has been signed and dated by the ordering physician must be kept on file by the supplier. A new prescription is required if there is a change in dose or frequency of administration.

Claims for the first month's supply of drugs must include a copy of the CMN form if filed hard copy.

If another immunosuppressive drug is added after the original CMN has been submitted, or if the code for a drug is changed (e.g., from a miscellaneous code to a specific J-code), another "initial" CMN form is required and must be submitted to the DME MAC. However, if there is a change in the dose or frequency of administration of an already approved drug, a revised CMN is not required, but the supplier must keep the new prescription on file. Providers must document this information in the patient's medical record.

Medicare Information
See chapter titled "Medicare Guidelines," under "Drugs, Biologicals, and Radiopharmaceuticals," for additional Medicare billing and documentation information.

J7509
J7509   Methylprednisolone, oral, per 4 mg

Lay Description
Methylprednisolone is a corticosteroid used to treat a variety of conditions. Indications include allergic disorders, arthritis, blood diseases, breathing problems, certain cancers, eye diseases, intestinal disorders, and collagen and skin diseases. Methylprednisolone may also be used with other medications as a replacement for certain hormones. Methylprednisolone works by decreasing the body's immune response to these diseases and reducing symptoms such as swelling and redness. Methylprednisolone may be administered orally, by intramuscular injection in the form of methylprednisolone acetate, or by intravenous infusion in the form of methylprednisolone sodium succinate. HCPCS Level II code J7509 represents 4 mg of oral methylprednisolone.

J7510
J7510   Prednisolone, oral, per 5 mg

Lay Description
Prednisolone is a synthetic adrenal corticosteroid. Corticosteroids are natural substances produced by the adrenal glands located adjacent to the kidneys. Corticosteroids are widely used to treat allergies, inflammation, and many disease processes. Prednisolone is used to treat a wide variety of conditions. Oral and injectable prednisolone is used to suppress inflammation in many inflammatory and allergic conditions. Examples include rheumatoid arthritis, systemic lupus, acute gouty arthritis, psoriatic arthritis, ulcerative colitis, and Crohn's disease. Severe allergic conditions that fail conventional treatment may also be treated with prednisolone. Examples include bronchial asthma, allergic rhinitis, drug-induced dermatitis, and contact and atopic dermatitis. Prednisolone is also used in the treatment of leukemia and lymphomas, idiopathic thrombocytopenia purpura, and autoimmune hemolytic anemia. Other miscellaneous conditions treated with this medication include thyroiditis and sarcoidosis. Prednisolone is used as a hormone replacement in patients whose adrenal glands are unable to produce sufficient amounts of corticosteroids. Prednisolone injection or sterile suspension can be injected into a muscle, joint, lesion, or soft tissue. HCPCS Level II code J7510 represents 5 mg of oral prednisolone.

Documentation Standards
A prescription (order) for the drug that has been signed and dated by the ordering physician must be kept on file by the supplier. A new prescription is required if there is a change in dose or frequency of administration.

Claims for the first month's supply of drugs must include a copy of the CMN form if filed hard copy.

If another immunosuppressive drug is added after the original CMN has been submitted, or if the code for a drug is changed (e.g., from a miscellaneous code to a specific J-code), another "initial" CMN form is required and must be submitted to the DME MAC. However, if there is a change in the dose or frequency of administration of an already approved drug, a revised CMN is not required, but the supplier must keep the new prescription on file. Providers must document this information in the patient's medical record.

Medicare Information
See chapter titled "Medicare Guidelines," under "Drugs, Biologicals, and Radiopharmaceuticals," for additional Medicare billing and documentation information.

J7511
J7511   Lymphocyte immune globulin, antithymocyte globulin, rabbit, parenteral, 25 mg

Lay Description
Lymphocyte immune globulin, antithymocyte globulin helps to prevent organ rejection in renal allograft transplant patients. It is given at the time of rejection or as an adjunct with other immunosuppressants to delay onset of the first rejection episode. It reduces the number of thymus-dependent lymphocytes. It changes the T lymphocyte immunity, which is partially responsible for cell-mediated immunity. Other medications may be prescribed to help prevent rejection of the transplanted kidney (e.g., corticosteroids, azathioprine) and/or prevent infection (e.g., antibiotics, antifungals, antivirals). It is also used for the treatment of moderate to severe aplastic anemia

Coders' Desk Reference for HCPCS

in patients who cannot undergo bone marrow transplantation. Lymphocyte immune globulin, antithymocyte globulin is administered via intravenous infusion over at least four hours. HCPCS Level II code J7511 represents 25 mg of lymphocyte immune globulin, antithymocyte globulin, rabbit.

Medicare Information

Lymphocyte immune globulin, anti-thymocyte globulin is covered under Medicare when used in the management of allograft rejection episodes in renal transplantation. It is covered when used to supplement conventional immunosuppressive drugs or as alternatives to elevated or accelerated dosing with conventional immunosuppressive agents.

J7513

J7513 Daclizumab, parenteral, 25 mg

Lay Description

Daclizumab is an immunosuppressive agent indicated to prevent organ rejection in kidney transplant patients. Immunosuppressive agents work to lower the body's natural immunity in patients who receive tissue and organ transplants. When a patient receives a kidney transplant, lymphocytes in the allograft recipient recognize the foreign tissue and attack the transplanted kidney. Daclizumab works by preventing lymphocytes from rejecting the allograft. More specifically, daclizumab works by inhibiting IL2 mediated activation of lymphocytes, a critical pathway in the cellular immune response involved in allograft rejection. The dose of daclizumab varies, but the recommended dose is 1 mg per kg (0.45 mg per pound) of body weight. Daclizumab is administered by intravenous infusion. HCPCS Level II code J7513 represents 25 mg of daclizumab.

J7515-J7516

J7515 Cyclosporine, oral, 25 mg
J7516 Cyclosporine, parenteral, 250 mg

Lay Description

Cyclosporine is used to prevent rejection of skin, pancreas, kidney, liver, heart, small intestine, and bone marrow transplants. When a patient receives an allogenic tissue or organ transplant, lympho-cytes in the allograft recipient recognize the foreign tissue and attack the transplanted tissue or organ. Cyclosporine can also be used to treat rheumatoid arthritis that is not responding to methotrexate and severe psoriasis. The exact mechanism of action is not known. T-lymphocytes are preferentially inhibited. The 1-helper cell is the primary target, but the 1-suppressor cell may also be suppressed. Cyclosporine also inhibits lymphokine production and release including interleukin-2 or 1-cell growth factor (TCGF). It should be administered with adrenal corticosteroids but not with other immunosuppressive agents. HCPCS Level II code J7515 represents 25 mg of oral cyclosporine; and J7516 represents 250 mg of parenteral cyclosporine.

J7517

J7517 Mycophenolate mofetil, oral, 250 mg

Lay Description

Mycophenolate mofetil is an immunosuppressive agent indicated to prevent organ rejection in kidney, heart, and liver transplant patients. Immunosuppressive agents work to lower the body's natural immunity in patients who receive tissue and organ transplants. When a patient receives an allogenic tissue or organ transplant, lymphocytes in the allograft recipient recognize the foreign tissue and attack the transplanted tissue or organ. Mycophenolate mofetil works in two ways to prevent rejection. First, it inhibits rejection by preventing the production of T-cells, lymphocytes, and development of antibodies from B-cells that stimulate rejection. Second, mycophenolate mofetil also inhibits mobilization of leukocytes to inflammatory sites. Mycophenolate mofetil is generally used in conjunction with cyclosporin and corticosteroids to prevent rejection. Mycophenolate mofetil may be administered orally by tablet (available in 250 mg or 500 mg doses) or in a liquid suspension (available in a dose of 200 mg/ml). Mycophenolate mofetil may also be administered by intravenous infusion in the form of mycophenolate mofetil hydrochloride (available in 500 mg vials) at a suggested rate not to exceed 500 mg over a two-hour period. HCPCS Level II code J7517 represents 250 mg of oral mycophenolate mofetil.

Documentation Standards

A prescription (order) for the drug that has been signed and dated by the ordering physician must be kept on file by the supplier. A new prescription is required if there is a change in dose or frequency of administration.

Claims for the first month's supply of drugs must include a copy of the CMN form if filed hard copy.

If another immunosuppressive drug is added after the original CMN has been submitted, or if the code for a drug is changed (e.g., from a miscellaneous code to a specific J-code), another "initial" CMN form is required and must be submitted to the DME MAC. However, if there is a change in the dose or frequency of administration of an already approved drug, a revised CMN is not required, but the supplier must keep the new prescription on file. Providers must document this information in the patient's medical record.

Medicare Information
See chapter titled "Medicare Guidelines," under "Drugs, Biologicals, and Radiopharmaceuticals," for additional Medicare billing and documentation information.

J7518
J7518   Mycophenolic acid, oral, 180 mg

Lay Description
Mycophenolic acid is a formulation of mycophenolate sodium. It acts by inhibiting lymphocyte proliferation and antibody production and is an immunosuppressive agent indicated to prevent organ rejection in kidney transplant patients. Mycophenolic acid is generally used in conjunction with cyclosporine and corticosteroids to prevent rejection. The recommended dose of mycophenolic acid is 720 mg orally twice a day on an empty stomach. HCPCS Level II code J7518 represents 180 mg of mycophenolic acid.

J7520
J7520   Sirolimus, oral, 1 mg

Lay Description
Sirolimus is an immunosuppressive agent formerly known as rapamycin. It is a macrocyclic lactone found in the soil of Easter Island. Sirolimus resembles tacrolimus and binds to the same intracellular binding protein or immunophilins known as FKBP-12. Sirolimus, in combination with cyclosporine or tacrolimus and steroids, is used for the prevention of acute kidney allograft rejection. Sirolimus is administered orally. HCPCS Level II code J7520 represents 1 mg of sirolimus.

Documentation Standards
A prescription (order) for the drug that has been signed and dated by the ordering physician must be kept on file by the supplier. A new prescription is required if there is a change in dose or frequency of administration.

Claims for the first month's supply of drugs must include a copy of the CMN form if filed hard copy.

If another immunosuppressive drug is added after the original CMN has been submitted, or if the code for a drug is changed (e.g., from a miscellaneous code to a specific J-code), another "initial" CMN form is required and must be submitted to the DME MAC. However, if there is a change in the dose or frequency of administration of an already approved drug, a revised CMN is not required, but the supplier must keep the new prescription on file. Providers must document this information in the patient's medical record.

Medicare Information
See chapter titled "Medicare Guidelines," under "Drugs, Biologicals, and Radiopharmaceuticals," for additional Medicare billing and documentation information.

J7525
J7525   Tacrolimus, parenteral, 5 mg

Lay Description
Tacrolimus is used to reduce the risk of rejection by the body of liver and kidney allogeneic transplants and of bone marrow transplants, usually used with corticosteroids. Recent trials show it to be effective in managing heart, pancreas, pancreatic island cell transplants, and small bowel disease patients. Tacrolimus prevents rejection by impeding T lymphocyte cells, cells that are in the immune system. A lower dose can be used than with cyclosporine because of its potency. Tacrolimus should not be used at the same time as cyclosporine. The current drug should be stopped at least 24 hours before beginning the other one. Tacrolimus can be administered orally, topically, or via intravenous infusion. HCPCS Level II code J7525 represents 5 mg of parenteral tacrolimus.

J7604, J7608
J7604   Acetylcysteine, inhalation solution, compounded product, administered through DME, unit dose form, per g
J7608   Acetylcysteine, inhalation solution, FDA-approved final product, noncompounded, administered through DME, unit dose form, per g

Lay Description
Acetylcysteine is a derivative of the naturally occurring amino acid L-cysteine. The drug is available in inhalation solution, oral, and injectable forms. It is a mucolytic agent when inhaled, used to lower the viscosity (i.e., thin) mucous secretions to allow easier expulsion or easier breathing. The oral and injectable forms are used as an antidote for acetaminophen overdose to prevent life-threatening liver damage. Acetylcysteine reacts with the acetaminophen, rendering some of the acetaminophen harmless. The inhaled form is indicated as an adjunct treatment for patients with acute and chronic bronchopulmonary diseases, cystic fibrosis, tracheostomies, pulmonary complications associated with surgery, post-traumatic chest conditions, and atelectasis due to mucous obstruction. It is also used during anesthesia and in diagnostic bronchial studies. As an antidote for acetaminophen poisoning, acetylcysteine should be administered as soon as possible, but within 24 hours after the overdose. The inhaled form is administered by nebulizer, tent, or as

Coders' Desk Reference for HCPCS

a compressed gas. The injectable form is administered by intravenous infusion over 60 minutes. The oral form should be administered after gastric lavage or emesis. The dosage depends on the indication and drug form. Code J7604 represents one gram of acetylcysteine inhalation solution administered through DME, unit dose form, compounded; J7408 represents one gram of the noncompounded version of the same.

J7605

J7605 Arformoterol, inhalation solution, FDA approved final product, noncompounded, administered through DME, unit dose form, 15 mcg

Lay Description

Arformoterol tartrate is a mirror image of the drug formoterol that exhibits slightly different properties. The drug, similar to formoterol, is a long-acting, selective, $beta_2$-adrenergic receptor agonist. Arformoterol has twice as much potency as formoterol. Inhaled arformoterol acts locally in the lung as a bronchodilator. Arformoterol tartrate inhalation solution is indicated for the long-term maintenance treatment of patients with chronic obstructive pulmonary disease (COPD), including chronic bronchitis and emphysema. The recommended dosage is 15 mcg administered twice a day (morning and evening) by nebulization. The drug is inhaled and should be administered by a standard nebulizer connected to an air compressor. Code J7605 represents 15 mcg of the drug.

J7607, J7609-J7615

J7607 Levalbuterol, inhalation solution, compounded product, administered through DME, concentrated form, 0.5 mg
J7609 Albuterol, inhalation solution, compounded product, administered through DME, unit dose, 1 mg
J7610 Albuterol, inhalation solution, compounded product, administered through DME, concentrated form, 1 mg
J7611 Albuterol, inhalation solution, FDA-approved final product, noncompounded, administered through DME, concentrated form, 1 mg
J7612 Levalbuterol, inhalation solution, FDA-approved final product, noncompounded, administered through DME, concentrated form, 0.5 mg
J7613 Albuterol, inhalation solution, FDA-approved final product, noncompounded, administered through DME, unit dose, 1 mg
J7614 Levalbuterol, inhalation solution, FDA-approved final product, noncompounded, administered through DME, unit dose, 0.5 mg
J7615 Levalbuterol, inhalation solution, compounded product, administered through DME, unit dose, 0.5 mg

Lay Description

Albuterol and levalbuterol are selective beta2-adrenergic receptor agonists that function as bronchodilators. The drugs block the actions of enzymes that cause the smooth muscles within the respiratory tract to contract. This relaxation of smooth muscles allows easier breathing. Albuterol and levalbuterol are indicated for the prevention and relief of bronchospasm in patients with reversible obstructive pulmonary disease and for the prevention of exercise-induced bronchospasm. Effects of the drug may last up to six hours after administration. The following HCPCS Level II codes represent the indicated version or form of the drug and all are administered through DME: J7607 represents 0.5 mg of levalbuterol in a concentrated form in a compounded product; J7609 represents 1 mg of albuterol in a compounded product in unit dose form with J7610 representing the same in a concentrated form; J7611 represents 1 mg of albuterol in a non-compounded FDA-approved final product in a concentrated form with J7613 representing the unit dose form of the same; J7612 represents 0.5 mg of levalbuterol in a non-compounded FDA-approved final product in a concentrated form with J7614 representing the unit dose form of the same; and J7615 represents 0.5 mg of levalbuterol in a unit dose form in a compounded product.

J7608

J7608 Acetylcysteine, inhalation solution, FDA-approved final product, noncompounded, administered through DME, unit dose form, per g

Lay Description

Please refer to code J7604 for the description, coding, and billing information.

J7609-J7610

J7609 Albuterol, inhalation solution, compounded product, administered through DME, unit dose, 1 mg

J7610 Albuterol, inhalation solution, compounded product, administered through DME, concentrated form, 1 mg

Lay Description

Please refer to code J7607 for the description, coding, and billing information.

J7615

J7615 Levalbuterol, inhalation solution, compounded product, administered through DME, unit dose, 0.5 mg

Lay Description

Please refer to code J7607 for the description, coding, and billing information.

J7620

J7620 Albuterol, up to 2.5 mg and ipratropium bromide, up to 0.5 mg, FDA-approved final product, noncompounded, administered through DME

Lay Description

Albuterol and ipratropium bromide is a combination bronchodilator used in inhalation solutions. Albuterol is a selective beta^2-adrenergic receptor agonist that blocks the actions of enzymes that cause the smooth muscles within the respiratory tract to contract. This relaxation of smooth muscles allows easier breathing. Ipratropium bromide is an anticholinergic agent that binds to receptors of vascular smooth muscle and endothelial cells and increases intracellular concentrations of guanosine cyclic monophosphate (cGMP), which creates smooth muscle cell relaxation. Albuterol and ipratropium bromide is indicated as a treatment for bronchospasms associated with chronic obstructive pulmonary disease (COPD). one vial usually contains 2.5 mg or albuterol combined with 0.5 mg of ipratropium bromide. The drug is available as a metered dose inhaler or in a solution for administration via a reusable nebulizer. Recommended dosage for inhalation is one vial four times a day administered administration via a reusable nebulizer. HCPCS Level II code J7620 represents combination drug composed of up to 2.5 mg of albuterol with up to 0.5 mg of ipratropium bromide inhalation solution, noncompounded, FDA-approved final product, administered through DME.

Medicare Information

See chapter titled "Medicare Guidelines," under "Drugs, Biologicals, and Radiopharmaceuticals," for Medicare billing and documentation information.

J7622

J7622 Beclomethasone, inhalation solution, compounded product, administered through DME, unit dose form, per mg

Lay Description

Beclomethasone is a corticosteroid. Beclomethasone is indicated for the treatment of bronchial asthma when administered as an oral inhalant. Beclomethasone controls symptoms of asthma and other lung diseases but does not cure them. HCPCS Level II code J7622 represents each mg of a compounded beclomethasone inhalation solution administered through DME in unit dose form.

J7624

J7624 Betamethasone, inhalation solution, compounded product, administered through DME, unit dose form, per mg

Lay Description

Betamethasone valerate is a corticosteroid with anti-inflammatory and immunosupressive abilities. The inhalation solution is used to prevent moderate to severe asthma. HCPCS Level II code J7624 represents each mg of a compounded betamethasone inhalation solution administered through DME in unit dose form.

J7626-J7627

J7626 Budesonide, inhalation solution, FDA-approved final product, noncompounded, administered through DME, unit dose form, up to 0.5 mg

J7627 Budesonide, inhalation solution, compounded product, administered through DME, unit dose form, up to 0.5 mg

Lay Description

Budesonide is a corticosteroid with anti-inflammatory and immunosupressive abilities. It is available as an inhalation solution in several formulations including a noncompounded unit dose form, a powder compounded for inhalation, and a concentrated form. The inhalation solution is used to prevent wheezing, shortness of breath, and difficulty breathing caused by severe asthma and other lung diseases. Budesonide controls symptoms of asthma and other lung diseases but does not cure them. Budesonide is usually inhaled once or twice a day. HCPCS Level II code J7626 represents up to 0.5 mg of budesonide inhalation solution, noncompounded unit dose form, FDA-approved final product, administered through DME; and J7627 represents up to 0.5 mg of budesonide inhalation solution, compounded unit dose form, administered through DME.

J7628-J7629

J7628 Bitolterol mesylate, inhalation solution, compounded product, administered through DME, concentrated form, per mg
J7629 Bitolterol mesylate, inhalation solution, compounded product, administered through DME, unit dose form, per mg

Lay Description

Bitolterol mesylate is a bronchodilator used in the treatment of bronchospasm associated with asthma. It may also be helpful in the treatment of emphysema and chronic bronchitis. Asthma is a condition that causes narrowing of the bronchial tubes due to muscle spasm and inflammation within the bronchial tubes. Bitolterol mesylate relaxes the smooth muscles surrounding these airway tubes, thereby increasing the diameter and ease of air flow through the tubes. Bitolterol mesylate is unique in that it is a "prodrug" because the body must first metabolize it before it becomes active. Biltolterol is administered in an aerosol inhaled by mouth. It usually is taken as needed to relieve symptoms or every eight hours to prevent symptoms. HCPCS Level II code J7628 represents 1 mg of bitolterol mesylate inhalation solution, compounded, concenetrated, administered through DME; J7629 represents 1 mg bitolterol mesylate inhalation solution, compounded, unit dose form, administered through DME.

J7631-J7632

J7631 Cromolyn sodium, inhalation solution, FDA-approved final product, noncompounded, administered through DME, unit dose form, per 10 mg
J7632 Cromolyn sodium, inhalation solution, compounded product, administered through DME, unit dose form, per 10 mg

Lay Description

Cromolyn sodium is a nonsteroidal anti-inflammatory that works by preventing the release of substances in the body that cause inflammation. More specifically, cromolyn sodium acts indirectly blocking calcium ions from entering the mast cell, thereby preventing mediator release. This prevents the release of substances that cause inflammation in the air passages of the lungs. Cromolyn sodium is used to prevent wheezing, shortness of breath, and difficulty breathing caused by asthma. It is also used to prevent breathing difficulties (bronchospasm) during exercise. Cromolyn comes as powder-filled capsules and solution to take by mouth, and an aerosol to inhale by mouth. The inhalant form is used to prevent asthma attacks and other conditions involving inflammation of the lung tissues. It is usually inhaled three or four times a day to prevent asthma attacks, or within an hour before activities to prevent breathing difficulties caused by exercise. Code J7631 represents 10 mg of inhalation solution that is an FDA-approved, final product, noncompounded and administered through DME; J7632 is the unit does form of the same.

J7633-J7634

J7633 Budesonide, inhalation solution, FDA-approved final product, noncompounded, administered through DME, concentrated form, per 0.25 mg
J7634 Budesonide, inhalation solution, compounded product, administered through DME, concentrated form, per 0.25 mg

Lay Description

Budesonide is a corticosteroid with anti-inflammatory and immunosupressive abilities. It is available as an inhalation solution in several formulations including a noncompounded unit dose form, a powder compounded for inhalation, and a concentrated form. The inhalation solution is used to prevent wheezing, shortness of breath, and difficulty breathing caused by severe asthma and other lung diseases. Budesonide controls symptoms of asthma and other lung diseases but does not cure them. Budesonide is usually inhaled once or twice a day. HCPCS Level II code J7633 represents up to 0.25 mg of budesonide inhalation solution, noncompounded concentrated form, FDA-approved final product, administered through DME, and J7634 represents 0.25 mg of budesonide inhalation solutio, compounded, and in concenetrated form, administered through DME.

J7635-J7636

J7635 Atropine, inhalation solution, compounded product, administered through DME, concentrated form, per mg

J7636 Atropine, inhalation solution, compounded product, administered through DME, unit dose form, per mg

Lay Description

Atropine is an extract of an alkaloid from the plants belladonna, hyoscyamus, or stramonium. It is also made synthetically. Atropine sulfate is a highly toxic compound of atropine and sulfuric acid that has the same uses and effects as atropine. It blocks the neurotransmitter acetylcholine in muscarinic receptors of the parasympathetic system. Muscarinic receptors occur throughout the nervous system including in the heart, smooth muscles of the blood vessels, lungs, salivary glands, gastrointestinal tract, and eye. Atropine sulfate in clinical doses counteracts the peripheral vessel dilatation and abrupt decrease in blood pressure produced by other drugs or biologicals. Atropine is used to reduce secretions in the respiratory tract. HCPCS Level II code J7635 represents 1 mg of the compounded concentrated inhalation form, administered through DME; and J7636 represents 1 mg of the compounded unit dose inhalation form, administered through DME.

J7637-J7638

J7637 Dexamethasone, inhalation solution, compounded product, administered through DME, concentrated form, per mg

J7638 Dexamethasone, inhalation solution, compounded product, administered through DME, unit dose form, per mg

Lay Description

Dexamethasone is a synthetic corticosteroid that is similar to a natural hormone produced by the adrenal gland. It is 25 times as potent as cortisol. Dexamethasone has anti-inflammatory, antiemetic and immunosuppressant properties. It is used to treat a wide variety of disorders. HCPCS Level II code J7637 represents a per mg dose of dexamethasone compounded concentrated inhalation solution, administered through DME; J7638 represents a per mg compounded unit dose form of dexamethasone inhalation solution, administered through DME.

J7639

J7639 Dornase alfa, inhalation solution, FDA-approved final product, noncompounded, administered through DME, unit dose form, per mg

Lay Description

Dornase alpha is an inhaled drug indicated for the treatment of cystic fibrosis. Healthy lungs continually secrete fluid into the airways to keep them moist. However, in cystic fibrosis, a reduced amount of water is present in the secretions making them thick and difficult to cough up or spit out. These thickened secretions block the airways, causing labored breathing and promoting the growth of bacteria and infection. These thickened secretions contain high concentrations of deoxyribonucleic acid (DNA) and dornase alpha, a genetically engineered form of the human enzyme deoxyribonuclease or DNAase. Dornase alpha works by breaking down the DNA, thereby reducing the thickness of the fluids. Dornase alpha is supplied in single-use ampules that contain 2.5 ml of a sterile, clear, colorless solution containing 1.0 mg/ml of dornase alpha. HCPCS Level II code J7639 represents 1 mg dornase alpha inhalation solution, unit dose form, administered through DME.

J7640

J7640 Formoterol, inhalation solution, compounded product, administered through DME, unit dose form, 12 mcg

Lay Description

Formoterol is a long-acting selective $beta_2$-adrenergic receptor agonist 33

($beta_2$-agonist). Inhaled formoterol acts locally in the lung as a bronchodilator. This is a long term medication used to treat asthma and to prevent exercise induced bronchospasm in adults and children over 12. It can also be used long term to treat Chronic Obstructive Pulmonary Disease (COPD) including bronchitis and emphysema. The usual dose is 12 micrograms every 12 hours through an inhaler. HCPCS Level II code J7640 represents 12 micrograms of compounded formoterol inhalation solution, unit dose form.

J7641

J7641 Flunisolide, inhalation solution, compounded product, administered through DME, unit dose, per mg

Lay Description

Flunisolide is a corticosteroid used as maintenance treatment for asthma. It is shown to be several hundred times stronger in animal anti-inflammatory assays than the cortisol standard. This may reduce or eliminate the need for oral corticosteroids. Corticosteroids reduce or eliminate inflammation in the lining of the airways. They may also reduce the reaction to inhaled allergen and can be used for the management of the nasal symptoms of seasonal or perennial rhinitis. The recommended dose varies depending on the treatment. HCPCS Level II code J7641 represents a per milligram dose of compounded flunisolide inhalation solution, administered through DME.

J7642-J7643

J7642 Glycopyrrolate, inhalation solution, compounded product, administered through DME, concentrated form, per mg

J7643 Glycopyrrolate, inhalation solution, compounded product, administered through DME, unit dose form, per mg

Lay Description

Glycopyrrolate is an anticholinergic drug. It inhibits the action of acetylcholine on structures innervated by postganglionic cholinergic nerves and on smooth muscles that respond to acetylcholine but lack cholinergic innervation. It reduces the amount of free acidity of gastric secretions and controls excessive pharyngeal, tracheal, and bronchial secretions. Glycopyrrolate inhalation solution is used for maintenance treatment for asthma and chronic obstructive pulmonary disease (COPD). It has been shown to be an effective bronchodilator when used once a day. HCPCS Level II code J7642 represents a per milligram dose of compounded glycopyrrolate concentrated inhalation solution, administered through DME and J7643 represents a per milligram dose of compounded glycopyrrolate inhalation solution, unit dose form, administered through DME.

J7644-J7645

J7644 Ipratropium bromide, inhalation solution, FDA-approved final product, noncompounded, administered through DME, unit dose form, per mg

J7645 Ipratropium bromide, inhalation solution, compounded product, administered through DME, unit dose form, per mg

Lay Description

Ipratropium bromide is an anticholinergic agent that functions as a bronchodilator when inhaled. The drug binds to receptors of vascular smooth muscle and endothelial cells and increases intracellular concentrations of guanosine cyclic monophosphate (cGMP), which creates smooth muscle cell relaxation. Inhaled ipratropium bromide, singularly or in combination with other bronchodilators, is for the treatment of bronchospasms associated with chronic obstructive pulmonary disease (COPD) including chronic bronchitis and emphysema. Recommended dosage for inhalation is 36 mcg four times a day. HCPCS Level II code J7644 represents one mg of ipratropium bromide inhalation solution, noncompounded, unit dose form, FDA-approved final product, administered through DME, and J7645 represents a mg of ipratropium bromide inhalation solution, compounded, unit dose form administered through DME.

Medicare Information

The following table represents the maximum milligrams/month of inhalation drugs through a nebulizer that would be billed. Claims for more than these amounts will be denied as not medically necessary, unless accompanied by documentation that justifies a larger amount:

- Ipratropium bromide up to 90 mg/month

See chapter titled "Medicare Guidelines," under "Drugs, Biologicals, and Radiopharmaceuticals," for additional Medicare billing and documentation information.

J7647, J7650

J7647 Isoetharine HCl, inhalation solution, compounded product, administered through DME, concentrated form, per mg

J7650 Isoetharine HCl, inhalation solution, compounded product, administered through DME, unit dose form, per mg

Lay Description

Isoetharine hydrochloride is a bronchodilator that relaxes the smooth muscles of the lungs that constrict due to inflammation or disease. It is used to treat asthma, emphysema, bronchitis, and chronic obstructive pulmonary disease (COPD). The medication comes in a solution that is used with a nebulizer and in a hand-held aerosol form. Report J7647 for the concentrated form, each mg; J7650 for the unit dose form, each mg.

J7648-J7649

J7648　Isoetharine HCl, inhalation solution, FDA-approved final product, noncompounded, administered through DME, concentrated form, per mg

J7649　Isoetharine HCl, inhalation solution, FDA-approved final product, noncompounded, administered through DME, unit dose form, per mg

Lay Description

Isoetharine hydrochloride (HCl) is a bronchodilator that relaxes the smooth muscles of the lungs that constrict due to inflammation or disease. It is used to treat asthma, emphysema, bronchitis, and chronic obstructive pulmonary disease (COPD). HCPCS Level II code J7648 represents a per milligram dose of noncompounded, concenetrated isoetharine HCl inhalation solution, FDA-approved final product, administered through DME and J7649 represents a per milligram dose of noncompounded, unit dose form, isoetharine HCl inhalation solution, FDA-approved final product, administered through DME.

J7650

J7650　Isoetharine HCl, inhalation solution, compounded product, administered through DME, unit dose form, per mg

Lay Description

Please refer to code J7647 for the description, coding, and billing information.

J7657-J7660

J7657　Isoproterenol HCl, inhalation solution, compounded product, administered through DME, concentrated form, per mg

J7658　Isoproterenol HCl, inhalation solution, FDA-approved final product, noncompounded, administered through DME, concentrated form, per mg

J7659　Isoproterenol HCl, inhalation solution, FDA-approved final product, noncompounded, administered through DME, unit dose form, per mg

J7660　Isoproterenol HCl, inhalation solution, compounded product, administered through DME, unit dose form, per mg

Lay Description

Isoproterenol hydrochloride (HCl) is a synthetic sympathometic amine that is similar to epinephrine but acts almost entirely on beta-receptors. It lowers peripheral vascular resistance in skeletal muscle, renal, and mesenteric vascular beds. Cardiac output is increased due to the lowered peripheral resistance. The inhalation form is used to treat bronchospasms. Commercial inhalation forms of isoproterenol have been discontinued.HCPCS Level II code J7657 represents a per milligram dose of compounded, concenetrated, isoprosterenol hydrochloride inhalation solution, administered through DME; J7658 represents a per milligram dose of noncompounded, concenetrated, FDA-approved final product, isoprosterenol hydrochloride inhalation solution, administered through DME; J7659 representsa per milligram dose of noncompounded, unit dose form, FDA-approved final product, isoprosterenol hydrochloride inhalation solution, administered through DME; and J7660 represents a per milligram dose of compounded, unit dose form, isoprosterenol hydrochloride inhalation solution, administered through DME.

J7667-J7670

J7667　Metaproterenol sulfate, inhalation solution, compounded product, concentrated form, per 10 mg

J7668　Metaproterenol sulfate, inhalation solution, FDA-approved final product, noncompounded, administered through DME, concentrated form, per 10 mg

J7669　Metaproterenol sulfate, inhalation solution, FDA-approved final product, noncompounded, administered through DME, unit dose form, per 10 mg

J7670　Metaproterenol sulfate, inhalation solution, compounded product, administered through DME, unit dose form, per 10 mg

Lay Description

Metaproterenol sulfate is a bronchodilator used to treat asthma, bronchitis, and emphysema. It acts on the beta-receptors in the bronchial smooth muscles to relax bronchospasms that cause difficulty breathing. The medication comes in a solution that is used with a nebulizer and in a hand-held aerosol and powder form. HCPCS Level II code J7668 represents 10 mg of a compounded, concentrated metaproterenol inhalation solution; J7668 represents 10 mg of a noncompounded, concentrated, FDA-approved final product, inhalation solution administered via DME; J7669 represents 10 mg of the noncompounded, FDA-approved final product, unit dose form, metaproterenol inhalation solution administered via DME; and J7670 represents 10 mg of compounded, unit dose form, metaproterenol inhalation solution administered via DME.

J7674

J7674　Methacholine chloride administered as inhalation solution through a nebulizer, per 1 mg

Lay Description

Methacholine chloride is a synthetic choline ester that acts to induce bronchoconstriction. This medication is used in a bronchospasm provocation test to diagnose asthma. This is often done when spirometry alone does not provide a definitive diagnosis. Two different dilution schedules are used in North America to perform the test. Both use 100 mg of methacholine. One is based on a two minute tidal breathing dosing protocol and the other is a five breath dosimeter protocol. Both methods utilize a nebulizer to administer the medication. HCPCS Level II code J7674 represents 1 mg of methacholine chloride.

J7676

J7676　Pentamidine isethionate, inhalation solution, compounded product, administered through DME, unit dose form, per 300 mg

Lay Description

Pentamidine isethionate is an aromatic diamidine that is an anti-protozoal. Its mechanism of action is not completely known. It is thought the drug interferes with the synthesis of DNA, RNA, and protein causing cell death. Pentamidine isethionate is indicated as a treatment for *Pneumocystis carinii*, trypanosomiasis, and leishmaniasis. The drug may be administered by intramuscular injection, inhalation, or intravenous infusion over one hour. The inhalation solution is inhaled through a special breathing unit that ensures the drug reaches deep into the lungs. The recommended dosage for the inhalation solution is 300 mg once a month and administered via a nebulizer. Treatment usually takes 30-45 minutes. Code J7676 represents 300 mg of the inhalation solution unit dose form.

J7680-J7681

J7680　Terbutaline sulfate, inhalation solution, compounded product, administered through DME, concentrated form, per mg

J7681　Terbutaline sulfate, inhalation solution, compounded product, administered through DME, unit dose form, per mg

Lay Description

Terbutaline sulfate is a beta$_2$ adrenergic agonist that functions as a bronchodilator. It works, in part, by stimulating the conversion of adenosine triphosphate (ATP) to cyclic 3',5'-adenosine monophosphate, which relaxes bronchial muscles. Terbutaline sulfate is indicated for the prevention and reversal of bronchospasm in asthma, bronchitis, and emphysema. Report J7680 for the concentrated form, each mg; J7681 for the unit dose form, each mg.

J7682

J7682　Tobramycin, inhalation solution, FDA-approved final product, noncompounded, unit dose form, administered through DME, per 300 mg

Lay Description

Tobramycin is an aminoglycoside antibiotic. Aminoglycoside antibiotics are those derived from various species of Streptomyces bacteria or produced synthetically. Aminoglycosides inhibit bacterial protein synthesis by binding with the 30S ribosomal subunit and are bactericidal. Streptomycin is derived from *Streptomyces tenebrarius*. It inhibits protein synthesis causing cell death. Susceptibility studies should be performed prior to the administration of tobramycin. It is indicated in the treatment of infections caused by gram-negative bacillary bacteria including *Pseudomonas aeruginosa, Staphylococcus aureus, Escherichia coli, Klebsiella* species, E*nterobacter* species, *Serretia* species, *Proteus* species, *Providencia* species, and *Citrobacter* species. The inhalation form is indicated in the treatment of *Pseudomonas aeruginosa* inpatients with cystic fibrosis. HCPCS Level II code J7682 represents 300 mg of noncompounded, FDA-approved final product, unit dose form of tobramycin inhalation solution administered via DME.

J7683-J7684

J7683　Triamcinolone, inhalation solution, compounded product, administered through DME, concentrated form, per mg

J7684　Triamcinolone, inhalation solution, compounded product, administered through DME, unit dose form, per mg

Lay Description

Triamcinolone is a synthetic corticosteroid, which is analogous to corticosteroids produced by the adrenal cortex. The drug is one to two times more potent than prednisone. Its mechanism of actions is not clearly defined. Triamcinolone does decrease inflammation by stabilizing leukocytes, suppress the chemicals normally released in immune response, and stimulate bone marrow. Inhaled triamcinolone is a local anti-inflammatory delivering the drug directly to the lungs. The drug has no effect on acute bronchospasms, but is indicated for prophylactic and maintenance therapy of asthma. HCPCS Level II code J7683 for the compounded concentrated form per 1 mg and J7684 for the compounded unit dose form represent 1 mg of the inhaled version of triamcinolone that is administered through DME.

J7685

J7685 Tobramycin, inhalation solution, compounded product, administered through DME, unit dose form, per 300 mg

Lay Description

Tobramycin is an aminoglycoside antibiotic. Aminoglycoside antibiotics are those derived from various species of Streptomyces bacteria or produced synthetically. Aminoglycosides inhibit bacterial protein synthesis by binding with the 30S ribosomal subunit and are bactericidal. Streptomycin is derived from *Streptomyces tenebrarius*. It inhibits protein synthesis causing cell death. Susceptibility studies should be performed prior to the administration of tobramycin. It is indicated in the treatment of infections caused by gram-negative bacillary bacteria including *Pseudomonas aeruginosa, Staphylococcus aureus, Escherichia coli, Klebsiella* species, *Enterobacter* species, *Serratia* species, *Proteus* species, *Providencia* species, and *Citrobacter* species. The inhalation form is indicated in the treatment of *Pseudomonas aeruginosa* inpatients with cystic fibrosis. HCPCS Level II code J7685 represents 300 mg of compounded for the unit dose form of tobramycin inhalation solution administered via DME.

J7699

J7699 NOC drugs, inhalation solution administered through DME

Lay Description

Use this code to represent an inhalation drug that has been administered through DME and is not represented by any other level I or level II HCPCS code.

J7799

J7799 NOC drugs, other than inhalation drugs, administered through DME

Lay Description

Use this code to represent a drug that has been administered through DME, but is not an inhalation drug. Be sure the drug does not have any other specified level I or level II HCPCS code to represent it.

J8498

J8498 Antiemetic drug, rectal/suppository, not otherwise specified

Lay Description

Antiemetic medication may be used in conjunction with anti-cancer drugs such as chemotherapeutic agents and acts to prevent or relieve nausea and vomiting. Antiemetics are antagonists for a specific serotonin subtype receptor located on the nerve terminals of the vagus in the small intestine. Report J8498 for rectal administration of an antiemetic drug that does not have a more specific code designated.

Medicare Information

See chapter titled "Medicare Guidelines," under "Drugs, Biologicals, and Radiopharmaceuticals," for Medicare billing and documentation information.

J8499

J8499 Prescription drug, oral, nonchemotherapeutic, NOS

Lay Description

Use this code to represent an oral prescription drug that has been taken as a form of chemotherapy, and is not represented by any other level I or level II HCPCS code.

J8501

J8501 Aprepitant, oral, 5 mg

Lay Description

Aprepitant is a chemical complex used as an oral antiemetic drug. It seeks cell receptors of human substance P/neurokinin 1 (NK1). NK1s are peptides found in the central and peripheral nerve systems involved in the transmission of a signal from outside the cell wall into the cell. Aprepitant blocks those transmissions. It is used in combination with a corticosteroid and a 5-HT3 antagonist to prevent acute and delayed nausea and vomiting associated with initial and repeat courses of certain chemotherapies, including high-dose cisplatin. The drug is self-administered orally. HCPCS Level II code J8501 represents 5 mg dose of oral aprepitant.

Medicare Information

Medicare will cover the oral antiemetic aprepitant when used in a three-drug combination of aprepitant, a 5-HT3 antagonist, and dexamethasone only when the patient is receiving one or more of the following drugs: carmustine, cisplatin, cyclophosphamide, dacarbazine, mechlorethamine, streptozocin, doxorubicin, epirubicin, or lomustine. The drug is only covered when administered in the three-drug combination. Aprepitant administered outside the three-drug combination or to patients who are not receiving the specified antineoplastic drugs will not be covered.

J8510

J8510   Busulfan; oral, 2 mg

Lay Description

Busulfan is an alkylating agent that is used to reduce tumor growth. It causes breaks in the DNA, which prevent replication, thus interfering with tumor cell reproduction. It is used in the treatment of chronic myelogenous leukemia, and disorders such as severe thrombocytosis and polycythemia vera. Side effects commonly reported from busulfan are brittle or thinned hair, dry skin, diarrhea, weight loss, fatigue, and blistering of the mouth. This code is for the oral administration per 2 mg.

J8515

J8515   Cabergoline, oral, 0.25 mg

Lay Description

Cabergoline is a chemical complex that binds to a dopamine receptor on cells and inhibits the secretion of prolactin. Prolactin is a hormone produced by the anterior pituitary gland that stimulates and sustains lactation. Cabergoline is indicated for the treatment of hyperprolactinemia, whether idiopathic or caused by a pituitary adenoma. The recommended initial dosage is 0.25 mg twice weekly increasing to 1 mg twice weekly depending upon the prolactin levels in the patient's blood. Cabergoline is available only as a self-administrable oral tablet. HCPCS Level II code J8515 represents 0.25 mg of cabergoline.

J8520-J8521

J8520   Capecitabine, oral, 150 mg
J8521   Capecitabine, oral, 500 mg

Lay Description

Capecitabine is an antineoplastic drug that is broken down in the liver into fluorouracil, also known as 5 FU. Fluorouracil is a fluorinated analogue of uracil. Uracil is a chemical compound found in nucleic acids that interferes with the synthesis of DNA and RNA causing cell death. Capecitabine, singularly or in combination with other chemotherapeutic drugs, is indicated as a treatment for colorectal cancer and metastatic breast cancer. The drug is self-administered orally. HCPCS Level II code J8520 represents 150 mg of capecitabine and J8521 represents 500 mg of capecitabine.

Medicare Information

See chapter titled "Medicare Guidelines," under "Drugs, Biologicals, and Radiopharmaceuticals," for additional Medicare billing and documentation information.

J8530

J8530   Cyclophosphamide; oral, 25 mg

Lay Description

Cyclophosphamide is a synthetic antineoplastic drug chemically related to the nitrogen mustards. The drug itself is inert and functions only after transformation in the liver to active alkylating metabolites. These metabolites interfere with the growth of susceptible rapidly proliferating malignant cells. The mechanism of action is thought to be its interference with the DNA of the tumor cell causing cell death. Cyclophosphamide is indicated singularly or in combination with other chemotherapeutic drugs, to treat a wide variety of cancers including Hodgkin's disease, lymphosarcoma, acute lymphocytic leukemia, Burkitt's lymphoma, carcinoma of the breast, multiple myeloma, chronic lymphocytic leukemia, bronchogenic carcinoma, neuroblastoma, ovarian carcinoma, and carcinoma of the uterine cervix. It is also used as an immunosuppressant to prevent transplant rejection and in the treatment of certain diseases with abnormal immune function, including severe lupus manifestations and vasculitis. Cyclophosphamide may be administered via intravenous injection or infusion, or may be injected intramuscularly, intraperitoneally, or intrapleurally. An oral version is also available. Dosage depends upon body weight and the disease being treated. The lyophilized version of cyclophosphamide is a freeze-dried version of the drug. HCPCS Level II code J8530 represents 25 mg of oral cyclophosphamide.

Medicare Information

See chapter titled "Medicare Guidelines," under "Drugs, Biologicals, and Radiopharmaceuticals," for additional Medicare billing and documentation information.

J8540

J8540   Dexamethasone, oral, 0.25 mg

Lay Description

Dexamethasone is a synthetic corticosteroid that is similar to a natural hormone produced by the adrenal gland. It is 25 times as potent as cortisol. Dexamethasone has anti-inflammatory, antiemetic and immunosuppressant properties. It is used to treat a wide variety of disorders. HCPCS Level II code J8540 represents a 0.25 mg oral dose.

J8560

J8560   Etoposide; oral, 50 mg

Lay Description

Etoposide is a semisynthetic derivative of podophyllotoxin, a toxic compound found in the rhizomes and roots of the mandrake plant. It is

HCPCS Lay Descriptions

believed to inhibit the repair of DNA causing cell death. Etoposide is an antineoplastic drug used in combination with other chemotherapeutic agents. It is available in injectable or oral versions. Injectable etoposide is indicated for the treatment of small cell lung cancer and refractory testicular cancer that has been previously treated with surgery, radiation, or other chemotherapy. The oral version is indicated for the treatment of small cell lung cancer. The recommended dosage of the injectable version ranges from 35 to 100 mg per m2 of body surface depending on which disease is being treated. The injectable version is administered by intravenous infusion over 30 to 60 minutes. The recommended dosage for the oral version is two times the intravenous version. HCPCS Level II code J8560 represents 50 mg of oral etoposide.

Medicare Information
See chapter titled "Medicare Guidelines," under "Drugs, Biologicals, and Radiopharmaceuticals," for additional Medicare billing and documentation information.

J8562
J8562 Fludarabine phosphate, oral, 10 mg

Lay Description
Fludarabine phosphate is an antineoplastic drug that is a fluorinated nucleotide analogue of the antiviral agent vidarabine. It is rapidly broken down into 2-fluoro-ara-A, which inhibits DNA synthesis and causes cell death. Fludarabine phosphate is indicated for the treatment of beta-cell chronic lymphocytic leukemia for patients who have not responded to an alkylating drug treatment. This drug is available in liquid form for IV infusions or in tablet form for oral administration. The recommended dose for oral administration is 40 mg per meter squared of body surface area.

J8565
J8565 Gefitinib, oral, 250 mg

Lay Description
Gefitinib is a chemical complex used as an antineoplastic drug. It inhibits forms of the amino acid tyrosine from binding to epidermal growth factor receptor (EGFR) sites. EGFR is expressed on the cell surface of many normal cells and cancer cells. Gefitinib is indicated for the treatment of patients with locally advanced or metastatic non-small cell lung cancer after failure of both platinum-based and docetaxel chemotherapies. It is available only as an oral self-administrable drug. The recommended dosage is 250 mg daily. Gefitinib has limited distribution under a risk management plan called the IRESSATM Access Program, to the following patient populations: patients currently receiving and benefiting from gefitinib; patients who have previously received and benefited from gefitinib; and previously enrolled patients or new patients in non-Investigational New Drug (IND) clinical trials approved by an institutional review board prior to June 17, 2005. New patients may also be able to obtain gefitinib if the manufacturer decides to make it available under IND and the patients meet the criteria for enrollment under the IND. HCPCS Level II code J8565 represents 250 mg of oral gefitinib.

Medicare Information
Medicare does not cover oral anti-cancer drugs or biologicals if the drug does not have an injectable or instillable version. This drug is available only in oral form and is not covered as it is a self-administrable drug.

J8597
J8597 Antiemetic drug, oral, not otherwise specified

Lay Description
This code is used to report the supply of oral antiemetic drugs that do not have another specific HCPCS Level II code. An antiemetic drug is given to prevent or relieve nausea and vomiting. An oral antiemetic may be indicated at the time of chemotherapy treatment to help allay the side effect of nausea and vomiting that often accompanies chemotherapy.

Medicare Information
See chapter titled "Medicare Guidelines," under "Drugs, Biologicals, and Radiopharmaceuticals," for Medicare billing and documentation information.

J8600
J8600 Melphalan; oral, 2 mg

Lay Description
Melphalan hydrochloride is a derivative of nitrogen mustard used as an antineoplastic drug. It interferes with RNA synthesis causing cell death. Melphalan is indicated for the treatment of multiple myeloma and advanced epithelial ovarian cancer. The injectable form is used for the treatment of multiple myeloma when the oral form is inappropriate. The recommended oral dosage for ovarian cancer is 0.2 mg pr kg of body weight for five days. The recommended oral dosage for multiple myeloma is 6 mg per day for two to three weeks. Each course can be repeated after four weeks. HCPCS Level II code J8600 represents 2 mg of oral melphalan hydrochloride.

Medicare Information

See chapter titled "Medicare Guidelines," under "Drugs, Biologicals, and Radiopharmaceuticals," for additional Medicare billing and documentation information.

J8610

J8610 Methotrexate; oral, 2.5 mg

Lay Description

Methotrexate sodium is a chemical complex that blocks cell metabolism. It works by hindering the production of an enzyme needed for the metabolism of dividing cells, like those involved in inflammation and the immune response. Methotrexate has been found useful in treating diseases linked with abnormally rapid cell growth. It is indicated singularly or in combination as a treatment for gestational choriocarcinoma, chorioadenoma destruens, hydatidiform mole, breast cancer, epidermoid cancers of the head and neck, advanced mycosis fungoides, squamous and small cell lung cancer, advanced non-Hodgkin's lymphoma, acute lymphocytic leukemia, Burkitt's lymphoma, and lymphosarcoma. It is also used to treat rheumatoid and psoriatic arthritis and severe psoriasis that is unresponsive to other treatments. HCPCS Level II code J8610 represents 2.5 mg of oral methotrexate sodium.

Medicare Information

See chapter titled "Medicare Guidelines," under "Drugs, Biologicals, and Radiopharmaceuticals," for additional Medicare billing and documentation information.

J8650

J8650 Nabilone, oral, 1 mg

Lay Description

Nabilone is a Schedule II, synthetic cannabinoid that is similar to the active ingredient found in the plant marijuana. Nabilone, like its natural counterpart, produces complex effects on the central nervous system, including alterations in mental status. It is suggested that the antiemetic effect of nabilone is caused by the cannabinoid receptor system in neural tissues. Nabilone is indicated for the treatment of nausea and vomiting associated with cancer chemotherapy in patients who have not adequately responded to conventional antiemetics. Patients should only use this drug when they are under the close supervision of another person. These restrictions are required as many of the patients treated with nabilone will experience altered mental states that not observed with other antiemetic drugs. Nabilone has the potential for abuse and misuse. This is an oral drug with a recommended dosage of one to two mg twice a day during each cycle of chemotherapy. Maximum recommended dosage is six mg per day. If needed, administration of the drug may continue for 48 hours after the last dose of each chemotherapy cycle. HCPCS Level II code J8650 represents 1mg dose of oral nabilone.

J8700

J8700 Temozolomide, oral, 5 mg

Lay Description

Temozolomide is a chemical complex that is broken down in the liver into monomethyltriazene, also known as MTIC. MTIC causes breaks in the DNA, which prevents replication, thus interfering with tumor cell reproduction. Temozolomide is indicated for the treatment of adult patients with newly diagnosed glioblastoma multiforme, and for the treatment of adult patients with refractory anaplastic astrocytoma. Temozolomide is available only as a self-administrable oral drug. The recommended dosage is 75 mg per m2 of body surface. HCPCS Level II code J8700 represents 5 mg of oral temozolomide.

Medicare Information

See chapter titled "Medicare Guidelines," under "Drugs, Biologicals, and Radiopharmaceuticals," for additional Medicare billing and documentation information.

J8705

J8705 Topotecan, oral, 0.25 mg

Lay Description

Topotecan hydrochloride is an antineoplastic drug that is a semisynthetic derivative of camptothecin, an alkaloid extract from plants such as Camptotheca acuminata. The drug works by causing breaks in DNA that the cell cannot repair leading to cell death. Topotecan hydrochloride is indicated as a treatment for metastatic carcinoma of the ovaries after failure of prior chemotherapy. It is also indicated as a treatment for small cell lung cancer that responded to chemotherapy, but subsequently progressed. The recommended dose is 2.3 mg per m2 of body surface once daily for five consecutive days. HCPCS Level II code J8705 represents 0.25 mg of oral topotecan hydrochloride.

J8999

J8999 Prescription drug, oral, chemotherapeutic, NOS

Lay Description

Use this code to represent an oral prescription drug that has been taken as a form of chemotherapy, and is not represented by any other level I or level II HCPCS code.

J9000-J9001

J9000 Injection, doxorubicin HCl, 10 mg
J9001 Injection, doxorubicin HCl, all lipid formulations, 10 mg

Lay Description

Doxorubicin hydrochloride is an anthracycline antibiotic antineoplastic drug isolated from the bacterium Streptomyces peucetius var. caesius. It binds to DNA and inhibits RNA synthesis creating cell death. It is utilized to treat many forms of cancer, such as bladder, breast, lung, stomach, thyroid, Hodgkin's and non-Hodgkin's disease, acute lymphoblastic (ALL) and myeloblastic (AML) leukemia, and Wilms' tumor. The liposome version is the doxorubicin hydrochloride enclosed in a spherical lipid bilayer membrane. Doxorubicin hydrochloride liposome is indicated as a treatment for patients with ovarian cancer whose disease has recurred or progressed after platinum-based chemotherapy, and for patients with AIDS-related Kaposi's sarcoma whose disease has progressed on prior combination chemotherapy or who are intolerant of such therapy. Both versions are administered via intravenous injection. HCPCS Level II code J9000 represents 10 mg of doxorubicin hydrochloride. HCPCS Level II code J9001 represents 10 mg of the liposome version of doxorubicin hydrochloride.

Medicare Information

See chapter titled "Medicare Guidelines," under "Drugs, Biologicals, and Radiopharmaceuticals," for Medicare billing and documentation information.

J9010

J9010 Injection, alemtuzumab, 10 mg

Lay Description

Alemtuzumab is a monoclonal antibody produced by recombinant DNA technology in Chinese hamster ovaries. This monoclonal antibody is directed against the CD52 antigen, which is found on the surface of normal and malignant B and T lymphocytes, NK cells, monocytes, macrophages, and tissues of the male reproductive system. Alemtuzumab is indicated for the treatment of chronic B cell lymphocytic leukemia in patients who have been treated with alkylating agents and who have failed fludarabine therapy. The recommended initial dose is 3 mg rising to 30 mg as a maintenance dose. The drug is administered as a two-hour intravenous infusion. HCPCS Level II code J9010 represents 10 mg of alemtuzumab.

J9015

J9015 Injection, aldesleukin, per single use vial

Lay Description

Aldesleukin is an interleukin-2 product produced by recombinant DNA technology using a strain of Escherichia coli bacterium. Interleukin-2 is a non-antibody protein produced by T cells in response to an antigen or mitogenic stimulation. It stimulates the production of other T cells, the growth and cytolytic function of NK cells to produce lymphokine-activated killer cells, and is a growth factor for and stimulates antibody synthesis in B cells. It is also thought to promote cell death in antigen-activated T cells. Aldesleukin is indicated for the treatment of adults with metastatic renal cell carcinoma and for the treatment of adults with metastatic melanoma. The recommended dosage is 600,000 IU per kg of body weight administered every eight hours by a 15-minute IV infusion for a maximum of 14 doses. Following nine days of rest, the schedule is repeated for another 14 doses, for a maximum of 28 doses per course. HCPCS Level II code J9015 represents a single use vial of aldesleukin.

J9017

J9017 Injection, arsenic trioxide, 1 mg

Lay Description

Arsenic trioxide is a toxic element used as an antineoplastic agent. The actions of the drug are not completely understood. It is known to cause structural cell changes and DNA fragmentation leading to cellular death. Arsenic trioxide is indicated for the induction of remission and consolidation in patients with relapsing or refractory acute promyelocytic leukemia who have undergone retinoid or anthracycline chemotherapy and whose disease has a specific gene expression. The drug must be diluted and administered via an intravenous infusion over one to two hours. The infusion may be extended up to four hours if the patient develops acute vasomotor reactions. Recommended dosage for induction of remission is 0.15 mg per kg of body weight daily until bone marrow remission. The total induction dose should not exceed 60 doses. Recommended dosage for consolidation treatment is 0.15 mg per kg daily for 25 doses over a period up to five weeks. Consolidation treatment should begin three to six weeks after completion of induction therapy. HCPCS Level II code J9017 represents 1 mg of arsenic trioxide.

J9020

J9020 Injection, asparaginase, 10,000 units

Lay Description

Asparaginase is a synthetic version of the enzyme L-asparaginase produced by recombinant DNA technology using a strain of Escherichia coli bacterium. The enzyme catalyzes the breakdown of asparagine, an amino acid. Leukemia cells cannot synthesize asparagine and depend upon exogenous sources. Asparaginase deletes asparagine throughout the body. This depletion kills the leukemia cells. Normal cells can synthesize the asparagine and are unaffected. Asparaginase is indicated in the treatment of acute lymphocytic leukemia for pediatric and adult patients. The dosage depends upon body weight and whether the use is for induction or maintenance therapy. The drug may be administered as an intravenous infusion via an existing IV over 30 minutes. Asparaginase can also be injected intramuscularly with the volume administered at each injection site limited to 2 ml. When used to induce remission, the drug is usually given in combination with other chemotherapeutic agents. HCPCS Level II code J9020 represents 10,000 units of asparaginase.

J9025

J9025 Injection, azacitidine, 1 mg

Lay Description

Azacitidine is a pyrimidine nucleoside used as an antineoplastic agent. The drug disrupts the chemistry of DNA and causes cellular death in rapidly dividing cells including cancer cells that no longer respond to normal growth control mechanism. Azacitidine is indicated for the treatment of myelodysplastic syndrome subtypes: refractory anemia or refractory anemia with sideroblasts (if accompanied by neutropenia, thrombocytopenia, or requiring transfusions), refractory anemia with excess blasts, refractory anemia with excess blasts in transformation, and chronic myelomonocytic leukemia. The recommended initial treatment therapy is 75 mg per m_2 of body surface subcutaneously injected daily for seven days, every four weeks. The dosage may be increased to 100 mg per m_2 if no beneficial effect is seen after two treatment cycles and if no side effects other than nausea and vomiting occur. A minimum of four treatment cycles is recommended. However, treatment can continue as long as beneficial effects are evident. HCPCS Level II code J9025 represents 1 mg of azacitidine.

J9027

J9027 Injection, clofarabine, 1 mg

Lay Description

Clofarabine is a purine nucleoside that is an antineoplastic agent. The drug inhibits DNA synthesis and cellular repair leading to cell death. Clofarabine is attracted to rapidly proliferating cells and quiescent cancer cell types. It is indicated for the treatment of pediatric patients, ages 1 to 21 years, with relapsed or refractory acute lymphoblastic leukemia who have undergone at least two prior treatment regimens. Recommended dosage is 52 mg per m2 of body surface infused intravenously over two hours for five consecutive days. This regimen may be repeated every two to six weeks. HCPCS Level II code J9027 represents 1 mg of clofarabine.

J9031

J9031 BCG (intravesical) per instillation

Lay Description

BCG live, intravesical is a freeze-dried preparation of Bacillus Calmette and Guerin, which is a weakened version of Mycobacterium bovis. Mycobacterium bovis is a form of tuberculous originally isolated from cattle. It is used as an antineoplastic agent. The BCG is reconstituted and administered intravesically into the urinary bladder. One dose is usually 81 mg of BCG reconstituted by a diluent and further diluted by 50 ml of sterile water. It causes a local acute inflammation with macrophage and lymphocyte infiltration of the bladder. The exact anti-tumor mechanism is unknown, but it is thought to be created by the lymphocyte reaction. BCG live, intravesical is indicated for the treatment and prophylaxis of carcinoma in situ of the urinary bladder, and for the prophylaxis of primary or recurrent stage Ta and/or stage T1 papillary tumors following transurethral resection. HCPCS Level II code J9031 represents one instillation of BCG live, which is one vial.

J9033

J9033 Injection, bendamustine HCl, 1 mg

Lay Description

Bendamustine HCl is an antineoplastic drug used to treat chronic lymphocytic leukemia. It is also used to treat indolent B-cell non-Hodgkin's lymphoma when the disease has progressed after being treated with rituximab. The recommended dose is 100 mg per square centimeter administered by IV adminisration on days one and two of a 28-day cycle, up to six cycles. HCPCS level II code J9033 represents 1 mg of bendamustine HCl.

J9035

J9035   Injection, bevacizumab, 10 mg

Lay Description

Bevacizumab is a monoclonal antibody produced by recombinant DNA technology in Chinese hamster ovaries. This monoclonal antibody binds to and inhibits the biologic activity of human vascular endothelial growth factor preventing the formation of new blood vessels. Bevacizumab, used in combination with intravenous 5-fluorouracil, is indicated for first-line treatment of patients with metastatic carcinoma of the colon or rectum. The recommended dose is 5 mg per kg of body weight administered once every 14 days disease progression is detected. Bevacizumab is administered by intravenous infusion. The initial dose infusion should be delivered over 90 minutes. If the first infusion is well tolerated, the second infusion may be administered over 60 minutes. If the 60-minute infusion is well tolerated, all subsequent infusions may be administered over 30 minutes. HCPCS Level II code J9035 represents 10 mg of bevacizumab.

Medicare Information

See the chapter titled "Medicare Guidelines," under "Drugs, Biologicals, and Radiopharmaceuticals," for Medicare information.

Medicare will cover off-label use of bevacizumab when used in one of nine clinical trials identified by CMS and sponsored by the National Cancer Institute. A list of clinical trials is available at http://cms.hhs.gov/coverage/download/id90b.pdf.

J9040

J9040   Injection, bleomycin sulfate, 15 units

Lay Description

Bleomycin sulfate is an antibiotic antineoplastic drug produced from a strain of Streptomyces verticillus. It is thought to cause cell death by the inhibition of DNA synthesis with some inhibition of RNA and protein synthesis. Bleomycin sulfate is indicated as a single agent or in combination with other therapeutic agents for squamous cell carcinoma, Hodgkin's disease, non-Hodgkin's lymphoma, testicular carcinoma, and for treatment of malignant pleural effusion. It can be administered as an intravenous, intramuscular, or subcutaneous injection. Bleomycin sulfate may also be administered into the pleural cavity. The recommended dosage for pleural cavity administration is 60 units. The recommended dosage for other administration is 0.25 to 0.50 units per kg of body weight administered once or twice a week. HCPCS Level II code J9040 represents 15 units of bleomycin sulfate.

Medicare Information

See chapter titled "Medicare Guidelines," under "Drugs, Biologicals, and Radiopharmaceuticals," for Medicare billing and documentation information.

J9041

J9041   Injection, bortezomib, 0.1 mg

Lay Description

Bortezomib is a modified form of boronic acid used as an antineoplastic agent. Boron is a nonmetallic element and boric acid is a form of boron. The drug inhibits the activity of a protein complex that regulates the intracellular concentration of specific proteins within a cell. This disruption of cell stability can lead to cell death. Bortezomib is indicated for the treatment of multiple myeloma in patients who have received at least two prior therapies and who have demonstrated disease progression on the last therapy. The recommended therapy is 1.3 mg per m2 of body surface injected intravenously twice weekly for two weeks with a subsequent 10-day rest period. This three-week period is considered one treatment cycle. Bortezomib may be administered for a maximum of eight treatment cycles. HCPCS Level II code J9041 represents 0.1 mg of bortezomib.

J9045

J9045   Injection, carboplatin, 50 mg

Lay Description

Carboplatin is a chemical complex containing the metal platinum used as an antineoplastic drug. It binds to DNA disrupting synthesis and causing cell death. Carboplatin is similar to, but more stable than cisplatin. It is indicated as an initial treatment for advanced ovarian cancer in combination with other chemotherapeutic agents. Carboplatin is also indicated as a secondary treatment of recurrent ovarian carcinoma after prior chemotherapy, including patients who have been previously treated with cisplatin. Dosage depends upon patient body surface, patient reactions to the drug, and whether it is used as a single agent or in combination. Carboplatin is administered by an intravenous infusion lasting 15 minutes or longer. Aluminum reacts with carboplatin causing a loss of potency, therefore, needles or intravenous sets containing aluminum parts that may come in contact with the drug must not be used for its preparation or administration. HCPCS Level II code J9045 represents 50 mg of carboplatin.

J9050

J9050 Injection, carmustine, 100 mg

Lay Description

Carmustine is one of the nitrosoureas, alkylating agents used as antineoplastic drugs. Nitrosoureas are a group of similar drugs that are highly lipid-soluble and cross the blood-brain barrier. Carmustine inhibits DNA repair causing cell death. It is indicated as a single agent or in combination therapy for the treatment of brain tumors, multiple myeloma, colorectal cancer, Hodgkin's disease, and non-Hodgkin's lymphoma. Dosage depends upon patient body surface, patient reactions to the drug, and whether it is used as a single agent or in combination. Carmustine is administered as an intravenous injection. HCPCS Level II code J9050 represents 100 mg of injectable carmustine.

J9055

J9055 Injection, cetuximab, 10 mg

Lay Description

Cetuximab is monoclonal antibody produced by recombinant DNA technology in a murine cell culture. This antibody binds specifically to the epidermal growth factor receptor (EGFR, HER1, c-ErbB-1) on both normal and tumor cells resulting in inhibition of cell growth and causing cell death. Cetuximab, used in combination with irinotecan, is indicated for the treatment of EGFR-expressing, metastatic colorectal carcinoma in patients who are refractory to irinotecan-based chemotherapy. Cetuximab, administered as a single agent, is also indicated for the treatment of EGFR-expressing, metastatic colorectal carcinoma in patients who are intolerant to irinotecan-based chemotherapy. The recommended initial dosage for combination or as a single agent is 400 mg per m2 of body surface administered as a 120-minute intravenous infusion. The recommended weekly maintenance dose is 250 mg per m2 of body surface infused intravenously over 60 minutes. HCPCS Level II code J9055 represents 10 mg of cetuximab.

Medicare Information

See the chapter titled "Medicare Guidelines," under "Drugs, Biologicals, and Radiopharmaceuticals," for Medicare information.

Medicare will cover off-label use of cetuximab when used in one of nine clinical trials identified by CMS and sponsored by the National Cancer Institute. A list of clinical trials is available at http://cms.hhs.gov/coverage/download/id90b.pdf.

J9060

J9060 Injection, cisplatin, powder or solution, 10 mg

Lay Description

Cisplatin is a chemical complex containing the metal platinum used as an antineoplastic drug. It binds to DNA disrupting synthesis and causing cell death. Cisplatin is indicated in combination therapy for treatment of metastatic testicular and ovarian cancer after surgical and radiation therapy. Cisplatin is indicated as a single agent treatment for advanced transitional cell bladder cancer that can no longer be treated locally, such as with surgery or radiation therapy. As a single agent, it may also be used as a secondary treatment for metastatic ovarian cancer that is refractory to standard chemotherapy where cisplatin has not been previously administered. Cisplatin is administered as an intravenous infusion. Dosage depends upon patient body surface, patient reactions to the drug, and whether it is used as a single agent or in combination. Aluminum reacts with cisplatin causing a loss of potency; therefore, needles or intravenous sets containing aluminum parts that may come in contact with the drug must not be used for its preparation or administration.

J9065

J9065 Injection, cladribine, per 1 mg

Lay Description

Cladribine is a synthetic version of adenosine used as an antineoplastic drug. Cladribine interferes with DNA repair and causes cell death. Cladribine is indicated as a treatment for active hairy cell leukemia. The recommended initial dosage is 0.9 mg per kg of body weight. It is administered by a continuous intravenous infusion over 24 hours. This continuous infusion is repeated daily for seven consecutive days. HCPCS Level II code J9065 represents 1 mg of cladribine.

Medicare Information

See chapter titled "Medicare Guidelines," under "Drugs, Biologicals, and Radiopharmaceuticals," for Medicare billing and documentation information.

J9070

J9070 Cyclophosphamide, 100 mg

Lay Description

Cyclophosphamide is a synthetic antineoplastic drug chemically related to the nitrogen mustards. The drug itself is inert and functions only after transformation in the liver to active alkylating metabolites. These metabolites interfere with the growth of susceptible rapidly proliferating malignant cells. The mechanism of action is thought to be its interference with the DNA of the tumor cell causing cell death. Cyclophosphamide is indicated singularly or in combination with other chemotherapeutic drugs, to treat a wide variety of cancers including Hodgkin's disease, lymphosarcoma, acute lymphocytic leukemia, Burkitt's lymphoma, carcinoma of the breast, multiple myeloma, chronic lymphocytic leukemia, bronchogenic carcinoma, neuroblastoma, ovarian carcinoma, and carcinoma of the uterine cervix. It is also used as an immunosuppressant to prevent transplant rejection and in the treatment of certain diseases with abnormal immune function, including severe lupus manifestations and vasculitis. Cyclophosphamide may be administered via intravenous injection or infusion, or may be injected intramuscularly, intraperitoneally, or intrapleurally. An oral version is also available. Dosage depends upon body weight and the disease being treated. The lyophilized version of cyclophosphamide is a freeze-dried version of the drug.

J9098-J9100

J9098 Injection, cytarabine liposome, 10 mg
J9100 Injection, cytarabine, 100 mg

Lay Description

Cytarabine is a synthetic nucleoside used as an antineoplastic drug. The drug interferes with DNA synthesis causing cell death. Cytarabine is indicated singularly or in combination with other chemotherapeutic drugs to induce remission in acute nonlymphocytic leukemia in adults and children and to treat acute lymphocytic leukemia and the blast phase of chronic myelocytic leukemia. Intrathecal cytarabine is indicated in the prophylaxis and treatment of meningeal leukemia. Cytarabine may be administered via intravenous injection or infusion, or may be injected intramuscularly, intraperitoneally, intrapleurally, or intrathecally. Dosage depends upon body weight and the disease being treated. The liposome version of cytarabine is a suspension of cytarabine encapsulated with liposomes. The liposome version is administered intrathecally to treat meningitis associated with lymphoma.

Medicare Information

See chapter titled "Medicare Guidelines," under "Drugs, Biologicals, and Radiopharmaceuticals," for Medicare billing and documentation information.

J9120

J9120 Injection, dactinomycin, 0.5 mg

Lay Description

Dactinomycin, also known as actinomycin D, is an antibiotic, produced by a strain of Streptomyces parvulus bacterium that is used as an antineoplastic agent. The drug inhibits RNA synthesis leading to cellular death. Dactinomycin is indicated in combination therapy for the treatment of Wilms' tumor, childhood rhabdomyosarcoma, Ewing's sarcoma, and metastatic nonseminomatous testicular cancer. The drug may be used as a single agent or in combination as a treatment for gestational trophoblastic neoplasia. Dactinomycin is also indicated as a part of a regional perfusion for the palliative and/or adjunctive treatment of locally recurrent or locoregional sarcoma, carcinoma, and adenocarcinoma. Recommended dosages vary by the type of neoplasm being treated and the patient's body surface or weight. The drug is highly toxic even in powdered form and is extremely corrosive to soft tissue. Dactinomycin is administered intravenously. HCPCS Level II code J9120 represents 0.5 mg of dactinomycin.

J9130

J9130 Dacarbazine, 100 mg

Lay Description

Dacarbazine, also known as DTIC, is a chemical complex that is an antineoplastic agent. The drug interferes with DNA synthesis causing cell death. Dacarbazine is indicated in the treatment of metastatic malignant melanoma. It is also used in combination with other chemotherapeutic agents as a treatment for Hodgkin's disease. The drug is administered by intravenous injection or infusion. The recommended dosage depends upon body surface, the disease being treated, and the treatment plan.

J9150-J9151

J9150 Injection, daunorubicin, 10 mg
J9151 Injection, daunorubicin citrate, liposomal formulation, 10 mg

Lay Description

Daunorubicin hydrochloride is an anthracycline antibiotic, produced by a strain of Streptomyces coeruleorubidus bacterium, that is used as an antineoplastic agent. The drug interrupts DNA synthesis creating breaks within the DNA strands leading to cellular death. Daunorubicin hydrochloride is indicated in combination with other chemotherapeutic agents for the remission induction of acute nonlymphocytic leukemia (myelogenous, monocytic, and erythroid) in adults and for acute lymphocytic leukemia in both children and adults. Recommended dosages are 25 to 30 mg per m^2 of body surface infused intravenously. In children younger than 2 years of age, it is recommended that the dose be based on body weight rather than body surface. The drug should never be given by intramuscular or subcutaneous injection. The length of a regimen and the subsequent courses of therapy depend upon the patient and type of leukemia being treated. Daunorubicin citrate liposome is indicted for the treatment of HIV-related advanced Kaposi's sarcoma. HCPCS Level II code J9150 represents 10 mg of daunorubicin hydrochloride. When the drug is encapsulated in lipid microspheres (liposome), it is represented by HCPCS Level II code J9151 in 10 mg units.

J9155

J9155   Injection, degarelix, 1 mg

Lay Description

Degarelix is a gonadotropin releasing hormone (GnRH) receptor inhibitor used to treat patients with advanced prostate cancer. It inhibits the testosterone, which retards the growth of cancer in the prostate. It's a synthetic mixture that contains seven amino acids. The recommended dose is 240 mg initially administered by two subcutaneous injections of 120 mg each. The recommended maintenance dose is 80 mg given as a single subcutaneous injection every 28 days.

J9160

J9160   Injection, denileukin diftitox, 300 mcg

Lay Description

Denileukin diftitox is a modified form of the diphtheria toxin produced from E. coli bacterium using recombinant DNA technology. This biological is used as an antineoplastic agent. It binds to IL-2 receptor sites on certain cells delivering the diphtheria toxin, which inhibits cellular protein synthesis causing the death of the cell. This receptor is usually highly active in activated B and T lymphocytes and macrophages. Denileukin diftitox is indicated for the treatment of persistent or recurrent cutaneous T cell lymphoma where the cells express the CD25 component of the IL-2 receptor. The biological is administered via an intravenous infusion of at least 15 minutes, daily for five consecutive days. This regimen should be administered every 21 days. The recommended dose is 9 or 18 mcg per kg of body weight. HCPCS Level II code J9160 represents 300 mcg of denileukin diftitox.

J9165

J9165   Injection, diethylstilbestrol diphosphate, 250 mg

Lay Description

Diethylstilbestrol (DES) diphosphate is a synthetic estrogen used as a hormone treatment for advanced prostate cancer. Estrogen is a hormone produced by the ovaries, adrenal gland, testis, and placenta. While small amounts are present in males, it is generally referred to as the female sex hormone. The high levels of estrogen within the body cause a decrease in testosterone production that can slow the growth of prostatic cancer cells. HCPCS Level II code J9165 represents 250 mg of the injectable version of DES.

J9171

J9171   Injection, docetaxel, 1 mg

Lay Description

Docetaxel is a semisynthetic antineoplastic drug created from the needles of the yew tree. The drug inhibits cell division, which stops the cancer cells from reproducing. Docetaxel is indicated as a single agent for the treatment of locally advanced or metastatic breast cancer after failure of prior chemotherapy and for locally advanced or metastatic nonsmall cell lung cancer after failure of prior platinum-based chemotherapy. In combination with other chemotherapeutic agents, it is indicated as adjuvant treatment of patients with operable node-positive breast cancer; patients with hormone refractory metastatic prostate cancer; patients with unresectable, locally advanced or metastatic nonsmall cell lung cancer who have not previously received chemotherapy for this condition; patient advanced gastric adenocarcinoma who have not received prior chemotherapy for advanced disease; and induction treatment of patients with inoperable locally advanced squamous cell carcinoma of the head and neck. Docetaxel is infused intravenously over one hour. Dosage depends upon m2 of patient body surface and the disease being treated. HCPCS Level II code J9171 represents 1 mg of docetaxel.

J9175

J9175   Injection, Elliotts' B solution, 1 ml

Lay Description

Elliotts B solution is a diluent of buffered electrolytes and dextrose that is comparable in pH, composition, and osmolarity to cerebrospinal fluid. Elliotts B solution is indicated as a diluent for the intrathecal administration of methotrexate sodium and cytarabine for the prevention or treatment of meningeal leukemia or lymphocytic lymphoma. HCPCS Level II code J9175 represents 1 ml of Elliotts B solution.

Medicare Information

See chapter titled "Medicare Guidelines," under "Drugs, Biologicals, and Radiopharmaceuticals," for Medicare billing and documentation information.

J9178

J9178   Injection, epirubicin HCl, 2 mg

Lay Description

Epirubicin hydrochloride (HCl) is an anthracycline, antibiotic, antineoplastic drug that is chemically similar to doxorubicin hydrochloride, but has a lower toxicity. It binds to DNA inhibiting RNA and protein synthesis creating cell death. Epirubicin hydrochloride is used as an adjunctive therapy for patients with primary breast cancer who have evidence of axillary node involvement following surgical resection. It is also indicated in the treatment of cancers of the lung, stomach, ovary, colon, and rectum, and for treatment of leukemia, lymphoma, and multiple myeloma. The initial recommended dosage is 100 to 120 mg per m2 of body surface administered as an intravenous infusion over 15 to 20 minutes. Dosages administered after the initial dose depend upon the patient's reaction and the infusion time for subsequent doses may be significantly decreased. HCPCS Level II code J9178 represents 2 mg of epirubicin hydrochloride.

J9181

J9181   Injection, etoposide, 10 mg

Lay Description

Etoposide is a semisynthetic derivative of podophyllotoxin, a toxic compound found in the rhizomes and roots of the mandrake plant. It is believed to inhibit the repair of DNA causing cell death. Etoposide is an antineoplastic drug used in combination with other chemotherapeutic agents. It is available in injectable or oral versions. Injectable etoposide is indicated for the treatment of small cell lung cancer and refractory testicular cancer that has been previously treated with surgery, radiation, or other chemotherapy. The oral version is indicated for the treatment of small cell lung cancer. The recommended dosage of the injectable version ranges from 35 to 100 mg per m2 of body surface depending on which disease is being treated. The injectable version is administered by intravenous infusion over 30 to 60 minutes. The recommended dosage for the oral version is two times the intravenous version. HCPCS Level II code J9181 represents 10 mg of injectable etoposide.

J9185

J9185   Injection, fludarabine phosphate, 50 mg

Lay Description

Fludarabine phosphate is an antineoplastic drug that is a fluorinated nucleotide analogue of the antiviral agent vidarabine. It is rapidly broken down into 2-fluoro-ara-A which inhibits DNA synthesis and causes cell death. Fludarabine phosphate is indicated for the treatment of beta-cell chronic lymphocytic leukemia for patients who have not responded to an alkylating drug treatment. It is administered through intravenous infusion over 30 minutes for five consecutive days. The recommended dosage is 25 mg per m2 of body surface. HCPCS Level II code J9185 represents 50 mg of fludarabine phosphate.

J9190

J9190   Injection, fluorouracil, 500 mg

Lay Description

Fluorouracil, also known as 5 FU, is an antineoplastic drug that is a fluorinated analogue of uracil. Uracil is a chemical compound found in nucleic acids. Once broken down, it interferes with the synthesis of DNA and RNA causing cell death. Fluorouracil is available in injectable and topical versions. The injectable version is indicated for the treatment of many different cancers, among them cancer of the breast, stomach, pancreas, and colon. The topical version is used to treat actinic or solar keratoses and superficial basal cell carcinomas. Dosage for the injectable version depends upon body weight and is administered by intravenous injection. HCPCS Level II code J9190 represents 500 mg of the injectable version of fluorouracil.

Medicare Information

See chapter titled "Medicare Guidelines," under "Drugs, Biologicals, and Radiopharmaceuticals," for Medicare billing and documentation information.

J9200

J9200   Injection, floxuridine, 500 mg

Lay Description

Floxuridine, also known as FUDR, is an antineoplastic drug that is broken down into the same substance as fluorouracil. It interferes with the synthesis of DNA and RNA causing cell death. Floxuridine is administered by continuous intra-arterial infusion using a pump. It is indicated as a palliative treatment of gastrointestinal adenocarcinoma that has metastasized to the liver in patients who are considered incurable by surgery or other means. The recommended dosage is 0.1 to 0.6 mg per kg of body weight per day. HCPCS Level II code J9200 represents 500 mg of floxuridine.

Medicare Information

See chapter titled "Medicare Guidelines," under "Drugs, Biologicals, and Radiopharmaceuticals," for Medicare billing and documentation information.

J9201

J9201   Injection, gemcitabine HCl, 200 mg

Lay Description

Gemcitabine hydrochloride is a nucleoside analogue used as an antineoplastic drug. It interferes with the synthesis of DNA and RNA causing cell death. Gemcitabine hydrochloride in combination with paclitaxel is indicated as a treatment for metastatic breast cancer after the failure of prior chemotherapy. It is indicated in combination with cisplatin in the treatment of inoperable locally advanced or metastatic non-small cell lung cancer. As a sole agent, gemcitabine hydrochloride is indicated as a treatment for inoperable locally advanced or metastatic pancreatic cancer previously treated with fluorouracil. The recommended initial dosage is from 1,000 to 1,250 mg per m2 of body surface administered by intravenous infusion over 30 minutes. HCPCS Level II code J9201 represents 200 mg of gemcitabine hydrochloride.

J9202

J9202   Goserelin acetate implant, per 3.6 mg

Lay Description

Goserelin acetate is a synthetic analogue of the luteinizing hormone-releasing hormone (LHRH) used as an antineoplastic drug. The implant is a biodegradable tube containing 3.6 mg of goserelin acetate that is slowly released over 28 days. This continued administration leads to suppression of pituitary gonadotropins and subsequently to lower levels of estrogen and testosterone. The goserelin acetate implant is indicated as a palliative treatment for advanced breast and prostatic cancer. In combination with flutamide, it is indicated for treatment of locally confined prostate cancer stage T2b-T4 (Stage B2-C). It may also be indicated as a treatment for endometriosis and as an endometrial-thinning agent prior to ablation. The goserelin acetate implant is injected subcutaneously into the upper abdominal wall every 28 days. HCPCS Level II code J9202 represents one 3.6 mg implant of goserelin acetate.

J9206

J9206   Injection, irinotecan, 20 mg

Lay Description

Irinotecan hydrochloride (HCL) is an antineoplastic drug that is a semisynthetic derivative of camptothecin, an alkaloid extract from plants such as Camptotheca acuminata. The drug works by causing strand breaks in DNA that the cell cannot repair leading to cell death. Irinotecan is indicated as a first line treatment in combination with fluorouracil and leucovorin for metastatic carcinoma of the colon or rectum. Irinotecan is also indicated for patients with metastatic carcinoma of the colon or rectum whose disease has recurred or progressed following initial fluorouracil-based therapy. The recommended dosage varies from 125 to 300 mg depending on the regimen. Irinotecan hydrochloride is administered by intravenous infusion over 90 minutes. HCPCS Level II code J9206 represents 20 mg of irinotecan hydrochloride.

Medicare Information

See the chapter titled "Medicare Guidelines," under "Drugs, Biologicals, and Radiopharmaceuticals," for Medicare information.

Medicare will cover off-label use of irinotecan when used in one of nine clinical trials identified by CMS and sponsored by the National Cancer Institute. A list of clinical trials is available at http://cms.hhs.gov/coverage/download/id90b.pdf.

J9207

J9207   Injection, ixabepilone, 1 mg

Lay Description

Ixabepilone is an antineoplastic drug used to treat metastatic or locally advanced breast cancer that is resistant to anthracycline and taxane or if those treatments are contraindicated. It inhibits cell division, which leads to cell death. The recommended dose is 40 mg/m2 by intravenous infusion over three hours. The treatment is administered every three weeks. HCPCS Level II code represents 1 milligram.

J9208

J9208   Injection, ifosfamide, 1 g

Lay Description

Ifosfamide is an antineoplastic that is a synthetic analogue of cyclophosphamide and is related to the nitrogen mustards. The drug functions only after transformation in the liver to active alkylating metabolites. These metabolites interfere with the DNA causing cell death. Ifosfamide is indicated as a third-line treatment for germ cell testicular cancer. The recommended dosage is 1.2 g per m2 of body surface administered by slow intravenous infusion over 30 minutes, through five consecutive days. Mesna is often given with ifosfamide as a prophylactic agent against hemorrhagic cystitis. HCPCS Level II code J9208 represents 1 gram of ifosfamide.

J9209

J9209   Injection, mesna, 200 mg

Lay Description

Mesna is a synthetic sulfur-hydrogen compound that is used as a detoxifying agent to inhibit the hemorrhagic cystitis caused by ifosfamide. Once broken down in the body, the drug combines with the urotoxic byproducts of ifosfamide rendering them harmless. Mesna is available in injectable and oral versions. The dosage is dependent upon the amount of ifosfamide givenÑcalculated at 20 percent the amount of ifosfamide. Mesna is administered as an intravenous injection at the time of ifosfamide administration, and then repeated at four and eight hours following the administration. Alternately, the first does may be by intravenous injection and the subsequent doses may be oral. HCPCS Level II code J9209 represents 200 mg of mesna.

J9211
J9211 Injection, idarubicin HCl, 5 mg

Lay Description
Idarubicin hydrochloride is an antineoplastic drug that is a semisynthetic analogue of daunorubicin. It interferes with DNA synthesis causing cell death. Idarubicin hydrochloride is indicated in combination with other chemotherapeutic drugs for the treatment of acute myeloid leukemia. The recommended dosage is 12 mg per m2 of body surface. Idarubicin hydrochloride is administered by intravenous infusion over 10 to 15 minutes. HCPCS Level II code J9211 represents 5 mg of idarubicin hydrochloride.

J9212
J9212 Injection, interferon alfacon-1, recombinant, 1 mcg

Lay Description
Interferon alfacon-1 is a non-natural form of human interferon alpha proteins that are produced by recombinant DNA technology. Interferons are small, naturally occurring proteins that bind to specific cell membranes and initial a series of events that include the inhibition of virus replication and the enhancement of macrophage and lymphocyte destruction of foreign cells. Interferon alfacon-1 is indicated for the treatment of chronic hepatitis C. The recommended dosage is 9 to 15 mcg administered as a subcutaneous injection every 48 hours for 24 weeks. HCPCS Level II code J9212 represents 1 mcg of interferon alfacon-1.

J9213
J9213 Injection, interferon, alfa-2a, recombinant, 3 million units

Lay Description
Interferon alfa-2a is a purified form of human interferon alpha proteins that are produced by recombinant DNA technology using Escherichia coli bacteria. Interferons are small, naturally occurring proteins that bind to specific cell membranes and initial a series of events that include the inhibition of virus replication and the enhancement of macrophage and lymphocyte destruction of foreign cells. Interferon alfa-2a is indicated for the treatment of AIDS-related Kaposi's sarcoma, hairy cell leukemia, chronic hepatitis C, and in Philadelphia chromosome-positive chronic myelogenous leukemia. The recommended dosage is 3 to 9 million IU depending upon the disease being treated.

Interferon alfa-2a is administered as an intramuscular or subcutaneous injection daily. Prefilled syringes are intended for subcutaneous injection only. HCPCS Level II code J9213 represents 3 million units of interferon alfa-2a.

J9214
J9214 Injection, interferon, alfa-2b, recombinant, 1 million units

Lay Description
Interferon alfa-2b is a purified form of human interferon alpha proteins that are produced by recombinant DNA technology using Escherichia coli bacteria. Interferons are small, naturally occurring proteins that bind to specific cell membranes and initial a series of events that include the inhibition of virus replication and the enhancement of macrophage and lymphocyte destruction of foreign cells. Interferon alfa-2b is indicated for the treatment of hairy cell leukemia, malignant melanoma, genital or venereal warts, Kaposi's sarcoma, and chronic hepatitis B and C. It is also indicated in combination with other chemotherapeutic agents as an initial treatment of clinically aggressive follicular non-Hodgkin's lymphoma. The recommended dosage varies from 5 to 25 million IU depending upon the disease being treated. Interferon alfa-2b can be administered as an intramuscular, subcutaneous, or intravenous infusion over 20 minutes or intralesional injection. HCPCS Level II code J9214 represents 1 million units of interferon alfa-2b.

J9215
J9215 Injection, interferon, alfa-N3, (human leukocyte derived), 250,000 IU

Lay Description
Interferon alfa-N3 is a purified form of human interferon alpha proteins that is derived from human leukocytes. The human leukocytes are induced by inoculation with a murine virus to produce the interferon alfa proteins. Interferons are small naturally occurring proteins that bind to specific cell membranes and initiate a series of events that include the inhibition of virus replication and the enhancement of macrophage and lymphocyte destruction of foreign cells. Interferon alfa-N3 is indicated for the treatment of condylomata acuminata (genital warts) where it is injected intralesionally. Interferon alfa-N3 has also been used off-label to treat multiple sclerosis, hepatitis C, and some cancers. HCPCS Level II code J9215 represents 250,000 IU of interferon alfa-N3.

J9216

J9216 Injection, interferon, gamma 1-b, 3 million units

Lay Description

Interferon gamma-1b is a purified form of human interferon gamma proteins that are produced by recombinant DNA technology using Escherichia coli bacteria. Interferons are small, naturally occurring proteins that bind to specific cell membranes and initial a series of events that include the inhibition of virus replication and the enhancement of macrophage and lymphocyte destruction of foreign cells. Interferon gamma-1b is indicated for the treatment of chronic granulomatous disease and severe malignant osteopetrosis. The recommended dosage varies from 1 to 1.5 million units per m2 of body surface. Interferon gamma-1b is administered as a subcutaneous injection. HCPCS Level II code J9216 represents 3 million units of interferon gamma-1b.

J9217-J9219

J9217 Leuprolide acetate (for depot suspension), 7.5 mg
J9218 Leuprolide acetate, per 1 mg
J9219 Leuprolide acetate implant, 65 mg

Lay Description

Leuprolide acetate is a synthetic analogue of the luteinizing hormone-releasing hormone (LHRH) that is used as an antineoplastic drug and a treatment for central precocious puberty, endometriosis, and uterine fibroids. It first stimulates and then suppresses follicle stimulating and luteinizing hormone release, resulting in suppression of testosterone and estrogen. A depot suspension is a drug that remains in the body long-term in storage and is slowly released into the blood. The leuprolide acetate depot suspension in dosages of 3.75 mg monthly and the 12.25 mg every three months are injected intramuscularly to treat endometriosis and uterine fibroids. When used to treat central precocious puberty, the dosage is individualized to the child and can range from 7.5 to 15 mg. Leuprolide acetate in doses of 7.5 mg and greater is injected subcutaneously and is used as a palliative treatment for advanced prostate cancer. The leuprolide acetate implant is a non-biodegradable tube containing 72 mg. The implant delivers the drug over a 12-month period. The implant is inserted subcutaneously in the inner portion of the upper arm. It must be removed or replaced when the drug is depleted. The leuprolide acetate implant is used as a palliative treatment of advanced prostate cancer. HCPCS Level II code J9217 represents 7.5 mg of leuprolide acetate in depot suspension. HCPCS Level II code J9218 represents 1 mg of leuprolide acetate and J9219 represents one 65 mg implant.

J9225-J9226

J9225 Histrelin implant (Vantas), 50 mg
J9226 Histrelin implant (Supprelin LA), 50 mg

Lay Description

A histrelin implant is a thin, flexible tube inserted subcutaneously that contains 50 mg of histrelin acetate, a synthetic version of luteinizing hormone-releasing hormone or gonadotropin-releasing hormone. Luteinizing hormone-releasing hormone is produced by the pituitary gland that stimulates the ovaries (to release an ovum), the release of estrogen, and certain cells in the testis. A histrelin implant is indicated as a palliative treatment for advanced prostate cancer. Histrelin decreases testosterone levels to castrate levels. A histrelin implant is also indicated for the treatment of children with central precocious puberty, who have an early onset of secondary sexual characteristics (earlier than 8 years of age in females and 9 years of age in males). They also show a significantly advanced bone age that can result in diminished adult height attainment. The implant contains 50 mg of histrelin, administered continuously over a 12-month period. When depleted, the implant must be removed and can be replaced with another implant. Code J9225 represents 50 mg of the Vantas® implant, and J9226 represents 50 mg of the Supprelin® implant.

J9230

J9230 Injection, mechlorethamine HCl, (nitrogen mustard), 10 mg

Lay Description

Mechlorethamine hydrochloride, also known as nitrogen mustard, is a highly toxic chemical complex used as an antineoplastic drug. In water or body fluids, it is rapidly transformed and acts by interfering with RNA synthesis causing an imbalance of growth, which then leads to cell death. Administered as an intravenous injection, mechlorethamine hydrochloride is indicated for the treatment of Hodgkin's disease, lymphosarcoma, polycythemia vera, chronic lymphocytic and myelocytic leukemias, mycosis fungoides, and bronchogenic cancers. When administered intrapleurally, intraperitoneally, or intrapericardially, it is used to treat malignant effusions. The recommended dosage is 0.4 mg per kg of body weight per day. The dosage may be divided into smaller doses. HCPCS Level II code J9230 represents 10 mg of mechlorethamine hydrochloride.

J9245
J9245 Injection, melphalan HCl, 50 mg

Lay Description
Melphalan hydrochloride is a derivative of nitrogen mustard used as an antineoplastic drug. It interferes with RNA synthesis causing cell death. Melphalan is indicated for the treatment of multiple myeloma and advanced epithelial ovarian cancer. The drug is available in oral and injectable form. The injectable form is used for the treatment of multiple myeloma when the oral form is inappropriate. The recommended oral dosage for ovarian cancer is 0.2 mg per kg of body weight for five days. The The recommended intravenous dosage is 16 mg per m^2 of body surface administered as a single infusion over 15 to 20 minutes. The intravenous dosage is administered at two-week intervals for four doses, then at four-week intervals. HCPCS Level II code J9245 represents 50 mg of injectable melphalan hydrochloride.

J9250-J9260
J9250 Methotrexate sodium, 5 mg
J9260 Methotrexate sodium, 50 mg

Lay Description
Methotrexate sodium is a chemical complex that blocks cell metabolism. It works by hindering the production of an enzyme needed for the metabolism of dividing cells, like those involved in inflammation and the immune response. Methotrexate has been found useful in treating diseases linked with abnormally rapid cell growth. It is indicated singularly or in combination as a treatment for gestational choriocarcinoma, chorioadenoma destruens, hydatidiform mole, breast cancer, epidermoid cancers of the head and neck, advanced mycosis fungoides, squamous and small cell lung cancer, advanced non-Hodgkin's lymphoma, acute lymphocytic leukemia, Burkitt's lymphoma, and lymphosarcoma. It is also used to treat rheumatoid and psoriatic arthritis and severe psoriasis that is unresponsive to other treatments. HCPCS Level II code J9250 represents 5 mg of injectable methotrexate sodium and J9260 represents 50 mg of injectable methotrexate sodium.

J9261
J9261 Injection, nelarabine, 50 mg

Lay Description
Nalarabine is an antineoplastic prodrug that is converted in the body into arabinofuranosylguanine (ara-G). Are-G accumulates in leukemic blast cells and is incorporated into cellular DNA. There ara-G inhabits synthesis and causes cell death. Nalarabine is indicated for the treatment of T-cell acute lymphoblastic leukemia and T-cell lymphoblastic lymphoma in patients who have not responded or relapsed following treatment with at least two chemotherapeutic regimens. The drug is administered by intravenous infusion. Recommended adult dosage is 1,500 mg per m^2 of body surface administered over two hours on days 1, 3, and 5. Recommended pediatric dosage is 650 mg per m^2 of body surface administered over one hour daily for five consecutive days. This chemotherapy cycle is repeated every 21 days until induction of complete response. HCPCS Level II code J9261 represents 50 mg of nalarabine.

J9263
J9263 Injection, oxaliplatin, 0.5 mg

Lay Description
Oxaliplatin is a chemical complex containing the metal platinum used as an antineoplastic drug. It binds to DNA disrupting synthesis and causing cell death. It is thought to have a greater cytotoxicity than cisplatin and carboplatin, which are other antineoplastic drugs containing platinum. The exact mechanism of action of oxaliplatin is not known. Oxaliplatin forms reactive platinum. Oxaliplatin is indicated with fluorouracil and leucovorin as a treatment for metastatic colon or rectum cancer that has recurred or progressed following irinotecan, fluorouracil, and leucovorin therapy. The recommended dosage is 85 mg per m^2 of body surface. Oxaliplatin is administered by intravenous infusion over two hours. It is administered in a separate bag, but simultaneously with leucovorin. HCPCS Level II code J9263 represents 0.5 mg of oxaliplatin.

Medicare Information
See the chapter titled "Medicare Guidelines," under "Drugs, Biologicals, and Radiopharmaceuticals," for Medicare information.

Medicare will cover off-label use of oxaliplatin when used in one of nine clinical trials identified by CMS and sponsored by the National Cancer Institute. A list of clinical trials is available at http://cms.hhs.gov/coverage/download/id90b.pdf.

J9264
J9264 Injection, paclitaxel protein-bound particles, 1 mg

Lay Description
Paclitaxel protein-bound particles are an albumin-bound form of paclitaxel, an antineoplastic agent. Paclitaxel protein-bound particles are indicated for the treatment of breast cancer after the failure of combination chemotherapy for metastatic disease, or relapse within six months of chemotherapy. The recommended therapy is 260mg

per m2 of body surface infused intravenously over 30 minutes every three weeks. Paclitaxel protein-bound particles are contraindicated in patients with baseline neutrophil counts of less than 1, 500. HCPCS Level II code J9264 represents 1 mg of paclitaxel protein-bound particles.

J9265

J9265   Injection, paclitaxel, 30 mg

Lay Description

Paclitaxel is a chemical compound isolated from the Pacific yew tree used as an antineoplastic drug. It disrupts intercellular functions causing cell death. Paclitaxel, either singularly or in combination with other chemotherapeutic drugs, is indicated as a treatment for Kaposi's sarcoma, advanced breast cancer, advanced ovarian cancer, and nonsmall cell lung cancer. Recommended dosage varies from 100 to 175 mg per m2 of body surface depending on the disease and treatment regimen. It is administered via intravenous infusion over three hours or over 24 hours depending on the treatment regimen. HCPCS Level II code J9265 represents 30 mg of paclitaxel.

J9266

J9266   Injection, pegaspargase, per single dose vial

Lay Description

Pegaspargase is a modified version of the enzyme L-asparaginase produced from E. coli bacterium and used as an antineoplastic agent. The enzyme catalyzes the breakdown of asparagine, an amino acid. Leukemia cells cannot synthesize asparagine and depend upon exogenous sources. Pegaspargase depletes asparagine throughout the body. This depletion kills the leukemia cells. Normal cells can synthesize the asparagine and are unaffected. Pegaspargase is indicated as a treatment for acute lymphoblastic leukemia in patients who have developed hypersensitivity to native forms of L-asparaginase. The drug is usually administered in combination with other chemotherapeutic agents and should only be administered as a single therapy when multi-agent therapy is inappropriate. The recommended dose is 2,500 IU per m2 of body surface via intravenous or intramuscular injection every 14 days. Lower doses of 82.5 IU per kg are recommended for children with a body surface of less than 0.6 m2. HCPCS Level II code J9266 represents a single dose vial of 3,750 IU of pegaspargase.

J9268

J9268   Injection, pentostatin, 10 mg

Lay Description

Pentostatin is an antibiotic isolated from the soil bacterium Streptomyces antibioticus used as antineoplastic drug. It interferes with enzyme activity preventing cellular reproduction. Pentostatin is indicated as a treatment for hairy cell leukemia refractory to alpha interferon. Pentostatin is given by intravenous injection or diluted in normal saline and infused over approximately 30 minutes. The recommended dosage is 4 mg per m2 of body surface. HCPCS Level II code J9268 represents 10 mg of pentostatin.

J9270

J9270   Injection, plicamycin, 2.5 mg

Lay Description

Plicamycin, also known as mithramycin, is an antibiotic with antineoplastic effects. The drug is derived from Streptomyces plicatus. It binds to DNA inhibiting RNA synthesis. Plicamycin is indicated for the treatment of testicular cancer in patients for whom surgery or radiotherapy is not an option. Plicamycin may also be considered in the treatment of symptomatic patients with hypercalcemia caused by chemotherapy for whom conventional therapy has failed. The drug may lower serum calcium by blocking the actions of vitamin D and inhibiting the effects of parathyroid hormone. The recommended antineoplastic dose is 25 to 30 mcg per kg of ideal body weight for a period of eight to 10 days. The recommended dose for hypercalcemia treatment is 25 mcg per kg of body weight for a period of three or four days. Plicamycin is administered via an intravenous infusion over four to six hours. The drug may cause severe thrombocytopenia and hemorrhagic syndrome. HCPCS Level II code J9270 represents 2.5 mg of plicamycin.

J9280

J9280   Mitomycin, 5 mg

Lay Description

Mitomycin is an antibiotic with antineoplastic effects. The drug is derived from Streptomyces caespitosus plicatus. It selectively inhibits DNA synthesis. Mitomycin is not recommended as a single agent primary therapy. Mitomycin is indicated for the treatment of disseminated adenocarcinoma of the stomach or pancreas in combination with other approved chemotherapeutic agents, or as a palliative treatment when other modalities have failed. The drug is not recommended as a replacement for surgery or radiotherapy. Mitomycin is administered intravenously via a catheter with a recommended dosage of 20 mg per m2 of body surface in six to eight week cycles. The patient must have a full hematological recovery from any previous therapy prior to the administration of mitomycin. The drug has a cumulative effect on bone marrow causing suppression and may cause hemolytic uremic syndrome at doses higher than 60 mg.

J9293

J9293   Injection, mitoxantrone HCl, per 5 mg

Lay Description

Mitoxantrone hydrochloride is a synthetic antineoplastic anthracenedione drug that disrupts the DNA of cells causing cell death The drug is used in combination with corticosteroids as an initial treatment for pain related to advanced hormone-refractory prostate cancer. Mitoxantrone hydrochloride is also indicated in combination with other approved drugs as the initial treatment for acute nonlymphocytic leukemia, including myelogenous, promyelocytic, monocytic, and erythroid leukemias. Mitoxantrone is also indicated for the treatment of secondary progressive, progressive relapsing, or worsening relapsing-remitting multiple sclerosis. The drug must be diluted and administered via an intravenous infusion. HCPCS Level II code J9293 represents 5 mg of mitoxantrone hydrochloride.

J9300

J9300   Injection, gemtuzumab ozogamicin, 5 mg

Lay Description

Gemtuzumab ozogamicin is a monoclonal antibody produced by recombinant DNA coupled with an antineoplastic antibiotic, calicheamicin. Calicheamicin is derived from the bacterium Micromonospora echinospora subsp. calichensis. The antibody portion of the drug binds specifically to the CD33 antigen, a protein found on the surface of leukemic blasts and immature normal cells of myelomonocytic lineage, but not on normal hematopoietic stem cells. Once bound with the CD33 antigen, the calicheamicin interferes with DNA replication and causes cell death. Gemtuzumab ozogamicin is indicated for the treatment of patients with CD33 positive acute myeloid leukemia in first relapse who are 60 years of age or older and who are not considered candidates for other chemotherapy. The recommended dosage is 9 mg per m2 of body surface administered by intravenous infusion over two hours. HCPCS Level II code J9300 represents 5 mg of gemtuzumab ozogamicin.

Medicare Information

See the chapter titled "Medicare Guidelines," under "Drugs, Biologicals, and Radiopharmaceuticals," for Medicare information.

J9302

J9302   Injection, ofatumumab, 10 mg

Lay Description

Ofatumumab is a human monoclonal antibody produced in murine cells. The drug binds specifically to the CD20 molecule contained in B lymphocytes, causing the breakdown of the cell. This drug is indicated for the treatment of patients who have chronic lymphocytic leukemia refractory to fludarabine and alemtuzumab. The drug is administered as a prolonged IV infusion. The recommended dosage is 2,000 mg after an initial 300 mg dose.

J9303

J9303   Injection, panitumumab, 10 mg

Lay Description

Panitumumab is a monoclonal antibody produced by recombinant DNA technology using Chinese hamster ovaries. The drug binds to human epidermal growth factor receptor (EGFR) sites inhibiting its effects. EGFR is a glycoprotein expressed in many normal epithelial cells including skin and hair follicles. Over-expression of EGFR usually accompanies many human epithelial cells including those of the colon and rectum. Panitumumab is indicated for the treatment of EGFR-expressing metastatic colorectal cancer in patients whose disease has progressed after treatment with fluoropyrimidine, oxaliplatin and irinotecan chemotherapy regimens. The drug is administered via an intravenous infusion over 60 minutes. Recommended dosage is 6 mg per kg of patient body weight every 14 days. Total dosages greater than 1000 mg should be administered over 90 minutes.

J9305

J9305   Injection, pemetrexed, 10 mg

Lay Description

Pemetrexed is a chemical complex used as an antineoplastic drug. It disrupts folate-dependent metabolic processes essential for cell reproduction. Pemetrexed in combination with cisplatin is indicated for the treatment of patients with malignant pleural mesothelioma whose disease is unresectable or who are otherwise not candidates for curative surgery metastatic lung cancer. As a singular agent, pemetrexed is indicated as a treatment for locally advanced or metastatic non-small cell lung cancer after prior chemotherapy. The recommended dosage is 500 mg per m^2 of body surface administered by intravenous injection. HCPCS Level II code J9305 represents 10 mg of pemetrexed.

Medicare Information

See the chapter titled "Medicare Guidelines," under "Drugs, Biologicals, and Radiopharmaceuticals," for Medicare information.

J9307

J9307   Injection, pralatrexate, 1 mg

Lay Description

Pralatrexate is a folate analogue that is a metabolic inhibitor that prevents the synthesis of thymidine. Thymidine is one of the nucleosides in DNA. This drug is used to treat patients with relapsed or refractory peripheral T-cell lymphoma. The drug is administered via an IV push over three to five minutes. The recommended dose is 30 mg per meter squared of body surface area.

J9310

J9310   Injection, rituximab, 100 mg

Lay Description

Rituximab is a monoclonal antibody produced by recombinant DNA in Chinese hamster ovaries used as an antineoplastic drug. It binds to the CD20 antigen on the surface of normal and malignant B-lymphocytes and causes cell death. This drug is used to treat the relapsed or refractory, low-grade, or follicular, CD20-positive, B-cell non-Hodgkin's lymphoma. In combination with other chemotherapeutic drugs, it is indicated as a treatment for diffuse large B-cell, CD20-positive non-Hodgkin's lymphoma. The recommended dosage is 375 mg per m^2 of body surface administered by intravenous infusion. HCPCS Level II code J9310 represents 100 mg of rituximab.

J9315

J9315   Injection, romidepsin, 1 mg

Lay Description

Romidepsin is a chemical compound that functions as a histone deacetylase inhibitor. Histone deacetylases are a class of enzymes that remove acetyl groups from an amino acid on a histone. Histones are strong alkaline proteins found in cell nuclei, which package and order the DNA into structural units. The accumulation of acetylated histones interrupts the cell cycle and induces death. Romidepsin is indicated in the treatment of cutaneous T-cell lymphoma in patients who have received at least one prior systemic therapy. The recommended dose is 14 mg per meter squared of body surface area administered as an IV infusion over a four-hour period.

J9320

J9320   Injection, streptozocin, 1 g

Lay Description

Streptozocin is a synthetic antineoplastic drug chemically related to other nitroureas that inhibits DNA synthesis causing cell death. Streptozocin is indicated for the treatment of metastatic islet cell carcinoma of the pancreas for both functioning and nonfunctioning carcinomas. Due to its renal toxicity, streptozocin should be limited to patients with symptomatic or progressive metastatic disease. The drug is administered intravenously by injection or via infusion. HCPCS Level II code J9320 represents 1 gram of streptozocin.

J9328

J9328   Injection, temozolomide, 1 mg

Lay Description

Temozolomide is a chemical complex that is broken down in the liver into monomethyl triazine, also known as MTIC. MTIC causes breaks in the DNA, which prevents replication, thus interfering with tumor cell reproduction. Temozolomide is indicated for the treatment of adult patients with newly diagnosed glioblastoma multiforme and for the treatment of adult patients with refractory anaplastic astrocytoma. Dosage is calculated based on the patient's body surface area. Temozolomide is administered by IV infusion.

J9330

J9330   Injection, temsirolimus, 1 mg

Lay Description

Temsirolimus is an antineoplastic drug used to treat advanced renal cancer. It inhibits mammalian target of rapamycin (mTOR) and binds to the protein that controls cell division. The recommended dose of temsirolimus is 25 mg administered by IV infusion over 30 to 60 minutes. The drug is usually administered once a week. HCPCS Level II code J9330 represents 1 mg of temsirolimus.

J9340

J9340   Injection, thiotepa, 15 mg

Lay Description

Thiotepa is a synthetic antineoplastic compound drug related chemically and pharmacologically to nitrogen mustard. The drug disrupts cell DNA producing cell death. Thiotepa may be administered intravenously, intracavitary, or intravesically. The drug has been tried in the treatment of a wide variety of neoplastic diseases with varying results. It has shown success in treating adenocarcinoma of the breast and ovary, superficial papillary carcinoma of the urinary bladder, and in controlling intracavity effusions secondary to diffuse or localized neoplastic diseases of various serosal cavities. While usually superseded by other treatments, thiotepa has been effective in the treatment of other lymphomas such as lymphosarcoma and Hodgkin's disease. HCPCS Level II code J9340 represents 15 mg of thiotepa.

J9351

J9351   Injection, topotecan, 0.1 mg

Lay Description

Topotecan hydrochloride is an antineoplastic drug that is a semisynthetic derivative of camptothecin, an alkaloid extract from plants such as Camptotheca acuminata. The drug works by causing breaks in DNA that the cell cannot repair leading to cell death. Topotecan hydrochloride is indicated as a treatment for metastatic carcinoma of the ovaries after failure of prior chemotherapy. It is also indicated as a treatment for small cell lung cancer that responded to chemotherapy, but subsequently progressed. The recommended dosage is 1.5 mg per m2 of body surface administered by intravenous infusion over 30 minutes for five consecutive days.

J9355

J9355   Injection, trastuzumab, 10 mg

Lay Description

Trastuzumab is a monoclonal antibody produced using recombinant DNA technology from Chinese hamster ovaries. The drug is an antineoplastic agent indicated for treatment of metastatic breast cancer that over expresses the HER2 protein. Trastuzumab selectively binds to the human epidermal growth factor receptor 2 protein (HER2) site and inhibits the production of cells that over express HER2. Trastuzumab is indicated as a treatment for HER2 over expressing breast cancer in patients who do not have heart failure or cardiomyopathy the following circumstances: as a single therapy for patients who have undergone one or more chemotherapy regimens for metastatic breast cancer; in combination therapy with doxorubicin, cyclophosphamide, and paclitaxel for node-positive breast cancer that has been surgically treated; and in combination with paclitaxel for patients who have not received chemotherapy for metastatic breast cancer. The drug is administered via an intravenous infusion and should not be given as an IV push or bolus. Recommended dosage for the initial infusion is 4 mg per kg of patient body weight infused over 90 minutes. Subsequent recommended dosage is 2 mg per kg of patient body weight infused over 30 minutes. The infusions are administered every seven days. HCPCS Level II code J9355 represents 10 mg of trastuzumab.

J9357

J9357   Injection, valrubicin, intravesical, 200 mg

Lay Description

Valrubicin intravesical is a synthetic version of anthracycline doxorubicin that is an antineoplastic agent instilled into the urinary bladder. The drug disrupts cell DNA causing chromosomal damage. Valrubicin is indicated for the intravesical treatment of BCG-refractory carcinoma in situ of the urinary bladder for those patients who cannot undergo an immediate cystectomy. HCPCS Level II code J9357 represents 200 mg of valrubicin.

J9360

J9360   Injection, vinblastine sulfate, 1 mg

Lay Description

Vinblastine sulfate is an antineoplastic drug that is an alkaloid extract from the herb known as Madagascar periwinkle or Vinca rosea Linn. It interferes with the cell metabolism of amino acids and nucleic acid synthesis causing cell death. Vinblastine sulfate, singularly or in combination, is indicated for the treatment of Hodgkin's disease, lymphocytic lymphoma, histiocytic lymphoma, mycosis fungoides, Kaposi's sarcoma, Letterer-Siwe disease, advanced carcinoma of the testis, choriocarcinoma resistant to other chemotherapeutic agents, and breast cancer that is unresponsive to surgery and hormonal therapy. The recommended dosage varies from 2.5 mg-18.5 mg per m² of body surface depending upon the patient's age and response. Vinblastine sulfate is administered by intravenous injection. HCPCS Level II code J9360 represents 1 mg of vinblastine sulfate.

Medicare Information

See chapter titled "Medicare Guidelines," under "Drugs, Biologicals, and Radiopharmaceuticals," for Medicare billing and documentation information.

J9370

J9370   Vincristine sulfate, 1 mg

Lay Description

Vincristine sulfate is an antineoplastic drug that is an alkaloid extract from the herb known as Madagascar periwinkle or Vinca rosea Linn. It interferes with the cell metabolism of amino acids and nucleic acid synthesis causing cell death. Vincristine sulfate, singularly or in combination, is indicated for the treatment of acute leukemia, non-Hodgkin's lymphoma, Hodgkin's disease, neuroblastoma, rhabdomyosarcoma, and Wilms' tumor. The recommended dosage varies from 0.5 to 1.4 mg per m2 of body surface depending upon the patient's age and response. Vincristine sulfate is administered by intravenous injection.

Medicare Information

See chapter titled "Medicare Guidelines," under "Drugs, Biologicals, and Radiopharmaceuticals," for Medicare billing and documentation information.

J9390

J9390   Injection, vinorelbine tartrate, 10 mg

Lay Description

Vinorelbine tartrate is an antineoplastic drug that is a semisynthetic derivative of vinblastine. Vinblastine is an alkaloid extract from the herb known as Madagascar periwinkle or Vinca rosea Linn. It interferes with the cell metabolism of amino acids and nucleic acid synthesis causing cell death. Vinorelbine tartrate, singularly or in combination with cisplatinum, is indicated for the treatment of unresectable, advanced nonsmall cell lung cancer. The recommended dosage is from 25 to 30 mg per m^2 of body surface depending upon the regimen. It is administered by intravenous injection over six to 10 minutes. HCPCS Level II code J9390 represents 10 mg of vinorelbine tartrate.

J9395

J9395   Injection, fulvestrant, 25 mg

Lay Description

Fulvestrant is an antineoplastic estrogen receptor antagonist. Many breast cancers have estrogen receptors and their growth can be stimulated by estrogen. Fulvestrant binds to the estrogen receptor preventing the estrogen from reaching the cells. It is indicated for the treatment of estrogen receptor, positive metastatic breast cancer in postmenopausal women who have not responded to other antiestrogen therapy. The recommended dosage is 250 mg. Fulvestrant is administered as a slow intramuscular injection into the buttocks. It may be administered as a single 5 ml injection or as two 2.5 ml injections. HCPCS Level II code J9395 represents 25 mg of fulvestrant.

Medicare Information

See the chapter titled "Medicare Guidelines," under "Drugs, Biologicals, and Radiopharmaceuticals," for Medicare information.

J9600

J9600   Injection, porfimer sodium, 75 mg

Lay Description

Porfimer sodium is a mixture of porphyrins that sensitizes cells to light. The drug is injected into neoplastic cells as step one of a two-step photodynamic treatment. Two to three days following injection, the neoplasm is irradiated with a laser light producing a cytotoxic reaction that destroys the cells. As the penetration of the light is limited, the photodynamic therapy is primarily used to treat small thin lesions on accessible surfaces. This type of photodynamic therapy is indicated for the palliative care of patients with completely obstructing esophageal cancer, patients with have partially obstructing esophageal cancer who cannot be satisfactorily treated with laser therapy alone, patients with partially or completely obstructive endobrachial nonsmall cell lung cancer, or patients who have microinvasive endobrachial nonsmall cell lung cancer for whom surgery and radiotherapy are not indicated. HCPCS Level II code J9600 represents 75 mg of porfimer sodium.

J9999

J9999   Not otherwise classified, antineoplastic drugs

Lay Description

Use this code to represent an antineoplastic drug that has been administered and is not represented by any other level I or level II HCPCS code.

K0001

K0001   Standard wheelchair

Lay Description

A standard wheelchair has a seat width of 16 (narrow) or 18 inches (adult), a seat depth of 16 inches, and 21 inches from seat to floor. It comes with a nonadjustable back height of 16 to 21 inches, a chrome plated frame, 24 inch molded rear wheels, 8 inch molded casters, nylon or vinyl upholstery, and fixed or swingaway detachable footrests. The footplate extension is between 16 and 21 inches. The standard wheelchair weighs more than 36 lbs.

Medicare Information

A standard wheelchair is characterized by the following:

- Weight: $\geq$ 36 lbs.
- Seat width: 16" (narrow), 18" (adult)
- Seat depth: 16"
- Seat height: $\geq$ 19" and $\leq$ 21"
- Back height: nonadjustable 16–17"
- Arm style: fixed or detachable
- Footplate extension: 16–21"
- Footrests: fixed or swingaway detachable

K0002

K0002 Standard hemi (low seat) wheelchair

Lay Description
This code reports a standard hemi (low seat) wheelchair. A hemi wheelchair has a seat height of 16 to 18 inches and is made for patients with a short stature or for patients who have an inability to place feet directly on the ground for propulsion. The hemi wheelchair has a weight capacity of 250 pounds and weighs 36 pounds or less. It comes with a chrome plated frame, 24-inch molded rear wheels, 8-inch molded casters, nylon or vinyl upholstery, and fixed or swing away detachable footrests.

K0003

K0003 Lightweight wheelchair

Lay Description
The lightweight wheelchair is indicated for patients requiring a chair for self-propulsion, and when the seat measurements required cannot be accommodated by a standard or hemi standard wheelchair. This device weighs less than 36 lbs, is fully reclining, and has swingaway detachable legrests. The seat width is 14, 16, or 18 inches, has a seat depth of 16 inches, and seat height between 17 and 21 inches. It has a nonadjustable back height of 16 to 17 inches, 24 inch molded rear wheels, 8 inch molded casters, nylon or vinyl upholstery, fixed-height detachable arms, and fixed or swingaway detachable footrests. The footplate extension is between 14 and 17 inches.

Medicare Information
A lightweight wheelchair is characterized by the following:

- Weight: ≤ 36 lbs.
- Seat width: 16" or 18"
- Seat depth: 16"
- Seat height: ≥ 17" and ≤ 21"
- Back height: non-adjustable 16–17"
- Arm height: fixed-height, detachable
- Footplate extension: 16–21"
- Footrests: fixed or swingaway detachable

A lightweight wheelchair is covered when a patient meets both of the following criteria:

- The patient cannot self-propel in a standard wheelchair using arms and/or legs
- The patient can and does self-propel in a lightweight wheelchair

K0004

K0004 High strength, lightweight wheelchair

Lay Description
The high strength, lightweight wheelchair is indicated for patients requiring a chair for self propulsion that is extra strong in frame construction, and when the seat measurements required cannot be accommodated by a standard or hemi standard wheelchair. This device weighs less than 34 lbs, with crossbraces. The seat width is 14, 16, or 18 inches, has a seat depth of 14 (child) or 16 inches (adult), and a seat height between 17 and 21 inches. It has a sectional or adjustable back height of 15 to 19 inches. It has 24 inch molded rear wheels, 8 inch molded casters, nylon upholstery, fixed-height detachable arms, and fixed or swingaway detachable footrests. The footplate extension is 16 to 21 inches.

Medicare Information
A high strength, lightweight wheelchair is characterized by the following:

- Lifetime warranty: on side frames and crossbraces
- Weight: ≤ 34 lbs.
- Seat width: 14", 16", or 18"
- Seat depth: 14" (child), 16" (adult)
- Seat height: ≥ 17" and ≤ 21"
- Back height: sectional or adjustable 15–19"
- Arm style: fixed or detachable
- Footplate extension: 16–21"
- Footrests: fixed or swingaway detachable

A high strength lightweight wheelchair is covered when a patient meets one or both of the following criteria:

- The patient self-propels the wheelchair while engaging in frequent activities that cannot be performed in a standard or lightweight wheelchair
- The patient requires a seat width, depth, or height that cannot be accommodated in a standard, lightweight, or hemi-wheelchair, and spends at least two hours per day in the wheelchair

K0005

K0005 Ultralightweight wheelchair

Lay Description
The ultra-lightweight wheelchair weighs less than 30 lbs, with crossbraces, has a seat width of 14, 16, or 18 inches, a seat depth of 14 (child) or 16 inches (adult), and a seat height between 17 and 21 inches. It has an adjustable rear axle position, nylon

upholstery, fixed or detachable arms, and fixed or swingaway detachable footrests. The footplate extension is 16 to 21 inches.

Medicare Information

An ultra-lightweight wheelchair is characterized by the following:

- Lifetime warranty: on side frames and crossbraces
- Weight: ≤ 30 lbs.
- Adjustable rear axle position
- Seat width: 14", 16", or 18"
- Seat depth: 14" (child), 16" (adult)
- Seat height: ≥ 17" and ≤ 21"
- Arm style: fixed or detachable
- Footplate extension: 16–21"
- Footrests: fixed or swingaway detachable

Coverage of an ultra-lightweight wheelchair is determined on an individual consideration basis. If an ultralightweight wheelchair base is determined to be not medically necessary, but criteria are met for a less costly wheelchair, payment will be based on the least costly alternative (K0001–K0004). However, since K0005 is in a different payment category, it will be denied as not medically necessary if billed as a purchase.

K0006-K0007

K0006 Heavy-duty wheelchair
K0007 Extra heavy-duty wheelchair

Lay Description

Wide, heavy-duty, and extra heavy-duty wheelchairs are indicated for obese patients when the seat measurements required cannot be accommodated by a standard wheelchair. The seat width is 18 inches, has a seat depth of 16 to 17 inches, and a seat height between 19 and 21 inches. It has a nonadjustable back height of 16 to 17 inches. It has reinforced back and seat upholstery, fixed-height detachable arms, and fixed or swingaway detachable footrests. The footplate extension is 16 to 21 inches. Report K0006 for a heavy-duty wheelchair that can support up to 300 lbs and K0007 for an extra heavy-duty wheelchair that can support more than 300 lbs.

Medicare Information

A heavy duty wheelchair (K0006) is characterized by the following:

- Seat width: 18"
- Seat depth: 16" or 17"
- Seat height: ≥ 19" and ≤ 21"
- Back height: Non-adjustable 16"—17"
- Arm style: fixed-height, detachable

A heavy-duty wheelchair is covered if the patient weighs more than 250 pounds or if the patient has severe spasticity.

An extra heavy-duty wheelchair (K0007) is covered if the patient weighs more than 300 pounds.

K0010-K0014

K0010 Standard-weight frame motorized/power wheelchair
K0011 Standard-weight frame motorized/power wheelchair with programmable control parameters for speed adjustment, tremor dampening, acceleration control and braking
K0012 Lightweight portable motorized/power wheelchair
K0014 Other motorized/power wheelchair base

Lay Description

Motorized (powered) wheelchairs are those not included in the manual wheelchair categories. They can be standard, lightweight, and customized, and can be fitted with a variety of accessories. These wheelchairs are generally slow-speed and fairly good at maneuvering and negotiating corners and certain inclines. They usually work from a battery power source. Motorized wheelchairs are not suited to patients who cannot operate the controls, such as stroke patients. Wheelchairs, in general, assist the patient in the activities of daily living (ADLs), both in and out of the home. They enable the patient to move about in both confined and open spaces. While some patients and/or their caretakers may prefer motorized wheelchairs, depending on the patient's clinical needs and ADL restrictions, payers' policies can differ widely in coverage. The patient's medical condition may dictate whether or not the patient can operate (maneuver and control) a motorized wheelchair alone or with limited assistance and/or observation. Report K0010 for a standard-weight frame motorized/power wheelchair; K0011 for a standard-weight frame motorized/power wheelchair with programmable control parameters for speed adjustment, tremor dampening, acceleration control, and braking; K0012 for a lightweight portable motorized/power wheelchair; and K0014 for a motorized/power wheelchair base that is not included in another code.

K0455

K0455 Infusion pump used for uninterrupted parenteral administration of medication, (e.g., epoprostenol or treprostinol)

Lay Description

Epoprostenol (Flolan) is a medication used primarily to treat pulmonary hypertension. Its brief half life typically requires continuous parenteral infusion.

The infusion pump is usually delivered through the subclavian or jugular veins, sometimes through a tunneled catheter that exits in an area maintainable by the patient. The pump is typically portable, worn on a harness or belt, and powered by either 9-volt or AA alkaline batteries. Often a second unit is worn, or immediately available, and alternated every 24 hours to ensure uninterrupted delivery.

Medicare Information
Medicare only pays for one pump for administering epoprostenol; the supplier is responsible for ensuring that there is an appropriate and acceptable contingency plan to address any emergency situations or mechanical failures of the equipment. A second pump provided as a backup will be denied as not medically necessary.

Note: See chapter titled "Medicare Guidelines," under "Infusion Pumps, External; Equipment and Supplies," for additional Medicare billing and documentation information.

K0606

K0606 Automatic external defibrillator, with integrated electrocardiogram analysis, garment type

Lay Description
Automatic external defibrillators are compact and portable devices that deliver an electrical shock to a person who has a sudden cardiac arrest. Automatic external defibrillator units use a microprocessor inside of a portable defibrillator to interpret a person's heart rhythm through electrodes. The computer recognizes ventricular fibrillation or ventricular tachycardia. Once recognized, the computer advises the operator/user that electrical defibrillation is needed or it will automatically deliver a counter shock.

Documentation Standards
An order for each item billed must be signed and dated by the treating physician, kept on file by the supplier, and made available to the DME MAC upon request.

Medicare Information
Non-wearable, automatic external defibrillators with integrated electrocardiogram capability are coded using E0617.

Wearable, automatic, external defibrillators with integrated electrocardiogram analysis are coded using K0606.

Other types of defibrillators are coded as A9270.

No separate payment is made for carrying cases or mounting hardware.

Medicare modifiers
Items billed to the DME MAC before a signed and dated order has been received by the supplier must be submitted with modifier EY added to each affected HCPCS code.

K0733

K0733 Power wheelchair accessory, 12 to 24 amp hour sealed lead acid battery, each (e.g., gel cell, absorbed glassmat)

Lay Description
A 12 to 24 amp hour lead-acid battery is a valve-regulated type that may be referred to as sealed or maintenance-free. This type of battery fixes the acid electrolyte in a gel or in an absorptive fiberglass mat. A gel cell suspends the electrolyte in a silica-based gel producing a thick pasty material. An absorbed glassmat (AGM) suspends the electrolyte in fiberglass matt separators that act as absorbent sponges. The battery needs no added water and can be safely operated in any position.

K0738

K0738 Portable gaseous oxygen system, rental; home compressor used to fill portable oxygen cylinders; includes portable containers, regulator, flowmeter, humidifier, cannula or mask, and tubing

Lay Description
A rented portable gaseous oxygen system is equipment that includes a home compressor used to fill portable oxygen cylinders. This type of system allows individuals to fill their own oxygen cylinders in their homes. This is accomplished by attaching the home compressor to an oxygen concentrator that provides the oxygen for the cylinders. The home compressor takes the oxygen and compresses it into the portable cylinders, which the patient uses when away from home. The home compressor can be used simultaneously to receive stationary oxygen while at the same time filling portable cylinders. This code includes all delivery hardware associated with use of the portable gaseous oxygen system, including portable containers, regulator, flowmeter, humidifier, cannula/mask, and tubing.

K0739-K0740

K0739 Repair or nonroutine service for durable medical equipment other than oxygen equipment requiring the skill of a technician, labor component, per 15 minutes

K0740 Repair or nonroutine service for oxygen equipment requiring the skill of a technician, labor component, per 15 minutes

Lay Description

This code reports the repair or non-routine service of durable medical equipment such as wheelchair repair or oxygen equipment, which requires the skill of a technician. This code reports the labor involved in the repair or service in units of 15-minute increments.

Medicare Information

This code excludes repairs on orthotic or prosthetic devices. For repairs on orthotic devices, see L4205 for labor and L4210 for parts. For repairs on prosthetic devices, see L7510 for parts and L7520 for labor. For repairs on maxillofacial prosthesis, see L8049.

K0800-K0812

K0800 Power operated vehicle, group 1 standard, patient weight capacity up to and including 300 pounds

K0801 Power operated vehicle, group 1 heavy-duty, patient weight capacity 301 to 450 pounds

K0802 Power operated vehicle, group 1 very heavy-duty, patient weight capacity 451 to 600 pounds

K0806 Power operated vehicle, group 2 standard, patient weight capacity up to and including 300 pounds

K0807 Power operated vehicle, group 2 heavy-duty, patient weight capacity 301 to 450 pounds

K0808 Power operated vehicle, group 2 very heavy-duty, patient weight capacity 451 to 600 pounds

K0812 Power operated vehicle, not otherwise classified

Lay Description

A power operated vehicle (POV) is a battery powered mobility device with tiller operated steering and three or four wheels. POVs may also be referred to as scooters. POVs are designed for a combination of indoor use with moderate outdoor capabilities on flat terrain and hard surfaces with minimal to moderate surface irregularity. A POV assists patients for whom a wheelchair is unsuitable in the activities of daily living, but POVs are not suited to all types of patients such as stroke victims or some quadriplegic and/or hemiplegic patients who cannot operate the controls nor be left alone while the vehicle is in operation. POVs are divided into two groups. Group 1 POVs have the following specifications: length 48 inches, width 28 inches, obstacle height 20 mm, minimum top end speed-flat 3 MPH, range 5 miles, and dynamic stability incline 6 degrees. Group 2 POVs have the following specifications: length 48 inches, width 28 inches, obstacle height 50 mm, minimum top end speed-flat 4 MPH, range 10 miles, and dynamic stability incline 7.5 degrees. POVs are further classified by weight capacity. Standard refers to a weight capacity up to and including 300 pounds. Heavy duty refers to a weight capacity of between 301 and 450 pounds. Very heavy duty refers to a weight capacity of between 451 and 600 pounds. Group 1 POVs are reported with K0800 (standard), K0801 (heavy duty), and K0802 (very heavy duty). Group 2 POVs are reported with K0806 (standard), K0807 (heavy duty), and K0808 (very heavy duty). Code K0812 should be reported for POVs that do not meet the above specifications.

K0813-K0816

K0813 Power wheelchair, group 1 standard, portable, sling/solid seat and back, patient weight capacity up to and including 300 pounds

K0814 Power wheelchair, group 1 standard, portable, captain's chair, patient weight capacity up to and including 300 pounds

K0815 Power wheelchair, group 1 standard, sling/solid seat and back, patient weight capacity up to and including 300 pounds

K0816 Power wheelchair, group 1 standard, captain's chair, patient weight capacity up to and including 300 pounds

Lay Description

These codes describe Group 1 standard power wheelchairs. Group 1 power wheelchairs have the following specifications: length 40 inches, width 24 inches, obstacle height 20 mm, minimum top end speed-flat 3 MPH, range 5 miles, dynamic stability incline 6 degrees, fatigue test on a level 200,000 cycles with 0.5 inch slats under all wheels, and 6,666 drop cycles. Standard wheelchairs have a maximum weight capacity of 300 pounds. Chairs represented by these four codes have been further subdivided by portability. Portable chairs (K0813 and K0814) are defined as being easily disassembled without the use of tools for transport in a vehicle whereas nonportable chairs cannot be easily disassembled (K0815 and K0816). Each of these subcategories has been further defined by the type of chair. Codes K0813 and K0815 report sling/solid seat/back chairs and K0814 and K0816 report captain's-type chairs.

K0820-K0823

K0820 Power wheelchair, group 2 standard, portable, sling/solid seat/back, patient weight capacity up to and including 300 pounds
K0821 Power wheelchair, group 2 standard, portable, captain's chair, patient weight capacity up to and including 300 pounds
K0822 Power wheelchair, group 2 standard, sling/solid seat/back, patient weight capacity up to and including 300 pounds
K0823 Power wheelchair, group 2 standard, captain's chair, patient weight capacity up to and including 300 pounds

Lay Description

These codes describe Group 2 standard power wheelchairs. Group 2 power wheelchairs have the following specifications: length 48 inches, width 34 inches, obstacle height 40 mm, minimum top speed-flat 3 MPH, range 7 miles, dynamic stability incline 6 degrees, fatigue test on a level 200,000 cycles with 0.5 inch slats under all wheels, and 6,666 drop cycles. Standard wheelchairs have a maximum weight capacity of 300 pounds. Chairs represented by these four codes have been further subdivided by portability. Portable chairs (K0820 and K0821) are defined as being easily disassembled without use of tools for transport in a vehicle whereas nonportable chairs cannot be easily disassembled (K0822 and K0823). Each of these subcategories has been further defined by the type of chair. Codes K0820 and K0822 report sling/solid seat/back chairs and K0821 and K0823 report captain's-type chairs.

K0824-K0825

K0824 Power wheelchair, group 2 heavy-duty, sling/solid seat/back, patient weight capacity 301 to 450 pounds
K0825 Power wheelchair, group 2 heavy-duty, captain's chair, patient weight capacity 301 to 450 pounds

Lay Description

These codes describe Group 2 heavy duty power wheelchairs. Group 2 power wheelchairs have the following specifications: length 48 inches, width 34 inches, obstacle height 40 mm, minimum top speed-flat 3 MPH, range 7 miles, dynamic stability incline 6 degrees, fatigue test on a level 200,000 cycles with 0.5 inch slats under all wheels, and 6,666 drop cycles. Heavy duty wheelchairs have a weight capacity of between 301 to 450 pounds. Chairs represented by these two codes have been further subdivided by type of chair. Code K0824 reports a sling/solid seat/back chair and K0825 reports a captain's-type chair.

K0826-K0827

K0826 Power wheelchair, group 2 very heavy-duty, sling/solid seat/back, patient weight capacity 451 to 600 pounds
K0827 Power wheelchair, group 2 very heavy-duty, captain's chair, patient weight capacity 451 to 600 pounds

Lay Description

These codes describe Group 2 very heavy duty power wheelchairs. Group 2 power wheelchairs have the following specifications: length 48 inches, width 34 inches, obstacle height 40 mm, minimum top speed-flat 3 MPH, range 7 miles, dynamic stability incline 6 degrees, fatigue test on a level 200,000 cycles with 0.5 inch slats under all wheels, and 6,666 drop cycles. Very heavy duty wheelchairs have a weight capacity of 451 to 600 pounds. Chairs represented by these two codes have been further subdivided by type of chair. Code K0826 reports a sling/solid seat/back chair and K0827 reports a captain's-type chair.

K0828-K0829

K0828 Power wheelchair, group 2 extra heavy-duty, sling/solid seat/back, patient weight capacity 601 pounds or more
K0829 Power wheelchair, group 2 extra heavy-duty, captain's chair, patient weight 601 pounds or more

Lay Description

These codes describe Group 2 extra heavy duty power wheelchairs. Group 2 power wheelchairs have the following specifications: length 48 inches, width 34 inches, obstacle height 40 mm, minimum top speed-flat 3 MPH, range 7 miles, dynamic stability incline 6 degrees, fatigue test on a level 200,000 cycles with 0.5 inch slats under all wheels, and 6,666 drop cycles. Extra heavy duty wheelchairs have a weight capacity of 601 pounds or more. Chairs represented by these two codes have been further subdivided by type of chair. Code K0828 reports a sling/solid seat/back chair and K0829 reports a captain's-type chair.

K0830-K0831

K0830 Power wheelchair, group 2 standard, seat elevator, sling/solid seat/back, patient weight capacity up to and including 300 pounds
K0831 Power wheelchair, group 2 standard, seat elevator, captain's chair, patient weight capacity up to and including 300 pounds

Lay Description

These codes describe Group 2 standard power wheelchairs with the added feature of a seat elevator. Seat elevators are used to assist with transfers and to reach items that would be out of reach from a standard wheelchair height. Group 2 power wheelchairs have the following specifications: length 48 inches, width 34 inches, obstacle height 40 mm, minimum top speed-flat 3 MPH, range 7 miles, dynamic stability incline 6 degrees, fatigue test on a level 200,000 cycles with 0.5 inch slats under all wheels, and 6,666 drop cycles. Standard wheelchairs have a maximum weight capacity of 300 pounds. Chairs represented by these two codes have been further subdivided by type of chair. Code K0830 reports a sling/solid seat/back chair and K0831 reports a captain's-type chair.

K0835-K0840

K0835   Power wheelchair, group 2 standard, single power option, sling/solid seat/back, patient weight capacity up to and including 300 pounds
K0836   Power wheelchair, group 2 standard, single power option, captain's chair, patient weight capacity up to and including 300 pounds
K0837   Power wheelchair, group 2 heavy-duty, single power option, sling/solid seat/back, patient weight capacity 301 to 450 pounds
K0838   Power wheelchair, group 2 heavy-duty, single power option, captain's chair, patient weight capacity 301 to 450 pounds
K0839   Power wheelchair, group 2 very heavy-duty, single power option sling/solid seat/back, patient weight capacity 451 to 600 pounds
K0840   Power wheelchair, group 2 extra heavy-duty, single power option, sling/solid seat/back, patient weight capacity 601 pounds or more

Lay Description

These codes describe Group 2 power wheelchairs with the added feature of a single power option. Group 2 power wheelchairs have the following specifications: length 48 inches, width 34 inches, obstacle height 40 mm, minimum top speed-flat 3 MPH, range 7 miles, dynamic stability incline 6 degrees, fatigue test on a level 200,000 cycles with 0.5 inch slats under all wheels, and 6,666 drop cycles. The single power option is available in all weight capacities, including standard (weight capacity up to and including 300 pounds), heavy duty (weight capacity 301 to 450 pounds), very heavy duty (weight capacity 451 to 600 pounds), and extra heavy duty (weight capacity 601 pounds or more). Standard and heavy duty weight capacity chairs with single power option are further classified by type of chair. Codes K0835 (standard) and K0836 (heavy duty) report sling/solid seat/back chairs. Codes K0836 (standard) and K0838 (heavy duty) report captain's-type chairs. Very heavy duty and extra heavy duty weight capacity chairs with a single power option are only available in sling/solid seat/back and are reported with K0839 and K0840 respectively.

K0841-K0843

K0841   Power wheelchair, group 2 standard, multiple power option, sling/solid seat/back, patient weight capacity up to and including 300 pounds
K0842   Power wheelchair, group 2 standard, multiple power option, captain's chair, patient weight capacity up to and including 300 pounds
K0843   Power wheelchair, group 2 heavy-duty, multiple power option, sling/solid seat/back, patient weight capacity 301 to 450 pounds

Lay Description

These codes describe Group 2 power wheelchairs with the added feature of a multiple power option. Group 2 power wheelchairs have the following specifications: length 48 inches, width 34 inches, obstacle height 40 mm, minimum top speed-flat 3 MPH, range 7 miles, dynamic stability incline 6 degrees, fatigue test on a level 200,000 cycles with 0.5 inch slats under all wheels, and 6,666 drop cycles. The multiple power option is available in only standard and heavy duty weight capacities. Standard weight capacity is defined as up to and including 300 pounds and heavy duty weight capacity is 301 to 450 pounds. Standard weight capacity chairs with single power option are further classified by type of chair. Code K0841 reports a standard sling/solid seat/back chair. Code K0842 reports a captain's-type chair. Heavy duty weight capacity chairs with a multiple power option are only available in sling/solid seat/back and are reported with K0843.

K0848-K0851

K0848   Power wheelchair, group 3 standard, sling/solid seat/back, patient weight capacity up to and including 300 pounds
K0849   Power wheelchair, group 3 standard, captain's chair, patient weight capacity up to and including 300 pounds
K0850   Power wheelchair, group 3 heavy-duty, sling/solid seat/back, patient weight capacity 301 to 450 pounds
K0851   Power wheelchair, group 3 heavy-duty, captain's chair, patient weight capacity 301 to 450 pounds

Lay Description

These codes describe standard and heavy duty Group 3 power wheelchairs. Group 3 power wheelchairs have the following specifications: length 48 inches, width 34 inches, obstacle height 60 mm, minimum top speed-flat 4.5 MPH, range 12 miles, dynamic stability incline 7.5 degrees, fatigue test on a level 200,000 cycles with 0.5 inch slats under all wheels, and 6,666 drop cycles. Standard weight capacity is defined as up to and including 300 pounds and heavy duty weight capacity is 301 to 450 pounds. Standard and heavy duty weight capacity chairs are further classified by type of chair. Codes K0848 (standard) and K0850 (heavy duty) report sling/solid seat/back chairs. Codes K0849 (standard) and K0851 (heavy duty) report captain's-type chairs.

K0852-K0855

K0852 Power wheelchair, group 3 very heavy-duty, sling/solid seat/back, patient weight capacity 451 to 600 pounds
K0853 Power wheelchair, group 3 very heavy-duty, captain's chair, patient weight capacity 451 to 600 pounds
K0854 Power wheelchair, group 3 extra heavy-duty, sling/solid seat/back, patient weight capacity 601 pounds or more
K0855 Power wheelchair, group 3 extra heavy duty, captain's chair, patient weight capacity 601 pounds or more

Lay Description

These codes describe very heavy duty and extra heavy duty Group 3 power wheelchairs. Group 3 power wheelchairs have the following specifications: length 48 inches, width 34 inches, obstacle height 60 mm, minimum top speed-flat 4.5 MPH, range 12 miles, dynamic stability incline 7.5 degrees, fatigue test on a level 200,000 cycles with 0.5 inch slats under all wheels, and 6,666 drop cycles. Very heavy duty weight capacity is 451 to 600 pounds and extra heavy duty is 601 pounds or more. Very heavy duty and extra heavy duty weight capacity chairs are further classified by type of chair. Codes K0852 (very heavy duty) and K0854 (extra heavy duty) report sling/solid seat/back chairs. Codes K0853 (very heavy duty) and K0855 (extra heavy duty) report captain's-type chairs.

K0856-K0860

K0856 Power wheelchair, group 3 standard, single power option, sling/solid seat/back, patient weight capacity up to and including 300 pounds
K0857 Power wheelchair, group 3 standard, single power option, captain's chair, patient weight capacity up to and including 300 pounds
K0858 Power wheelchair, group 3 heavy-duty, single power option, sling/solid seat/back, patient weight 301 to 450 pounds
K0859 Power wheelchair, group 3 heavy-duty, single power option, captain's chair, patient weight capacity 301 to 450 pounds
K0860 Power wheelchair, group 3 very heavy-duty, single power option, sling/solid seat/back, patient weight capacity 451 to 600 pounds

Lay Description

These codes describe Group 3 power wheelchairs with the added feature of a single power option. Group 3 power wheelchairs have the following specifications: length 48 inches, width 34 inches, obstacle height 60 mm, minimum top speed-flat 4.5 MPH, range 12 miles, dynamic stability incline 7.5 degrees, fatigue test on a level 200,000 cycles with 0.5 inch slats under all wheels, and 6,666 drop cycles. The single power option is available in standard (weight capacity up to and including 300 pounds), heavy duty (weight capacity 301 to 450 pounds), and very heavy duty (weight capacity 451 to 600 pounds). Standard and heavy duty weight capacity chairs are further classified by type of chair. Codes K0856 (standard) and K0858 (heavy duty) report sling/solid seat/back chairs. Codes K0857 (standard) and K0859 (heavy duty) report captain's-type chairs. Very heavy duty weight capacity chairs with a single power option are only available in sling/solid seat/back and are reported with K0860.

K0861-K0864

K0861 Power wheelchair, group 3 standard, multiple power option, sling/solid seat/back, patient weight capacity up to and including 300 pounds
K0862 Power wheelchair, group 3 heavy-duty, multiple power option, sling/solid seat/back, patient weight capacity 301 to 450 pounds
K0863 Power wheelchair, group 3 very heavy-duty, multiple power option, sling/solid seat/back, patient weight capacity 451 to 600 pounds
K0864 Power wheelchair, group 3 extra heavy-duty, multiple power option, sling/solid seat/back, patient weight capacity 601 pounds or more

Lay Description

These codes describe Group 3 power wheelchairs with the added feature of a multiple power option. Group 3 power wheelchairs have the following specifications: length 48 inches, width 34 inches, obstacle height 60 mm, minimum top speed-flat 4.5 MPH, range 12 miles, dynamic stability incline 7.5 degrees, fatigue test on a level 200,000 cycles with 0.5 inch slats under all wheels, and 6,666 drop cycles. The multiple power option is available with sling/solid seat/back in all weight capacities. Report K0861 for standard weight capacity (up to and including 300 pounds), K0862 for heavy duty (301 to 450 pounds), K0863 for very heavy duty (451 to 600 pounds), and K0864 for extra heavy duty (601 pounds or more).

K0868-K0871

K0868 Power wheelchair, group 4 standard, sling/solid seat/back, patient weight capacity up to and including 300 pounds
K0869 Power wheelchair, group 4 standard, captain's chair, patient weight capacity up to and including 300 pounds
K0870 Power wheelchair, group 4 heavy-duty, sling/solid seat/back, patient weight capacity 301 to 450 pounds
K0871 Power wheelchair, group 4 very heavy-duty, sling/solid seat/back, patient weight capacity 451 to 600 pounds

Lay Description

These codes describe Group 4 power wheelchairs. Group 4 power wheelchairs have the following specifications: length 48 inches, width 34 inches, obstacle height 75 mm, minimum top speed-flat 6 MPH, range 16 miles, dynamic stability incline 9 degrees, fatigue test on a level 200,000 cycles with 0.5 inch slats under all wheels, and 6,666 drop cycles. Group 4 power wheelchairs are available in three weight capacities, including standard (up to and including 300 pounds), heavy duty (301 to 450 pounds), and very heavy duty (450 to 600 pounds). Standard weight capacity chairs are further classified by type of chair. Codes K0870 reports a sling/solid seat/back chair and K0871 reports a captain's-type chair. Heavy duty and very heavy duty chairs are available only as sling/solid seat/back and are reported with K0872 and K0873 respectively.

K0877-K0880

K0877 Power wheelchair, group 4 standard, single power option, sling/solid seat/back, patient weight capacity up to and including 300 pounds
K0878 Power wheelchair, group 4 standard, single power option, captain's chair, patient weight capacity up to and including 300 pounds
K0879 Power wheelchair, group 4 heavy-duty, single power option, sling/solid seat/back, patient weight capacity 301 to 450 pounds
K0880 Power wheelchair, group 4 very heavy-duty, single power option, sling/solid seat/back, patient weight 451 to 600 pounds

Lay Description

These codes describe Group 4 power wheelchairs with the added feature of a single power option. Group 4 power wheelchairs have the following specifications: length 48 inches, width 34 inches, obstacle height 75 mm, minimum top speed-flat 6 MPH, range 16 miles, dynamic stability incline 9 degrees, fatigue test on a level 200,000 cycles with 0.5 inch slats under all wheels, and 6,666 drop cycles. The single power option is available in three weight capacities, including standard (up to and including 300 pounds), heavy duty (301 to 450 pounds), and very heavy duty (450 to 600 pounds). Standard weight capacity chairs with a single power option are further classified by type of chair. Codes K0877 reports a sling/solid seat/back chair and K0878 reports a captain's-type chair. Heavy duty and very heavy duty chairs are available only as sling/solid seat/back and are reported with K0879 and K0880 respectively.

K0884-K0886

K0884 Power wheelchair, group 4 standard, multiple power option, sling/solid seat/back, patient weight capacity up to and including 300 pounds

K0885 Power wheelchair, group 4 standard, multiple power option, captain's chair, patient weight capacity up to and including 300 pounds

K0886 Power wheelchair, group 4 heavy-duty, multiple power option, sling/solid seat/back, patient weight capacity 301 to 450 pounds

Lay Description

These codes describe Group 4 power wheelchairs with the added feature of a multiple power option. Group 4 power wheelchairs have the following specifications: length 48 inches, width 34 inches, obstacle height 75 mm, minimum top speed-flat 6 MPH, range 16 miles, dynamic stability incline 9 degrees, fatigue test on a level 200,000 cycles with 0.5 inch slats under all wheels, and 6,666 drop cycles. Group 4 power wheelchairs with a multiple power option are available in standard (up to and including 300 pounds) and heavy duty (301 to 450 pounds) weight capacities. Standard weight capacity chairs are further classified by type of chair. Code K0884 reports a sling/solid seat/back chair and K0885 reports a captain's-type chair. Heavy duty chairs are available only as sling/solid seat/back and are reported with K0886.

K0890-K0891

K0890 Power wheelchair, group 5 pediatric, single power option, sling/solid seat/back, patient weight capacity up to and including 125 pounds

K0891 Power wheelchair, group 5 pediatric, multiple power option, sling/solid seat/back, patient weight capacity up to and including 125 pounds

Lay Description

These codes describe Group 5 power wheelchairs, which are pediatric wheelchairs with a patient weight capacity up to and including 125 pounds. Group 5 power wheelchairs have the following specifications: length 48 inches, width 28 inches, obstacle height 60 mm, minimum top speed-flat 4.5 MPH, range 12 miles, dynamic stability incline 7.5 degrees, fatigue test on a level 200,000 cycles with 0.5 inch slats under all wheels, and 6,666 drop cycles. Group 5 power wheelchairs are available with single and multiple power options in a sling/solid seat/back chair. Report K0890 for a single power option and K0891 for a multiple power option.

K0898-K0899

K0898 Power wheelchair, not otherwise classified

K0899 Power mobility device, not coded by DME PDAC or does not meet criteria

Lay Description

Power wheelchairs and power mobility device codes are assigned based on specific criteria related to length, width, obstacle height, minimum top end speed on a flat surface, range, dynamic stability on incline, fatigue tests on a level with 0.5-inch slats, and drop cycles. Criteria were defined by Statistical Analysis Durable Medical Equipment Regional Carrier (SADMERC), a national entity that provides services under contract to CMS related to DMEPOS HCPCS coding and pricing. Report K0898 for power wheelchairs that do not meet the specifications listed in the power wheelchair groups (Groups 1 to 5). Report K0899 for power mobility devices that are not coded by SADMERC or that do not meet the specific criteria provided by SADMERC.

L0112

L0112 Cranial cervical orthotic, congenital torticollis type, with or without soft interface material, adjustable range of motion joint, custom fabricated

Lay Description

A custom fabricated cranial cervical orthosis for congenital muscular torticollis (CMT) is used to treat infants with CMT complicated by plagiocephaly. CMT is a postural deformity that results primarily from unilateral shortening and fibrosis of the sternocleidomastoid muscle. This causes the head to tilt to one side. Plagiocephaly, manifested as deformities of the skull base, cranium, or face, may occur in infants with CMT. These deformities may be the result of intrauterine compression or may occur after birth due to consistent positioning of the head to one side during sleep. Code L0112 reports a cranial cervical orthosis designed to treat both the torticollis and any resulting plagiocephaly. The cranial orthosis consists of a custom fabricated helmet that may be lined with a soft interface material. The helmet remolds the skull to a more normal shape. The helmet is attached to an adjustable cervical orthosis that supports the neck and relieves the tilting of the head. The cervical component can be adjusted as the sternocleidomastoid muscle lengthens and the head tilt becomes less severe.

L0113

L0113 Cranial cervical orthotic, torticollis type, with or without joint, with or without soft interface material, prefabricated, includes fitting and adjustment

Lay Description

A prefabricated cranial cervical orthosis for muscular torticollis is used to treat patints with torticollis. Torticollis is a postural deformity that results primarily from unilateral shortening and fibrosis of the sternocleidomastoid muscle. This causes the head to tilt to one side. The cranial orthosis consists of a prefabricated helmet that may be lined with a soft interface material. The helmet is attached to an adjustable cervical orthosis that supports the neck and relieves the tilting of the head. The cervical component can be adjusted as the sternocleidomastoid muscle lengthens and the head tilt becomes less severe.

L0120-L0130

L0120 Cervical, flexible, nonadjustable (foam collar)
L0130 Cervical, flexible, thermoplastic collar, molded to patient

Lay Description

Cervical collars are used to limit the range of motion in the head and neck. By having the jaws and chin supported, the angle between the chin and the chest is maintained, which alleviates stress on the posterior neck/nuchal and suboccipital areas. This reduces the potential for cervical root irritation and adds an extra measure of head/neck immobilization. There is still a minute degree of mobilization capability while the patient is in the cervical collar. Codes L0120 and L0130 report flexible cervical collars. Cervical foam collars coded with L0120 are nonadjustable in terms of collar width but can be easily adjusted to the circumference of the patient's neck by simply pulling the collar closed and securing it in an overlapping fashion using the Velcro anchor at the back of the collar. Some collars can be obtained in low, medium, or high contour styles, depending on the collar width and degree of head and/or neck immobilization desired. Cervical thermoplastic collars reported with L0130 are molded to the patient.

L0140-L0160

L0140 Cervical, semi-rigid, adjustable (plastic collar)
L0150 Cervical, semi-rigid, adjustable molded chin cup (plastic collar with mandibular/occipital piece)
L0160 Cervical, semi-rigid, wire frame occipital/mandibular support

Lay Description

Cervical collars are used to limit the range of motion in the head and neck. By having the jaws and chin supported, the angle between the chin and the chest is maintained, which alleviates stress on the posterior neck/nuchal and suboccipital areas. This reduces the potential for cervical root irritation and adds an extra measure of head/neck immobilization. There is still a minute degree of mobilization capability while the patient is in the cervical collar. Codes L0140, L0150, and L0160 report semi-rigid cervical collars. Semi-rigid collars are typically constructed from plastic or like materials, with padded inner surfaces and may have an added jaw/chin support. Report L0140 for a cervical, semi-rigid, plastic, adjustable collar and L0150 when the plastic collar has a mandibular/occipital piece (molded chin cup). Code L0160 is reported for a semi-rigid, wire frame cervical collar with an occipital/mandibular support.

L0170

L0170 Cervical, collar, molded to patient model

Lay Description

Cervical collars are used to limit the range of motion in the head and neck. By having the jaws and chin supported, the angle between the chin and the chest is maintained, which alleviates stress on the posterior neck/nuchal and suboccipital areas. This reduces the potential for cervical root irritation and adds an extra measure of head/neck immobilization. There is still a minute degree of mobilization capability while the patient is in the cervical collar. Report L0170 for a cervical collar that has been molded to a patient model.

L0172

L0172 Cervical, collar, semi-rigid thermoplastic foam, 2 piece

Lay Description

Cervical collars are used to limit the range of motion in the head and neck. By having the jaws and chin supported, the angle between the chin and the chest is maintained, which alleviates stress on the posterior neck/nuchal and suboccipital areas. This reduces the potential for cervical root irritation and adds an extra measure of head/neck immobilization. There is still a minute degree of mobilization capability while the patient is in the cervical collar. The collar coded with L0172 has two pieces, is semi-rigid, is usually light in weight though constructed from sturdy plastics, and also has padded or lined surfaces so as not to chafe the patient's skin. Sizes vary according to source.

Documentation Standards

It is expected that the patient's medical records will reflect the need for the care provided. The patient's medical records include the physician's office records, hospital records, nursing home records, home health agency records, records from other health care professionals, and test reports. This documentation must be available to the contractor upon request.

An order for each new or full replacement item must be signed and dated by the treating physician, kept on file by the supplier, and made available to the DME MAC upon request. Items billed to the DME MAC before a signed and dated order has been received by the supplier must be submitted with modifier EY added to each affected HCPCS code.

The order must list the unique features of the base code that is billed plus every addition that will be billed on a separate claim line. The medical record must contain information that supports the medical necessity of the item and all additions that are ordered. An order is not necessary for the repair of an orthosis.

L0174

L0174   Cervical, collar, semi-rigid, thermoplastic foam, 2 piece with thoracic extension

Lay Description

This code reports the supply of a specific type of two-piece cervical collar. Cervical orthoses are used to restrict motion to prevent pain, to protect spinal instability before or after surgery, and as emergency protection from the effects of trauma. The cervical spine (neck) offers the ability for a wide range of motion. The head normally rotates almost 180 degrees; about 145 degrees of flexion and extension is considered a clinical base as is about 90 degrees of lateral flexion. This type of orthosis restricts these movements by immobilizing the head. The design reported by this code has two semi-rigid pieces. One piece may be a chin support component that drops into the support collar. Other models may feature front and back components. Velcro closures are used to close and adjust the two pieces. The design reported by this code also features an extension to the thoracic region to further stabilize the cervical spine. This may be an upper waistband connected by rigid bars (front and back) to the cervical collar. The thoracic component essentially converts the device to a cervical thoracic orthosis. Report L0174 for supply of a two-piece, semi-rigid thermoplastic foam cervical orthosis with thoracic extension.

Documentation Standards

It is expected that the patient's medical records will reflect the need for the care provided. The patient's medical records include the physician's office records, hospital records, nursing home records, home health agency records, records from other health care professionals, and test reports. This documentation must be available to the contractor upon request.

An order for each new or full replacement item must be signed and dated by the treating physician, kept on file by the supplier, and made available to the DME MAC upon request. Items billed to the DME MAC before a signed and dated order has been received by the supplier must be submitted with modifier EY added to each affected HCPCS code.

The order must list the unique features of the base code that is billed plus every addition that will be billed on a separate claim line. The medical record must contain information that supports the medical necessity of the item and all additions that are ordered. An order is not necessary for the repair of an orthosis.

L0180-L0200

L0180   Cervical, multiple post collar, occipital/mandibular supports, adjustable
L0190   Cervical, multiple post collar, occipital/mandibular supports, adjustable cervical bars (SOMI, Guilford, Taylor types)
L0200   Cervical, multiple post collar, occipital/mandibular supports, adjustable cervical bars, and thoracic extension

Lay Description

These codes report the supply of multiple post cervical collars. Cervical orthoses are used to restrict motion to prevent pain or to address spinal instability before or after surgery. The healthy cervical spine (neck) offers a wide range of motion. The head normally rotates almost 180 degrees; about 145 degrees of flexion and extension is considered a clinical base as is about 90 degrees of lateral flexion. These types of orthoses restrict these movements by immobilizing the head. All collars will have more than one bar or post to support and immobilize the cervical spine. The Somi brace is named as an acronym for sternal occipital mandibular immobilizer. The Somi brace features three adjustable vertical bars on the front of the device that connects a rigid upper sternal band to the cervical and head support. The head and neck component supports against the mandible (lower jaw) and occiput (back of head). The Guilford brace is an eponym for the designer and features two adjustable posts (front and back) that extend from a shoulder harness to a ring that supports the head. Some designs may also feature an extension to the thoracic region to further stabilize the cervical spine. This may be a rigid extension to the thoracic region. The thoracic component essentially converts the device to a cervical thoracic orthosis. Report L0180 for supply of an adjustable multiple post-cervical collar. Report L0190 for supply of a multiple post-cervical collar with adjustable cervical bars. Report L0200 for supply of an adjustable multiple post-cervical collar with a thoracic extension.

Documentation Standards

It is expected that the patient's medical records will reflect the need for the care provided. The patient's medical records include the physician's office records, hospital records, nursing home records, home health agency records, records from other health care professionals, and test reports. This documentation must be available to the contractor upon request.

An order for each new or full replacement item must be signed and dated by the treating physician, kept on file by the supplier, and made available to the DME MAC upon request. Items billed to the DME MAC before a signed and dated order has been received by the supplier must be submitted with modifier EY added to each affected HCPCS code.

The order must list the unique features of the base code that is billed plus every addition that will be billed on a separate claim line. The medical record must contain information that supports the medical necessity of the item and all additions that are ordered. An order is not necessary for the repair of an orthosis.

L0220

L0220   Thoracic, rib belt, custom fabricated

Lay Description

A thoracic rib belt is an elastic belt used to support the thoracic area and rib cage following injury. These belts may be custom fabricated for the patient.

Documentation Standards

It is expected that the patient's medical records will reflect the need for the care provided. The patient's medical records include the physician's office records, hospital records, nursing home records, home health agency records, records from other health care professionals, and test reports. This documentation must be available to the contractor upon request.

An order for each new or full replacement item must be signed and dated by the treating physician, kept on file by the supplier, and made available to the DME MAC upon request. Items billed to the DME MAC before a signed and dated order has been received by the supplier must be submitted with modifier EY added to each affected HCPCS code.

The order must list the unique features of the base code that is billed plus every addition that will be billed on a separate claim line. The medical record must contain information that supports the medical necessity of the item and all additions that are ordered. An order is not necessary for the repair of an orthosis.

L0430

L0430   Spinal orthotic, anterior-posterior-lateral control, with interface material, custom fitted (DeWall Posture Protector only)

Lay Description

A postural support system provides integrated support for the spine and trunk with anterior, posterior, and lateral control. It reduces motion by limiting side-bending, flexion, extension, and to some extent rotation. It is indicated to reduce pain and facilitate healing following injury or surgery to the thoracic spine or thoracic soft tissues; to support weak spinal muscles; to treat spinal deformities, such as idiopathic scoliosis; and to immobilize the thoracic spine in individuals with unstable spinal disorders of T3 to L3 or compression fracture due to osteoporosis This orthosis is a vest type garment composed of a sturdy, stretch fabric, such as Lycra, with Velcro fasteners. The vest is custom fitted to the individual. Code L0430 should be reported only for a DeWall type postural support system.

L0450-L0490

L0450   Thoracic-lumbar-sacral orthotic (TLSO), flexible, provides trunk support, upper thoracic region, produces intracavitary pressure to reduce load on the intervertebral disks with rigid stays or panel(s), includes shoulder straps and closures, prefabricated, includes fitting and adjustment

L0452   Thoracic-lumbar-sacral orthotic (TLSO), flexible, provides trunk support, upper thoracic region, produces intracavitary pressure to reduce load on the intervertebral disks with rigid stays or panel(s), includes shoulder straps and closures, custom fabricated

L0454   Thoracic-lumbar-sacral orthotic (TLSO) flexible, provides trunk support, extends from sacrococcygeal junction to above T-9 vertebra, restricts gross trunk motion in the sagittal plane, produces intracavitary pressure to reduce load on the intervertebral disks with rigid stays or panel(s), includes shoulder straps and closures, prefabricated, includes fitting and adjustment

L0456 Thoracic-lumbar-sacral orthotic (TLSO), flexible, provides trunk support, thoracic region, rigid posterior panel and soft anterior apron, extends from the sacrococcygeal junction and terminates just inferior to the scapular spine, restricts gross trunk motion in the sagittal plane, produces intracavitary pressure to reduce load on the intervertebral disks, includes straps and closures, prefabricated, includes fitting and adjustment

L0458 Thoracic-lumbar-sacral orthotic (TLSO), triplanar control, modular segmented spinal system, 2 rigid plastic shells, posterior extends from the sacrococcygeal junction and terminates just inferior to the scapular spine, anterior extends from the symphysis pubis to the xiphoid, soft liner, restricts gross trunk motion in the sagittal, coronal, and transverse planes, lateral strength is provided by overlapping plastic and stabilizing closures, includes straps and closures, prefabricated, includes fitting and adjustment

L0460 Thoracic-lumbar-sacral orthotic (TLSO), triplanar control, modular segmented spinal system, 2 rigid plastic shells, posterior extends from the sacrococcygeal junction and terminates just inferior to the scapular spine, anterior extends from the symphysis pubis to the sternal notch, soft liner, restricts gross trunk motion in the sagittal, coronal, and transverse planes, lateral strength is provided by overlapping plastic and stabilizing closures, includes straps and closures, prefabricated, includes fitting and adjustment

L0462 Thoracic-lumbar-sacral orthotic (TLSO), triplanar control, modular segmented spinal system, 3 rigid plastic shells, posterior extends from the sacrococcygeal junction and terminates just inferior to the scapular spine, anterior extends from the symphysis pubis to the sternal notch, soft liner, restricts gross trunk motion in the sagittal, coronal, and transverse planes, lateral strength is provided by overlapping plastic and stabilizing closures, includes straps and closures, prefabricated, includes fitting and adjustment

L0464 Thoracic-lumbar-sacral orthotic (TLSO), triplanar control, modular segmented spinal system, 4 rigid plastic shells, posterior extends from sacrococcygeal junction and terminates just inferior to scapular spine, anterior extends from symphysis pubis to the sternal notch, soft liner, restricts gross trunk motion in sagittal, coronal, and transverse planes, lateral strength is provided by overlapping plastic and stabilizing closures, includes straps and closures, prefabricated, includes fitting and adjustment

L0466 Thoracic-lumbar-sacral orthotic (TLSO), sagittal control, rigid posterior frame and flexible soft anterior apron with straps, closures and padding, restricts gross trunk motion in sagittal plane, produces intracavitary pressure to reduce load on intervertebral disks, includes fitting and shaping the frame, prefabricated, includes fitting and adjustment

L0468 Thoracic-lumbar-sacral orthotic (TLSO), sagittal-coronal control, rigid posterior frame and flexible soft anterior apron with straps, closures and padding, extends from sacrococcygeal junction over scapulae, lateral strength provided by pelvic, thoracic, and lateral frame pieces, restricts gross trunk motion in sagittal, and coronal planes, produces intracavitary pressure to reduce load on intervertebral disks, includes fitting and shaping the frame, prefabricated, includes fitting and adjustment

L0470 Thoracic-lumbar-sacral orthotic (TLSO), triplanar control, rigid posterior frame and flexible soft anterior apron with straps, closures and padding, extends from sacrococcygeal junction to scapula, lateral strength provided by pelvic, thoracic, and lateral frame pieces, rotational strength provided by subclavicular extensions, restricts gross trunk motion in sagittal, coronal, and transverse planes, produces intracavitary pressure to reduce load on the intervertebral disks, includes fitting and shaping the frame, prefabricated, includes fitting and adjustment

L0472 Thoracic-lumbar-sacral orthotic (TLSO), triplanar control, hyperextension, rigid anterior and lateral frame extends from symphysis pubis to sternal notch with 2 anterior components (one pubic and one sternal), posterior and lateral pads with straps and closures, limits spinal flexion, restricts gross trunk motion in sagittal, coronal, and transverse planes, includes fitting and shaping the frame, prefabricated, includes fitting and adjustment

L0480 Thoracic-lumbar-sacral orthotic (TLSO), triplanar control, 1 piece rigid plastic shell without interface liner, with multiple straps and closures, posterior extends from sacrococcygeal junction and terminates just inferior to scapular spine, anterior extends from symphysis pubis to sternal notch, anterior or posterior opening, restricts gross trunk motion in sagittal, coronal, and transverse planes, includes a carved plaster or CAD-CAM model, custom fabricated

L0482 Thoracic-lumbar-sacral orthotic (TLSO), triplanar control, 1 piece rigid plastic shell with interface liner, multiple straps and closures, posterior extends from sacrococcygeal junction and terminates just inferior to scapular spine, anterior extends from symphysis pubis to sternal notch, anterior or posterior opening, restricts gross trunk motion in sagittal, coronal, and transverse planes, includes a carved plaster or CAD-CAM model, custom fabricated

L0484 Thoracic-lumbar-sacral orthotic TLSO, triplanar control, 2 piece rigid plastic shell without interface liner, with multiple straps and closures, posterior extends from sacrococcygeal junction and terminates just inferior to scapular spine, anterior extends from symphysis pubis to sternal notch, lateral strength is enhanced by overlapping plastic, restricts gross trunk motion in the sagittal, coronal, and transverse planes, includes a carved plaster or CAD-CAM model, custom fabricated

L0486 Thoracic-lumbar-sacral orthotic (TLSO), triplanar control, 2 piece rigid plastic shell with interface liner, multiple straps and closures, posterior extends from sacrococcygeal junction and terminates just inferior to scapular spine, anterior extends from symphysis pubis to sternal notch, lateral strength is enhanced by overlapping plastic, restricts gross trunk motion in the sagittal, coronal, and transverse planes, includes a carved plaster or CAD-CAM model, custom fabricated

L0488 Thoracic-lumbar-sacral orthotic (TLSO), triplanar control, 1 piece rigid plastic shell with interface liner, multiple straps and closures, posterior extends from sacrococcygeal junction and terminates just inferior to scapular spine, anterior extends from symphysis pubis to sternal notch, anterior or posterior opening, restricts gross trunk motion in sagittal, coronal, and transverse planes, prefabricated, includes fitting and adjustment

L0490 Thoracic-lumbar-sacral orthotic (TLSO), sagittal-coronal control, 1 piece rigid plastic shell, with overlapping reinforced anterior, with multiple straps and closures, posterior extends from sacrococcygeal junction and terminates at or before the T-9 vertebra, anterior extends from symphysis pubis to xiphoid, anterior opening, restricts gross trunk motion in sagittal and coronal planes, prefabricated, includes fitting and adjustment

Lay Description

A thoracic-lumbar-sacral orthosis (TLSO) is a brace that is a rigid or semirigid device used for the purpose of supporting weak or deformed areas of the spine, or for restricting or eliminating motion (immobilization) in diseased or injured areas of the spine. An orthosis can be either prefabricated (custom fitted) or custom fabricated. These particular orthoses can have various features and can be constructed or have component parts of different types of materials. The benefits from orthotics use, specifically during convalescence from an injury or illness (useful to the weak or deformed body area) or as a postoperative treatment measure can include the following: Restricted range of motion of the affected area (immobilization), support of the affected area, and/or protection from injury, reinjury, suture tearing, and/or wound dehiscence. A prefabricated or custom fitted orthosis is one that the manufacturer has produced in quantity, without a specific patient in mind. A prefabricated orthosis may be trimmed, bent, molded (with or without heat), or otherwise modified for use by a specific patient (i.e., custom fitted). An orthosis that is assembled from prefabricated components is considered prefabricated. Any orthosis that does not meet the definition of a custom fabricated orthosis is considered prefabricated. A custom fabricated orthosis is one that is individually made for a specific patient, starting with basic materials including, but not limited to, plastic, metal, leather, or cloth in the form of sheets, bars, and so forth. It involves substantial work, such as cutting, bending, molding, sewing, and so forth. It may involve the incorporation of some prefabricated components. It involves more than trimming, bending, or making other modifications to a substantially prefabricated item. A molded-to-patient-model orthosis is a particular type of custom fabricated orthosis in which an impression of the specific body part is made (by means of a plaster cast, CAD-CAM technology, etc.). This impression is then used to make a positive model (of plaster or other material) of the body part to be braced. The orthosis is then molded on this positive model to be fit exactly to the patient's body part. Codes L0452, L0478, L0480, L0482, L0484, and L0486 describe custom fabricated orthoses.

Documentation Standards

If the item is furnished secondary to a fracture (traumatic or nontraumatic, such as due to severe osteoporosis), a copy of the x-ray study confirming the fracture should be easily accessible within the medical record. If the device is furnished post-surgery, a copy of the operative report should be contained in the medical record. This information should be made available to the contractor upon request.

For custom fabricated orthoses, there must be documentation in the supplier's records to support the medical necessity of that type of device rather than a prefabricated orthosis. This information does not have to be routinely submitted with the claim, but must be available to the DME MAC on request.

Providers should have a national supplier identification number to allow for billing of the item to the DME MAC, if appropriate. No special forms, such as CMNs, are required to be completed for any of these items.

Medicare Information

Thoracic-lumbar-sacral orthoses (TLSO) described by L0450–L0490 and lumbar-sacral orthoses have the following characteristics:

- They are used to immobilize the specified areas of the spine
- They have an intimate fit and are generally designed to be worn under clothing
- They are not specifically designed for patients in wheelchairs

In addition to the first and second bullet points, the body jacket type orthoses (L0458–L0466, L0480–L0490) are characterized by a rigid plastic shell that encircles the trunk and provides a high degree of immobility.

Thoracic-lumbar-sacral orthoses are covered when they are ordered by a provider to reduce pain by restricting mobility of the trunk, to facilitate healing following an injury to and/or a surgical procedure performed on the spine or related soft tissues, or to otherwise support weak spinal muscles and/or a deformed spine.

Evaluation of the patient and measurement and/or casting and fitting of the orthosis are included in the allowance for the orthosis. There is no separate payment for these services.

L0491-L0492

L0491   Thoracic-lumbar-sacral orthotic (TLSO), sagittal-coronal control, modular segmented spinal system, 2 rigid plastic shells, posterior extends from the sacrococcygeal junction and terminates just inferior to the scapular spine, anterior extends from the symphysis pubis to the xiphoid, soft liner, restricts gross trunk motion in the sagittal and coronal planes, lateral strength is provided by overlapping plastic and stabilizing closures, includes straps and closures, prefabricated, includes fitting and adjustment

L0492   Thoracic-lumbar-sacral orthotic (TLSO), sagittal-coronal control, modular segmented spinal system, 3 rigid plastic shells, posterior extends from the sacrococcygeal junction and terminates just inferior to the scapular spine, anterior extends from the symphysis pubis to the xiphoid, soft liner, restricts gross trunk motion in the sagittal and coronal planes, lateral strength is provided by overlapping plastic and stabilizing closures, includes straps and closures, prefabricated, includes fitting and adjustment

Lay Description

A thoracic-lumbar-sacral orthosis (TLSO) is a brace that is a rigid or semirigid device used for the purpose of supporting weak or deformed areas of the spine, or for restricting or eliminating motion (immobilization) in diseased or injured areas of the spine. An orthosis can be prefabricated (custom fitted) or custom fabricated. These particular orthoses can have various features and can be constructed or have component parts of different types of materials. The benefits from orthotics use, specifically during convalescence from an injury or illness or as a postoperative treatment measure, can include the following: restricted range of motion of the affected area (immobilization), support of the affected area (useful to the weak or deformed body area), and/or protection from injury, reinjury, suture tearing, and/or wound dehiscence. A prefabricated (also known as custom fitted) orthosis is one that the manufacturer has produced in quantity, without a specific patient in mind. A prefabricated orthosis may be trimmed, bent, molded (with or without heat), or otherwise modified for use by a specific patient (i.e., custom fitted). An orthosis that is assembled from prefabricated components is considered prefabricated. Any orthosis that does not meet the definition of a custom fabricated orthosis is considered prefabricated. In contrast to a prefabricated orthosis, a custom fabricated orthosis is one that is individually made for a specific patient, starting with basic materials including, but not limited to, plastic, metal, leather, or cloth in the form of sheets, bars, and so forth. It involves substantial work, such as cutting, bending, molding, sewing, and so forth. It may involve the incorporation of some prefabricated components. It involves more than trimming, bending, or making other modifications to a prefabricated item. A molded-to-patient-model orthosis is a particular type of custom fabrication orthosis in which an impression of the specific body part is made (by means of a plaster cast, CAD-CAM technology, etc.). This impression is then used to make a positive model (of plaster or other material) of the body part to be braced. The orthosis is then molded on this positive model to be fit exactly to the patient's body part. Codes L0491 and L0492 report prefabricated TLSOs that provide control in the coronal-sagittal planes by use of a modular segmented system. Code L0491 has two rigid plastic shells and L0492 has three.

Medicare Information
See chapter titled "Medicare Guidelines," under "Prostheses and Orthotics," for Medicare billing and documentation information.

L0621-L0624

L0621　Sacroiliac orthotic, flexible, provides pelvic-sacral support, reduces motion about the sacroiliac joint, includes straps, closures, may include pendulous abdomen design, prefabricated, includes fitting and adjustment

L0622　Sacroiliac orthotic, flexible, provides pelvic-sacral support, reduces motion about the sacroiliac joint, includes straps, closures, may include pendulous abdomen design, custom fabricated

L0623　Sacroiliac orthotic, provides pelvic-sacral support, with rigid or semi-rigid panels over the sacrum and abdomen, reduces motion about the sacroiliac joint, includes straps, closures, may include pendulous abdomen design, prefabricated, includes fitting and adjustment

L0624　Sacroiliac orthotic, provides pelvic-sacral support, with rigid or semi-rigid panels placed over the sacrum and abdomen, reduces motion about the sacroiliac joint, includes straps, closures, may include pendulous abdomen design, custom fabricated

Lay Description
Sacroiliac orthoses may be flexible, rigid, or semi-rigid. These orthoses provide support for the lower portion of the torso, including the pelvic region, and reduce motion about the sacroiliac joint. Because of the narrow width of theses types of orthoses, they are commonly referred to as belts or corsets. An orthosis can be prefabricated or custom fabricated. A prefabricated (also known as custom fitted) orthosis is one that the manufacturer has produced in quantity, without a specific patient in mind. A prefabricated orthosis may be trimmed, bent, molded (with or without heat), or otherwise modified for use by a specific patient (i.e., custom fitted). An orthosis that is assembled from prefabricated components is considered prefabricated. In contrast, a custom-fabricated orthosis is one that is individually made for a specific patient, starting with basic materials, including plastic, metal, leather, or cloth in the form of sheets, bars, and so forth. It involves substantial work, such as cutting, bending, molding, sewing, and so forth. It may involve the incorporation of some prefabricated components. It involves more than trimming, bending, or making other modifications to a prefabricated item. Sacroiliac orthoses are usually prescribed to reduce sacroiliac diastasis or to reduce pelvic symphysis separation, and can even be given on a prophylactic basis to workers whose day-to-day tasks involve heavy lifting. Codes L0621 and L0622 represent the flexible type of sacroiliac orthosis, and L0623 and L0624 represent the rigid or semi-rigid type of sacroiliac orthosis.

L0625-L0627

L0625　Lumbar orthotic, flexible, provides lumbar support, posterior extends from L-1 to below L-5 vertebra, produces intracavitary pressure to reduce load on the intervertebral discs, includes straps, closures, may include pendulous abdomen design, shoulder straps, stays, prefabricated, includes fitting and adjustment

L0626　Lumbar orthotic, sagittal control, with rigid posterior panel(s), posterior extends from L-1 to below L-5 vertebra, produces intracavitary pressure to reduce load on the intervertebral discs, includes straps, closures, may include padding, stays, shoulder straps, pendulous abdomen design, prefabricated, includes fitting and adjustment

L0627　Lumbar orthotic, sagittal control, with rigid anterior and posterior panels, posterior extends from L-1 to below L-5 vertebra, produces intracavitary pressure to reduce load on the intervertebral discs, includes straps, closures, may include padding, shoulder straps, pendulous abdomen design, prefabricated, includes fitting and adjustment

Lay Description

Lumbar orthoses may be flexible, rigid, or semi-rigid. These orthoses provide support to the lumbar (L1-L5) spinal area. They function by producing pressure within the abdominal and body cavities, creating space between the vertebrae, and allowing the intervertebral disk enough space to comfortably fit between the vertebrae. An orthosis can be prefabricated (custom fitted) or custom fabricated. A prefabricated (also known as custom fitted) orthosis is one that the manufacturer has produced in quantity, without a specific patient in mind. A prefabricated orthosis may be trimmed, bent, molded (with or without heat), or otherwise modified for use by a specific patient (i.e., custom fitted). An orthosis that is assembled from prefabricated components is considered prefabricated. In contrast to a prefabricated orthosis, a custom fabricated orthosis is one that is individually made for a specific patient, starting with basic materials including, but not limited to, plastic, metal, leather, or cloth in the form of sheets, bars, and so forth. It involves substantial work, such as cutting, bending, molding, sewing, and so forth. It may involve the incorporation of some prefabricated components. Flexible lumbar orthoses are used to treat mild spinal instability, painful arthritis, vertebral fractures of the lumbar and lower thoracic spine, and may be used immediately after lumbar surgery (e.g., discectomy, fusion) to provide back support. The rigid lumbar orthoses are used postfracture to reduce risk of further injury, or postoperatively for complex spinal surgeries when increased support is required. Rigid devices are also recommended for the treatment of scoliosis. HCPCS Level II code L0625 represents the flexible type of lumbar orthotic and L0626-L0627 represent the rigid type of lumbar orthotic.

L0628-L0640

L0628　Lumbar-sacral orthotic, flexible, provides lumbo-sacral support, posterior extends from sacrococcygeal junction to T-9 vertebra, produces intracavitary pressure to reduce load on the intervertebral discs, includes straps, closures, may include stays, shoulder straps, pendulous abdomen design, prefabricated, includes fitting and adjustment

L0629　Lumbar-sacral orthotic, flexible, provides lumbo-sacral support, posterior extends from sacrococcygeal junction to T-9 vertebra, produces intracavitary pressure to reduce load on the intervertebral discs, includes straps, closures, may include stays, shoulder straps, pendulous abdomen design, custom fabricated

L0630　Lumbar-sacral orthotic, sagittal control, with rigid posterior panel(s), posterior extends from sacrococcygeal junction to T-9 vertebra, produces intracavitary pressure to reduce load on the intervertebral discs, includes straps, closures, may include padding, stays, shoulder straps, pendulous abdomen design, prefabricated, includes fitting and adjustment

L0631　Lumbar-sacral orthotic (LSO), sagittal control, with rigid anterior and posterior panels, posterior extends from sacrococcygeal junction to T-9 vertebra, produces intracavitary pressure to reduce load on the intervertebral discs, includes straps, closures, may include padding, shoulder straps, pendulous abdomen design, prefabricated, includes fitting and adjustment

L0632　Lumbar-sacral orthotic (LSO), sagittal control, with rigid anterior and posterior panels, posterior extends from sacrococcygeal junction to T-9 vertebra, produces intracavitary pressure to reduce load on the intervertebral discs, includes straps, closures, may include padding, shoulder straps, pendulous abdomen design, custom fabricated

L0633　Lumbar-sacral orthotic (LSO), sagittal-coronal control, with rigid posterior frame/panel(s), posterior extends from sacrococcygeal junction to T-9 vertebra, lateral strength provided by rigid lateral frame/panels, produces intracavitary pressure to reduce load on intervertebral discs, includes straps, closures, may include padding, stays, shoulder straps, pendulous abdomen design, prefabricated, includes fitting and adjustment

L0634 Lumbar-sacral orthotic (LSO), sagittal-coronal control, with rigid posterior frame/panel(s), posterior extends from sacrococcygeal junction to T-9 vertebra, lateral strength provided by rigid lateral frame/panel(s), produces intracavitary pressure to reduce load on intervertebral discs, includes straps, closures, may include padding, stays, shoulder straps, pendulous abdomen design, custom fabricated

L0635 Lumbar-sacral orthotic (LSO), sagittal-coronal control, lumbar flexion, rigid posterior frame/panel(s), lateral articulating design to flex the lumbar spine, posterior extends from sacrococcygeal junction to T-9 vertebra, lateral strength provided by rigid lateral frame/panel(s), produces intracavitary pressure to reduce load on intervertebral discs, includes straps, closures, may include padding, anterior panel, pendulous abdomen design, prefabricated, includes fitting and adjustment

L0636 Lumbar-sacral orthotic (LSO), sagittal-coronal control, lumbar flexion, rigid posterior frame/panels, lateral articulating design to flex the lumbar spine, posterior extends from sacrococcygeal junction to T-9 vertebra, lateral strength provided by rigid lateral frame/panels, produces intracavitary pressure to reduce load on intervertebral discs, includes straps, closures, may include padding, anterior panel, pendulous abdomen design, custom fabricated

L0637 Lumbar-sacral orthotic (LSO), sagittal-coronal control, with rigid anterior and posterior frame/panels, posterior extends from sacrococcygeal junction to T-9 vertebra, lateral strength provided by rigid lateral frame/panels, produces intracavitary pressure to reduce load on intervertebral discs, includes straps, closures, may include padding, shoulder straps, pendulous abdomen design, prefabricated, includes fitting and adjustment

L0638 Lumbar-sacral orthotic (LSO), sagittal-coronal control, with rigid anterior and posterior frame/panels, posterior extends from sacrococcygeal junction to T-9 vertebra, lateral strength provided by rigid lateral frame/panels, produces intracavitary pressure to reduce load on intervertebral discs, includes straps, closures, may include padding, shoulder straps, pendulous abdomen design, custom fabricated

L0639 Lumbar-sacral orthotic (LSO), sagittal-coronal control, rigid shell(s)/panel(s), posterior extends from sacrococcygeal junction to T-9 vertebra, anterior extends from symphysis pubis to xyphoid, produces intracavitary pressure to reduce load on the intervertebral discs, overall strength is provided by overlapping rigid material and stabilizing closures, includes straps, closures, may include soft interface, pendulous abdomen design, prefabricated, includes fitting and adjustment

L0640 Lumbar-sacral orthotic (LSO), sagittal-coronal control, rigid shell(s)/panel(s), posterior extends from sacrococcygeal junction to T-9 vertebra, anterior extends from symphysis pubis to xyphoid, produces intracavitary pressure to reduce load on the intervertebral discs, overall strength is provided by overlapping rigid material and stabilizing closures, includes straps, closures, may include soft interface, pendulous abdomen design, custom fabricated

Lay Description

A lumbosacral orthotic can be flexible, rigid, or semi-rigid. An LSO provides lumbosacral support from the sacrococcygeal junction to the T-9 vertebrae. It is a device that is used for the purpose of supporting weak or deformed areas of the spine, or for restricting or eliminating motion (immobilization) in diseased or injured areas of the spine. An orthosis can be prefabricated or custom fabricated. A prefabricated (also known as custom fitted) orthosis is one that the manufacturer has produced in quantity, without a specific patient in mind. A prefabricated orthosis may be trimmed, bent, molded (with or without heat), or otherwise modified for use by a specific patient (i.e., custom fitted). An orthosis that is assembled from prefabricated components is considered prefabricated. In contrast, a custom-fabricated orthosis is one that is individually made for a specific patient, starting with basic materials including plastic, metal, leather, or cloth in the form of sheets, bars, and so forth. It involves substantial work, such as cutting, bending, molding, sewing, and so forth. It may involve the incorporation of some prefabricated components. It involves more than trimming, bending, or making other modifications to a prefabricated item. The benefits of orthotics use, specifically during convalescence from an injury or illness (useful to the weak or deformed body area) or as a postoperative treatment measure, can include the following: Restricted range of motion of the affected area (immobilization); support of the affected area; and/or protection from injury, reinjury, suture tearing, and/or wound dehiscence. An LSO can be designed to control movement of both the trunk and between the segments of the vertebrae in one or more planes of motion. The most common planes are coronal/frontal, sagittal, and transverse. Codes L0628 and L0629 represent the flexible type of LSO; L0630-L0632 represent one type of rigid LSO that controls motion in the sagittal plane only; L0633-L0640 represent other types of rigid LSOs that control motion in both the sagittal and coronal planes.

L0700-L0710

L0700   Cervical-thoracic-lumbar-sacral orthosis (CTLSO), anterior-posterior-lateral control, molded to patient model, (Minerva type)
L0710   Cervical-thoracic-lumbar-sacral orthotic (CTLSO), anterior-posterior-lateral-control, molded to patient model, with interface material, (Minerva type)

Lay Description

These codes report a specific type of cervical thoracic lumbar sacral orthosis (CTLSO). These orthoses control all spinal movement, lateral as well as anterior and posterior. Since the unit has a cervical component, the patient's head and neck are also immobilized. In addition to immobilization, the orthosis reduces compression load on the affected area of the spine. These devices are usually prepared ahead of a planned surgery. Measurements, scans, and moldings are taken by an orthotist. The orthosis is fashioned out of plastic polymers based on the patient data. The orthosis is bivalved, or cut into front and back pieces for donning and adjustment. Ventilation holes may be cut into the body of the orthosis, since they are typically worn over the course of the day. The Minerva component is an extension from the body of the orthosis that supports the mandible and occiput and stabilizes the cervical spine. Report L0700 for supply of a custom fabricated CTLSO. Report L0710 for supply of a custom fabricated CTLSO with interface material between the orthosis and the patient's skin.

L0810-L0861

L0810   Halo procedure, cervical halo incorporated into jacket vest
L0820   Halo procedure, cervical halo incorporated into plaster body jacket
L0830   Halo procedure, cervical halo incorporated into Milwaukee type orthotic
L0859   Addition to halo procedure, magnetic resonance image compatible systems, rings and pins, any material
L0861   Addition to halo procedure, replacement liner/interface material

Lay Description

This system represents the non-conductive halo traction ring and skull pins. These component parts represent pieces of what is commonly called the halo system. The halo system consists of a metal ring that is secured to the upper part of the skull (mid-forehead area) with pins. A cervical halo is used to immobilize the cervical spine usually due to an odontoid fracture (fracture of the second cervical vertebrae). Two metal rods extend from the halo along the sides of the head to the shoulder area and are attached to a well-fitted plastic vest, jacket, or other type of orthotic. While the patient is wearing the halo system, the patient may be required to have diagnostic imaging such as MRI or CT procedures. These additions to the halo system ensure patient safety by eliminating the risk of scalp burns, while also allowing for a clearer, higher-quality image. If the metal rods are attached to a plastic vest/jacket, report L0810; if attached to a plaster body jacket, report L0820; if attached to a Milwaukee type orthosis, report L0830. Code L0859 represents the rings, pins, and all other materials that come with the halo system.

L0970-L0976

L0970   Thoracic-lumbar-sacral orthotic (TLSO), corset front
L0972   Lumbar-sacral orthotic (LSO), corset front
L0974   Thoracic-lumbar-sacral orthotic (TLSO), full corset
L0976   Lumbar-sacral orthotic (LSO), full corset

Lay Description

This range of codes reports specific corset additions to spinal orthoses. Some spinal orthoses, such as the "chair back" designs, require a closure addition for the anterior of the device. The corset front is attached to this type of posterior orthosis and provides a means to close and adjust tension of the device. The corset closure is a lace-and-eyelet configuration. Some designs feature a full corset design. These devices will have a stiff fabric body, sometimes with semi-rigid ribbing, and a corset closure, usually on the front. Report L0970 for supply of a corset front addition to a thoracic lumbar sacral orthosis (TLSO). Report L0972 for supply of a corset front addition to a lumbar sacral orthosis (LSO). Report L0974 for supply of a full corset TLSO. Report L0976 for supply of a full corset LSO.

L0978

L0978   Axillary crutch extension

Lay Description

This code reports the supply of an axillary crutch extension. The axillary crutch is the most common type of crutch in use today. A pad under the armpit, or axilla, bears most of the user's weight over the length of double uprights that extend to the floor. An extra upright piece makes the crutch adjustable (extension crutch). A handle bridges the double uprights about one-third the length down the crutch. Report L0978 for supply of an axillary crutch extension.

L0980

L0980   Peroneal straps, pair

Lay Description

This code reports the supply of each pair of perineal straps. These straps, or belts, are used occasionally with spinal orthoses that tend to migrate upward as the wearer engages in activities. The belt connects to the lower aspect of the orthosis, front to rear, by passing in a criss-cross fashion under the groin, or perineum. Report L0980 for supply of each pair of perineal straps. Note that many Level II listings misspell perineal as "peroneal." Certain ankle straps used to provide traction during endoscopic surgery may be referred to as peroneal straps, but are not reported by this spinal orthosis code.

L0984

L0984   Protective body sock, each

Lay Description

A protective body sock is a garment made up of soft, cushiony fabric that is used under spinal orthotics and body jackets. This item does not meet the definition of a brace and is considered more as a convenience item for the patient. Code L0984 represents the supply of one body sock.

L1000

L1000   Cervical-thoracic-lumbar-sacral orthotic (CTLSO) (Milwaukee), inclusive of furnishing initial orthotic, including model

Lay Description

This code reports the supply of a Milwaukee-style cervical thoracic lumbar sacral orthosis (CTLSO). This is among the oldest designs of spinal braces still in use today, most commonly as treatment for idiopathic scoliosis, a lateral curvature of the spine that usually presents around puberty. A variety of brace configurations are seen, but all reported by this code will have a component that supports the head, limiting movement of the cervical spine (neck). Traditional braces were made of rigid leather, although most modern versions are constructed of thermoplastic and natural and artificial padding. The classic model features rigid waist and upper torso components. Metal rods, front and back, connect these components and the cervical support. Various padding may be placed to further manipulate the spine. Computer models based on detailed patient measurements and radiographs are used to calculate spinal geometries and loading. Several initial orthoses may be generated before a long-term brace is fabricated. Report L1000 for supply of a Milwaukee-style CTLSO, including initial orthosis and model.

L1001

L1001   Cervical-thoracic-lumbar-sacral orthotic (CTLSO), immobilizer, infant size, prefabricated, includes fitting and adjustment

Lay Description

This is a cervical thoracic lumbar sacral orthosis (CTLSO) that is intended for use on infants with suspected or diagnosed spinal injury resulting from trauma or delivery complications or a tumor impinging on the spine, or it can be used for temporary immobilization for IV placement. This orthotic stabilizes the child's head and spine, and its unique shape keeps the child's spine aligned with the airway to promote an optimal healing process. Code L1001 represents the supply of one infant-sized CTLSO immobilizer.

HCPCS Lay Descriptions

L1005

L1005 Tension based scoliosis orthotic and accessory pads, includes fitting and adjustment

Lay Description

This code reports the supply of a tension based scoliosis orthosis. Idiopathic scoliosis is a lateral curvature of the spine that usually presents by adolescence. Girls are affected at a ratio of five to one over boys. The classic nonsurgical approach is to stabilize the spine and manipulate development toward normal anatomy through the use of cervical thoracic lumbar sacral orthoses (CTLSO) or TLSOs. Tension based orthoses address scoliosis by exerting correctional forces on the spine through use of elastic fabrics and bands. Fabrics with elastic properties, pads, and elastic bands are fitted on the patient, often in configurations that change as development occurs. The orthosis is worn over the trunk, without a cervical component. Report L1005 for supply of a tension based scoliosis orthosis, including fitting and adjustment.

L1010

L1010 Addition to cervical-thoracic-lumbar-sacral orthotic (CTLSO) or scoliosis orthotic, axilla sling

Lay Description

This code reports the addition of an axilla sling to a scoliosis orthosis. Idiopathic scoliosis is a lateral curvature of the spine that usually presents by adolescence. Girls are affected at a ratio of five to one over boys. The classic nonsurgical approach is to stabilize the spine and manipulate development toward normal anatomy through the use of cervical thoracic lumbar sacral orthoses (CTLSO) or TLSOs. An axilla sling may be added to an orthosis to provide corrective leverage on the upper spine, usually in combination with fabric pads elsewhere on the apparatus. As the name implies, the sling runs under the armpit and connects the anterior and posterior components of the orthosis. It may be added to either a CTLSO or TLSO. Report L1010 for supply of an axilla sling to a scoliosis orthosis.

Documentation Standards

It is expected that the patient's medical records will reflect the need for the care provided. The patient's medical records include the physician's office records, hospital records, nursing home records, home health agency records, records from other health care professionals, and test reports. This documentation must be available to the contractor upon request.

An order for each new or full replacement item must be signed and dated by the treating physician, kept on file by the supplier, and made available to the DME MAC upon request. Items billed to the DME MAC before a signed and dated order has been received by the supplier must be submitted with modifier EY added to each affected HCPCS code.

The order must list the unique features of the base code that is billed plus every addition that will be billed on a separate claim line. The medical record must contain information that supports the medical necessity of the item and all additions that are ordered. An order is not necessary for the repair of an orthosis.

L1020-L1025

L1020 Addition to cervical-thoracic-lumbar-sacral orthotic (CTLSO) or scoliosis orthotic, kyphosis pad

L1025 Addition to cervical-thoracic-lumbar-sacral orthotic (CTLSO) or scoliosis orthotic, kyphosis pad, floating

Lay Description

These codes report the addition of pads to a scoliosis orthosis. Idiopathic scoliosis is a lateral curvature of the spine that usually presents by adolescence. Girls are affected at a ratio of five to one over boys. The classic non-surgical approach is to stabilize the spine and manipulate development toward normal anatomy through the use of cervical thoracic lumbar sacral orthoses (CTLSO) or TLSOs. Fabric pads are often added to an orthosis, often at the area of greatest thoracic curve (kyphosis) and usually in combination with a thoracic strap or axilla sling. When a pad is suspended from the apparatus on a movable strap, it is known as a "floating" pad, as opposed to one that is mounted onto the rigid shell. Maximum pad adjustment is ideal to adjust the amount of pressure and angle of applied force. Report L1020 for supply of a kyphosis pad to a scoliosis orthosis. Report L1025 for supply of a floating kyphosis pad to a scoliosis orthosis

L1030-L1040

L1030 Addition to cervical-thoracic-lumbar-sacral orthotic (CTLSO) or scoliosis orthotic, lumbar bolster pad

L1040 Addition to cervical-thoracic-lumbar-s acral orthotic (CTLSO) or scoliosis orthotic, lumbar or lumbar rib pad

Lay Description

These codes report addition of specific types of pads to a scoliosis orthosis. Idiopathic scoliosis is a lateral curvature of the spine that usually presents by adolescence. Girls are affected at a ratio of five to one over boys. The classic non-surgical approach is to stabilize the spine and manipulate development toward normal anatomy through the use of cervical thoracic lumbar sacral orthoses (CTLSO). Fabric or foam pads are often added to an orthosis, often at the area of lumbar curve. The pads are considered accessories to flexible corset-style orthoses and occasionally to rigid models. The pads are typically rectangular shaped and may be referred to informally as a "shingle." The actual pad may be fabric-based, urethane, closed cell foam, or other material. Lumbar pads may be available as inflatable units. The addition may be made to a CTLSO or other type of scoliosis orthosis. Report L1030 for supply of a lumbar bolster pad. Report L1040 for supply of a lumbar pad or lumbar rib pad.

L1050

L1050 Addition to cervical-thoracic-lumbar-sacral orthotic (CTLSO) or scoliosis orthotic, sternal pad

Lay Description

This code reports the addition of a sternal pad to a scoliosis orthosis. Idiopathic scoliosis is a lateral curvature of the spine that usually presents by adolescence. Girls are affected at a ratio of five to one over boys. The classic non-surgical approach is to stabilize the spine and manipulate development toward normal anatomy through the use of cervical thoracic lumbar sacral orthoses (CTLSO). Other forms of scoliosis may be treated with orthoses as well. The padded sternal component reported by this code may be added to a scoliosis orthosis to provide a pressure point against the sternal bone. Some may be applied and held in place by straps. But most models feature an integrated pad and rigid outer shell, sometimes including a tension hinge on an armature to adjust pressure on the sternum. The actual pad may be fabric-based, urethane, closed cell foam, or other material. The addition may be made to a CTLSO or other type of scoliosis orthosis. Report L1050 for supply of each sternal pad added to a scoliosis orthosis.

L1060

L1060 Addition to cervical-thoracic-lumbar-sacral orthotic (CTLSO) or scoliosis orthotic, thoracic pad

Lay Description

This code reports the addition of a thoracic pad to a scoliosis orthosis. Idiopathic scoliosis is a lateral curvature of the spine that usually presents by adolescence. Girls are affected at a ratio of five to one over boys. The classic non-surgical approach is to stabilize the spine and manipulate development toward normal anatomy through the use of cervical thoracic lumbar sacral orthoses (CTLSO). These devices rely on pressure points to manipulate spinal development and strategically placed padding provides this pressure. Other forms of scoliosis may be treated with orthoses as well. Thoracic pads may be applied and held in place by straps. Others are integrated into the rigid shell that comprises the thoracic component of the orthosis. Report L1060 for supply of each thoracic pad added to a scoliosis orthosis.

L1070

L1070 Addition to cervical-thoracic-lumbar-sacral orthotic (CTLSO) or scoliosis orthotic, trapezius sling

Lay Description

This code reports the addition of a trapezius sling to a scoliosis orthosis. Idiopathic scoliosis is a lateral curvature of the spine that usually presents by adolescence. Girls are affected at a ratio of five to one over boys. The classic non-surgical approach is to stabilize the spine and manipulate development toward normal anatomy through the use of cervical thoracic lumbar sacral orthoses (CTLSO). These devices rely on pressure points to manipulate spinal development and strategically placed padding provides this pressure. Other forms of scoliosis may be treated with orthoses as well. The trapezius muscle is on the upper back and works to move the shoulder blade. A trapezius sling is an addition to the anterior and posterior thoracic components that cross high on the shoulder near the neck. Padding on the sling provides a pressure point, usually to address the upper thoracic and lower cervical vertebra. Report L1070 for supply of a trapezius sling added to a scoliosis orthosis.

L1080-L1085

L1080 Addition to cervical-thoracic-lumbar-sacral orthotic (CTLSO) or scoliosis orthotic, outrigger

L1085 Addition to cervical-thoracic-lumbar-sacral orthotic (CTLSO) or scoliosis orthotic, outrigger, bilateral with vertical extensions

Lay Description

These codes report outrigger additions to scoliosis orthoses. Idiopathic scoliosis is a lateral curvature of the spine that usually presents by adolescence. Girls are affected at a ratio of five to one over boys. The classic non-surgical approach is to stabilize the spine and manipulate development toward normal anatomy through the use of cervical thoracic lumbar sacral orthoses (CTLSO). These devices rely on pressure points to manipulate spinal development. Other forms of scoliosis may be treated with orthoses as well. Outriggers are components added to the rigid portion of the orthosis. They are most often associated with Milwaukee-style orthoses. Outriggers themselves are often stainless steel bars and attachment may be to a vertical bar of the orthosis. The outrigger usually contributes leverage for pressure points. Report L1080 for supply of an outrigger addition to a scoliosis orthosis. Report L1085 for supply of a bilateral outrigger addition to a scoliosis orthosis with vertical extension.

L1090

L1090 Addition to cervical-thoracic-lumbar-sacral orthotic (CTLSO) or scoliosis orthotic, lumbar sling

Lay Description

A lumbar sling is an addition to a scoliosis orthotic device. Scoliosis is an abnormal curvature of the spine frrom side to side giving the spine an "S" shape. The sling addition is a padded strap or sling used used to put pressure on the spine for to hold or put pressure on the lumbar spine. HCPCS L1090 represents a lumbar sling addition to a cervical-thoracic-lumbar-sacral orthotic device.

L1100-L1110

L1100 Addition to cervical-thoracic-lumbar-sacral orthotic (CTLSO) or scoliosis orthotic, ring flange, plastic or leather

L1110 Addition to cervical-thoracic-lumbar-sacral orthotic (CTLSO) or scoliosis orthotic, ring flange, plastic or leather, molded to patient model

Lay Description

This code reports the addition of a custom molded ring flange to a scoliosis orthosis. This device supports the mandible and occiput of a cervical thoracic lumbar sacral orthoses (CTLSO). Idiopathic scoliosis is a lateral curvature of the spine that usually presents by adolescence. Girls are affected at a ratio of five to one over boys. The classic nonsurgical approach is to stabilize the spine and manipulate development toward normal anatomy through the use of CTLSO. Certain CTLSO models employ a plastic ring to immobilize the cervical spine and head, which is less visible than the larger supports seen on some models. Report L1100 for the addition of a prefabricated ring flange, supplied in either plastic or leather. Report L1110 for the addition of a custom-molded ring flange, supplied in either plastic or leather.

L1200

L1200 Thoracic-lumbar-sacral orthotic (TLSO), inclusive of furnishing initial orthotic only

Lay Description

This code reports the supply of a thoracic lumbar sacral orthosis (TLSO). These devices are sometimes referred to as "low profile" because they lack the "high profile" of a cervical component and many designs fit unobtrusively under clothing. These braces are not specifically limited to correction of scoliosis. Some may be prescribed following certain surgeries or to treat symptoms of trauma. Numerous fittings may be required, as idiopathic scoliosis requires adjustments as the patient's spine develops. Report L1200 for the supply of an initial TLSO only.

L1230

L1230 Addition to thoracic-lumbar-sacral orthotic (TLSO), (low profile), Milwaukee type superstructure

Lay Description

This code reports addition of a Milwaukee type superstructure to a thoracic lumbar sacral orthosis (TLSO). The Milwaukee brace is among the oldest designs of spinal braces still in use today, most commonly as treatment for idiopathic scoliosis, a lateral curvature of the spine that usually presents around puberty. A variety of Milwaukee brace configurations are seen, but the classic model features rigid waist and upper torso components. Vertical metal rods, front and back, connect these components. Various padding arrangements and slings may be placed to further manipulate the spine. Report L1230 for addition of a Milwaukee type superstructure to a low profile TLSO.

Documentation Standards

It is expected that the patient's medical records will reflect the need for the care provided. The patient's medical records include the physician's office records, hospital records, nursing home records, home health agency records, records from other health care professionals, and test reports. This documentation must be available to the contractor upon request.

An order for each new or full replacement item must be signed and dated by the treating physician, kept on file by the supplier, and made available to the DME MAC upon request. Items billed to the DME MAC before a signed and dated order has been received by the supplier must be submitted with modifier EY added to each affected HCPCS code.

The order must list the unique features of the base code that is billed plus every addition that will be billed on a separate claim line. The medical record must contain information that supports the medical necessity of the item and all additions that are ordered. An order is not necessary for the repair of an orthosis.

L1250

L1250 Addition to thoracic-lumbar-sacral orthotic (TLSO), (low profile), anterior ASIS pad

Lay Description
This code reports the addition of an anterior ASIS pad to a thoracic lumbar sacral orthosis (TLSO). The acronym ASIS stands for anterior sacroiliac spine, which is the prominence of the hipbone at the front of the waist. This type of pad typically is used to provide a pressure point across the lower abdomen. Pressure here raises intraabdominal pressure, which in turn supports the lumbosacral spine. Report L1250 for addition of an anterior ASIS pad to a TLSO.

Documentation Standards
It is expected that the patient's medical records will reflect the need for the care provided. The patient's medical records include the physician's office records, hospital records, nursing home records, home health agency records, records from other health care professionals, and test reports. This documentation must be available to the contractor upon request.

An order for each new or full replacement item must be signed and dated by the treating physician, kept on file by the supplier, and made available to the DME MAC upon request. Items billed to the DME MAC before a signed and dated order has been received by the supplier must be submitted with modifier EY added to each affected HCPCS code.

The order must list the unique features of the base code that is billed plus every addition that will be billed on a separate claim line. The medical record must contain information that supports the medical necessity of the item and all additions that are ordered. An order is not necessary for the repair of an orthosis.

L1280

L1280 Addition to thoracic-lumbar-sacral orthotic (TLSO), (low profile), rib gusset (elastic), each

Lay Description
A rib gusset is an addition to a spinal orthotic. It is an elastic support used to provide structural integrity and to lower the pressure on the ribs. HCPCS level II code L1280 represents each addition to thoracic-lumbar-sacral orthotic (TLSO), (low profile), rib gusset (elastic).

L1300-L1310

L1300 Other scoliosis procedure, body jacket molded to patient model
L1310 Other scoliosis procedure, postoperative body jacket

Lay Description
These codes report the supply of a body jacket to treat scoliosis. Idiopathic scoliosis is a lateral curvature of the spine that usually presents by adolescence. Girls are affected at a ratio of five to one over boys. The non-surgical approach to idiopathic scoliosis is to stabilize the spine and manipulate development toward normal anatomy, and may include use of a body jacket. Body jackets may also be used for other cases of scoliosis. Preparation of a body jacket entails taking a plaster mold of the patient's body. Radiography, body scans, and computer modeling may also be employed. A plastic shell is prepared from the modeling and manipulated for optional therapy. The jacket may be bi-valved, or split into front and back halves for entry. The shell is vented and lined with cushion material. In some instances, a body jacket is required for recovery from surgery. In these cases, the casting and measurements are usually, but not always, taken prior to surgery. Report L1300 for supply of a custom molded body jacket. Report L1310 for supply of a postoperative body jacket.

L1500-L1520

L1500 Thoracic-hip-knee-ankle orthotic (THKAO), mobility frame (Newington, Parapodium types)
L1510 Thoracic-hip-knee-ankle orthotic (THKAO), standing frame, with or without tray and accessories
L1520 Thoracic-hip-knee-ankle orthotic (THKAO), swivel walker

Lay Description
These codes report supply of orthoses specific to paraplegic patients or those with compromised function of the lower extremities. A thoracic hip knee ankle orthosis (THKAO) is a supportive apparatus worn by the patient. Each zone is fully supported by the orthosis. Some units simply provide the patient with a means to stand, which improves muscle tone and assists bowel and bladder motility. Some models provide hand or arm controls to assist the patient in movement of the lower extremities, thus affording a level of ambulation. The Parapodium is a particular design of THKAO that offers hand and arm assisted steps. The devices may be used to assist paraplegics in walking or in rehabilitation efforts for patients addressing paralysis in the lower limbs. The THKAO can assist certain patients in relearning step and gait. The patient enters and exits the Parapodium orthosis from a

wheelchair; some designs may require assistance. Swivel walkers are a special THKAO designed primarily for children. The ankle, knee, hip, and trunk supporting structure is mounted on swiveling footplates. To ambulate, the wearer rocks alternatively onto each footplate, typically twisting the upper torso and swinging the arms. Report L1500 for supply of a THKAO support frame. Report L1510 for supply of a THKAO standing frame without accessories. Report L1520 for supply of a swivel walker.

L1600-L1650

L1600   Hip orthotic (HO), abduction control of hip joints, flexible, Frejka type with cover, prefabricated, includes fitting and adjustment

L1610   Hip orthotic (HO), abduction control of hip joints, flexible, (Frejka cover only), prefabricated, includes fitting and adjustment

L1620   Hip orthosis (HO), abduction control of hip joints, flexible, (Pavlik harness), prefabricated, includes fitting and adjustment

L1630   Hip orthotic (HO), abduction control of hip joints, semi-flexible (Von Rosen type), custom fabricated

L1640   Hip orthotic (HO), abduction control of hip joints, static, pelvic band or spreader bar, thigh cuffs, custom fabricated

L1650   Hip orthotic (HO), abduction control of hip joints, static, adjustable, (Ilfled type), prefabricated, includes fitting and adjustment

Lay Description

This range of codes reports supply of flexible hip orthoses designed to control hip abduction (spreading the legs). Many of these designs address congenital anomalies such as hip dysplasia in infants and pretoddlers. The Frejka orthosis is a pillow like device that separates and immobilizes the legs. The Pavlik harness features cuffs that fit to the femurs; a front and back harness arrangement fits over the shoulders and chest and may be adjusted to maintain the desired leg position. Like the Frejka device, this design also immobilizes the upper legs in a flexed and abducted position. The Von Rosen orthosis is a cross-shaped, semi-rigid pad that is custom fitted to the baby and then fixed into the desired position. The Ilfeld-style device uses a spreader bar fitted to cuffs on the baby's thighs and is either prefabricated or custom fabricated. Either is adjustable and the degree of abduction is controlled by adjusting the length of the cross bar. A waistband is generally used to hold the splint in place more securely. None of the above devices completely immobilize the legs and hips. All prefabricated devices include fitting and adjustment. Report L1600 for supply of a Frejka-type orthosis with cover. Report L1610 for supply of a Frejka-type orthosis cover only. Report L1620 for supply of a prefabricated Pavlik-style harness. Report L1630 for supply of a custom fitted Von Rosen-style orthosis. Report L1640 for a custom fabricated Ilfeld-type device. Report L1650 for a prefabricated Ilfeld-type device.

L1652-L1686

L1652   Hip orthotic, bilateral thigh cuffs with adjustable abductor spreader bar, adult size, prefabricated, includes fitting and adjustment, any type

L1660   Hip orthotic (HO), abduction control of hip joints, static, plastic, prefabricated, includes fitting and adjustment

L1680   Hip orthotic (HO), abduction control of hip joints, dynamic, pelvic control, adjustable hip motion control, thigh cuffs (Rancho hip action type), custom fabricated

L1685   Hip orthosis (HO), abduction control of hip joint, postoperative hip abduction type, custom fabricated

L1686   Hip orthotic (HO), abduction control of hip joint, postoperative hip abduction type, prefabricated, includes fitting and adjustment

Lay Description

These codes report supply of prefabricated hip orthoses designed to control hip abduction (spreading the legs) in adults. Such devices may be for any number of disorders, following certain surgeries, or to treat symptoms of trauma.

L1690

L1690   Combination, bilateral, lumbo-sacral, hip, femur orthotic providing adduction and internal rotation control, prefabricated, includes fitting and adjustment

Lay Description

This code represents a type of assistive technology often referred to as SWASH (standing, walking, and sitting hip orthosis). A SWASH is most commonly used on children with cerebral palsy, who often have difficulties with dystonia, hip migration, and a scissoring gait that interferes with ambulation and limits independent sitting. When properly fitted, the SWASH stabilizes the hip and prevents excessive adduction and internal rotation. This ultimately helps the child with stability while standing and gait during walking. When the child sits, the orthosis dictates continuous abduction, resulting in a wider base. This allows for a balanced posture and keeps the child from having to use their hands for support. Because of the technical nature of the SWASH orthosis, providers interested in using the device are required to attend a specialized training course. Code L1690 represents the supply, fitting, and adjustment of a SWASH.

L1700-L1755

L1700 Legg Perthes orthotic, (Toronto type), custom fabricated
L1710 Legg Perthes orthotic, (Newington type), custom fabricated
L1720 Legg Perthes orthotic, trilateral, (Tachdijan type), custom fabricated
L1730 Legg Perthes orthotic, (Scottish Rite type), custom fabricated
L1755 Legg Perthes orthotic, (Patten bottom type), custom fabricated

Lay Description

These codes report supply of a specific type of custom fabricated orthosis used to treat Legg Calve Perthes disease (LCPD or, more commonly, Legg Perthes). Legg Perthes disease is an osteonecrosis of the femoral head and hip socket found only in children, usually boys between the ages of 2 and 12. Bone death occurs in the ball of the hip due to interruption in blood flow. The disease is of unknown etiology. The Toronto type orthosis addresses the disorder with an unusual splint design. Each leg is secured by cuffs high on the thigh. A single vertical tube is connected to these thigh cuffs near the crotch. The lower end is connected to horizontal spreader bars fixed to special shoes. A ball joint between the vertical tube and the spreader bar allows knee flexibility. Shoe blocks are attached to the shoes to maintain alignment.

L1810-L1832

L1810 Knee orthotic (KO), elastic with joints, prefabricated, includes fitting and adjustment
L1820 Knee orthotic, elastic with condylar pads and joints, with or without patellar control, prefabricated, includes fitting and adjustment
L1830 Knee orthotic (KO), immobilizer, canvas longitudinal, prefabricated, includes fitting and adjustment
L1831 Knee orthotic, locking knee joint(s), positional orthotic, prefabricated, includes fitting and adjustment
L1832 Knee orthotic, adjustable knee joints (unicentric or polycentric), positional orthotic, rigid support, prefabricated, includes fitting and adjustment

Lay Description

Knee orthotics (braces) come in a variety of sizes and shapes, and are made differently depending on their intended use. A prophylactic brace is use to prevent or reduce the severity of knee ligament injuries. A rehabilitative brace allows protected movement of the injured knee, and usually has hinges that allow the knee to be locked into certain positions. A functional brace is used to support an unsteady knee during daily activities or is used during a sporting activity. A derotation brace is used after an injury to a ligament and typically has bars, straps, and hinges; it is used during sporting activities and is most often made up of lightweight materials so that it allows significant motion and speed. An unloader brace is specifically designed for patients suffering from pain and disability due to osteoarthritis. This brace works by keeping the knee in the valgus position, which allows unloading of the compressive forces on the medial compartment.

L1836

L1836 Knee orthotic, rigid, without joint(s), includes soft interface material, prefabricated, includes fitting and adjustment

Lay Description

This code reports the supply of a prefabricated rigid knee orthosis. Certain knee orthoses (KOs) are designed to immobilize the knee completely and therefore do not feature a joint system. Such devices may be applied to a knee injury to facilitate healing, or to protect the joint following surgery. The orthosis holds the knee in a fixed position, usually slightly flexed. Cushion material to interface between the rigid orthosis and the patient's skin is included in the code description as are fitting sessions. Report L1836 for supply of a prefabricated rigid knee orthosis.

L1840

L1840 Knee orthotic (KO), derotation, medial-lateral, anterior cruciate ligament, custom fabricated

Lay Description

This code reports supply of a custom made knee orthosis that limits medial and lateral rotation of the knee for patients with compromised anterior cruciate ligament function. This is a dynamic rigid body orthosis, meaning that muscle actions against the orthosis work to stabilize the joint. The anterior cruciate ligament (ACL) is the most often injured ligament in the knee, often without external contact. The ACL limits forward motion and rotation of the tibia. Patients with compromised ACL exhibit muscle movement abnormalities in activities as simple as walking on level surfaces. Stopping, landing from a jump, running downhill, or making rapid lateral maneuvers causes a sense of instability. Most knee orthoses that address ACL instability exert pressures to prevent the knee from coming into full extension. Devices such as the Lenox-Hill orthosis also work to control torque, or twisting, actions of the tibia. Report L1840 for supply of a custom made derotation knee orthosis.

L1843-L1846

L1843 Knee orthotic (KO), single upright, thigh and calf, with adjustable flexion and extension joint (unicentric or polycentric), medial-lateral and rotation control, with or without varus/valgus adjustment, prefabricated, includes fitting and adjustment

L1844 Knee orthotic (KO), single upright, thigh and calf, with adjustable flexion and extension joint (unicentric or polycentric), medial-lateral and rotation control, with or without varus/valgus adjustment, custom fabricated

L1845 Knee orthotic, double upright, thigh and calf, with adjustable flexion and extension joint (unicentric or polycentric), medial-lateral and rotation control, with or without varus/valgus adjustment, prefabricated, includes fitting and adjustment

L1846 Knee orthotic, double upright, thigh and calf, with adjustable flexion and extension joint (unicentric or polycentric), medial-lateral and rotation control, with or without varus/valgus adjustment, custom fabricated

Lay Description

Knee orthotics (braces) come in a variety of sizes and shapes, and are made differently depending on their intended use. A prophylactic brace is use to prevent or reduce the severity of knee ligament injuries. A rehabilitative brace allows protected movement of the injured knee, and usually has hinges that allow the knee to be locked into certain positions. A functional brace is used to support an unsteady knee during daily activities or is used during a sporting activity. A derotation brace is used after an injury to a ligament and typically has bars, straps, and hinges; it is used during sporting activities and is most often made up of lightweight materials so that it allows significant motion and speed. An unloader brace is specifically designed for patients suffering from pain and disability due to osteoarthritis. This brace works by keeping the knee in the valgus position, which allows unloading of the compressive forces on the medial compartment.

L1847

L1847 Knee orthotic (KO), double upright with adjustable joint, with inflatable air support chamber(s), prefabricated, includes fitting and adjustment

Lay Description

This code reports the supply of a specific type of prefabricated knee orthosis that uses air support chambers. A great variety of knee brace orthoses are available, and many feature a lateral and medial upright and an adjustable joint. The type reported by this code, however, also supports the knee with air filled chambers rather than cushion material alone. This type of orthosis may be used to initially stabilize the joint following trauma. Report L1847 for supply of a prefabricated, double upright knee orthosis with adjustable joint and air support chambers.

L1850

L1850 Knee orthotic (KO), Swedish type, prefabricated, includes fitting and adjustment

Lay Description

This code reports the supply of a particular design of knee orthosis (KO) known as the Swedish cage, or Swedish type. A great variety of knee brace orthoses are available, and many feature a lateral and medial upright and an adjustable joint. The Swedish cage design also features a posterior support piece to further stabilize the joint and prevent hyperextension. The Swedish style brace is further distinguished by its longer length. The thigh and calf cuffs are generally positioned at a further extreme than similar hinged KOs. This type of orthosis is "off-the-shelf," or prefabricated. Report L1850 for supply of each Swedish type, prefabricated KO.

L1860

L1860 Knee orthotic (KO), modification of supracondylar prosthetic socket, custom fabricated (SK)

Lay Description

This code reports a custom fabricated modification to a knee orthosis (KO) that is fitted in combination with a specific type of prosthetic socket. A prosthetic socket is the device that secures to the residual limb. The prosthetic leg attaches to the socket. In this instance, the socket is a variety that fits above the bony protuberance, or condyles, that constitute the distal end of the femur and the proximal end of the tibia (supracondylar). A KO may be required in patients with lower limb prosthetics to stabilize the joint, particularly during training in the use of an artificial limb. Report L1860 for supply of a custom fabricated KO modification to a supracondylar socket.

L1900

L1900 Ankle-foot orthotic (AFO), spring wire, dorsiflexion assist calf band, custom fabricated

Lay Description

This code reports the supply of a custom made, specialty ankle foot orthosis (AFO). Most AFOs employ medial and lateral upright bars attached from a calf band to an orthotic shoe or footplate. This device uses heavy gauge stainless steel spring wire rather than upright bars. The coiled spring action is at the attachment to the shoe or footplate and assists in dorsiflexion of the ankle joint (raising the foot at the ankle). These devices hold an advantage in being lightweight while offering good dorsiflexion assistance. Report L1900 for supply of a custom fabricated, spring wire AFO.

L1902-L1906

L1902 Ankle-foot orthotic (AFO), ankle gauntlet, prefabricated, includes fitting and adjustment

L1904 Ankle-foot orthotic (AFO), molded ankle gauntlet, custom fabricated

L1906 Ankle-foot orthosis (AFO), multiligamentus ankle support, prefabricated, includes fitting and adjustment

Lay Description

Ankle orthotics, gauntlets, and supports are generalized under the heading ankle-foot orthosis (AFO). (An exception within this range is the simple, prefabricated neoprene sock-type device reported by L1901.) AFOs within this range are prescribed for a variety of conditions for ambulatory patients, including congenital anomalies, pronation of the ankle, tendon problems, arthritis, and amputation. These devices generally extend well above the ankle, often to the upper calf, and may accommodate multiple planes of ankle movement. Some devices also limit ankle movement. The units may be built from standardized molds or custom fabricated from a plaster impression taken of the patient's foot and ankle. The units themselves may be made of metal, plastic polymers, or leather, sometimes in combination, and usually with various fabrics, cushions, and closure systems. A custom-fabricated orthosis involves substantial work, such as cutting, bending, molding, or sewing. It may involve the incorporation of some prefabricated components. It involves more than trimming, bending, or making other modifications to a substantially prefabricated item. Polypropylene models are close fitting and are often worn inside the shoe. Gauntlets usually feature lateral and medial stabilizers to address eversion and inversion, arch support, heel lock, padded tongue to facilitate application, and side panels for additional reinforcement. Fitting and adjustment is included in the supply of the product. Report L1902 and L1904 describe custom fabricated orthoses. Some gauntlets use natural heat therapy to gently warm troubled areas on the ankle and foot. They consist of stabilizers (usually plastic) on either side to help resist inversion and eversion. Other features usually offered are arch support and complete heel lock, elastic back section to eliminate blistering, padded tongue to facilitate application, and side panels for more reinforcement. In L1904, a molded-to-patient-model orthosis is a particular type of custom fabricated orthosis in which an impression of the foot is taken, by means of a plaster cast, CAD-CAM technology, etc. This impression is then used to make a positive model (of plaster or other material) of the body part to be braced. The orthosis is then molded on this positive model to be fit exactly to the patient's foot. It may require several castings and fittings by an orthotist/MD. Code L1906 reports a prefabricated ankle support for multiple ligaments.

Medicare Information

AFOs described by L1900–L1990 and L2106–L2116 are covered for ambulatory patients with weakness or deformity of the foot and ankle who require stabilization for medical reasons and who have the potential to benefit functionally.

See chapter titled "Medicare Guidelines," under "Ankle-Foot Orthosis (AFO) and Knee-Ankle-Foot Orthosis (KAFO); Related Additions and Replacements; Repairs," for additional Medicare billing and documentation information.

L1910

L1910 Ankle-foot orthotic (AFO), posterior, single bar, clasp attachment to shoe counter, prefabricated, includes fitting and adjustment

Lay Description

This code reports the supply of a prefabricated single bar ankle foot orthosis (AFO). This type of AFO involves a single upright bar that attaches to a cuff near the top of the back of the calf and spans to an attachment that fits at the heel of the foot with a clasp attachment. The bar is shaped to the curve of the back of the calf and ankle. The AFO is available "off-the-shelf," and fitting and adjustment to a specific patient is required. Report L1910 for supply of each prefabricated, posterior, single upright AFO.

L1920

L1920 Ankle-foot orthotic (AFO), single upright with static or adjustable stop (Phelps or Perlstein type), custom fabricated

Lay Description

The type of ankle-foot orthosis (AFO) reported by L1920 involves a single upright bar that attaches to a band near the top of the calf and spans to an attachment that fits at the ankle-foot. The bar is usually on the lateral side of the orthotic and its length may be adjustable. The AFO is custom fabricated to address a specific disorder and to fit a specific patient. Report L1920 for supply of each custom fabricated single upright AFO of the Phelps or Peristein type.

L1930-L1940

L1930 Ankle-foot orthotic (AFO), plastic or other material, prefabricated, includes fitting and adjustment

L1932 AFO, rigid anterior tibial section, total carbon fiber or equal material, prefabricated, includes fitting and adjustment

L1940 Ankle-foot orthotic (AFO), plastic or other material, custom fabricated

Lay Description

Ankle-foot orthoses extend well above the ankle (usually to near the top of the calf) and are fastened around the lower leg above the ankle. A prefabricated ankle-foot orthosis (AFO), code L1930, involves producing many generic AFOs from a single mold. This device is constructed for many patients and is generic in design, made of plastic or other material. Code L1930 also includes the fitting and adjustment of the prefabricated AFO. Code L1940 is for a custom fabricated (molded to patient model) AFO and involves taking a mold of the patient first and fabricating an AFO from that mold. This device is constructed for only one patient and is not generic in design, made of plastic or other material.

Medicare Information

AFOs described by L1900–L1990 and L2106–L2116 are covered for ambulatory patients with weakness or deformity of the foot and ankle who require stabilization for medical reasons and who have the potential to benefit functionally.

Codes L1900, L1920, L1940–L2030, L2036–L2108, and L2126–L2128 describe custom fabricated orthoses. These codes must not be used for prefabricated orthoses.

See chapter titled "Medicare Guidelines," under "Ankle-Foot Orthosis (AFO) and Knee-Ankle-Foot Orthosis (KAFO); Related Additions and Replacements; Repairs," for additional Medicare billing and documentation information.

L1945

L1945 Ankle-foot orthotic (AFO), plastic, rigid anterior tibial section (floor reaction), custom fabricated

Lay Description

This code reports the supply of a specific type of custom-made ankle foot orthosis (AFO). Typically a plaster mold is made of the patient's calf, ankle, and foot, although scans and computer modeling may also be used. A thermoplastic orthosis is created based on the patient's image. The device reported by this code features an anterior plastic upright piece, known as floor reaction. This upright is integrated into a solid footplate. A floor reaction AFO is often used for patients with lower limb weaknesses, since it prevents dorsiflexion collapse at the ankle. It is ordinarily prescribed bilaterally. The orthosis is rear-entry with Velcro or strap closures. Report L1945 for supply of each custom made plastic floor reaction-style plastic AFO.

L1950

L1950 Ankle-foot orthotic (AFO), spiral, (Institute of Rehabilitative Medicine type), plastic, custom fabricated

Lay Description

This code reports supply of a specific type of custom-made ankle foot orthosis (AFO). The IRM is typically a single-piece AFO. The calf cuff is integrated into a single upright that spirals around the lower calf to join a footplate. Some designs are hemi-spiral, others make a full spiral. This thermoplastic component is based on patient specific measurements or moldings. Report L1950 for supply of each spiral-type custom AFO.

L1960

L1960 Ankle-foot orthotic (AFO), posterior solid ankle, plastic, custom fabricated

Lay Description

A custom fabricated (molded to patient model) ankle-foot orthosis (AFO), code L1960, involves taking a mold of a patient first and fabricating an AFO from that mold. This device is constructed of plastic for only one patient and has a posterior solid ankle.

Medicare Information

AFOs described by L1900–L1990 and L2106–L2116 are covered for ambulatory patients with weakness or deformity of the foot and ankle who require stabilization for medical reasons and who have the potential to benefit functionally.

Codes L1900, L1920, L1940–L2030, L2036–L2108, and L2126–L2128 describe custom fabricated orthoses. These codes must not be used for prefabricated orthoses.

See chapter titled "Medicare Guidelines," under "Ankle-Foot Orthosis (AFO) and Knee-Ankle-Foot Orthosis (KAFO); Related Additions and Replacements; Repairs," for additional Medicare billing and documentation information.

L1970

L1970 Ankle-foot orthotic (AFO), plastic with ankle joint, custom fabricated

Lay Description

A custom-fabricated orthosis is one that is individually made for a specific patient starting with basic materials including, but not limited to, plastic, metal, leather, or cloth in the form of sheets, bars, and so forth. It involves substantial work, such as cutting, bending, molding, sewing, and so forth. It may involve the incorporation of some prefabricated components. It involves more than trimming, bending, or making other modifications to a substantially prefabricated item. A molded-to-patient-model orthosis is a particular type of custom fabricated orthosis in which an impression of the ankle joint is made by means of a plaster cast, CAD-CAM technology, etc. This impression is then used to make a model of plastic of the ankle joint to be braced. The orthosis is then molded on this model to be fit exactly to the ankle. This provides for free limited motion, or assist in dorsiflexion and plantar flexion while limiting inversion and eversion of the ankle. The plastic design is lightweight and allows the patient to interchange shoes. It may provide critical foot and arch support. Neutral arch position promotes healing of injured ligaments. Side supports helps position the brace correctly and tightly to move in harmony with the foot and ankle and assures full time protection and support.

Medicare Information

AFOs described by L1900–L1990 and L2106–L2116 are covered for ambulatory patients with weakness or deformity of the foot and ankle who require stabilization for medical reasons and who have the potential to benefit functionally.

Codes L1900, L1920, L1940–L2030, L2036–L2108, and L2126–L2128 describe custom fabricated orthoses. These codes must not be used for prefabricated orthoses.

See chapter titled "Medicare Guidelines," under "Ankle-Foot Orthosis (AFO) and Knee-Ankle-Foot Orthosis (KAFO); Related Additions and Replacements; Repairs," for additional Medicare billing and documentation information.

L1980-L1990

L1980 Ankle-foot orthotic (AFO), single upright free plantar dorsiflexion, solid stirrup, calf band/cuff (single bar 'BK' orthotic), custom fabricated

L1990 Ankle-foot orthotic (AFO), double upright free plantar dorsiflexion, solid stirrup, calf band/cuff (double bar 'BK' orthotic), custom fabricated

Lay Description

The type of ankle-foot orthosis (AFO) reported by L1980 and L1990 involves use of upright bars that attach to a band near the top of the calf and spans to a stirrup attachment that fits at the ankle-foot. A single bar (L1980) is usually on the lateral side of the orthotic. The double bar (L1990) model has upright supports on the medial and lateral sides of the AFO. Both models allow for free plantarflexion and dorsiflexion (movement to raise and lower the foot) at the hinged stirrup. The AFO is custom fabricated to address a specific disorder and to fit a specific patient. Report L1980 for supply of each custom fabricated single-bar "BK" AFO and report L1990 for supply of each custom fabricated double-bar "BK" AFO.

L2000-L2034

L2000 Knee-ankle-foot orthotic (KAFO), single upright, free knee, free ankle, solid stirrup, thigh and calf bands/cuffs (single bar 'AK' orthotic), custom fabricated

L2005 Knee-ankle-foot orthotic (KAFO), any material, single or double upright, stance control, automatic lock and swing phase release, mechanical activation, includes ankle joint, any type, custom fabricated

L2010 Knee-ankle-foot orthotic (KAFO), single upright, free ankle, solid stirrup, thigh and calf bands/cuffs (single bar 'AK' orthotic), without knee joint, custom fabricated

L2020 Knee-ankle-foot orthotic (KAFO), double upright, free ankle, solid stirrup, thigh and calf bands/cuffs (double bar 'AK' orthotic), custom fabricated

L2030 Knee-ankle-foot orthotic (KAFO), double upright, free ankle, solid stirrup, thigh and calf bands/cuffs, (double bar 'AK' orthotic), without knee joint, custom fabricated

L2034 Knee-ankle-foot orthotic (KAFO), full plastic, single upright, with or without free motion knee, medial-lateral rotation control, with or without free motion ankle, custom fabricated

Lay Description

These codes report the supply of specific custom fabricated knee-ankle-foot orthotics (KAFO). Designs for KAFO devices are similar to ankle-foot devices. Similar materials are employed. Some units may be built from standardized molds, but most are custom fabricated for a specific patient based on plaster molds and measurements. In addition to the solid stirrup ankle-foot features reported by this range of codes, a KAFO will have an upper thigh band or plastic shell and a hinged apparatus to eliminate (static) or limit knee movement. Codes L2010 and L2030 report a static knee joint, however. As with AFOs, single upright bars are usually on the lateral side of the orthosis and double uprights are medial and lateral. All KAFOs reported by this range feature free, or jointed, ankle components. Many KAFOs offer a variety of adjustments for knee flexion and most allow the patient to manually release the knee hinge to facilitate comfortable sitting. Report L2000 for supply of a custom made, single upright design with free knee. Report L2010 for supply of a custom fabricated, single upright model without knee joint features. Report L2020 for supply of a custom fabricated, double upright model with free knee features. Report L2030 for supply of a custom fabricated double upright design without knee joint. Report L2034 for a single upright design with or without free knee features.

L2106-L2116

L2106 Ankle-foot orthotic (AFO), fracture orthotic, tibial fracture cast orthotic, thermoplastic type casting material, custom fabricated

L2108 Ankle-foot orthotic (AFO), fracture orthotic, tibial fracture cast orthotic, custom fabricated

L2112 Ankle-foot orthotic (AFO), fracture orthotic, tibial fracture orthotic, soft, prefabricated, includes fitting and adjustment

L2114 Ankle-foot orthosis (AFO), fracture orthosis, tibial fracture orthosis, semi-rigid, prefabricated, includes fitting and adjustment

L2116 Ankle-foot orthotic (AFO), fracture orthotic, tibial fracture orthotic, rigid, prefabricated, includes fitting and adjustment

Lay Description

Certain tibial fractures may be treated with ankle-foot orthoses (AFOs). These devices generally extend well above the ankle, often to the upper calf. Ankle movement may be locked or limited, or multiple planes of ankle movement allowed. The units may be built from standardized prefabricated molds or custom fabricated from a plaster impression taken of the patient's foot, ankle, and lower leg. The units themselves may be made of metal, plastic polymers, or leather, sometimes in combination, and usually with various fabrics, cushions, and closure systems. Some models are "thermoplastic," which means shape can be adjusted by application of heat. Fracture AFOs may also be custom built from rigid materials such as plaster or synthetic polymers, as well as from prefabricated and easily manipulated semi-rigid (polypropylene) and soft materials (rubber, plastic foam). Fitting and adjustment is included in the supply of the product. Report L2106 for supply of a custom fabricated thermoplastic-type tibial fracture orthosis; L2108 for supply of a custom fabricated tibial fracture orthosis; L2112 for supply of a prefabricated soft tibial fracture orthosis; L2114 for supply of a prefabricated semi-rigid tibial fracture orthosis; and L2116 for supply of a prefabricated rigid tibial fracture orthosis.

L2126-L2136

L2126 Knee-ankle-foot orthotic (KAFO), fracture orthotic, femoral fracture cast orthotic, thermoplastic type casting material, custom fabricated
L2128 Knee-ankle-foot orthotic (KAFO), fracture orthotic, femoral fracture cast orthotic, custom fabricated
L2132 Knee-ankle-foot orthotic (KAFO), fracture orthotic, femoral fracture cast orthotic, soft, prefabricated, includes fitting and adjustment
L2134 Knee-ankle-foot orthotic (KAFO), fracture orthotic, femoral fracture cast orthotic, semi-rigid, prefabricated, includes fitting and adjustment
L2136 KAFO, fracture orthotic, femoral fracture cast orthotic, rigid, prefabricated, includes fitting and adjustment

Lay Description

These codes report the supply of specific femoral fracture cast orthoses. Codes are differentiated by casting material and rigidity and whether the device is custom made or prefabricated. Custom fabricated orthoses are generally manufactured for a specific patient based on measurements, castings, and sometimes computer modeling. Prefabricated orthoses are generally produced in volume, with variations only for size, and are intended for use by any patient in need of such a device. Prefabricated devices require fitting and adjustment sessions. Knee ankle foot orthotics (KAFOs) typically extend well above the knee, and in these instances address fractures of the femur. Thermoplastic is shaped and contoured by application of heat. Report L2126 for a custom fabricated orthosis of thermoplastic material. Report L2128 for a custom fabricated orthosis of any other type of material. Report L2132 for supply of a soft prefabricated orthosis; L2134 for supply of a semi-rigid prefabricated orthosis; and L2136 for supply of a rigid prefabricated orthosis.

L2200

L2200 Addition to lower extremity, limited ankle motion, each joint

Lay Description

This code reports an addition to a previously provided orthosis. Report L2200 for the supply of a device or service to limit ankle motion on an ankle-foot orthosis. The ankle joint moves the foot in flexion (plantarflexion is the dropping of the foot downward and dorsiflexion moves the foot upward) as well as inversion and eversion. A previously supplied orthosis is adjusted to limit ankle motion. This may entail molding a block to the interface of the ankle/foot parts of the orthosis, or otherwise manipulating the orthosis to limit movement.

L2210-L2265

L2210 Addition to lower extremity, dorsiflexion assist (plantar flexion resist), each joint
L2220 Addition to lower extremity, dorsiflexion and plantar flexion assist/resist, each joint
L2230 Addition to lower extremity, split flat caliper stirrups and plate attachment
L2232 Addition to lower extremity orthotic, rocker bottom for total contact ankle-foot orthotic (AFO), for custom fabricated orthotic only
L2240 Addition to lower extremity, round caliper and plate attachment
L2250 Addition to lower extremity, foot plate, molded to patient model, stirrup attachment
L2260 Addition to lower extremity, reinforced solid stirrup (Scott-Craig type)
L2265 Addition to lower extremity, long tongue stirrup

Lay Description

This range of codes reports additions to previously provided orthoses. Dorsiflexion assist (as well as plantarflexion assist/resist) devices involve the application of a small spring-loaded cylinder on the ankle portion of the orthosis that works against a piston rod on the foot section. The spring tension assists or resists the flexing action of the foot as prescribed. (Plantarflexion is the dropping of the foot downward; dorsiflexion moves the foot upward.) Certain devices, such as caliper plates, stirrup plates, and stirrups can be mounted to an existing orthosis. Others may be molded directly to a plastic polymer orthosis. These additions are used to manipulate the flexion mobility of the ankle joint. Report L2210 for the supply of dorsiflexion assist or plantarflexion resist additions to an orthosis of the ankle, per joint; L2210 for the supply of dorsiflexion and plantarflexion assist/resist additions to an orthosis of the ankle, per joint; L2230 for supply of a split flat caliper stirrup and plate attachment added to an orthosis of the ankle; L2240 for supply of a round caliper and plate attachment added to an orthosis of the ankle; L2250 for supply of a footplate molded to an existing orthosis of the ankle; L2260 for supply of a reinforced solid stirrup to an existing orthosis of the ankle; and L2265 for supply of a long tongue stirrup to an existing orthosis of the ankle.

L2270-L2275

L2270 Addition to lower extremity, varus/valgus correction (T) strap, padded/lined or malleolus pad

L2275 Addition to lower extremity, varus/valgus correction, plastic modification, padded/lined

Lay Description

Varus/valgus is usually a congenital condition (or pathological condition, such as in poliomyelitis). Varus is the condition where the joint is bent outward; valgus is the condition where the joint is bent inward, or medially. Treatment may entail an ankle-foot orthosis (AFO). Valgus of the ankle, or inversion, might be treated by an AFO with a bar on the medial side and a t-strap on the lateral side. Varus, or eversion, might be treated by an AFO with a bar on the lateral side and a t-strap on the medial side. Report L2270 for supply of a correction strap or pad for varus/valgus to an existing orthosis of the ankle and L2275 for supply of a plastic modification correction for varus/valgus to an existing orthosis of the ankle.

L2280

L2280 Addition to lower extremity, molded inner boot

Lay Description

Report L2280 for the supply of a molded inner boot added to an orthosis of the lower extremity. These units may be polypropylene vacuum formed to a plaster mold of the patient's foot and ankle.

L2300-L2310

L2300 Addition to lower extremity, abduction bar (bilateral hip involvement), jointed, adjustable

L2310 Addition to lower extremity, abduction bar, straight

Lay Description

These codes report the supply of abduction bars added to a fracture orthosis. Code L2300 by description entails bilateral hip involvement. The fracture bar added to the orthosis maintains abduction (legs spread) during healing. The bar is jointed and adjustable. Report L2310 for a straight abduction bar added to a fracture orthosis.

L2370

L2370 Addition to lower extremity, Patten bottom

Lay Description

This code reports the addition to a lower extremity orthosis of a Patten bottom. A Patten bottom is a type of strike boot added to the bottom of a knee ankle foot orthosis (KAFO). The Patten bottom is connected to the rigid outer shell of the orthotic so that with the limb slightly flexed, weight is transferred to the orthosis and upper leg rather than on the foot and ankle. Report L2370 for addition of a Patten bottom to an orthosis of the lower extremity.

L2397

L2397 Addition to lower extremity orthotic, suspension sleeve

Lay Description

Orthoses of the lower extremities are sometimes attached by a suspension sleeve. These interface devices often feature a soft silicone or neoprene liner that makes a non-slip suction-type contact to the skin. Report L2397 for supply of each suspension sleeve.

L2405-L2492

L2405 Addition to knee joint, drop lock, each

L2415 Addition to knee lock with integrated release mechanism (bail, cable, or equal), any material, each joint

L2425 Addition to knee joint, disc or dial lock for adjustable knee flexion, each joint

L2430 Addition to knee joint, ratchet lock for active and progressive knee extension, each joint

L2492 Addition to knee joint, lift loop for drop lock ring

Lay Description

This range of codes addresses additions to external knee joint orthoses used to treat knee dysfunctions. The codes report additions or adaptations to the joint mechanism of a base orthosis. Many of these types of orthoses minimally feature a manual adjustment that locks the joint for walking and another to release the knee for comfortable sitting. The traditional manual drop lock system requires the patient to lift a locking mechanism to release the fixed walking position. More advanced adaptations automatically lock and unlock the joint as the patient goes through gait motions (swing-phase or pendulum lock systems). Some adaptations add a release mechanism, such as a bail or cable, or a dial lock. A polycentric joint works like a cam, offering more rigidity as the joint is extended and less during flexion. A ratchet joint features a series of locking positions that can be selected or skipped over by the wearer, either for active use or as a means to progressively increase range of motion. A lift loop is a gripping device for the wearer to raise the locking ring of a drop lock mechanism. Report L2405 for supply of each drop lock device, each joint; L2415 for supply of an integrated release mechanism, each joint; L2425 for supply of a disc or dial lock, each joint; L2430 for supply of a ratchet lock, each joint; L2435 for supply of each polycentric joint; and L2492 for supply of each lift loop for each drop lock ring.

L2755

L2755 Addition to lower extremity orthotic, high strength, lightweight material, all hybrid lamination/prepreg composite, per segment, for custom fabricated orthotic only

Lay Description

This code reports supply of a segmental addition to a lower extremity orthosis of high strength, lightweight material, such as carbon graphite laminates. These high-end materials are extremely lightweight yet posses good torsional and structural properties. This additional segment is for custom fabricated orthosis only.

L2760-L2780

L2760 Addition to lower extremity orthotic, extension, per extension, per bar (for lineal adjustment for growth)
L2768 Orthotic side bar disconnect device, per bar
L2780 Addition to lower extremity orthotic, noncorrosive finish, per bar

Lay Description

This range of codes reports supply of additions to lower extremity orthoses support bars and associated devices. These bars are usually paired medially and laterally on the orthosis, although single-bar units are also used. Growth in children necessitates regular changing of bars and disconnect devices may be added to facilitate bar change out and adjustment. Report L2760 for supply of each additional extension bar; L2768 for supply of each disconnect device added to an orthosis; and L2780 for supply of a noncorrosive finish added to an orthosis bar.

L2795-L2810

L2795 Addition to lower extremity orthotic, knee control, full kneecap
L2800 Addition to lower extremity orthotic, knee control, knee cap, medial or lateral pull, for use with custom fabricated orthotic only
L2810 Addition to lower extremity orthotic, knee control, condylar pad

Lay Description

This range of codes reports supply of additions to lower extremity orthoses designed to improve knee stability and control through manipulative padding and coverings. These additions may allow for greater loading or unloading of a side of the joint, possibly relieving pressure on an arthritic or injured site. Report L2795 for supply of a full kneecap covering added to an orthosis; L2800 for supply of a kneecap addition to an orthosis that offers medial or lateral pull; and L2810 for supply of condylar pad addition to an orthosis.

L2820-L2830

L2820 Addition to lower extremity orthotic, soft interface for molded plastic, below knee section
L2830 Addition to lower extremity orthotic, soft interface for molded plastic, above knee section

Lay Description

These codes report supply of soft interface additions to lower extremity orthoses. This is padding against the skin for molded plastic pieces. A great deal of orthosis design engineering focuses on above-the-joint and below-the-joint supports. These supports must work through the skin surface to stabilize skeletal bone as well as softer-tissue structures such as ligaments, cartilage, and musculature. Report L2820 for supply of soft interface additions below the knee and L2830 for supply of soft interface additions above the knee.

L2840-L2850

L2840 Addition to lower extremity orthotic, tibial length sock, fracture or equal, each
L2850 Addition to lower extremity orthotic, femoral length sock, fracture or equal, each

Lay Description

These codes report supply of fracture socks, or the equivalent. These are highly elastic stockings, often with a natural fabric liner on the skin contact side. The stockings are often made of a closed mesh that can be trimmed for length. Fracture socks may be applied for certain types of closed fractures of the lower extremity, usually in combination with a rigid orthosis. The sock/orthosis combination holds certain advantages over traditional plaster casting in that patients often experience less muscle shrinkage. Report L2840 for supply of a tibial length sock and L2850 for femoral length.

L2861

L2861 Addition to lower extremity joint, knee or ankle, concentric adjustable torsion style mechanism for custom fabricated orthotics only, each

Lay Description

This code describes concentric adjustable torsion style mechanisms used for the lower extremity joint, knee or ankle, for custom fabricated orthotics only. These components incorporate adjustable and removable dynamic power assist. The power assist add-on component is mounted to a conventionally functioning knee or ankle component within a custom orthotic and adds the prescribed function to dynamic assist/resist as required. These additions are used to improve stability and walking functions.

L2999

L2999 Lower extremity orthoses, not otherwise specified

Lay Description

This code reports the supply of an orthosis of the lower extremity that is not defined elsewhere in the HCPCS listing. Certain wraps, splints, shoes, or other supplies may be reported by the code. Generally speaking, a Medicare claim for L2999 must include "a narrative description of the item, the brand name and model name/number of the item, and a statement defining the medical necessity of the item for the particular patient."

L3000-L3030

L3000 Foot insert, removable, molded to patient model, UCB type, Berkeley shell, each
L3001 Foot, insert, removable, molded to patient model, Spenco, each
L3002 Foot insert, removable, molded to patient model, Plastazote or equal, each
L3003 Foot insert, removable, molded to patient model, silicone gel, each
L3010 Foot insert, removable, molded to patient model, longitudinal arch support, each
L3020 Foot insert, removable, molded to patient model, longitudinal/metatarsal support, each
L3030 Foot insert, removable, formed to patient foot, each

Lay Description

This range of codes reports supply of a variety of prescription orthosis shoe inserts, differentiated largely by product type, construction material, and method of preparation and fitting. These devices fit inside the shoe. Most are molded to a plaster or foam replica of the patient's foot, but some are modeled to electronic images of the foot. Inserts molded to the patient's foot directly (L3030) are often made of thermo-formable materials that can be heat softened, custom applied, and trimmed in a single session. The UCB (also known as UCBL or "Berkeley shell") is named for the University of California Biomechanics Laboratories, the developer of several types of rigid inserts. Materials for this range of codes include high and low heat plastic, leather, and various synthetics.

Plastazote is a type of closed cell polyethylene foam and Spenco is manufactured from closed cell neoprene. Most inserts will address a variety of corrections to the foot. Report L3000 for supply of each Berkeley shell-type of shoe insert; L3001 for a Spenco insert; L3002 for a Plastazote or equivalent insert; L3003 for supply of a silicone gel insert; L3010 for a simple longitudinal arch support insert; L3020 for supply of an insert that provides longitudinal arch support as well as support to the transverse metatarsal arch at the ball of the foot; and L3030 for supply of an insert that is formed to the patient's foot.

Medicare Information

Inserts and other shoe modifications (L3000–L3170, L3300–L3450, L3465–L3520, L3550–L3595) are covered if they are on a shoe that is an integral part of a covered brace and if they are medically necessary for the proper functioning of the brace.

Medicare modifiers

Shoes and related modifications, inserts, heel/sole replacements, or shoe transfers billed without modifier KX will be denied as noncovered because coverage is statutorily excluded. According to a national policy determination, a shoe and related modifications, inserts, and heel/sole replacements are covered only when the shoe is an integral part of a brace. A matching shoe that is not attached to a brace and items related to that shoe must not be billed with modifier KX and will be denied as noncovered because coverage is statutorily excluded.

L3040-L3060

L3040 Foot, arch support, removable, premolded, longitudinal, each
L3050 Foot, arch support, removable, premolded, metatarsal, each
L3060 Foot, arch support, removable, premolded, longitudinal/metatarsal, each

Lay Description

This range of codes reports the supply of arch support products that are available premolded and not modeled to a replica of the patient's foot. These prefabricated "stock" devices may still require a custom fitting, however. Materials are usually various synthetics. Report L3040 for supply of an insert to provide simple longitudinal arch support; L3050 for supply of an insert to provide support to the transverse metatarsal arch at the ball of the foot; and L3060 for supply of an insert to provide longitudinal arch support as well as support to the transverse metatarsal arch at the ball of the foot.

Medicare Information

Inserts and other shoe modifications (L3000–L3170, L3300–L3450, L3465–L3520, L3550–L3595) are

L3070-L3090

L3070 Foot, arch support, nonremovable, attached to shoe, longitudinal, each
L3080 Foot, arch support, nonremovable, attached to shoe, metatarsal, each
L3090 Foot, arch support, nonremovable, attached to shoe, longitudinal/metatarsal, each

Lay Description
These codes report the supply of nonremovable arch support products that are attached to the patient's shoe. Materials are usually various synthetics. Report L3070 for supply of an insert to provide simple longitudinal arch support. Report L3080 for supply of an insert to provide support to the transverse metatarsal arch at the ball of the foot. Report L3090 for supply of an insert to provide longitudinal arch support as well as support to the transverse metatarsal arch at the ball of the foot.

Medicare Information
Inserts and other shoe modifications (L3000–L3170, L3300–L3450, L3465–L3520, L3550–L3595) are covered if they are on a shoe that is an integral part of a covered brace and if they are medically necessary for the proper functioning of the brace.

L3100

L3100 Hallus-valgus night dynamic splint

Lay Description
This type of night splint addresses poor alignment of the base joint of the great toe (hallux-valgus) through strapping, padding, and rigid splinting. A slip-on type splint is applied to the great toe and straps are applied to correctly align the toe while the patient sleeps. Report L3100 for supply of each night splint.

Medicare Information
Inserts and other shoe modifications (L3000–L3170, L3300–L3450, L3465–L3520, L3550–L3595) are covered if they are on a shoe that is an integral part of a covered brace and if they are medically necessary for the proper functioning of the brace.

L3140-L3150

L3140 Foot, abduction rotation bar, including shoes
L3150 Foot, abduction rotation bar, without shoes

Lay Description
These codes report the supply of abduction rotation bars. Abduction is the movement away from the median plane, in this case of the foot outward. These bars maintain the position of the feet and, consequently, the femoral head in a fixed position. The abduction bar is often prescribed to treat cases of talipes (clubfoot) and genu varus (pigeon toe-in) and certain types of hip dysplasia in toddlers. The prototypical orthosis is the Denis-Browne splint, which is an abduction rotation bar that attaches either to the footplate of a baby shoe or is wrapped to the foot. The variety that attaches to a shoe may be adjusted with a special wrench. Report L3140 for supply of abduction rotation bars with shoes. Report L3150 for supply of abduction rotation bars only.

Medicare Information
Inserts and other shoe modifications (L3000–L3170, L3300–L3450, L3465–L3520, L3550–L3595) are covered if they are on a shoe that is an integral part of a covered brace and if they are medically necessary for the proper functioning of the brace.

L3170

L3170 Foot, plastic, silicone or equal, heel stabilizer, each

Lay Description
Report L3170 for supply of prefabricated plastic silicone or equivalent heel stabilizer bars to control abduction and rotation. Ordinarily, this is an insert or modification to a shoe that is part of a lower extremity orthosis system.

Medicare Information
Inserts and other shoe modifications (L3000–L3170, L3300–L3450, L3465–L3520, L3550–L3595) are covered if they are on a shoe that is an integral part of a covered brace and if they are medically necessary for the proper functioning of the brace.

L3201-L3203

L3201 Orthopedic shoe, Oxford with supinator or pronator, infant
L3202 Orthopedic shoe, Oxford with supinator or pronator, child
L3203 Orthopedic shoe, Oxford with supinator or pronator, junior

Lay Description

These codes report supply of specific orthopedic footwear. The codes are differentiated by whether the footwear is modeled for infants, children, or juniors. The shoes reported by this range of codes are oxford style. The shoes are fitted with adjustment for supination or pronation. Supination is bowing out of the foot and adjustment is usually to raise the lateral edge of the shoe or to lower the medial edge. Pronation is a "flat foot" or bowing in of the foot. Adjustment is usually to raise the medial edge or lower the lateral edge of the shoe. Report L3201 for supply of oxford-style orthopedic shoes for an infant; L3202 for a child; and L3203 for a junior.

Medicare modifiers

According to a national policy determination, a shoe and related modifications, inserts, and heel/sole replacements are covered only when the shoe is an integral part of a brace. A matching shoe that is not attached to a brace and items related to that shoe must not be billed with modifier KX and will be denied as noncovered because coverage is statutorily excluded.

Shoes that are incorporated into a brace must be billed by the same supplier billing for the brace. Shoes that are billed separately (i.e., not as part of a brace) will be denied as noncovered. Modifier KX must not be used in this situation.

L3204-L3207

L3204 Orthopedic shoe, hightop with supinator or pronator, infant
L3206 Orthopedic shoe, hightop with supinator or pronator, child
L3207 Orthopedic shoe, hightop with supinator or pronator, junior

Lay Description

These codes report supply of specific orthopedic footwear. The codes are differentiated by whether the footwear is modeled for infants, children, or juniors. The shoes reported by this range of codes are hightop style. The shoes are fitted with adjustment for supination or pronation. Supination is bowing out of the foot and adjustment is usually to raise the lateral edge of the shoe or to lower the medial edge. Pronation is a "flat foot" or bowing in of the foot. Adjustment is usually to raise the medial edge or lower the lateral edge of the shoe. Report L3204 for supply of hightop-style shoes for an infant; L3206 for a child; and L3207 for a junior.

L3208-L3211

L3208 Surgical boot, each, infant
L3209 Surgical boot, each, child
L3211 Surgical boot, each, junior

Lay Description

A surgical boot or shoe is a special type of footwear, usually high-top style, designed to accommodate post-surgical wrappings and dressings and to allow the patient a degree of mobility. Ordinarily these boots are manufactured without left-foot or right-foot design considerations and are sold as single units. Report L3208 for supply of each surgical boot or shoe for an infant; L3209 for a child; and L3211 for a junior.

L3212

L3212 Benesch boot, pair, infant

Lay Description

L3215-L3230

L3215 Orthopedic footwear, ladies shoe, oxford, each
L3216 Orthopedic footwear, ladies shoe, depth inlay, each
L3217 Orthopedic footwear, ladies shoe, hightop, depth inlay, each
L3219 Orthopedic footwear, mens shoe, oxford, each
L3221 Orthopedic footwear, mens shoe, depth inlay, each
L3222 Orthopedic footwear, mens shoe, hightop, depth inlay, each
L3224 Orthopedic footwear, woman's shoe, oxford, used as an integral part of a brace (orthotic)
L3225 Orthopedic footwear, man's shoe, oxford, used as an integral part of a brace (orthotic)
L3230 Orthopedic footwear, custom shoe, depth inlay, each

Lay Description

This range of codes reports supply of orthopedic footwear. The codes are differentiated by whether the footwear is modeled for men or women, whether the shoe is an integral part of a lower extremity orthosis, and the style of the shoe. Depth inlay is a design feature to accommodate an in-the-shoe component of a lower extremity orthosis. The inlay may be removable for use of the shoe with or without the brace component. Shoes that are an integral part of a lower extremity orthosis generally feature a stirrup or caliper and plate attachment system to an external brace. Custom shoes are made for a specific patient.

Generally, a code reports supply of a single shoe when sold as a single unit. For supply of each woman's orthopedic shoe, report L3215 for an oxford shoe, L3216 for a shoe with depth inlay, and L3217 for a high-top shoe with depth inlay. For supply of each man's orthopedic shoe, report L3219 for an oxford shoe, L3221 for a shoe with depth inlay, L3222 for a high-top shoe with depth inlay. Report L3224 and L3225 for respective supply of women and men's models of orthopedic oxford shoes that are an integral part of an orthosis system and L3230 for supply of each custom shoe with depth inlay.

Medicare Information
Oxford shoes that are an integral part of a brace are billed using codes L3224 or L3225 with modifier KX. For these codes, one unit of service is billed for each shoe. Oxford shoes that are not part of a leg brace must be billed with codes L3215 or L3219 without modifier KX.

Medicare modifiers
Shoes and related modifications, inserts, heel/sole replacements, or shoe transfers billed without modifier KX will be denied as noncovered because coverage is statutorily excluded.

L3250
L3250 Orthopedic footwear, custom molded shoe, removable inner mold, prosthetic shoe, each

Lay Description
Report L3250 for each prosthetic shoe that is custom molded for a patient and has a removable inner mold and a custom fabricated insert designed for toe or distal partial foot amputation.

Medicare modifiers
Shoes and related modifications, inserts, heel/sole replacements, or shoe transfers billed without modifier KX will be denied as noncovered because coverage is statutorily excluded.

The right (RT) and left (LT) modifiers must be used with footwear codes. When bilateral items are provided on the same date of service, bill both on the same claim line using modifiers LT and RT and two units of service.

L3260
L3260 Surgical boot/shoe, each

Lay Description
A surgical boot or shoe is a special type of footwear, usually high-top style, designed to accommodate post-surgical wrappings and dressings and to allow the patient a degree of mobility. Ordinarily these boots are manufactured without left-foot or right-foot design considerations and are sold as single units. Report L3260 for supply of each surgical boot or shoe.

Documentation Standards
If the item is furnished secondary to a fracture, a copy of the x-ray study that confirmed the fracture should be easily accessible within the medical record.

L3265
L3265 Plastazote sandal, each

Lay Description
Plastazote is a type of closed cell polyethylene foam and L3265 reports supply of each Plastazote sandal. This type of footwear is often prescribed for patients who have undergone surgery of the toes or metatarsal area or who have problems in the forefoot zone. The sole of the sandal is manufactured from polyethylene foam to protect and cushion the plantar surface. Closures are usually Velcro strapping.

L3300-L3334
L3300 Lift, elevation, heel, tapered to metatarsals, per in
L3310 Lift, elevation, heel and sole, neoprene, per in
L3320 Lift, elevation, heel and sole, cork, per in
L3330 Lift, elevation, metal extension (skate)
L3332 Lift, elevation, inside shoe, tapered, up to one-half in
L3334 Lift, elevation, heel, per in

Lay Description
This range of codes reports lift modification to shoes. The codes are differentiated largely by type of material, style, and application in the shoe. Report L3300 for supply of a tapered heel lift, per inch of height; L3310 for supply of a neoprene heel and sole lift, per inch of height; L3320 for supply of cork heel and sole lift, per inch of height; L3330 for supply of a metal extension lift; L3332 for supply of any type of tapered inside-the-shoe lift, up to one-half inch; and L3334 for any type of heel elevation lift, per inch.

L3340-L3350
L3340 Heel wedge, SACH
L3350 Heel wedge

Lay Description
Heel wedges are modifications to shoes to lift medial or lateral aspects of the foot (pronation or supination) or otherwise address foot or posture problems. SACH is an acronym for solid ankle, cushioned heel. Report L3340 for supply of a

SACH-type wedge modification and L3350 for a simple heel wedge.

L3360-L3370
L3360 Sole wedge, outside sole
L3370 Sole wedge, between sole

Lay Description
Heel wedges are modifications to shoes to lift medial or lateral aspects of the foot (pronation or supination) or otherwise address foot or posture problems. Report L3360 for a wedge placed on the outside sole of the shoe. Report L3370 for a wedge placed between the outside sole and the shoe itself.

L3380
L3380 Clubfoot wedge

Lay Description
This code reports a shoe modification wedge to address clubfoot. Talipes equinovarus is the Latin-based medical term for clubfoot. Equino is a reference to horse and varus means to "toe-in." Babies born with clubfoot exhibit extreme plantarflexion, which, as in horses, means weight is born on the extreme forefoot and toes. The feet are also characteristically turned inward. Talipes refers to the talus bone of the foot, which is not fully developed in clubfoot. Optimally, cases of clubfoot are aggressively addressed early in life. Shoe wedges may be of some benefit to those patients who still exhibit characteristics as children, teens, and adults. The wedge is usually fitted to fill the extreme arch of the foot seen in these patients. Report L3380 for supply of a clubfoot wedge shoe modification.

L3400
L3400 Metatarsal bar wedge, rocker

Lay Description
Bar wedges and rockers are used to transfer and alleviate pressure and improve the gait. Rocker soles assist in the burring of energy that forces the body forward after the center of gravity goes over the peak of the rocker. The rockers also assist in cases of limited range of motion with regards to the ankle or metatarsophalangeal joints. Rockers are created by adding extra crepe to the midsole portion of the shoe and then beveling it away just proximal to the point of pressure. There are different types of rockers, but they should all have a stable flat area at mid-stance. There are also many styles of rockers. There are also metatarsophalangeal bars that refer to specific shoe modifications. All metatarsophalangeal bars are to help metatarsalgia and relieve plantar pressure by adding a wedge of firm material across the sole of the shoe. By placing the bar to the metatarsophalangeal heads it unloads the pressure from the metatarsophalangeal heads, which allows transfer from the shafts of the metatarsals to the distal end of the toes.

L3465-L3470
L3465 Heel, Thomas with wedge
L3470 Heel, Thomas extended to ball

Lay Description
These codes report modifications to a shoe heel known as the Thomas wedge. This is a bar applied to the exterior of the sole of the shoe posterior to the metatarsal heads. The bar is shaved at either end. The wedge provides pressure relief off the metatarsal heads, or ball of the foot. Report L3465 for supply of a Thomas wedge mounted to the heel of a shoe. Report L3470 for supply of a Thomas wedge that extends to the ball of the foot.

L3480-L3485
L3480 Heel, pad and depression for spur
L3485 Heel, pad, removable for spur

Lay Description
Bone spurs often form on the bones of the feet, particularly on the calcaneus or heel bone. These spurs can be extremely painful, particularly as pressure is placed against them. Report L3480 for supply of a heel pad with a depression for treatment of a bone spur and L3485 for supply of a removable heel pad for a bone spur.

L3600-L3610
L3600 Transfer of an orthotic from one shoe to another, caliper plate, existing
L3610 Transfer of an orthotic from one shoe to another, caliper plate, new

Lay Description
These codes report the transfer or replacement of caliper plates from one shoe to another. The caliper plate is the footplate of an ankle foot orthosis (AFO) or knee ankle foot orthosis (KAFO). The plate features short, integrated medial and lateral uprights that connect to the upper portion of the AFO. The caliper plate is usually incorporated into a shoe, typically by cutting or splitting the sole. These plates are subject to some wear and occasionally need to be replaced. More commonly, though, the shoe becomes worn and the caliper plate is switched to a new shoe. Report L3600 when an existing caliper plate is transferred from one shoe to the other. Report L3610 when a new caliper plate is transferred from one shoe to the other.

L3620-L3630

L3620 Transfer of an orthotic from one shoe to another, solid stirrup, existing
L3630 Transfer of an orthotic from one shoe to another, solid stirrup, new

Lay Description

These codes report the transfer or replacement of solid stirrups from one shoe to another. The solid stirrup is a particular design component of many ankle foot orthoses (AFO) or knee ankle foot orthoses (KAFO). Stirrups usually are attached directly to the shoe between the sole and heel, although the footplate inside the shoe occasionally is used. A solid stirrup reported by these codes integrates the upright with the footplate portion. A medial and lateral upright connects to the upper portion of the AFO. The stirrup may be subject to some wear and occasionally needs to be replaced. More commonly, though, the shoe becomes worn and the stirrup is switched to a new shoe. Report L3620 when an existing solid stirrup is transferred from one shoe to the other. Report L3630 when a new solid stirrup is transferred from one shoe to the other.

L3640

L3640 Transfer of an orthotic from one shoe to another, Dennis Browne splint (Riveton), both shoes

Lay Description

This code reports the transfer of a specific type of orthosis from one shoe to another. The Denis Browne splint is named for the British pediatric surgeon who invented the device early in the last century. It is a static orthotic device used to treat babies and young children with congenital disorders such as hip dysplasia and congenital genu varus (toe-in). An abduction bar is attached to a special footplate of the patient's baby shoes. The bar and footplates fix the patient's feet and, therefore, the femoral heads into a therapeutic position. Adjustment on the footplate allows for positioning of the feet. In infancy, the splint may be left on for long periods. In toddlers, the splint may be used only at night and during nap times. As the patient grows, new shoes must be fitted. The Denis Browne splint can be detached from the old pair of shoes and mounted to the new pair. Report L3640 for transfer of a Denis Browne-type splint from one pair of shoes to another.

L3650-L3677

L3650 Shoulder orthotic (SO), figure of eight design abduction restrainer, prefabricated, includes fitting and adjustment
L3671 Shoulder orthotic (SO), shoulder joint design, without joints, may include soft interface, straps, custom fabricated, includes fitting and adjustment
L3674 Shoulder orthotic (SO), abduction positioning (airplane design), thoracic component and support bar, with or without nontorsion joint/turnbuckle, may include soft interface, straps, custom fabricated, includes fitting and adjustment
L3677 Shoulder orthotic (SO), shoulder joint design, without joints, may include soft interface, straps, prefabricated, includes fitting and adjustment

Lay Description

A shoulder orthosis (SO) or shoulder immobilizer is a support device (usually not rigid or semirigid) used for sustaining injured, postsurgical, and/or weak or deformed areas of the shoulder girdle and for restricting or eliminating motion (immobilization). The benefits from orthotic and immobilizer use, specifically during convalescence from an injury (strain, chip fracture with strain, fracture) or illness or as a postoperative treatment measure, can include the following: restricted range of motion of the affected area (immobilization), support of the affected area, and/or protection from injury, reinjury, suture tearing, and/or wound dehiscence. Some of the devices support the shoulder while limiting most ranges of motion, particularly abduction, which is the movement that raises the arm. All of these items usually require the assistance of a person other than the patient for appropriate application. Most of these items can be adjusted to fit the patient and come in a variety of sizes.

Documentation Standards

If the item is furnished secondary to a fracture (traumatic or nontraumatic, such as due to severe osteoporosis), a copy of the x-ray study confirming the fracture should be easily accessible within the medical record. If the device is furnished post-surgery, a copy of the operative report should be contained in the medical record. This information should be made available to the payer upon request.

L3710

L3710 Elbow orthotic (EO), elastic with metal joints, prefabricated, includes fitting and adjustment

Lay Description

This code reports supply of a simple, prefabricated elastic elbow orthotic with metal joints. The device is prefabricated, which means the orthotist selects from mass produced products based on the size of the patient and fits the device accordingly. These devices may be neoprene or Lycra sleeves pulled over the elbow or wrapped around the elbow and closed with Velcro straps. Incorporated into the fabric of the orthosis are rigid, jointed bars, typically on the medial and lateral sides. Report L3710 for supply of a prefabricated elastic style elbow orthosis with metal joints.

L3762

L3762 Elbow orthotic (EO), rigid, without joints, includes soft interface material, prefabricated, includes fitting and adjustment

Lay Description

This code reports the supply of a prefabricated, rigid elbow orthosis. In certain instances the elbow must be immobilized as completely as possible, such as following trauma or during recovery from a surgery of the joint capsule. This type of orthosis acts much like a cast in that the joint is locked in position, usually in several degrees of flexion. The brace is rigid and includes cushion material between the hard structure and the patient's skin. The device is prefabricated, which means the orthotist selects from mass produced products based on the size of the patient and fits the device accordingly. Report L3762 for supply of a prefabricated, rigid elbow orthosis.

L3763-L3764

L3763 Elbow-wrist-hand orthotic (EWHO), rigid, without joints, may include soft interface, straps, custom fabricated, includes fitting and adjustment

L3764 Elbow-wrist-hand orthotic (EWHO), includes one or more nontorsion joints, elastic bands, turnbuckles, may include soft interface, straps, custom fabricated, includes fitting and adjustment

Lay Description

Fracture orthoses may be similar in design, depending on the manufacturer and the intended application. These are bracing devices, typically containing hardware such as aluminum or other lightweight arm supports for the desired degree of abduction, as well as plastic, polyethylene, or foam. These devices may use the patient torso or neck as an anchor as well as the phalanges. There may be hinges at certain points in the device to allow for a certain degree of elbow or wrist motion. The treating provider must initially apply these items, but a person other than the patient can be instructed in the proper application when/if the patient removes the device during specified intervals. Sizes can vary according to the manufacturer (there may be pediatric sizes as well). The items are generally manufactured in right and left models. Shoulder braces, with arm, elbow, and wrist immobilization, support and control the range of motion of the upper extremity, including the upper arm, scapula, clavicle, elbow, forearm, and/or wrist. They also support most muscles and ligamentous tissues related to the movement of the upper extremity. They maintain a degree of abduction between the patient's torso and the affected upper limb, at the degree desired (usually 45-90 degrees). Each of these devices will typically leave the fingers free, but grasping heavy items is usually unable to be accomplished and is not advised. They are used post-traumatically for severe fractures. Code L3985 is for the forearm, and has a hand with a wrist hinge; L3986 is for a combination of the humerus and the radius and/or ulna (e.g., Colles' fracture). Both of these orthoses are custom made for the patient.

L3806-L3808, L3900-L3925, L3929-L3935

L3806 Wrist-hand-finger orthotic (WHFO), includes one or more nontorsion joint(s), turnbuckles, elastic bands/springs, may include soft interface material, straps, custom fabricated, includes fitting and adjustment

L3807 Wrist-hand-finger orthotic (WHFO), without joint(s), prefabricated, includes fitting and adjustments, any type

L3808 Wrist-hand-finger orthotic (WHFO), rigid without joints, may include soft interface material; straps, custom fabricated, includes fitting and adjustment

L3900 Wrist-hand-finger orthotic (WHFO), dynamic flexor hinge, reciprocal wrist extension/ flexion, finger flexion/extension, wrist or finger driven, custom fabricated

L3901 Wrist-hand-finger orthotic (WHFO), dynamic flexor hinge, reciprocal wrist extension/ flexion, finger flexion/extension, cable driven, custom fabricated

L3904 Wrist-hand-finger orthotic (WHFO), external powered, electric, custom fabricated

L3905 Wrist-hand orthotic (WHO), includes one or more nontorsion joints, elastic bands, turnbuckles, may include soft interface, straps, custom fabricated, includes fitting and adjustment

L3906 Wrist-hand orthosis (WHO), without joints, may include soft interface, straps, custom fabricated, includes fitting and adjustment

L3908 Wrist-hand orthotic (WHO), wrist extension control cock-up, nonmolded, prefabricated, includes fitting and adjustment

L3912 Hand-finger orthotic (HFO), flexion glove with elastic finger control, prefabricated, includes fitting and adjustment

L3913 Hand finger orthotic (HFO), without joints, may include soft interface, straps, custom fabricated, includes fitting and adjustment

L3915 Wrist hand orthotic (WHO), includes one or more nontorsion joint(s), elastic bands, turnbuckles, may include soft interface, straps, prefabricated, includes fitting and adjustment

L3917 Hand orthotic (HO), metacarpal fracture orthotic, prefabricated, includes fitting and adjustment

L3919 Hand orthotic (HO), without joints, may include soft interface, straps, custom fabricated, includes fitting and adjustment

L3921 Hand finger orthotic (HFO), includes one or more nontorsion joints, elastic bands, turnbuckles, may include soft interface, straps, custom fabricated, includes fitting and adjustment

L3923 Hand finger orthotic (HFO), without joints, may include soft interface, straps, prefabricated, includes fitting and adjustment

L3925 Finger orthotic (FO), proximal interphalangeal (PIP)/distal interphalangeal (DIP), nontorsion joint/spring, extension/flexion, may include soft interface material, prefabricated, includes fitting and adjustment

L3929 Hand-finger orthotic (HFO), includes one or more nontorsion joint(s), turnbuckles, elastic bands/springs, may include soft interface material, straps, prefabricated, includes fitting and adjustment

L3931 Wrist-hand-finger orthotic (WHFO), includes one or more nontorsion joint(s), turnbuckles, elastic bands/springs, may include soft interface material, straps, prefabricated, includes fitting and adjustment

L3933 Finger orthotic (FO), without joints, may include soft interface, custom fabricated, includes fitting and adjustment

L3935 Finger orthotic, nontorsion joint, may include soft interface, custom fabricated, includes fitting and adjustment

Lay Description

A wrist-hand-finger orthosis (WHFO) is typically a rigid or semirigid device used for the purpose of supporting injured, post-surgical, and/or weak or deformed areas of the wrist, hand, and metacarpal regions (phalanges are usually freely mobile with these types of devices) and for restricting or eliminating motion (immobilization) of the affected structure. While orthoses are usually prefabricated (custom fitted) or custom fabricated, these types of orthoses are generally not customized. Many of these items appear as sleeves or stockinette types of items. The benefits from WHFO use, specifically during convalescence from an injury or illness or as a postoperative treatment measure, can include the following: Restricted range of motion of the affected area (immobilization), support of the affected area and/or protection from injury, reinjury, suture tearing, and/or wound dehiscence.

L3891

L3891 Addition to upper extremity joint, wrist or elbow, concentric adjustable torsion style mechanism for custom fabricated orthotics only, each

Lay Description

This code describes concentric adjustable torsion style mechanisms used for the upper extremity joint, wrist or elbow, for custom fabricated orthotics only. Each component is used to describe the removable components used with custom orthotics. These components incorporate adjustable and removable dynamic power assist. The power assist add-on component is mounted to a conventionally functioning wrist or elbow within a custom orthotic and they add the prescribed function to dynamic assist/resist as required. These additions are used to improve reach, grasp, and pinching functions.

L3960-L3962

L3960 Shoulder-elbow-wrist-hand orthotic (SEWHO), abduction positioning, airplane design, prefabricated, includes fitting and adjustment

L3961 Shoulder elbow wrist hand orthotic (SEWHO), shoulder cap design, without joints, may include soft interface, straps, custom fabricated, includes fitting and adjustment

L3962 Shoulder-elbow-wrist-hand orthotic (SEWHO), abduction positioning, Erb's palsy design, prefabricated, includes fitting and adjustment

Lay Description

A shoulder-elbow-wrist-hand orthosis (SEWHO) is used for the purpose of supporting injured, post-surgical, and/or weak or deformed areas of the shoulder, elbow, wrist, or hand. These codes may be similar in design, depending on the manufacturer and the intended application. These are bracing devices used on wheelchairs, typically containing hardware such as aluminum or other lightweight arm supports for the desired degree of abduction, as well as plastic, polyethylene, or foam. These devices may use the patient torso or neck as an anchor as well as the phalanges. There may be hinges at certain points in the device to allow for a certain degree of elbow or wrist motion. The treating provider must initially apply these items, but a person other than the patient can be instructed in the proper application when/if the patient removes the device during specified intervals. Sizes can vary according to the manufacturer (there may be pediatric sizes as well). The items are generally manufactured in right and left models. Shoulder braces, with arm, elbow, and wrist immobilization, support and control the range of motion of the upper extremity, including the upper arm, scapula, clavicle, elbow, forearm, and/or wrist. They also support most muscles and ligamentous tissues related to the movement of the upper extremity. They maintain a degree of abduction between the patient's torso and the affected upper limb, at the degree desired (usually 45-90 degrees). Each of these devices will typically leave the fingers free, but grasping heavy items is usually unable to be accomplished and is not advised. They are used post-traumatically for severe fractures and for certain types of surgical procedures, such as partial or total shoulder replacement. A prefabricated or custom fitted orthosis is one that the manufacturer has produced in quantity, without a specific patient in mind. A prefabricated orthosis may be trimmed, bent, molded (with or without heat), or otherwise modified for use by a specific patient (i.e., custom fitted). An orthosis that is assembled from prefabricated components is considered prefabricated. Any orthosis that does not meet the definition of a custom fabricated orthosis is considered prefabricated. A custom fabricated orthosis is one that is individually made for a specific patient, starting with basic materials including, but not limited to, plastic, metal, leather, or cloth in the form of sheets, bars, and so forth. It involves substantial work, such as cutting, bending, molding, sewing, and so forth. It may involve the incorporation of some prefabricated components. It involves more than trimming, bending, or making other modifications to a substantially prefabricated item. A molded-to-patient-model orthosis is a particular type of custom fabricated orthosis in which an impression of the specific body part is made (by means of a plaster cast, CAD-CAM technology, etc.). Code L3960 is an airplane design with abduction positioning, or positioning that is away from the median and is prefabricated, or not custom made for the patient. Code L3962 is Erb's palsy design with abduction positioning, and is also prefabricated.

Documentation Standards

If one of the devices described is furnished secondary to a fracture (traumatic or nontraumatic, such as due to severe osteoporosis), a copy of the x-ray study that confirmed the fracture should be easily accessible within the medical record. If the device is furnished postsurgery, a copy of the operative report should be contained in the medical record.

L3964-L3969

L3964 Shoulder-elbow orthotic (SEO), mobile arm support attached to wheelchair, balanced, adjustable, prefabricated, includes fitting and adjustment

L3965 Shoulder-elbow orthotic (SEO), mobile arm support attached to wheelchair, balanced, adjustable Rancho type, prefabricated, includes fitting and adjustment

L3966 Shoulder-elbow orthotic (SEO), mobile arm support attached to wheelchair, balanced, reclining, prefabricated, includes fitting and adjustment

L3967 Shoulder-elbow-wrist-hand orthotic (SEWHO), abduction positioning (airplane design), thoracic component and support bar, without joints, may include soft interface, straps, custom fabricated, includes fitting and adjustment

L3968 Shoulder-elbow orthotic (SEO), mobile arm support attached to wheelchair, balanced, friction arm support (friction dampening to proximal and distal joints), prefabricated, includes fitting and adjustment

L3969 Shoulder-elbow orthotic (SEO), mobile arm support, monosuspension arm and hand support, overhead elbow forearm hand sling support, yoke type suspension support, prefabricated, includes fitting and adjustment

Lay Description

A shoulder-elbow-wrist-hand orthosis (SEWHO) is used for the purpose of supporting injured, post-surgical, and/or weak or deformed areas of the shoulder, elbow, wrist, or hand. These codes may be similar in design, depending on the manufacturer and the intended application. These are bracing devices attached to wheelchairs, typically containing hardware such as aluminum or other lightweight arm supports for the desired degree of abduction, as well as plastic, polyethylene, or foam. These devices may use the patient torso or neck as an anchor as well as the phalanges. There may be hinges at certain points in the device to allow for a certain degree of elbow or wrist motion. The treating provider must initially apply these items, but a person other than the patient can be instructed in the proper application when/if the patient removes the device during specified intervals. Sizes can vary according to the manufacturer (there may be pediatric sizes as well). The items are generally manufactured in right and left models. Shoulder braces, with arm, elbow, and wrist immobilization, support and control the range of motion of the upper extremity, including the upper arm, scapula, clavicle, elbow, forearm, and/or wrist. They also support most muscles and ligamentous tissues related to the movement of the upper extremity. They maintain a degree of abduction between the patient's torso and the affected upper limb, at the degree desired (usually 45-90 degrees). Each of these devices will typically leave the fingers free, but grasping heavy items is usually unable to be accomplished and is not advised. They are used post-traumatically for severe fractures and for certain types of surgical procedures, such as partial or total shoulder replacement. A prefabricated or custom fitted orthosis is one that the manufacturer has produced in quantity, without a specific patient in mind. A prefabricated orthosis may be trimmed, bent, molded (with or without heat), or otherwise modified for use by a specific patient (i.e., custom fitted). An orthosis that is assembled from prefabricated components is considered prefabricated. Any orthosis that does not meet the definition of a custom fabricated orthosis is considered prefabricated. A custom fabricated orthosis is one that is individually made for a specific patient, starting with basic materials including, but not limited to, plastic, metal, leather, or cloth in the form of sheets, bars, and so forth. It involves substantial work, such as cutting, bending, molding, sewing, and so forth. It may involve the incorporation of some prefabricated components. It involves more than trimming, bending, or making other modifications to a substantially prefabricated item. A molded-to-patient-model orthosis is a particular type of custom fabricated orthosis in which an impression of the specific body part is made (by means of a plaster cast, CAD-CAM technology, etc.). These codes describe shoulder-elbow-wrist-hand orthoses that are supports attached to a wheelchair. Report L3964 if it is adjustable; L3965 is Rancho adjustable; L3966 reclines; L3967 has abduction positioning (airplane design); L3968 has a friction arm support; and L3969 has monosuspension arm and hand support. These are not custom made for the patient.

Documentation Standards

If one of the devices described is furnished secondary to a fracture (traumatic or nontraumatic, such as due to severe osteoporosis), a copy of the x-ray study that confirmed the fracture should be easily accessible within the medical record. If the device is furnished postsurgery, a copy of the operative report should be contained in the medical record.

L3980-L3984

L3980 Upper extremity fracture orthotic, humeral, prefabricated, includes fitting and adjustment

L3982 Upper extremity fracture orthotic, radius/ulnar, prefabricated, includes fitting and adjustment

L3984 Upper extremity fracture orthotic, wrist, prefabricated, includes fitting and adjustment

Lay Description

Fracture orthoses may be similar in design, depending on the manufacturer and the intended application. These are bracing devices, typically containing hardware such as aluminum or other lightweight arm supports for the desired degree of abduction, as well as plastic, polyethylene, or foam. These devices may use the patient torso or neck as an anchor as well as the phalanges. There may be hinges at certain points in the device to allow for a certain degree of elbow or wrist motion. The treating provider must initially apply these items, but a person other than the patient can be instructed in the proper application when/if the patient removes the device during specified intervals. Sizes can vary according to the manufacturer (there may be pediatric sizes as well). The items are generally manufactured in right and left models. Shoulder braces, with arm, elbow, and wrist immobilization, support and control the range of motion of the upper extremity, including the upper arm, scapula, clavicle, elbow, forearm, and/or wrist. They also support most muscles and ligamentous tissues related to the movement of the upper extremity. They maintain a degree of abduction between the patient's torso and the affected upper limb, at the degree desired (usually 45-90 degrees). Each of these devices will typically leave the fingers free, but grasping heavy items is usually unable to be accomplished and is not advised. They are used post-traumatically for severe fractures. A prefabricated or custom fitted orthosis is one that the manufacturer has produced in quantity, without a specific patient in mind. A prefabricated orthosis may be trimmed, bent, molded (with or without heat), or otherwise modified for use by a specific patient (i.e., custom fitted). An orthosis that is assembled from prefabricated components is considered prefabricated. Any orthosis that does not meet the definition of a custom fabricated orthosis is considered prefabricated. A custom fabricated orthosis is one that is individually made for a specific patient, starting with basic materials including, but not limited to, plastic, metal, leather, or cloth in the form of sheets, bars, and so forth. It involves substantial work, such as cutting, bending, molding, sewing, and so forth. It may involve the incorporation of some prefabricated components. It involves more than trimming, bending, or making other modifications to a substantially prefabricated item. A molded-to-patient-model orthosis is a particular type of custom fabricated orthosis in which an impression of the specific body part is made (by means of a plaster cast, CAD-CAM technology, etc.). Code L3980 is for the humerus; L3982 is for the radius/ulna; L3984 is for the wrist, all of which are prefabricated or not custom made for the patient.

Documentation Standards

If one of the devices described is furnished secondary to a fracture (traumatic or nontraumatic, such as due to severe osteoporosis), a copy of the x-ray study that confirmed the fracture should be easily accessible within the medical record. If the device is furnished postsurgery, a copy of the operative report should be contained in the medical record.

L4040-L4055

L4040 Replace molded thigh lacer, for custom fabricated orthotic only

L4045 Replace nonmolded thigh lacer, for custom fabricated orthotic only

L4050 Replace molded calf lacer, for custom fabricated orthotic only

L4055 Replace nonmolded calf lacer, for custom fabricated orthotic only

Lay Description

These codes report the replacement of molded lacers. Lacers are cuff-like devices that fit around a portion of a limb. They have a slit opening on one side to don the device and a lace-string corset-style closure of gussets and eyelets. Often they are of thermoplastic material with cushion liners built from patient molds, but many are still manufactured of leather, or have leather incorporated into the design. An orthotic device may attach to this device. Many are used for suspension of a prosthetic attachment. Report L4040 for replacement of a molded thigh lacer and L4045 for replacing a non-molded thigh lacer. Report L0450 for replacement of a molded calf lacer and L4055 for a non-molded calf lacer. These codes are all for a custom fabricated orthosis only.

L4205

L4205 Repair of orthotic device, labor component, per 15 minutes

Lay Description

Code L4205 is used for the labor component of repair of a previously provided orthosis except for any labor involved in the replacement of an orthotic component that has a specific L code. Report the time in 15-minute increments.

Medicare Information

Code L4205 is used for the labor component or repair of a previously provided orthosis, except for any labor involved in the replacement of an orthotic component that has a specific L-code. It may only be billed for the actual time involved in the repair of an orthosis. It must not be used for any labor involved in the evaluation, fabrication, or fitting of a new or full replacement orthosis.

A claim for L4205 must include an explanation of exactly what is under repair for the orthosis. A claim for L4210 must include a description of each item that is billed. This information should be attached to a hard copy claim.

Note: See chapter titled "Medicare Guidelines," under "Ankle-Foot Orthosis (AFO) and Knee-Ankle-Foot Orthosis (KAFO); Related Additions and Replacements; Repairs," for additional Medicare billing and documentation information.

L4370-L4380

L4370 Pneumatic full leg splint, prefabricated, includes fitting and adjustment
L4380 Pneumatic knee splint, prefabricated, includes fitting and adjustment

Lay Description

These codes report the supply of pneumatic splints, or air splints. These devices immobilize the limb by compressing air in chambers between the rigid outer shell and the patient's leg. These orthoses are used commonly in first response situations to trauma. But some models may be prescribed for more extended use to support the knee joint. The devices reported by these codes are prefabricated and may require fitting and adjustment sessions to suit individual patient needs. Typically, the chambers are inflated by a hand pump or electric pump until the desired level of pressure against the limb is attained. Report L4370 for supply of a pneumatic full leg splint and L4380 for a pneumatic knee splint.

Documentation Standards

An order for each new or full replacement item must be signed and dated by the treating physician, kept on file by the supplier, and made available to the DME MAC upon request. Items billed to the DME MAC before a signed and dated order has been received by the supplier must be submitted with modifier EY added to each affected HCPCS code.

The order must list the unique features of the base code that is billed plus every addition that will be billed on a separate claim line. The medical record must contain information that supports the medical necessity of the item and all additions that are ordered. An order is not necessary for the repair of an orthosis.

Medicare Information

Knee-ankle-foot orthoses (KAFO) described by codes L2000–L2039, L2126–L2136, and L4370 are covered for ambulatory patients for whom an ankle-foot orthosis is covered and for whom additional knee stability is required.

If the basic coverage criteria for an AFO or KAFO are not met, the orthosis will be denied as not medically necessary.

L4392-L4394

L4392 Replacement, soft interface material, static AFO
L4394 Replace soft interface material, foot drop splint

Lay Description

These codes represent replacements of softer interface materials for static ankle foot orthotics and foot drop splints. Ankle flexion contracture is a condition in which there is shortening of the muscles and/or tendons that plantarflex the ankle with the resulting inability to bring the ankle to 0 degrees by passive range of motion (0 degrees ankle position is when the foot is perpendicular to the lower leg). "Foot drop" is a condition in which there is weakness and/or lack of use of the muscles that dorsiflex the ankle, but there is the ability to bring the ankle to 0 degrees by passive range of motion. A foot drop splint/recumbent positioning device is a prefabricated ankle-foot orthosis, with a soft interface, that has all of the following characteristics: designed to maintain the foot at a fixed position of 0 degrees (i.e., perpendicular to the lower leg), not designed to accommodate an ankle with a plantar flexion contracture, and used by a patient who is nonambulatory. Report L4392 for a soft interface material replacement of a static ankle foot orthosis. Report L4394 for the replaced soft interface material of a foot drop splint.

Documentation Standards

If an ankle contracture splint (L4396) or foot drop splint/recumbent positioning device (L4398) is used solely for the prevention or treatment of a heel pressure ulcer, modifier GY must be added to the base code and to the code for the replacement liner (L4392, L4394). When modifier GY is added to a code, there must be a short narrative statement indicating why modifier GY is reported, such as "Used to prevent pressure ulcer," "Used to treat pressure ulcer," or "Used to treat edema." This statement should be attached to a hard copy claim.

Medicare Information

If an ankle contracture splint is covered, a replacement interface is covered as long as the patient continues to meet indications and other coverage rules for the splint. Coverage of a replacement interface is limited to a maximum of one per six months. Additional interfaces will be denied as not medically necessary.

Note: See chapter titled "Medicare Guidelines," under "Ankle-Foot Orthosis (AFO) and Knee-Ankle-Foot Orthosis (KAFO); Related Additions and Replacements; Repairs," for additional Medicare billing and documentation information.

L4396

L4396 Static or dynamic ankle-foot orthotic (AFO), including soft interface material, adjustable for fit, for positioning, may be used for minimal ambulation, prefabricated, includes fitting and adjustment

Lay Description

A static ankle foot orthosis (AFO) is a prefabricated AFO that may be adjustable for fit and positioning and is designed to accommodate an ankle with a plantar flexion contracture up to 45 degrees. It applies a dorsiflexion force to the ankle, allows pressure reduction, is used by a patient who is minimally ambulatory or nonambulatory, and has a soft interface. AFOs extend well above the ankle (usually to near the top of the calf) and are fastened around the lower leg above the ankle. A dynamic AFO allows a more gradual stretch, and allows the patient to progress as their tolerance is increased. The low-load stretching also allows the patient to maintain their gains in range of motion. The dynamic AFO has an adjustable cord and articulating dorsal shell that assists in controlling the degree of stretch, while at the same time allowing for an adjustment of the cords tension. This code includes the fitting, adjustment, and supply of a static or dynamic ankle foot orthosis.

Documentation Standards

If an ankle contracture splint (L4396) or foot drop splint/recumbent positioning device (L4398) is used solely for the prevention or treatment of a heel pressure ulcer, modifier GY must be added to the base code and to the code for the replacement liner (L4392, L4394). When modifier GY is added to a code, there must be a short narrative statement indicating why modifier GY is reported, such as "Used to prevent pressure ulcer," "Used to treat pressure ulcer," or "Used to treat edema." This statement should be attached to a hard copy claim.

Medicare Information

If an ankle contracture splint is used for the treatment of a plantar flexion contracture, the pretreatment passive range of motion must be measured with a goniometer and documented in the medical record. There must be documentation of an appropriate stretching program carried out by professional staff (in a nursing facility) or caregiver (at home).

An ankle contracture splint is covered if all of the following criteria are met:

- There is plantar flexion contracture of the ankle (ICD-9-CM diagnosis code 718.47) with dorsiflexion on passive range of motion testing of at least 10–degrees (i.e., a nonfixed contracture)
- There is reasonable expectation of the ability to correct the contracture
- Contracture is interfering or expected to interfere significantly with the patient's functional abilities
- It is used as a component of a therapy program that includes active stretching of the involved muscles and/or tendons

Note: See chapter titled "Medicare Guidelines," under "Ankle-Foot Orthosis (AFO) and Knee-Ankle-Foot Orthosis (KAFO); Related Additions and Replacements; Repairs," for additional Medicare billing and documentation information.

L4398

L4398 Foot drop splint, recumbent positioning device, prefabricated, includes fitting and adjustment

Lay Description

A foot drop splint/recumbent positioning device is a prefabricated ankle-foot orthosis that is designed to maintain the foot at a fixed position of 0 degrees (i.e., perpendicular to the lower leg), but not designed to accommodate an ankle with a plantar flexion contracture. The foot drop splint is used by a patient who is nonambulatory and has a soft interface. This code includes the fitting and adjustment as well as the supply of the static ankle foot orthosis.

Documentation Standards

If an ankle contracture splint (L4396) or foot drop splint/recumbent positioning device (L4398) is used solely for the prevention or treatment of a heel pressure ulcer, modifier GY must be added to the base code and to the code for the replacement liner (L4392, L4394). When modifier GY is added to a code, there must be a short narrative statement indicating why modifier GY is reported, such as "Used to prevent pressure ulcer," "Used to treat pressure ulcer," or "Used to treat edema." This statement should be attached to a hard copy claim.

Medicare Information

See chapter titled "Medicare Guidelines," under "Ankle-Foot Orthosis (AFO) and Knee-Ankle-Foot Orthosis (KAFO); Related Additions and

Replacements; Repairs," for Medicare billing and documentation information.

L5000-L5020

L5000 Partial foot, shoe insert with longitudinal arch, toe filler
L5010 Partial foot, molded socket, ankle height, with toe filler
L5020 Partial foot, molded socket, tibial tubercle height, with toe filler

Lay Description

These codes report the supply of partial foot orthoses. Partial amputations of the foot often entail disarticulation of the forefoot (phalanges and metatarsals), leaving the heel (calcaneus) intact. Prosthesis preparation for partial foot amputations is complicated by several factors, including socket fitting to the foot remnant and filler material for the amputation. Typically, a toe filler is prepared from artificial materials to resemble the size and shape of the missing toes and metatarsal pad. This is designed to fit into a conventional shoe. Based on moldings or castings taken before amputation, a flexible sleeve is custom fabricated from rubber or other material with elastic properties. The fore end is designed to attach to the toe filler. The proximal end may be fitted with a zipper that closes up the back of the ankle in the general area over the Achilles tendon. This design is usually fitted up to the tibial tubercle—the bony prominence at the ankle. Other designs simply fit over the residual foot/ankle by elastic compression. This constitutes the molded socket that interfaces between the residual foot/ankle and the toe filler. The prosthesis is designed to fit into a conventional or orthotic shoe. Report L5000 for supply of a partial foot prosthesis shoe insert with longitudinal arch. Report L5010 for supply of a partial foot prosthesis with an ankle height molded socket and toe filler. Report L5020 for supply of a partial foot prosthesis with a tibial tubercle height molded socket and toe filler.

L5050-L5060

L5050 Ankle, Symes, molded socket, SACH foot
L5060 Ankle, Symes, metal frame, molded leather socket, articulated ankle/foot

Lay Description

These codes report the supply of specific prostheses for Symes-type amputations. The Symes amputation is a disarticulation at the ankle joint with preservation of the fatty heel pad, which is rotated over the distal closure. The heel pad becomes the most distal part of the residual limb and an interface for a prosthesis. Based on moldings or castings taken before or after amputation, a flexible sleeve is custom fabricated from rubber or other material with elastic properties. This constitutes the molded socket that interfaces between the residual ankle and the prosthetic foot. A solid ankle, cushioned heel (SACH) foot prosthesis is a basic passive device. Report L5050 for supply of a SACH foot prosthesis on a molded socket. Report L5060 for supply of a SACH prosthesis with metal frame, molded leather socket, and articulated ankle/foot.

L5100-L5105

L5100 Below knee, molded socket, shin, SACH foot
L5105 Below knee, plastic socket, joints and thigh lacer, SACH foot

Lay Description

These codes report the supply of specific prostheses for below-the-knee amputations. Based on moldings or castings taken before or after amputation, a flexible sleeve is custom fabricated from rubber or other material with elastic properties. This constitutes the molded socket that interfaces between the residual limb and the prosthesis that attaches to it. Plastic sockets are typically custom fabricated, sometimes from thermoplastic materials that are molded and shaped as heat is applied. A thigh lacer is a cuff-like device that fits around that portion of the residual limb. It has a slit opening on the front side to don the device and a lace-string corset-style closure of gussets and eyelets. Often lacers are of thermoplastic material with cushion liners built from patient molds, but many are still manufactured of leather, or have leather incorporated into the design. The thigh lacer supports and suspends the below-the-knee prosthesis from above. A solid ankle, cushioned heel (SACH) foot prosthesis is a basic passive device. Report L5100 for supply of a below-the-knee prosthetic system of a molded socket, shin component, and SACH foot. Report L5105 for supply of a below-the-knee prosthetic system of a plastic socket, joints and thigh lacer, and SACH foot.

L5200

L5200 Above knee, molded socket, single axis constant friction knee, shin, SACH foot

Lay Description

This code reports the supply of a specific above-the-knee prosthetic system. Based on moldings or castings taken before or after amputation, a flexible sleeve is custom fabricated from rubber or other material with elastic properties. This constitutes the molded socket that interfaces between the residual limb and the prosthetic system that attaches to it. Plastic sockets may be custom fabricated from moldings as well, sometimes from thermoplastic materials that are molded and shaped as heat is applied. A single-axis friction knee is a prosthetic component to replace the knee joint. This type of joint is among the oldest designs and consists of a simple axle connecting the thigh and shank segments. The joint is capable of flexion and extension, but cannot bear the users weight unless locked in an extended position. Constant friction is applied to the joint hinge to keep it from swinging too freely, particularly in gait. A solid ankle, cushioned heel (SACH) foot prosthesis is a basic passive device. These prostheses are considered inexpensive and simple to manufacture. Report L5200 for supply of an above-the-knee molded socket prosthesis system with single axis constant friction knee, shin, and SACH foot components.

L5250-L5270

L5250 Hip disarticulation, Canadian type; molded socket, hip joint, single axis constant friction knee, shin, SACH foot

L5270 Hip disarticulation, tilt table type; molded socket, locking hip joint, single axis constant friction knee, shin, SACH foot

Lay Description

These codes report the supply of prostheses for patients who have had hip disarticulation amputations (removal of the entire leg at the juncture of the hip socket and femoral head). The Canadian type prosthesis consists of a plastic waistband at the trunk line of the iliac crests. Any residual stump may also be utilized for prosthesis attachment and a molded plastic socket encloses the ischial tuberosity to bear weight. The artificial hip joint is toward the anterior of the prosthesis and is unlocked, as is the knee joint. The "tilt table" type prosthesis refers to a specific device that takes the patient's weight off the fresh incisions during early rehabilitation following disarticulation. Based on moldings or castings taken before or after amputation, a flexible sleeve is custom fabricated from rubber or other material with elastic properties. This constitutes the molded socket that interfaces between the residual limb and the prosthetic system that attaches to it. Plastic sockets may be custom fabricated from moldings as well, sometimes from thermoplastic materials that are molded and shaped as heat is applied. A single-axis friction knee is a prosthetic component to replace the knee joint. This type of joint is among the oldest designs and consists of a simple axle connecting the thigh and shank segments. The joint is capable of flexion and extension, but cannot bear the users weight unless locked in an extended position. Constant friction is applied to the joint hinge to keep it from swinging too freely, particularly in gait. A solid ankle, cushioned heel (SACH) foot prosthesis is a basic passive device. The knee and foot components are considered inexpensive and simple to manufacture. Report L5250 for supply of a Canadian-type prosthesis for hip disarticulation with molded socket and locking hip joint with single axis friction knee joint and SACH foot. Report L5270 for supply of tilt table-type prosthesis for hip disarticulation with molded socket and locking hip joint with single axis friction knee joint and SACH foot.

L5311

L5311 Knee disarticulation (or through knee), molded socket, external knee joints, shin, SACH foot, endoskeletal system

Lay Description

The type of prosthetic system reported by this code is for disarticulations at the knee joint. Based on moldings or castings taken before or after amputation, a flexible sleeve is custom fabricated from rubber or other material with elastic properties. This constitutes the molded socket that interfaces between the residual limb and the prosthetic system that attaches to it. Plastic sockets may be custom fabricated from moldings as well, sometimes from thermoplastic materials that are molded and shaped as heat is applied. The artificial knee components are external to the larger device, which is an endoskeletal system. Rather than an internal rigid shaft, this type of prosthesis uses the external hard shell to transfer the patient's weight from the knee to the foot component. A solid ankle, cushioned heel (SACH) foot prosthesis is a basic passive device. Report L5311 for supply of an endoskeletal, external knee joint prosthesis for knee disarticulation with SACH foot.

L5321

L5321 Above knee, molded socket, open end, SACH foot, endoskeletal system, single axis knee

Lay Description

The type of prosthetic system reported by this code is an above-the-knee amputation. Based on moldings or castings taken before or after amputation, a flexible sleeve is custom fabricated from rubber or other material with elastic properties. This constitutes the molded socket that interfaces between the residual limb and the prosthetic system that attaches to it. Plastic sockets may be custom fabricated from moldings as well, sometimes from thermoplastic materials that are molded and shaped as heat is applied. The artificial knee component is single axis, which means the joint is capable of simple flexion and extension actions only. Rather than internal rigid supports, this type of prosthesis uses the external hard shell to transfer the patient's weight from the thigh and knee to the foot component. A solid ankle, cushioned heel (SACH) foot prosthesis is a basic passive device. Report L5321 for supply of an endoskeletal, single axis knee joint prosthesis for above-the-knee amputation with SACH foot.

L5331

L5331   Hip disarticulation, Canadian type, molded socket, endoskeletal system, hip joint, single axis knee, SACH foot

Lay Description

This code reports a prosthetic system for patients who have undergone a hemipelvectomy (removal of half of the pelvic girdle and an entire leg). This type of amputation presents numerous problems for the prosthetist, since there is no residual limb with which to anchor a device. The socket is based on moldings and castings taken before or after amputation and may extend well up the torso. The Canadian type prosthesis features a molded plastic socket to enclose the remaining ischial tuberosity to bear weight. An artificial hip joint is toward the anterior of the prosthesis and is unlocked, as is the knee joint, which is single axis. This means the joint is capable of simple flexion and extension actions only. Rather than internal rigid supports, this type of leg prosthesis uses the external hard shell to transfer the patient's weight from the thigh and knee to the foot component (endoskeletal). A solid ankle, cushioned heel (SACH) foot prosthesis is a basic passive device. Report L5331 for supply of a Canadian type prosthesis with endoskeletal support, hip joint, single axis knee, and SACH foot.

L5400-L5430

L5400   Immediate postsurgical or early fitting, application of initial rigid dressing, including fitting, alignment, suspension, and one cast change, below knee

L5410   Immediate postsurgical or early fitting, application of initial rigid dressing, including fitting, alignment and suspension, below knee, each additional cast change and realignment

L5420   Immediate postsurgical or early fitting, application of initial rigid dressing, including fitting, alignment and suspension and one cast change AK or knee disarticulation

L5430   Immediate postsurgical or early fitting, application of initial rigid dressing, including fitting, alignment and suspension, AK or knee disarticulation, each additional cast change and realignment

Lay Description

These codes report supply of early fittings and dressings following below-the-knee amputation or disarticulation at the knee joint. A major consideration for prosthetists is the constantly changing size and shape of the residual limb, or stump, which is the attachment site for a prosthesis. Following amputation of the limb, post-surgical or "early" dressings are applied to the surgical stump, sometimes during the same operative session. These early applications are designed to compress and prepare the distal tissues in anticipation of fitting a test socket and later a permanent socket. Early applications may be known as immediate post-surgical fittings (IPSFs). The accepted plan for most lower limb amputations is to transition the patient as quickly as possible to use of a prosthesis. This minimizes muscle atrophy and limb weakness seen in longer convalescences. In some instances, a plaster cast or other rigid dressing is hand molded to the residual limb as the amputation session is completed. In other instances, the initial dressing is applied up to several days following surgery. As swelling diminishes and also to access the surgical closure, the dressing must be periodically changed out. These early dressings may be fitted to interface with test prosthetic devices. Report L5400 for supply of an initial rigid dressing and one subsequent cast change to a below-the-knee amputation. Report L5410 for each additional cast change to a below-the-knee amputation. Report L5420 for supply of an initial rigid dressing and one subsequent cast change to an amputation at the knee or a knee disarticulation. Report L5430 for supply of each additional cast change to an amputation at the knee or a knee disarticulation.

L5450-L5460

L5450   Immediate postsurgical or early fitting, application of nonweight bearing rigid dressing, below knee

L5460   Immediate postsurgical or early fitting, application of nonweight bearing rigid dressing, above knee

Lay Description

These codes report supply of early non-weight bearing fittings and dressings following amputation of a lower limb. Following amputation of the limb, post-surgical or "early" dressings are applied to the surgical stump, sometimes during the same operative session. These early applications are designed to compress and prepare the distal tissues in anticipation of fitting a test socket and later a permanent socket. In some instances, a plaster cast or other rigid dressing is hand molded to the residual limb as the amputation session is completed. In other instances, the initial dressing is applied up to several days following surgery. As swelling diminishes and also to access the surgical closure, the dressing must be periodically changed out. For plaster and rigid dressings, this entails cutting off the cast and reapplying the dressing. In some cases, removable casts or caps are devised. These devices may be removed and reapplied several times. The dressings reported by these codes are never fitted to interface with test prostheses. Report L5450 for supply of an initial non-weight bearing rigid dressing for a below-the-knee amputation. Report L5460 for supply of an initial non-weight bearing rigid dressing for an above-the-knee amputation.

L5500-L5505

L5500 Initial, below knee PTB type socket, nonalignable system, pylon, no cover, SACH foot, plaster socket, direct formed

L5505 Initial, above knee, knee disarticulation, ischial level socket, nonalignable system, pylon, no cover, SACH foot, plaster socket, direct formed

Lay Description

These codes report the supply of initial hand molded plaster socket systems for amputation of a lower limb. These are initial sockets that are the transition between the initial rigid dressings applied post-surgery and the test socket systems that prepare the patient for a long-term prosthesis. A patella tendon bearing (PTB) type socket generally features an adjustable cuff worn just above the knee joint. This cuff suspends the lower components, comprised in this instance of the direct-formed plaster socket over the stump, the pylon, and foot components. Plaster sockets may be directly formed from bandages saturated with plaster of paris. Once fitted, the plaster socket cannot be aligned. A pylon is a post-like structure fitted to the plaster socket on one end and the prosthetic foot component on the other. It is a feature of most lower limb prosthetic designs. The pylon may be a tube made of aluminum, titanium, steel, or carbon fiber reinforced plastic and in early fittings is usually adjustable for length. Unlike many long-term prostheses, this unit will not feature a cosmetic covering. A solid ankle, cushioned heel (SACH) foot prosthesis is a basic passive device. Report L5500 for supply of an initial direct formed, plaster PTB-style socket, pylon, and SACH foot. A high, above-the-knee amputation or disarticulation at the femoral head presents numerous challenges for the prosthetist, since there is very little residual limb to attach the prosthesis. An ischial level socket in this instance is a direct-formed plaster encasement of the ischial tuberosity, to bear the patient's weight. Once fitted, it cannot be aligned. A pylon is fitted to the plaster socket on one end and the prosthetic foot component on the other. Report L5505 for supply of an initial direct formed, plaster ischial level socket, pylon, and SACH foot.

L5510-L5540

L5510 Preparatory, below knee PTB type socket, nonalignable system, pylon, no cover, SACH foot, plaster socket, molded to model

L5520 Preparatory, below knee PTB type socket, nonalignable system, pylon, no cover, SACH foot, thermoplastic or equal, direct formed

L5530 Preparatory, below knee PTB type socket, nonalignable system, pylon, no cover, SACH foot, thermoplastic or equal, molded to model

L5535 Preparatory, below knee PTB type socket, nonalignable system, no cover, SACH foot, prefabricated, adjustable open end socket

L5540 Preparatory, below knee PTB type socket, nonalignable system, pylon, no cover, SACH foot, laminated socket, molded to model

Lay Description

These codes report a variety of non-alignable preparatory prostheses for below-the-knee amputations. Preparatory prostheses are transition devices between the initial rigid dressings and pylons applied post-surgery and the finished long-term prosthetic system. The codes are differentiated by the style of socket and the material used in its fabrication. As is typical with preparatory sockets, none can be aligned once fitted. A patella tendon bearing (PTB) type socket generally features an adjustable cuff worn just above the knee joint. This cuff suspends the socket, which can be made of any of a variety of materials. A plaster socket, in this instance, is formed from bandages saturated with plaster of paris applied over a previously cast model of the stump. A thermoplastic socket, may be formed by applying heat to the rough-formed socket and modeling it to either the patient's stump directly or to a previously cast model of the stump. Another style of preparatory socket involves laminating together two or more resin-saturated materials over a previously cast model of the stump. Other preparatory sockets are prefabricated—selected from mass produced components based only on patient size. This type of preparatory socket is adjustable. A pylon is a post-like structure fitted to the plaster socket on one end and the prosthetic foot component on the other. It is a feature of most lower limb prosthetic designs. The pylon may be a tube made of aluminum, titanium, steel, or carbon fiber reinforced plastic and in early fittings is usually adjustable for length. Unlike many long-term prostheses, none of these units will feature cosmetic coverings. A solid ankle, cushioned heel (SACH) foot prosthesis is a basic passive device. Report L5510 for supply of a preparatory PTB style plaster socket molded to model with pylon and SACH foot.

Report L5520 for supply of a direct-formed thermoplastic preparatory socket with pylon and SACH foot. Report L5530 for supply of a thermoplastic preparatory socket molded to model with pylon and SACH foot. Report L5535 for supply of an adjustable prefabricated preparatory socket with pylon and SACH foot. Report L5540 for supply of laminated-to-model preparatory socket with pylon and SACH foot.

L5560-L5590

L5560 Preparatory, above knee, knee disarticulation, ischial level socket, nonalignable system, pylon, no cover, SACH foot, plaster socket, molded to model

L5570 Preparatory, above knee — knee disarticulation, ischial level socket, nonalignable system, pylon, no cover, SACH foot, thermoplastic or equal, direct formed

L5580 Preparatory, above knee, knee disarticulation, ischial level socket, nonalignable system, pylon, no cover, SACH foot, thermoplastic or equal, molded to model

L5585 Preparatory, above knee — knee disarticulation, ischial level socket, nonalignable system, pylon, no cover, SACH foot, prefabricated adjustable open end socket

L5590 Preparatory, above knee, knee disarticulation, ischial level socket, nonalignable system, pylon, no cover, SACH foot, laminated socket, molded to model

Lay Description

These codes report preparatory prostheses for knee disarticulations with ischial level sockets. Preparatory prostheses are transition devices between the initial rigid dressings and pylons applied post-surgery and the finished long-term prosthetic system. The codes are differentiated by the style of socket and the material used in its fabrication. Ischial level sockets embrace the thigh to the level of the ischial tuberosity, or so-called "sit bones." Preparatory sockets extending to this level are for transition and are unsuitable for aggressive ambulation. Permanent sockets for knee disarticulations are usually three-quarter-thigh length. As is typical with preparatory sockets, none can be aligned once fitted. A plaster socket, in this instance, is formed from bandages saturated with plaster of paris applied over a previous cast model of the stump and ischium. A thermoplastic socket may be formed by applying heat to the rough-formed socket and modeling it to either the patient's stump and ischium directly or to a previously cast model of the stump. Another style of preparatory socket involves laminating together two or more resin-saturated materials over a previously cast model of the stump. Other preparatory sockets are prefabricated—selected from mass produced components based only on patient size. This type of preparatory socket is adjustable. A pylon is a post-like structure fitted to the socket on one end and the prosthetic foot component on the other. It is a feature of most lower limb prosthetic designs. The pylon may be a tube made of aluminum, titanium, steel, or carbon fiber reinforced plastic and in early fittings is usually adjustable for length. Unlike many long-term prostheses, none of these units will feature cosmetic coverings. None of the units reported by this range of codes feature knee joints. A solid ankle, cushioned heel (SACH) foot prosthesis is a basic passive device. Report L5560 for supply of a preparatory plaster socket molded to model with pylon and SACH foot. Report L5570 for supply of a direct-formed thermoplastic preparatory socket with pylon and SACH foot. Report L5580 for supply of a thermoplastic preparatory socket molded to model with pylon and SACH foot. Report L5585 for supply of an adjustable prefabricated preparatory socket with pylon and SACH foot. Report L5590 for supply of laminated-to-model preparatory socket with pylon and SACH foot.

L5611-L5614

L5611 Addition to lower extremity, endoskeletal system, above knee, knee disarticulation, 4-bar linkage, with friction swing phase control

L5613 Addition to lower extremity, endoskeletal system, above knee, knee disarticulation, 4-bar linkage, with hydraulic swing phase control

L5614 Addition to lower extremity, exoskeletal system, above knee-knee disarticulation, 4 bar linkage, with pneumatic swing phase control

Lay Description

These codes report the addition of specific types of swing control devices to knee joints fitted to patients who have undergone above-the-knee amputation or disarticulation at the knee joint. The codes report supply of polycentric-type knee joints. Single axis knee joints are capable of simple flexion and extension only. The polycentric joint offers greater range of motion. The center of rotation for a polycentric knee joint varies as the flexion angle changes. This feature offers the patient better toe clearance during the swing phase of gait. A common type of polycentric knee is known as the four-bar linkage. This device has four axes of rotation connected by four rigid linkages and all codes in this range describe this type of knee component. Friction control over the knee joint means that the joint adjustments are tightened down to prevent unwanted movement during gait. Hydraulic swing phase control means the joint is fitted with a fluid filled piston to damper unwanted movement during gait. Pneumatic swing phase control means the joint is fitted with an air filled piston to damper unwanted movement during gait. All codes in the range report an endoskeletal prosthesis. In this type of design, a pylon, or pole, bears most of the weight load from the thigh to the prosthetic foot, rather than the exterior prosthetic shell in exoskeletal systems. Report L5611 for addition to a lower extremity prosthesis of a friction swing phase control polycentric knee joint. Report L5613 for addition to a lower extremity prosthesis of a hydraulic swing phase control polycentric knee joint. Report L5614 for addition to a lower extremity prosthesis of a pneumatic swing phase control polycentric knee joint.

L5616

L5616 Addition to lower extremity, endoskeletal system, above knee, universal multiplex system, friction swing phase control

Lay Description

This code reports an addition to an endoskeletal above-the-knee prosthesis of a specific design of knee joint. There are two major design differences for the shank component of a leg prosthesis. Endoskeletal shank designs transfer most of the weight from the residual limb to the prosthetic foot through a pylon, a post-like structure fitted to the socket on one end and the prosthetic foot component on the other. The pylon may be a tube made of aluminum, titanium, steel, or carbon fiber reinforced plastic. The pylon may be adjustable and may feature shock absorption characteristics. Most endoskeletal systems are modular and components can be fairly easily upgraded. The endoskeletal pylon system may be covered with an entirely cosmetic outer shell that resembles an actual leg. Exoskeletal designs feature a rigid and structural outer shell that transfers most of the weight from the residual limb to the prosthetic foot. Exoskeletal designs also usually have a pylon, but most of the weight is distributed by the shell. Exoskeletal systems are usually covered and painted to resemble an actual leg. In general, exoskeletal systems are considered durable and easy to maintain. Both systems offer special versions for active and athletic amputees. The universal multiplex is a particular design suited for moderately active use. This code reports friction swing phase control, which means the joint may be adjusted more tightly to control unwanted movement during gait. Report L5616 for addition of a universal multiplex system with friction swing phase control to an existing endoskeletal above-the-knee prosthesis.

L5630

L5630 Addition to lower extremity, Symes type, expandable wall socket

Lay Description

This code reports addition of a Symes type expandable wall socket to a test socket. A socket is the portion of a prosthesis that fits around the residual limb (or stump) and to which prosthetic components are attached. Test sockets are typically soft and often have transparent fittings that allow the prosthetist to visualize the fit. A test socket tests the interface between the prosthesis and the residual limb. The eponym Symes is an association to the Scottish surgeon James Syme, who introduced many orthopedic procedures in the early 19th Century. The Symes disarticulation at the ankle joint remains in common use. Report L5630 for supply of an expandable wall socket to a test socket for a Symes-type ankle disarticulation.

L5631

L5631 Addition to lower extremity, above knee or knee disarticulation, acrylic socket

Lay Description

This code reports the addition of a specific variation to a test socket for knee disarticulations or above-the-knee amputations. A socket is the portion of a prosthesis that fits around the residual limb (or stump) and to which prosthetic components are attached. A test socket, also known as a "check" socket, tests the interface between the prosthesis and the residual limb. The type of socket reported by this code is of acrylic material and many will be clear. A clear socket allows the prosthetist to visualize the fit and see points of contact and potential problem areas. Report L5631 for supply of an acrylic test socket for knee disarticulations or above-the-knee amputations.

L5632-L5636

L5632 Addition to lower extremity, Symes type, PTB brim design socket
L5634 Addition to lower extremity, Symes type, posterior opening (Canadian) socket
L5636 Addition to lower extremity, Symes type, medial opening socket

Lay Description

These codes report the addition of specific alterations to test sockets. A socket is the portion of a prosthesis that fits around the residual limb (or stump) and to which prosthetic components are attached. Test sockets are typically soft and often have transparent fittings that allow the prosthetist to visualize the fit. A test socket tests the interface between the prosthesis and the residual limb. The eponym Symes is an association to the Scottish surgeon James Syme, who introduced many orthopedic procedures in the early 19th Century. The Symes disarticulation at the ankle joint remains in common use. Among prostheses, however, Symes refers to a particular design where a door is cut into the prosthetic device or, in this instance, the test socket. A patella tendon bearing (PTB) brim design is a socket that extends up to the area above the knee joint; the stump is held in place by the brim shape of the socket. Report L5632 for addition of a PTB brim style socket. Report L5634 for addition of a Symes style socket with a posterior opening. Report L5636 for addition of a Symes style socket with a medial opening.

L5637-L5639

L5637　Addition to lower extremity, below knee, total contact

L5638　Addition to lower extremity, below knee, leather socket

L5639　Addition to lower extremity, below knee, wood socket

Lay Description

These codes address socket variations for below-the-knee prostheses. A socket is the portion of a prosthesis that fits around the residual limb and to which prosthetic components are attached. Several test sockets may be required as the dimensions of the residual limb stabilize following amputation and as the musculature changes over time. A total contact socket, also known as a total surface bearing, is one that fully interfaces with the entire residual limb (or stump). Traditionally, a test socket is donned with a bit of space between the stump and the contact area of the socket. This space is accessed and injected with a substance that dries to a gel-like consistency, conforming exactly to the shape of the stump and the socket. A total contact interface allows more surface area to bear weight against the prosthesis. Report L5637 for supply of a total contact addition to a below-the-knee prosthesis; L5638 for supply of a leather socket addition to a below-the-knee prosthesis; and L5639 for supply of a wood socket addition to a below-the-knee prosthesis.

L5645-L5653

L5645　Addition to lower extremity, below knee, flexible inner socket, external frame

L5646　Addition to lower extremity, below knee, air, fluid, gel or equal, cushion socket

L5647　Addition to lower extremity, below knee, suction socket

L5648　Addition to lower extremity, above knee, air, fluid, gel or equal, cushion socket

L5649　Addition to lower extremity, ischial containment/narrow M-L socket

L5650　Additions to lower extremity, total contact, above knee or knee disarticulation socket

L5651　Addition to lower extremity, above knee, flexible inner socket, external frame

L5652　Addition to lower extremity, suction suspension, above knee or knee disarticulation socket

L5653　Addition to lower extremity, knee disarticulation, expandable wall socket

Lay Description

This range of codes addresses additions to lower extremity prostheses of test sockets. Above and below the knee amputations are addressed. A socket is the portion of a prosthesis that fits around the residual limb and to which prosthetic components are attached. Amputees consistently report that the comfort and fit of the socket is crucial to the success of the prosthesis. Test sockets are used to determine optimal interface between the patient's skin at the residual limb and the artificial material of the prosthesis. Several test sockets may be required as the dimensions of the residual limb stabilize following amputation and as the musculature changes over time. Some socket designs feature a flexible inner socket combined with an external frame and/or strapping. Air cushion sockets were developed for aggressive ambulation and running. Suction sockets usually employ a silicone interface. The vacuum is created by the natural properties of the silicone as the socket is donned and weight placed against the interface. Some systems feature a release button to aid in removal. An ischial containment socket is a traditional above-the-knee design where the ischial tuberosity is contained within the walls of the socket (also known as "plug fit" or anatomical fit). The M-L socket is another variety of anatomical fit, above-the-knee designs. The M-L (medial-lateral) socket is tight fitting with most of the squeezing taking place on the lateral side followed by the medial side. Report L5645 for supply of a flexible inner socket with an external frame for a below-the-knee prosthesis. Report L5646 for supply of an air cushion socket for a below-the-knee prosthesis. Report L5647 for supply of a suction socket for a below-the-knee prosthesis. Report L5648 for supply of an air cushion socket for an above-the-knee prosthesis. Report L5649 for supply of an ischial containment or narrow M-L socket for an above-the-knee prosthesis. Report L5650 for supply of a total contact socket for an above-the-knee or knee disarticulation prosthesis. Report L5651 for supply of a flexible inner socket with external frame for an above-the-knee prosthesis. Report L5652 for supply of a suction suspension socket for an above-the-knee or knee disarticulation prosthesis. Report L5653 for supply of an expandable wall socket for a knee disarticulation prosthesis.

L5654-L5658

L5654 Addition to lower extremity, socket insert, Symes, (Kemblo, Pelite, Aliplast, Plastazote or equal)
L5655 Addition to lower extremity, socket insert, below knee (Kemblo, Pelite, Aliplast, Plastazote or equal)
L5656 Addition to lower extremity, socket insert, knee disarticulation (Kemblo, Pelite, Aliplast, Plastazote or equal)
L5658 Addition to lower extremity, socket insert, above knee (Kemblo, Pelite, Aliplast, Plastazote or equal)

Lay Description

These codes report supply of specific types of socket inserts. Socket inserts help to protect the fragile skin of the residual limb while compensating for daily changes in limb volume. Some manufacturers of prostheses require socket inserts. Other designs can be comfortably fit without use of an insert. Irregular or bony residual limbs present complications that can be addressed by inserts. The codes in this range are differentiated by type of amputation and length of residual limb. Symes-type disarticulation occurs at the ankle joint with the fat pad of the heel preserved and rotated over the closure. Specific insert materials are mentioned in the code description. Kemblo is a durable rubber-like synthetic that traditionally is used alone or laminated to leather. Pelite is a thermoplastic—a semirigid synthetic that can be molded and shaped when heat is applied. Plastazote is a closed-cell foam product. Report L5654 for supply of a socket insert for a Symes-type disarticulation. Report L5655 for supply of a socket insert for a below-knee amputation. Report L5656 for supply of a socket insert for a knee disarticulation. Report L5658 for supply of a socket insert for an above-the-knee amputation.

L5661-L5665

L5661 Addition to lower extremity, socket insert, multidurometer Symes
L5665 Addition to lower extremity, socket insert, multidurometer, below knee

Lay Description

These codes report the supply of multidurometer socket inserts for either a Symes-type disarticulation at the ankle or a below-the-knee amputation. Some manufacturers of prostheses require socket inserts. Other designs can be comfortably fit without use of an insert. A durometer is a device to measure surface resiliency of material and a firmness scale is used by fabricators of prosthetic devices. Multidurometer, in this context, is used to define an insert material made up of three or more materials, each with a different firmness rating. Combinations may include laminates of Plastazote, Poron, or other materials. Report L5661 for supply of a multidurometer socket insert for a Symes disarticulation. Report L5665 for supply of a multidurometer socket insert for a below-the-knee amputation.

L5666

L5666 Addition to lower extremity, below knee, cuff suspension

Lay Description

This code reports supply of a specific type of suspension socket for patients who have had below-the-knee amputation. A cuff is a gripping device that fits, in this instance, around the residual limb below the knee. A cuff is smaller than a corset or "lacer," but works in a similar fashion. It is made of rigid or semi-rigid material lined on the inside with cushioning material. The cuff may be closed snugly around the limb by straps, Velcro, or eyelet and gusset lacing. The socket and prosthesis may make full contact with the residual limb, particularly when weight is brought to bear, but the attachment integrity of the system is the suspension from the cuff. Report L5666 for supply of a cuff suspension addition to a below-the-knee socket and prosthesis.

L5668

L5668 Addition to lower extremity, below knee, molded distal cushion

Lay Description

This code reports supply of a molded distal cushion addition to a prosthesis liner. These types of cushions are now made of viscoelastic materials—gel-like substances that may be molded or provided off-the-shelf. In this instance, the cushion is molded to a positive image of the residual distal stump for precise fit. Report L5668 for supply of a molded distal cushion addition.

L5670-L5672

L5670 Addition to lower extremity, below knee, molded supracondylar suspension (PTS or similar)
L5671 Addition to lower extremity, below knee / above knee suspension locking mechanism (shuttle, lanyard, or equal), excludes socket insert
L5672 Addition to lower extremity, below knee, removable medial brim suspension

Lay Description

These codes report suspension style additions to lower extremity prostheses. A patella tendon bearing (PTB) type of prosthesis may have already been fitted to a below-the-knee amputation. Above-the-knee amputations may require the addition of a suspension-locking device to hold the prosthesis. The PTS is a prosthesis that suspends from the prominence of the condyles of the tibial plateau just distal to the knee joint. The prosthesis is allowed to hang from just below the knee joint until weight is placed upon it. A shuttle system incorporates a pin and lock at the bottom of the socket to suspend the prosthesis and may be used for amputations above or below the knee. Report L5670 for supply of an addition of a molded supracondylar suspension device for a below-the-knee prosthesis. Report L5671 for supply of a locking mechanism for a below-the-knee or above-the-knee prosthesis. Code L5671 includes both the part of the suspension locking mechanism that is integrated into the lower extremity prosthesis socket and the pin, lanyard, or other component that is attached to the socket insert. Code L5671 does not include the socket insert itself. Report L5672 for supply of a below knee removable medial brim suspension.

L5680, L5682

L5680 Addition to lower extremity, below knee, thigh lacer, nonmolded
L5682 Addition to lower extremity, below knee, thigh lacer, gluteal/ischial, molded

Lay Description

These codes report supply of so-called thigh lacers, or corsets, for patients who have undergone below-the-knee amputations. These corset-like cuffs are often made of leather or composites and may be custom manufactured or off-the-shelf. Custom-made devices are usually molded to a positive image of the leg. Closure is usually lacing through eyelets and gussets along the anterior face. A lower leg prosthesis is attached to the corset, usually by two vertical metal sidebars, thus forming a type of suspension system. At one time thigh lacers were a common form of suspension for transtibial prostheses. With the rise of total contact sockets, however, thigh lacer suspension has seen diminishing use. Thigh lacers still offer an advantage in that much of the weight is distributed from the thigh to the lower leg over the vertical sidebars and may be prescribed for patients who do not tolerate full contact pressure on the residual limb. Report L5680 for supply of a non-molded thigh lacer for a below-the-knee amputation. Report L5682 for supply of a molded thigh lacer designed for attachment at the extreme upper thigh for a below-the-knee amputation.

L5686

L5686 Addition to lower extremity, below knee, back check (extension control)

Lay Description

This code reports the supply of a device that, when added to a lower prosthesis, prevents the knee joint from hyperextension, or bending backward. This device may be a strap, blocking, or locking mechanism that prevents the artificial knee from moving beyond the position needed for normal standing. Report L5686 for supply of each back check device.

L5692-L5695

L5692 Addition to lower extremity, above knee, pelvic control belt, light
L5694 Addition to lower extremity, above knee, pelvic control belt, padded and lined
L5695 Addition to lower extremity, above knee, pelvic control, sleeve suspension, neoprene or equal, each

Lay Description

These codes report additions of pelvic control systems to above-the-knee amputation prosthetics. These are often belt systems worn around the lower waist. A light belt is a simple fabric belt worn around the lower waist. The Silesian belt consists of a broad, and often padded belt that fits around the lower back and half way around the hips. A thinner cinch belt fits over the broad portion and closes and adjusts the system. The belt systems partially suspend the prosthesis, usually from a single location on the lateral side. A sleeve suspension is pulled over the residual limb, and in this instance extends over the ischium and pelvis. Neoprene is specifically cited in the code description, but gel-like materials made from silicon are probably used most often today. Report L5692 for supply of a light pelvic control belt added to an above-the-knee prosthetic system. Report L5694 for supply of a padded and lined pelvic control belt added to an above-the-knee prosthetic system. Report L5695 for supply of a sleeve suspension pelvic control added to an above-the-knee prosthetic system.

L5696

L5696 Addition to lower extremity, above knee or knee disarticulation, pelvic joint

Lay Description

This code reports the addition of a pelvic joint to an above-the-knee amputation or pelvic joint disarticulation. The pelvic joint may be single or multiple axes and typically is mounted at the anterior of the prosthesis. A variety of designs and features are available. The joint allows for flexibility at the hip and may allow ambulation. Report L5696 or supply of a pelvic joint added to an above-the-knee amputation or pelvic joint disarticulation.

L5697-L5698

L5697 Addition to lower extremity, above knee or knee disarticulation, pelvic band
L5698 Addition to lower extremity, above knee or knee disarticulation, Silesian bandage

Lay Description

These codes report the supply of additional supports to an above-the-knee amputation or pelvic joint disarticulation prosthetic system. Most modern femoral amputation prostheses are designed to attach and hold firmly to the residual limb without use of hip belts or additional supports. In some instances, however, patients may require additional support or suspension in the form of pelvic bands or bandages. These are typically broad, padded bands or wrappings worn around the lower waist and from which the prosthesis can be attached. The site of attachment is usually at a lateral and/or anterior location on the prosthesis. Report L5697 for supply of a pelvic band addition to an above-the-knee amputation or pelvic joint disarticulation prosthetic system. Report L5698 for supply of a Silesian bandage addition to an above-the-knee amputation or pelvic joint disarticulation prosthetic system.

L5699

L5699 All lower extremity prostheses, shoulder harness

Lay Description

This code reports the supply of a shoulder harness support to an above-the-knee amputation or a pelvic joint disarticulation prosthetic system. Most modern femoral amputation prostheses are designed to attach and hold firmly to the residual limb without use of hip belts or additional supports at the shoulder. In some instances, however, patients may require additional support or suspension in the form of a shoulder harness. This type of device may involve both shoulders or be a more simple single shoulder harness-sling. The site of attachment is usually at a lateral and/or anterior location on the prosthesis.

Report L5699 for supply of a shoulder harness addition to an above-the-knee amputation or pelvic joint disarticulation prosthetic system.

L5700-L5703

L5700 Replacement, socket, below knee, molded to patient model
L5701 Replacement, socket, above knee/knee disarticulation, including attachment plate, molded to patient model
L5702 Replacement, socket, hip disarticulation, including hip joint, molded to patient model
L5703 Ankle, Symes, molded to patient model, socket without solid ankle cushion heel (SACH) foot, replacement only

Lay Description

These codes report replacement for molded sockets for lower limb prosthetic systems. The codes are differentiated by the level of amputation. Amputation patients routinely see significant daily changes in the volume and physical dimensions of the residual limb, or stump. This challenge is addressed as best as possible by fitting test or "check" sockets during the early phase of adjustment to a prosthetic limb. The use of liners and stockings of varying thickness also addresses volume change in the stump. Terminal sockets designed for extended use have limited life spans and must be changed out for any of a variety of reasons, including changes in stump volume. These codes report supply of a replacement socket molded to a plaster positive model taken of the residual limb. Changes in the limb may require that a new model be prepared, or an earlier model may still be workable. Increasingly, computer models and scans are used. The socket material may be heat molded or otherwise shaped to conform precisely to the patient model. Report L5700 for supply of a replacement molded socket for a below-the-knee (BK) prosthetic system. Report L5701 for supply of a replacement molded socket for an above-the-knee (AK) or knee disarticulation prosthetic system. Report L5702 for supply of a replacement molded socket with hip joint for a hip disarticulation prosthetic system. Report L5703 for supply of a replacement socket for a Symes ankle prosthetic system.

L5704-L5707

L5704 Custom shaped protective cover, below knee
L5705 Custom shaped protective cover, above knee
L5706 Custom shaped protective cover, knee disarticulation
L5707 Custom shaped protective cover, hip disarticulation

Lay Description

A custom shaped protective covering for a prosthesis is one of two general varieties. Prostheses with internal supports (endoskeletal) usually feature an outer protective cover made of closed cell foam and a skin-color finish. Externally supported prostheses (exoskeletal) usually feature a hard, synthetic shell, also usually finished to resemble human skin. Both varieties may start out from an off-the-shelf blank, but are carefully customized to match the size and length, thickness, and coloring of an opposing or lost limb. This range of codes reports the replacement of these protective outer surface cover systems (POSCS). Report L5704 for supply of a custom shaped protective cover for a below-the-knee prosthesis. Report L5705 for supply of a custom shaped protective cover for an above-the-knee prosthesis. Report L5706 for supply of a custom shaped protective cover for a knee disarticulation prosthesis. Report L5707 for supply of a custom shaped protective cover for a hip disarticulation prosthesis.

L5781-L5782

L5781 Addition to lower limb prosthesis, vacuum pump, residual limb volume management and moisture evacuation system
L5782 Addition to lower limb prosthesis, vacuum pump, residual limb volume management and moisture evacuation system, heavy-duty

Lay Description

These codes report a specialized vacuum system for the socket. Amputation patients routinely see significant daily changes in the volume and physical dimensions of the residual limb, or stump. This volume can change significantly in the course of a day and some suction socket systems are believed to exacerbate short-term volume loss. The vacuum system reported by these codes is designed to create a greater vacuum between the liner and the wall of the socket than is found in standard suction socket systems. Moisture trapped between the liner and socket is also removed. The system purportedly stabilizes volume fluctuation in the residual limb. Report L5781 for supply of a vacuum pump to a lower limb prosthesis. Report L5782 for supply of a heavy-duty vacuum pump to a lower limb prosthesis.

L5785-L5795

L5785 Addition, exoskeletal system, below knee, ultra-light material (titanium, carbon fiber or equal)
L5790 Addition, exoskeletal system, above knee, ultra-light material (titanium, carbon fiber or equal)
L5795 Addition, exoskeletal system, hip disarticulation, ultra-light material (titanium, carbon fiber or equal)

Lay Description

These codes report the addition of ultra-light weight material components to an exoskeletal lower limb prosthesis. The codes are differentiated by level of amputation. Two major types of lower limb prostheses are currently offered. Endoskeletal shank designs transfer most of the weight from the residual limb to the prosthetic foot through a pylon, a post-like structure fitted to the socket on one end and the prosthetic foot component on the other. The pylon may be a tube made of aluminum, titanium, steel, or carbon fiber-reinforced plastic. Most endoskeletal systems are modular and components can be fairly easily upgraded. The endoskeletal pylon system may be covered with an entirely cosmetic outer shell that resembles an actual leg. Exoskeletal designs feature a rigid and structural outer shell that transfers most of the weight from the residual limb to the prosthetic foot. Exoskeletal designs also often have a pylon, but most of the weight is distributed by the shell. Exoskeletal systems are usually covered and painted to resemble an actual leg. In general, exoskeletal systems are considered durable and easy to maintain. Both systems offer special versions for active and athletic amputees. These codes report modification to an exoskeletal system by the addition of carbon fiber, titanium, or other lightweight materials, either to the pylon component, the exoskeletal shell, or both. Report L5785 for the addition of ultra-light weight material components to an exoskeletal below-the-knee (BK) lower limb prosthesis. Report L5790 for the addition of ultra-light weight material components to an exoskeletal above-the-knee (AK) lower limb prosthesis. Report L5790 for the addition of ultra-light weight material components to an exoskeletal hip disarticulation lower limb prosthesis.

L5810-L5812

L5810 Addition, endoskeletal knee-shin system, single axis, manual lock
L5811 Addition, endoskeletal knee-shin system, single axis, manual lock, ultra-light material
L5812 Addition, endoskeletal knee-shin system, single axis, friction swing and stance phase control (safety knee)

Lay Description

These codes report additions to endoskeletal prosthetic systems of single axis knees. Endoskeletal shank designs transfer most of the weight from the residual limb to the prosthetic foot through a pylon, a post-like structure fitted to the socket on one end and the prosthetic foot component on the other. The pylon may be a tube made of aluminum, titanium, steel, or carbon fiber-reinforced plastic. Most endoskeletal systems are modular and components can be easily upgraded. The endoskeletal pylon system may be covered with a cosmetic outer shell that resembles an actual leg. Addition of a single axis knee joint to an endoskeletal system entails proper interface with the upper component and the pylon (shin) component. A single axis joint is capable of straight-on flexion and extension only. The type reported by L5810 features a locking pin that maintains the standing position. The device must be manually released for the patient to flex the joint and to sit down. Report L5811 for a similar device made out of ultra-light weight material. Report L5812 for a single axis friction control adjustable joint. Friction control over the knee joint means that the adjustments can be tightened down to prevent unwanted joint movement, especially during gait. The joint also features a braking or locking mechanism to maintain proper standing position and to prevent overextension of the joint.

L5814-L5818

L5814 Addition, endoskeletal knee-shin system, polycentric, hydraulic swing phase control, mechanical stance phase lock
L5816 Addition, endoskeletal knee-shin system, polycentric, mechanical stance phase lock
L5818 Addition, endoskeletal knee/shin system, polycentric, friction swing and stance phase control

Lay Description

These codes report additions to endoskeletal prosthetic systems of multiple axis, or polycentric knee joints. These knees flex and extend like single axis joints, but also offer limited lateral movement and twisting action. Endoskeletal shank designs transfer most of the weight from the residual limb to the prosthetic foot through a pylon, a post-like structure fitted to the socket on one end and the prosthetic foot component on the other. The pylon may be a tube made of aluminum, titanium, steel, or carbon fiber-reinforced plastic. Most endoskeletal systems are modular and components can be easily upgraded. The endoskeletal pylon system may be covered with a cosmetic outer shell that resembles an actual leg. Addition of a single axis knee joint to an endoskeletal system entails proper interface with the upper component and the pylon (shin) component. A hydraulic cylinder may be used to assist joint movement, especially during the swing phase of gait. A locking mechanism or a friction brake may be added to support the system as the patient stands. Report L5814 for addition of a polycentric joint with hydraulic swing phase control to an endoskeletal prosthetic system. Report L5816 for addition of a polycentric joint with mechanical stance lock to an endoskeletal prosthetic system. Report L5818 for addition of a polycentric joint with friction swing and stance control to an endoskeletal prosthetic system.

L5822-L5830

L5822 Addition, endoskeletal knee-shin system, single axis, pneumatic swing, friction stance phase control
L5824 Addition, endoskeletal knee-shin system, single axis, fluid swing phase control
L5826 Addition, endoskeletal knee-shin system, single axis, hydraulic swing phase control, with miniature high activity frame
L5828 Addition, endoskeletal knee-shin system, single axis, fluid swing and stance phase control
L5830 Addition, endoskeletal knee/shin system, single axis, pneumatic/swing phase control

Lay Description

These codes report additions to endoskeletal prosthetic systems of single axis knee joints. Specific devices are added to the joints to assist the swing phase of gait and sometimes to control stance, or standing. Single axis knee joints are capable of simple flexion and extension only. Endoskeletal shank designs transfer most of the weight from the residual limb to the prosthetic foot through a pylon, a post-like structure fitted to the socket on one end and the prosthetic foot component on the other. The pylon may be a tube made of aluminum, titanium, steel, or carbon fiber-reinforced plastic. Most endoskeletal systems are modular and components can be easily upgraded. The endoskeletal pylon system may be covered with a cosmetic outer shell that resembles an actual leg. Friction control over the knee joint means that adjustments can be tightened down to slow down joint movement, especially during gait. Consequently, friction control joints may be fitted with assistance devices to help extend the joint during the swing phase of gait. These devices may employ a cylinder filled with air or gas (pneumatic) or fluids such as oil (hydraulic). Pressure in the cylinder forces a piston to assist movement of the joint while dampening impact during heel strike. The pressure may also be employed to act as a brake to control joint movement while standing. A high activity frame is a supportive structure around the knee joint and is designed for high levels of activity and uneven terrain. The framework may assist in special functions such as shortening the shin component for better heel and toe clearance over uneven terrain. Report L5822 for addition of a single axis joint with pneumatic swing phase and friction stance control. Report L5824 for addition of a single axis joint with fluid swing phase control. Report L5826 for addition of a single axis joint with hydraulic swing phase control with miniature high activity frame. Report L5828 for addition of a single axis joint with fluid swing and stance phase control. Report L5830 for addition of a single axis joint with pneumatic swing phase control.

L5840

L5840 Addition, endoskeletal knee/shin system, 4-bar linkage or multiaxial, pneumatic swing phase control

Lay Description

This code reports addition of a specific endoskeletal knee-shin system known as multiaxial features. Endoskeletal shank designs transfer most of the weight from the residual limb to the prosthetic foot through a pylon, a post-like structure fitted to the socket on one end and the prosthetic foot component on the other. The pylon may be a tube made of aluminum, titanium, steel, or carbon fiber-reinforced plastic. Most endoskeletal systems are modular and components can be easily upgraded. The endoskeletal pylon system may be covered with a cosmetic outer shell that resembles an actual leg. As the name denotes, a four-bar joint system features four vertical bars—paired anterior and posterior, superior and inferior hinges linked together— that pivot the joint. The additional bars affect the center of gravity and provide for a stable joint. Other multi-axial joints may feature bearings or other innovations to provide additional movement. Certain joints may be fitted with assistance devices to help extend and/or flex the joint during the swing phase of gait. These devices may employ a cylinder filled with air or gas (pneumatic). Pressure in the cylinder forces a piston to assist movement of the joint while dampening impact during heel strike. Report L5840 for addition of a four-bar linkage or multiaxial joint with pneumatic swing phase control.

L5845

L5845 Addition, endoskeletal knee/shin system, stance flexion feature, adjustable

Lay Description

This code reports addition to an endoskeletal knee-shin system of an adjustable stance flexion feature. Endoskeletal shank designs transfer most of the weight from the residual limb to the prosthetic foot through a pylon, a post-like structure fitted to the socket on one end and the prosthetic foot component on the other. The pylon may be a tube made of aluminum, titanium, steel, or carbon fiber-reinforced plastic. Most endoskeletal systems are modular and components can be easily upgraded. The endoskeletal pylon system may be covered with a cosmetic outer shell that resembles an actual leg. This code reports addition of an adjustable device that limits movement of the knee joint while standing, but still assisting the bending, or flexion, of the joint during gait. This type of device may be piston-driven, either pneumatic or hydraulic. Some models activate stance control as the patient "bounces" weight on the knee, which locks and unlocks the device for prolonged standing. Report L5845 for addition of an adjustable stance flexion feature to an endoskeletal knee-shin system.

L5848

L5848 Addition to endoskeletal knee-shin system, fluid stance extension, dampening feature, with or without adjustability

Lay Description

This code reports the addition to a knee-shin endoskeletal system of an adjustable fluid stance extension with dampening feature, with or without adjustability addition. Endoskeletal shank designs transfer most of the weight from the residual limb to the prosthetic foot through a pylon, a post-like structure fitted to the socket on one end and the prosthetic foot component on the other. The pylon may be a tube made of aluminum, titanium, steel, or carbon fiber-reinforced plastic. Most endoskeletal systems are modular and components can be easily upgraded. The endoskeletal pylon system may be covered with a cosmetic outer shell that resembles an actual leg. This type of addition is to a knee joint prosthesis and involves the use of a hydraulic driven device. Fluid such as oil is compressed in a chamber. As the joint moves, the oil is further compressed or relaxed, which governs the stance phase of the prosthesis. The compression chamber further works to dampen shock as weight is placed on the fully extended joint to engage the stance phase. Most of these designs are integrated into the joint interior. Adjustments allow the patient to open and close valves to control fluid movement through the chambers. Report L5848 for addition of an adjustable fluid stance extension with dampening feature to a knee-shin endoskeletal system, with or without an adjustability addition.

L5850-L5855

L5850 Addition, endoskeletal system, above knee or hip disarticulation, knee extension assist

L5855 Addition, endoskeletal system, hip disarticulation, mechanical hip extension assist

Lay Description

These codes report the addition of mechanical joint assists to prosthetic joints of the knee or hip. A variety of prosthetic joint designs are available, particularly for endoskeletal systems with knee components. Almost all feature some type of control to temper joint movement when not needed. Constant friction control involves adjusting tension against the joint pivot, essentially making it more difficult to move throughout its range. Other designs may involve external brakes that slow or stop joint action, particularly in the full extension stance phase. Mechanical assist devices are often added to prosthetic joints to make them move more easily in one direction, particularly during the swing phase of gait. These devices may feature an air-filled or fluid filled cylinder and piston design that helps to push the knee joint into extension. Others may entail spring action to operate the mechanical assistance. Prosthetic hip joints are usually on the anterior side near the top of the femoral pylon—somewhat removed from the natural anatomic location. Disarticulation of the hip constitutes only about 2 percent of lower limb amputations. Several types of mechanical assistance designs are used for hip joints. Some employ cords with elastic properties to assist flexion. More modern designs entail spring-driven assistance devices with components integrated into the joint. Report L5850 for addition of a knee extension assist to an endoskeletal system (above-the-knee amputation or hip disarticulation). Report L5855 for addition of a mechanical hip extension assist to an endoskeletal system (hip disarticulation).

L5910-L5920

L5910 Addition, endoskeletal system, below knee, alignable system

L5920 Addition, endoskeletal system, above knee or hip disarticulation, alignable system

Lay Description

An addition of an alignable system for lower extremity endoskeletal prostheses is reported by these codes. Alignment of the prosthesis usually occurs during the latter phases of the manufacturing process. Endoskeletal systems feature internal supports. Preliminary alignment of an above-the-knee prosthesis may occur at a fitting session before the protective covering is applied. Ordinarily, however, alignment is performed at the time of final fitting. Below-the-knee systems sometimes feature alignment settings for the foot/ankle component that can be adjusted by the wearer. Report L5910 for supply of an alignable system to a below-the-knee endoskeletal prosthesis. Report L5920 for supply of an alignable system to an above-the-knee or hip disarticulation endoskeletal prosthesis.

L5925

L5925 Addition, endoskeletal system, above knee, knee disarticulation or hip disarticulation, manual lock

Lay Description

This code reports the addition of a manual lock to a hip or knee joint of an endoskeletal system for above-the-knee amputation or hip disarticulation. A manual lock to a joint prosthesis is usually designed to be easily engaged and disengaged by the wearer. Some may feature a ring or lever that pulls a cable triggering locking mechanism. The lock itself may be a simple drop-pin design that engages the two main components of the joint, usually in full extension. This allows the patient to confidently stand without worry that the joint will collapse into flexion or hyperextend backward. The wearer must actively disengage the lock to allow the joint to flex for sitting. For some prostheses, the lock is engaged for walking as well as standing. Some manual locks can be engaged while the joint is in any variety of positions as needed by the user. Report L5925 for the addition of a manual lock.

L5930

L5930 Addition, endoskeletal system, high activity knee control frame

Lay Description

This code reports the addition of a high activity knee control frame to an endoskeletal prosthesis. Lower limb prosthesis users are usually classified in some manner according to their physical abilities. Those with good prospects for high activity levels and athletes may be fitted with special adaptations to accommodate additional stresses on the knee prosthesis. A knee control frame is usually employed in more advanced prostheses and is most often used to support high-end joint components to accommodate extreme use. These typically include a polycentric knee joint with hydraulic features and possibly microprocessor controls. Report L5930 for the addition of a high activity knee control frame to an endoskeletal prosthesis.

L5968

L5968 Addition to lower limb prosthesis, multiaxial ankle with swing phase active dorsiflexion feature

Lay Description

This code reports the addition of a specific design of multiaxial ankle to a lower limb prosthesis. A multiaxial ankle prosthesis is capable of dorsiflexion and plantarflexion (the single axis movement of the foot up and down) as well as limited twisting motion and medial and lateral movement. This offers stability and allows the user to better negotiate uneven terrain. In addition, this prosthesis automatically moves the foot into dorsiflexion (foot up) during the swing phase of gait to prepare for heel strike. This feature may be accomplished several ways. A spring-loaded cylinder acting on a piston rod is one approach. Spring tension pushes the heel down and raises the forefoot into dorsiflexion. Other designs may be activated by energy storing capabilities as weight is released from the foot. Report L5968 for addition of a multiaxial ankle with swing phase active dorsiflexion feature.

L5970-L5972

L5970 All lower extremity prostheses, foot, external keel, SACH foot

L5971 All lower extremity prosthesis, solid ankle cushion heel (SACH) foot, replacement only

L5972 All lower extremity prostheses, flexible keel foot (SAFE, STEN, Bock Dynamic or equal)

Lay Description

These codes report the supply of a variety of prosthetic feet types. The keel of a prosthetic foot is the rigid (or spring-like) section that generally runs from heel to toe near the footplate. It may serve merely as a structural piece, as in designs using wooden or rigid keels. In other designs, the keel absorbs impact and transfers energy as weight rolls from heel strike to "toe-off"—the moment when weight is released from the forefoot. The keel may be made of wood, plastic, carbon-reinforced fibers, or metal. An external keel, as the name implies, is exposed and the prosthesis may be hollow, or exoskeletal. A solid ankle, cushion heel type foot is known by the acronym SACH and a variety of models are available. In some, the external keel is part of the shell. Flexible keels are integral components of many energy storing prosthetic feet. A stationary ankle, flexible exoskeleton type of foot is known by the acronym SAFE. These types of prosthetic feet have flexible keels, either internally or as external components of the shell. The SAFE foot is known for ability to slightly invert and evert and to absorb shock. Some designs of SACH and SAFE feet have a pylon-type bolt that penetrates through the prosthesis and connects to the ankle component and pylon. The STEN foot is named for "STored ENergy," which is largely accomplished through use of a flexible keel and other resilient materials. Report L5970 for supply of any type of external keel type of SACH foot prosthesis. Report L5971 for supply of a solid ankle cushion heel (SACH) replacement component for lower extremity prosthesis. Report L5972 for supply of any type of flexible keel foot such as SAFE, STEN, or other types of dynamic foot designs.

L5973

L5973 Endoskeletal ankle foot system, microprocessor controlled feature, dorsiflexion and/or plantar flexion control, includes power source

Lay Description

Endoskeletal ankle foot system, microprocessor controlled feature, dorsiflexion and/or plantar flexion control, includes power source is an electronic, microprocessor controlled prosthetic ankle-foot system. This system was designed to assist lower extremity amputees with walking on level ground or on uneven terrain, up and down inclines and declines, up and down stairs, and standing up from a sitting position. The system permits a more dynamic, real-time adjustment of the prosthetic as the patient takes a step.

L5974-L5975

L5974 All lower extremity prostheses, foot, single axis ankle/foot

L5975 All lower extremity prosthesis, combination single axis ankle and flexible keel foot

Lay Description

These codes report the supply of specific types of prosthetic feet. A single axis ankle is capable of dorsiflexion and plantarflexion (the movement of the foot up and down) only. This is among the more fundamental designs of prosthetic feet. The keel is the component of a prosthetic foot that generally runs from heel to toe near the footplate. A flexible keel may be made of carbon reinforced fibers, metal, or resilient materials. The flexible keel absorbs impact and transfers energy as weight rolls from heel strike to "toe-off"— the moment when weight is released from the forefoot. Flexible keels are integral components of many energy storing prosthetic feet. Report L5974 for supply of a single axis ankle and foot prosthesis. Report L5975 for supply of a single axis ankle and flexible keel foot prosthesis.

L5976

L5976 All lower extremity prostheses, energy storing foot (Seattle Carbon Copy II or equal)

Lay Description

This code reports the supply of a specific level of energy storing prosthetic feet. The hallmark of energy storing prosthetic feet is some type of material that deforms with weight pressure then resumes its original shape as pressure is removed with a consequent release of energy. The keel is the component of a prosthetic foot that generally runs from heel to toe near the footplate. A flexible keel may be made of carbon-reinforced fibers, metal, or resilient materials. The flexible keel absorbs impact and transfers energy as weight rolls from heel strike to "toe-off"— the moment when weight is released from the forefoot. Flexible keels are integral components of many energy storing prosthetic feet. The type of foot reported by L5976 is designed for athletic users who wish to run on the prosthesis. The energy storing demands are somewhat higher than other prostheses with energy storing features. Most of these active use designs incorporate some type of recurve carbon fiber spring. The Carbon Copy II, FlexFoot, and SpringLight are all high-end energy storing prostheses. Report L5976 for supply of an energy storing foot prosthesis.

L5978-L5979

L5978 All lower extremity prostheses, foot, multiaxial ankle/foot
L5979 All lower extremity prostheses, multiaxial ankle, dynamic response foot, one piece system

Lay Description

These codes report the supply of a specific type of foot prosthesis. A multi-axial ankle is capable of dorsiflexion and plantarflexion (the movement of the foot up and down), as well as limited twisting motion, medial and lateral movement, and internal and external rotation. This offers stability and allows the user to better negotiate uneven terrain. The dynamic response foot is a type of energy storing prosthetic foot. It falls well within the range of active use, but somewhat short of the high-end athletic prostheses. The keel in this type of foot is energy absorbing with good transfer upon "toe-off." Sure-Flex, Genesis II, and Seattle Lite are considered in this category. Report L5978 for supply of a foot prosthesis with multi-axial ankle. Report L5979 for multi-axial ankle integrated with dynamic response foot as a single unit.

L5980-L5981

L5980 All lower extremity prostheses, flex-foot system
L5981 All lower extremity prostheses, flex-walk system or equal

Lay Description

These codes report the supply of a specific type of foot prosthesis. The original flex-foot system was a unique design to accommodate active users. The foot was developed in the early 1980s using a single L-shaped strip of carbon fiber, which at the time was a material new to prosthesis fabrication. The lower horizontal portion was fitted to sole material and the upper vertical part was attached to the pylon. A separate strip was attached to the rear of the footplate like a leaf spring to act as the heel. The design provides spring-like compression action, as well as some torque and flexibility properties. The foot is known for high flexibility and good energy storing capabilities and remains in widespread use. The flex-walk system is a second generation of the flex-foot design and addresses the needs of amputees with longer residual limbs with moderate activity levels, as well as pediatric applications. Both versions adapt well to both endoskeletal and exoskeletal shank designs. Report L5980 for supply of any flex-foot system. Report L5981 for supply of any flex-walk system or its equal.

L5985

L5985 All endoskeletal lower extremity prostheses, dynamic prosthetic pylon

Lay Description

This code reports the supply of a dynamic pylon for a lower extremity prosthesis system. A pylon is a post-like structure fitted to the residual limb socket on one end and the prosthetic foot component on the other. The pylon may be a tube made of aluminum, titanium, steel, or carbon fiber-reinforced plastic. A dynamic pylon has energy storing properties, typically provided by an internal spring or series of springs. Some models, such as the Endolite telescopic torsion pylon, also allow for some twisting movement. The energy return feature absorbs shock and in some users provides gait efficiency with less energy outlay. Report L5985 for supply of a dynamic pylon to a lower extremity prosthesis system.

L5988

L5988 Addition to lower limb prosthesis, vertical shock reducing pylon feature

Lay Description

This code reports the supply of a vertical shock-reducing pylon for a lower extremity prosthesis system. A pylon is a post-like structure fitted to the residual limb socket on one end and the prosthetic foot component on the other. The pylon may be a tube made of aluminum, titanium, steel, or carbon fiber-reinforced plastic. A pylon may be fitted with a device to absorb vertical shock, as occurs during heel strike. These additions have energy storing properties, typically provided by an internal spring or series of springs. This feature absorbs shock and in some users provides gait efficiency with less energy outlay. The Ossur Re-Flex VSP is perhaps the prototypical design for vertical shock pylons. Report L5988 for supply of a vertical shock-reducing pylon to a lower extremity prosthesis system.

L6000-L6020

L6000   Partial hand, Robin-Aids, thumb remaining (or equal)
L6010   Partial hand, Robin-Aids, little and/or ring finger remaining (or equal)
L6020   Partial hand, Robin-Aids, no finger remaining (or equal)

Lay Description

This range of codes reports the supply of a traditional type of shoulder-powered hand prosthesis known as the Robin-Aids. Fabricated by United States Manufacturing Company (USMC) in California, the Robin-Aids were designed for patients with partial hand amputation. The prosthesis is functional through use of a simple mechanical shoulder harness with a cable extending to the prosthesis. The length of socket depends on the amputation and the types of tasks demanded of the prosthesis. Heavy-duty use typically requires a deeper socket. A cosmetic glove-like covering may finish the prosthesis. A two-position prosthetic thumb is used when that digit is missing. Other digits may feature single or multiple joints. Report L6000 for supply of a Robin-Aids prosthesis for partial hand with thumb remaining. Report L6010 for supply of a Robin-Aids prosthesis for partial hand with little finger and/or ring finger remaining. Report L6020 for supply of a Robin-Aids prosthesis for partial hand with no finger remaining.

L6025

L6025   Transcarpal/metacarpal or partial hand disarticulation prosthesis, external power, self-suspended, inner socket with removable forearm section, electrodes and cables, 2 batteries, charger, myoelectric control of terminal device

Lay Description

A myoelectric prosthesis of the hand is an electronic device used as a replacement for an amputation at the transcarpal or metacarpal area. This type of prosthesis uses an external battery pack to supply power to electric motors and microprocessors that control the movement of the device in different directions. The myoelectric prosthetic has a more realistic appearance and provides the patient with increased function. Control of the device is through skin electrodes inside the socket of the prosthetic. They are able to detect and amplify the electrical activity of muscle groups left in the hand. These impulses are cycled though the microprocessor units and result in movement of the hand through electric motors. HCPCS Level II code L6025 includes an external power, self-suspended, inner socket with removable forearm section; electrodes and cables; two batteries and a charger; and myoelectric control of the terminal device.

L6050-L6055

L6050   Wrist disarticulation, molded socket, flexible elbow hinges, triceps pad
L6055   Wrist disarticulation, molded socket with expandable interface, flexible elbow hinges, triceps pad

Lay Description

These codes report the supply of hand prostheses for disarticulations at the wrist. As is typical of traditional below-the-elbow prostheses, an upper arm harness assists the mechanical operation. Movement is transferred by cable from the harness to the prosthesis. A cuff or half-cuff is situated over the tricep muscle. Paired medial and lateral elbow hinges act as leverage points to assist movement. The socket is the interface between the residual limb and the prosthesis. Traditionally, a plaster mold is taken of the residual stump and a positive replica is made. The socket is then vacuum fitted to the replica. A socket may be made from any variety of materials, although modern ones are increasingly fabricated from thermoplastic resins or elastic sleeves. Many are designed for use with gel liners. Patients with wrist disarticulation amputations can retain a great level of pronation and supination movement. An expandable interface at the socket end may be fashioned to accommodate limb growth in children or for interchangeable prostheses. Report L6050 for supply of a molded socket with flexible elbow hinges and a triceps pad. Report L6055 for supply of a molded socket with an expandable interface and flexible elbow hinges and a triceps pad.

L6100-L6110

L6100   Below elbow, molded socket, flexible elbow hinge, triceps pad
L6110   Below elbow, molded socket (Muenster or Northwestern suspension types)

Lay Description

These codes report two types of sockets for below-the-elbow or transradial amputations. A cuff or half-cuff is situated over the tricep muscle. Paired medial and lateral elbow hinges act as leverage points to assist movement. The socket is the interface between the residual limb and the prosthesis. Traditionally, a plaster mold is taken of the residual stump and a positive replica is made. The socket is then vacuum fitted to the replica. A socket may be made from any variety of materials, although modern ones are increasingly fabricated from thermoplastic resins or elastic sleeves. Many are designed for use with gel liners. The Muenster and Northwestern style sockets traditionally extend proximally to the elbow condyles. The Muenster fits snugly on the anterior and posterior aspects; the Northwestern on the medial and lateral sides. Modified versions of both are available, often with the upper posterior side cut away for movement and breathability. Both styles are suspension sockets, which hold snugly to the residual limb and suspend the prosthetic components. Report L6100 for supply of a molded socket with flexible elbow hinges and a triceps pad. Report L6110 for supply of a Muenster or Northwestern style molded socket with flexible elbow hinges and a triceps pad.

L6703-L6704

L6703   Terminal device, passive hand/mitt, any material, any size
L6704   Terminal device, sport/recreational/work attachment, any material, any size

Lay Description

A terminal device is an addition to an upper extremity prosthesis that replaces a missing hand in function, appearance, or both. The device attaches to a base wrist unit. Terminal devices are interchangeable and a patient may use different versions at different times. Terminal devices may be passive or active. Passive devices more cosmetically resemble a hand and are usually less functional. L6703 represents a paasive hand or mitt of any material or size. L6704 represents specialized devices for sport, recreation or work, of any material or size.

L6706-L6714

L6706   Terminal device, hook, mechanical, voluntary opening, any material, any size, lined or unlined
L6707   Terminal device, hook, mechanical, voluntary closing, any material, any size, lined or unlined
L6708   Terminal device, hand, mechanical, voluntary opening, any material, any size
L6709   Terminal device, hand, mechanical, voluntary closing, any material, any size
L6711   Terminal device, hook, mechanical, voluntary opening, any material, any size, lined or unlined, pediatric
L6712   Terminal device, hook, mechanical, voluntary closing, any material, any size, lined or unlined, pediatric
L6713   Terminal device, hand, mechanical, voluntary opening, any material, any size, pediatric
L6714   Terminal device, hand, mechanical, voluntary closing, any material, any size, pediatric

Lay Description

A terminal device is an addition to an upper extremity prosthesis that replaces a missing hand in function, appearance, or both. The device attaches to a base wrist unit. Terminal devices are interchangeable and a patient may use different versions at different times. Terminal devices may be passive or active. Passive devices more cosmetically resemble a hand and are usually less functional. Active devices provide some of the normal hand functions. These active terminal devices may be in the form of a hook or a hand. A hook is a metal device with two fingers that can be opened or closed and are usually made of aluminum or steel. Hands are more esthetic and allow finger position control. Body powered or manual prostheses use cables and gross limb movement to control the device. They are usually of moderate weight and cost. Active devices may have voluntary opening or closing mechanisms. The more common, voluntary opening mechanisms are closed at relaxation and open when the patient exerts control. Control may be mechanical or electric using patient muscle contractions. Relaxation of the muscles allows the device to close around the object. Voluntary closing mechanisms are open at rest. Residual forearm flexors control the grasp of the desired object. Report L6706 for voluntary opening mechanical hooks of any material or size, lined or unlined and L6707 for voluntary closing mechanical hooks of any material or size, lined or unlined. Report L6711 for pediatric voluntary opening mechanical hooks of any material or size, lined or unlined and L6712 for pediatric voluntary closing mechanical hooks of any material or size, lined or unlined. Report L6708 for a voluntary opening mechanical hand of any material or size and L6709 for a voluntary closing mechanical hand of any material or size. Report L6713 for a pediatric voluntary opening mechanical hand of any material or size and L6714 pediatric voluntary closing mechanical hand of any material or size.

L6925

L6925 Wrist disarticulation, external power, self-suspended inner socket, removable forearm shell, Otto Bock or equal electrodes, cables, 2 batteries and one charger, myoelectronic control of terminal device

Lay Description

A myoelectric prosthesis is an electronic device used as a replacement for an amputation at the wrist. This type of prosthesis uses an external battery pack to supply power to electric motors and microprocessors that control the movement of the device in different directions. The myoelectric prosthetic has a more realistic appearance and provides the patient with increased function. Control of the device is through skin electrodes inside the socket of the prosthetic. They are able to detect and amplify the electrical activity of muscle groups left in the limb. These impulses are cycled though the microprocessor units and result in movement through electric motors. HCPCS Level II code L6925 includes external power, self-suspended inner socket, removable forearm shell, Otto Bock or equal electrode, cables, two batteries, one charger, and myoelectronic control of the terminal device.

L6935

L6935 Below elbow, external power, self-suspended inner socket, removable forearm shell, Otto Bock or equal electrodes, cables, 2 batteries and one charger, myoelectronic control of terminal device

Lay Description

A myoelectric prosthesis is an electronic device used as a replacement for a below elbow amputation. This type of prosthesis uses an external battery pack to supply power to electric motors and microprocessors that control the movement of the device in different directions. The myoelectric prosthetic has a more realistic appearance and provides the patient with increased function. Control of the device is through skin electrodes inside the socket of the prosthetic. They are able to detect and amplify the electrical activity of muscle groups left in the limb. These impulses are cycled though the microprocessor units and result in movement through electric motors. HCPCS Level II code L6935 includes external power, self-suspended inner socket, removable forearm shell, Otto Bock or equal electrode, cables, two batteries, one charger, and myoelectronic control of the terminal device.

L6945

L6945 Elbow disarticulation, external power, molded inner socket, removable humeral shell, outside locking hinges, forearm, Otto Bock or equal electrodes, cables, 2 batteries and one charger, myoelectronic control of terminal device

Lay Description

A myoelectric prosthesis is an electronic device used as a replacement for an amputation at the elbow. This type of prosthesis uses an external battery pack to supply power to electric motors and microprocessors that control the movement of the device in different directions. The myoelectric prosthetic has a more realistic appearance and provides the patient with increased function. Control of the device is through skin electrodes inside the socket of the prosthetic. They are able to detect and amplify the electrical activity of muscle groups left in the limb. These impulses are cycled though the microprocessor units and result in movement through electric motors. HCPCS Level II code L6945 includes external power, molded inner socket, removable humeral shell, outside locking hinges, forearm, Otto Bock or equal electrode, cables, two batteries, one charger, and myoelectronic control of the terminal device.

L7007-L7009

L7007 Electric hand, switch or myoelectric controlled, adult
L7008 Electric hand, switch or myoelectric, controlled, pediatric
L7009 Electric hook, switch or myoelectric controlled, adult

Lay Description

A terminal device is an addition to an upper extremity prosthesis that replaces a missing hand in function, appearance, or both. The device attaches to a base wrist unit. Terminal devices are interchangeable and a patient may use different versions at different times. Terminal devices may be passive or active. Passive devices more cosmetically resemble a hand and are usually less functional. Active devices provide some of the normal hand functions. These active terminal devices may be in the form of a hook or a hand. A hook is a metal device with two fingers that can be opened or closed and are usually made of aluminum or steel. Hands are more esthetic and allow finger position control. Body powered or manual prostheses use cables and gross limb movement to control the device. They are usually of moderate weight and cost. Electric hands may be switch activated or myoelectric. Myoelectric prostheses transmit electrical impulses from electrodes on the surface of the residual muscles to an electric motor that operates the terminal device. Myoelectric devices are heavier and more expensive than manual prostheses. Myoelectric devices can have one or two electrodes. The two electrode version has separate electrodes for flexion and extension. The one electrode version uses only one electrode for both flexion and extension with differing muscle contraction strength controlling each function. Report L7007 for an adult electric hand with either switch or myoelectric control, and L7008 for the pediatric version of the same. Report L7009 for an adult electric hook with either switch or myoelectric control with L7045 represnting the pediatric version.

L7045

L7045   Electric hook, switch or myoelectric controlled, pediatric

Lay Description

A terminal device is an addition to an upper extremity prosthesis that replaces a missing hand in function, appearance, or both. The device attaches to a base wrist unit. Terminal devices are interchangeable and a patient may use different versions at different times. Terminal devices may be passive or active. Passive devices more cosmetically resemble a hand and are usually less functional. Active devices provide some of the normal hand functions. These active terminal devices may be in the form of a hook or a hand. A hook is a metal device with two fingers that can be opened or closed and are usually made of aluminum or steel. Hands are more esthetic and allow finger position control. Body powered or manual prostheses use cables and gross limb movement to control the device. They are usually of moderate weight and cost. Electric hands may be switch activated or myoelectric. Myoelectric prostheses transmit electrical impulses from electrodes on the surface of the residual muscles to an electric motor that operates the terminal device. Myoelectric devices are heavier and more expensive than manual prostheses. Myoelectric devices can have one or two electrodes. The two electrode version has separate electrodes for flexion and extension. The one electrode version uses only one electrode for both flexion and extension with differing muscle contraction strength controlling each function. This code represents the pediatric version of an electric hook either switch or myoelectric control. This code represents the pediatric version of an electric hook. Report L7009 for the adult version.

L7510

L7510   Repair of prosthetic device, repair or replace minor parts

Lay Description

Report L7510 for any minor materials (those without specific HCPCS codes) used as replacement parts, or to achieve the adjustment and/or repair of a prosthetic device.

Medicare Information

Adjustments and repairs (but not replacements) are billed as a labor charge using L7520 (one unit of service representing 15 minutes of labor time). Documentation should exist in the supplier's records indicating the precise adjustments and/or repairs performed and actual time involved. The time reported for L7520 should only be for laboratory repair time and associated prosthetic evaluation. Evaluation not associated with repair or adjustment is noncovered and should not be coded with L7520. The time for patient evaluation, gait instruction, and other general education should not be reported with L7520.

Code L7510 is used to bill for any minor materials (those without HCPCS definitions) used to achieve the adjustment and/or repair.

Note: See chapter titled "Medicare Guidelines," under "Lower Limb Prostheses; Related Additions and Replacements; Miscellaneous Prostheses and Services," for additional Medicare billing and documentation information.

L7520

L7520   Repair prosthetic device, labor component, per 15 minutes

Lay Description

Adjustments and repairs made to prostheses are billed as a labor charge using HCPCS code L7520 with one unit of service representing 15 minutes of labor time. The time reported for L7520 must only be for laboratory repair time and associated prosthetic evaluation.

Medicare Information

Adjustments and repairs (but not replacements) are billed as a labor charge using L7520 (one unit of service representing 15 minutes of labor time). Documentation should exist in the supplier's records indicating the precise adjustments and/or repairs performed and actual time involved. The time reported for L7520 should only be for laboratory repair time and associated prosthetic evaluation. Evaluation not associated with repair or adjustment is noncovered and should not be coded with L7520. The time for patient evaluation, gait instruction, and

Coders' Desk Reference for HCPCS

other general education should not be reported with L7520.

Code L7510 is used to bill for any minor materials (those without HCPCS definitions) used to achieve the adjustment and/or repair.

Note: See chapter titled "Medicare Guidelines," under "Lower Limb Prostheses; Related Additions and Replacements; Miscellaneous Prostheses and Services," for additional Medicare billing and documentation information.

L7900

L7900 Male vacuum erection system

Lay Description

Vacuum erection systems are used to treat erectile dysfunction in men. In normal circumstances, sexual arousal in men causes blood to flow into the corpus cavernosum, the blood storage columns of the penis, which creates an erection for sexual activity. Erectile dysfunction occurs when blood flow is inadequate, sometimes in combination with defects in the natural blood trapping mechanism that allows an erection to be sustained. A vacuum device is usually a clear silastic cylinder that fits externally over the penis. A vacuum is created, either manually or by an electronic pump, causing blood to be drawn into the penis. Typically a release valve on the device prevents too much vacuum pressure from building. A special elastic, metal, or leather ring is slipped around the base of the member, holding the blood within the erect penis. The vacuum pump is then removed. The ring is left on during intercourse and removed immediately afterward. Report L7900 for supply of each vacuum erection system.

L8000-L8002

L8000 Breast prosthesis, mastectomy bra
L8001 Breast prosthesis, mastectomy bra, with integrated breast prosthesis form, unilateral
L8002 Breast prosthesis, mastectomy bra, with integrated breast prosthesis form, bilateral

Lay Description

Mastectomy bras come in a variety of materials and sizes to fit patients who have undergone a mastectomy. They support and shape the patient, usually in the same way she was prior to the mastectomy. Report L8000 for a mastectomy bra without inserts; L8001 for a mastectomy bra for a patient who has had only one breast removed; L8002 for patients who have had both breasts removed.

Medicare Information

An external breast prosthesis garment, with mastectomy form (L8015) is covered for use in the postoperative period prior to a permanent breast prosthesis or as an alternative to a mastectomy bra and breast prosthesis.

L8010-L8031

L8010 Breast prosthesis, mastectomy sleeve
L8015 External breast prosthesis garment, with mastectomy form, post mastectomy
L8020 Breast prosthesis, mastectomy form
L8030 Breast prosthesis, silicone or equal, without integral adhesive
L8031 Breast prosthesis, silicone or equal, with integral adhesive

Lay Description

This range of codes reports the supply of specific breast prosthetics. A mastectomy sleeve is a full-length elastic support sleeve for the upper arm and axilla. Removal of lymph nodes during mastectomy surgery can cause lymphedema, a fluid retention and swelling, in this instance in the axilla and upper arm region. Mastectomy sleeves address this condition. Some may feature a shoulder cap and support straps around the upper torso; others just fit the arm and are held in place by the tensor properties of the fabric. Forms are external cosmetic breast devices that fit on the skin, or onto garments, following a patient's mastectomy surgery. Certain lightweight models may be made of silicone or other synthetics. Many designs adhere to the skin while others feature tabs to attach to bras or other garments. Report L8010 for supply of a mastectomy sleeve; L8015 for supply of a breast prosthesis garment with mastectomy form used prior to permanent breast prosthesis or as an alternative to a mastectomy bra and breast prosthesis. This is a camisole type undergarment with polyester fill. L8020 for a simple mastectomy form; and L8030 for a silicone breast prosthesis, or equal.

Documentation Standards

The supplier must keep on file an order for the breast prosthesis that shows the type of prosthesis. The order must be signed and dated by the treating physician.

If a patient's medical condition changes, the patient's physician must submit a new order that explains the need for a different type of breast prosthesis. The order must be kept in the supplier's files but does not need to be submitted with the claim.

Medicare Information

An external breast prosthesis garment, with mastectomy form is covered for use in the postoperative period prior to a permanent breast prosthesis or as an alternative to a mastectomy bra and breast prosthesis.

A breast prosthesis is covered for a patient who has had a mastectomy (ICD-9-CM diagnosis codes V45.71, 174.0–174.9).

The useful lifetime expectancy for silicone breast prostheses is two years. For fabric, foam, or fiber filled breast prostheses, the useful lifetime expectancy is six months. Replacement sooner than the useful lifetime expectancy because of ordinary wear-and-tear will be denied as noncovered.

An external breast prosthesis of the same type can be replaced at any time if it is lost or is irreparably damaged (this does not include ordinary wear-and-tear). An external breast prosthesis of a different type can be covered at any time if there is a change in the patient's medical condition necessitating a different type of item.

L8035-L8039

L8035   Custom breast prosthesis, post mastectomy, molded to patient model
L8039   Breast prosthesis, not otherwise specified

Lay Description

A custom fabricated breast prosthesis is one that is individually made for a patient who is post-mastectomy status, starting with basic materials. Code L8035 describes a molded to patient model custom breast prosthesis. This particular type of custom fabricated prosthesis is one in which an impression is made of the chest wall first and the impression is then used to make a positive model of the chest wall. The breast prosthesis is molded on this positive model. Report L8039 for a breast prosthesis that is not otherwise specified.

L8040

L8040   Nasal prosthesis, provided by a nonphysician

Lay Description

A nasal prosthesis is a removable superficial prosthesis that restores all or part of the nose. It may include the nasal septum. Report L8040 when a non-physician provides the prosthesis.

Medicare Information

The following services and items are included in the allowance for a facial prosthesis and should not be separately billed to Medicare:

- Evaluation of the patient
- Preoperative planning
- Cost of materials

- Labor involved in the fabrication and fitting of the prosthesis
- Modifications to the prosthesis made at the time of delivery or within 90 days thereafter
- Repair due to normal wear or tear within 90 days of delivery
- Follow-up visits within 90 days of delivery of the prosthesis

Note: See chapter titled "Medicare Guidelines," under "Facial Prostheses," for additional Medicare billing and documentation information.

L8041

L8041   Midfacial prosthesis, provided by a nonphysician

Lay Description

A midfacial prosthesis is a removable superficial prosthesis that restores part or all of the nose plus significant adjacent facial tissue/structures, but does not include the orbit or any intraoral maxillary component. Adjacent facial tissue/structures include one or more of the following: soft tissue of the cheek, upper lip, or forehead. Report L8041 when a non-physician provides the prosthesis.

Medicare Information

The following services and items are included in the allowance for a facial prosthesis and should not be separately billed to Medicare:

- Evaluation of the patient
- Preoperative planning
- Cost of materials
- Labor involved in the fabrication and fitting of the prosthesis
- Modifications to the prosthesis made at the time of delivery or within 90 days thereafter
- Repair due to normal wear or tear within 90 days of delivery
- Follow-up visits within 90 days of delivery of the prosthesis

Note: See chapter titled "Medicare Guidelines," under "Facial Prostheses," for additional Medicare billing and documentation information.

L8042

L8042   Orbital prosthesis, provided by a nonphysician

Lay Description

An orbital prosthesis is a removable superficial prosthesis that restores the eyelids and the hard and soft tissue of the orbit. It may also include the eyebrow. This code does not include the ocular prosthesis component. Report L8042 when a non-physician provides the prosthesis.

Medicare Information

The following services and items are included in the allowance for a facial prosthesis and should not be separately billed to Medicare:

- Evaluation of the patient
- Preoperative planning
- Cost of materials
- Labor involved in the fabrication and fitting of the prosthesis
- Modifications to the prosthesis made at the time of delivery or within 90 days thereafter
- Repair due to normal wear or tear within 90 days of delivery
- Follow-up visits within 90 days of delivery of the prosthesis

Note: See chapter titled "Medicare Guidelines," under "Facial Prostheses," for additional Medicare billing and documentation information.

L8043

L8043   Upper facial prosthesis, provided by a nonphysician

Lay Description

An upper facial prosthesis is a removable superficial prosthesis that restores the orbit plus significant adjacent facial tissue/structures, but does not include the nose or any intraoral maxillary component. Adjacent facial tissue/structures include one or more of the following: soft tissue of the cheek or forehead. This code does not include the ocular prosthesis component. Report L8043 when a non-physician provides the prosthesis.

Medicare Information

The following services and items are included in the allowance for a facial prosthesis and should not be separately billed to Medicare:

- Evaluation of the patient
- Preoperative planning
- Cost of materials
- Labor involved in the fabrication and fitting of the prosthesis
- Modifications to the prosthesis made at the time of delivery or within 90 days thereafter
- Repair due to normal wear or tear within 90 days of delivery
- Follow-up visits within 90 days of delivery of the prosthesis

Note: See chapter titled "Medicare Guidelines," under "Facial Prostheses," for additional Medicare billing and documentation information.

L8044

L8044   Hemi-facial prosthesis, provided by a nonphysician

Lay Description

A hemi-facial prosthesis is a removable superficial prosthesis that restores part or all of the nose plus the orbit and significant adjacent facial tissue/structures, but does not include any intraoral maxillary component. This code does not include the ocular prosthesis component. Report L8044 when a non-physician provides the prosthesis.

Medicare Information

The following services and items are included in the allowance for a facial prosthesis and should not be separately billed to Medicare:

- Evaluation of the patient
- Preoperative planning
- Cost of materials
- Labor involved in the fabrication and fitting of the prosthesis
- Modifications to the prosthesis made at the time of delivery or within 90 days thereafter
- Repair due to normal wear or tear within 90 days of delivery
- Follow-up visits within 90 days of delivery of the prosthesis

Note: See chapter titled "Medicare Guidelines," under "Facial Prostheses," for additional Medicare billing and documentation information.

L8045

L8045   Auricular prosthesis, provided by a nonphysician

Lay Description

An auricular prosthesis is a removable superficial prosthesis that restores all or part of the ear. Report L8045 when a non-physician provides the prosthesis.

Medicare Information

The following services and items are included in the allowance for a facial prosthesis and should not be separately billed to Medicare:

- Evaluation of the patient
- Preoperative planning
- Cost of materials
- Labor involved in the fabrication and fitting of the prosthesis

- Modifications to the prosthesis made at the time of delivery or within 90 days thereafter
- Repair due to normal wear or tear within 90 days of delivery
- Follow-up visits within 90 days of delivery of the prosthesis

Note: See chapter titled "Medicare Guidelines," under "Facial Prostheses," for additional Medicare billing and documentation information.

L8046

L8046 Partial facial prosthesis, provided by a nonphysician

Lay Description
A partial facial prosthesis is a removable superficial prosthesis that restores a portion of the face but does not specifically involve the nose, orbit, or ear. Report L8046 when a non-physician provides the prosthesis.

Medicare Information
The following services and items are included in the allowance for a facial prosthesis and should not be separately billed to Medicare:

- Evaluation of the patient
- Preoperative planning
- Cost of materials
- Labor involved in the fabrication and fitting of the prosthesis
- Modifications to the prosthesis made at the time of delivery or within 90 days thereafter
- Repair due to normal wear or tear within 90 days of delivery
- Follow-up visits within 90 days of delivery of the prosthesis

Note: See chapter titled "Medicare Guidelines," under "Facial Prostheses," for additional Medicare billing and documentation information.

L8047

L8047 Nasal septal prosthesis, provided by a nonphysician

Lay Description
A nasal septal prosthesis is a removable prosthesis that occludes a hole in the nasal septum but does not include superficial nasal tissue. Report L8047 when a non-physician provides the prosthesis.

Medicare Information
The following services and items are included in the allowance for a facial prosthesis and should not be separately billed to Medicare:

- Evaluation of the patient
- Preoperative planning
- Cost of materials
- Labor involved in the fabrication and fitting of the prosthesis
- Modifications to the prosthesis made at the time of delivery or within 90 days thereafter
- Repair due to normal wear or tear within 90 days of delivery
- Follow-up visits within 90 days of delivery of the prosthesis

Note: See chapter titled "Medicare Guidelines," under "Facial Prostheses," for additional Medicare billing and documentation information.

L8048

L8048 Unspecified maxillofacial prosthesis, by report, provided by a nonphysician

Lay Description
Report L8048 for any materials used for repair or modification of a maxillofacial prosthesis provided by a non-physician. Code L8048 is also used for a facial prosthesis that is not described by a specific code.

Medicare Information
Covered modifications or repairs are billed using L8049 for the labor components and L8048 for any materials used. Time reported using L8049 should only be for laboratory modification/repair time and associated prosthetic evaluation. It is used only for services after 90 days from the date of delivery of the prosthesis. Evaluation not associated with repair or modification is noncovered and should not be coded as L8049.

If a facial prosthesis has a component that is used to attach it to a bone-anchored implant or to an internal prosthesis (e.g., maxillary obturator), that component should be billed separately using L8048. This code should not be used for implanted prosthesis anchoring components.

See chapter titled "Medicare Guidelines," under "Facial Prostheses," for additional Medicare billing and documentation information.

L8049

L8049 Repair or modification of maxillofacial prosthesis, labor component, 15 minute increments, provided by a nonphysician

Lay Description
Modifications or repairs of a maxillofacial prosthesis are reported using L8049 for the labor component by a non-physician provider. Report the time in 15-minute increments. Time reported using L8049 should only be for laboratory modification/repair

time and associated prosthetic evaluation used only for services after 90 days from the date of delivery of the prosthesis.

Medicare Information

Covered modifications or repairs are billed using L8049 for the labor components and L8048 for any materials used. Time reported using L8049 should only be for laboratory modification/repair time and associated prosthetic evaluation. It is used only for services after 90 days from the date of delivery of the prosthesis. Evaluation not associated with repair or modification is noncovered and should not be coded as L8049.

See chapter titled "Medicare Guidelines," under "Facial Prostheses," for additional Medicare billing and documentation information.

L8400-L8417

L8400 Prosthetic sheath, below knee, each
L8410 Prosthetic sheath, above knee, each
L8415 Prosthetic sheath, upper limb, each
L8417 Prosthetic sheath/sock, including a gel cushion layer, below knee or above knee, each

Lay Description

This range of codes reports supply of prosthetic sheaths. Many wearers of prostheses use nylon (or other artificial or natural fabric) sleeves over the residual limb to interface between skin and the socket material. The sheath may be a stocking in the case of ankle/foot prostheses, although the term prosthetic sock refers to a sleeve that is closed on one end and may be used on either upper or lower extremity amputations. A special gel cushion layer may be used to assist the attachment capabilities of the socket. Sheaths and socks play an important role in adjusting for volume changes in the residual limb, and many products provide thickness padding against the socket. Report L8400 for supply of each below-the-knee sheath; L8410 for supply of each above-the-knee sheath; L8415 for supply of each upper limb sheath; and L8417 for supply of each above-the knee or below-the-knee sheath or sock, including a gel cushion layer.

L8420-L8435

L8420 Prosthetic sock, multiple ply, below knee, each
L8430 Prosthetic sock, multiple ply, above knee, each
L8435 Prosthetic sock, multiple ply, upper limb, each

Lay Description

The term prosthetic sock refers to a sleeve that is closed on one end and may be used on either upper or lower extremity amputations. The sock may be nylon, wool, or other artificial or natural fabric or blends. The sock plays an important role in adjusting for volume changes in the residual limb, and many products provide thickness padding against the socket. This thickness is expressed as a ply rating; generally one to six ply socks are most commonly available. By selecting a ply rating, usually in combination with liners, the wearer can adjust for changes in the size of the residual limb. Report L8420 for supply of each below-the-knee multiple ply prosthetic sock; L8430 for supply of each above-the-knee multiple ply prosthetic sock; and L8435 for supply of each upper limb multiple ply prosthetic sock.

L8440-L8465

L8440 Prosthetic shrinker, below knee, each
L8460 Prosthetic shrinker, above knee, each
L8465 Prosthetic shrinker, upper limb, each

Lay Description

This range of codes reports the supply of prosthetic shrinkers, or stump shrinkers. These elastic stockings are usually applied shortly after amputation to control swelling of the residual limb and to prepare the site for a temporary prosthesis. Most shrinkers are made of elastic material and the devices may be strapped on or simply held in place by the tensor properties of the fabric. Most devices are designed to mold and shape the site in preparation for eventual fitting of a prosthesis. Report L8440 for supply of each below-the-knee prosthetic shrinker; L8460 for supply of each above-the-knee prosthetic shrinker; and L8465 for supply of each upper limb prosthetic shrinker.

L8470-L8485

L8470 Prosthetic sock, single ply, fitting, below knee, each
L8480 Prosthetic sock, single ply, fitting, above knee, each
L8485 Prosthetic sock, single ply, fitting, upper limb, each

Lay Description

This range of codes reports the fitting of single ply prosthetic socks. The term prosthetic sock refers to a sleeve that is closed on one end and may be used on either upper or lower extremity amputations. The sock may be nylon, wool, or other artificial or natural fabric or blends. The sock plays an important role in adjusting for volume changes in the residual limb, and many products provide thickness padding against the socket. This thickness is expressed as a ply rating. This range of codes reports only single ply thickness fittings. Report L8470 for fitting of each single ply prosthetic of a below-the-knee amputation; L8480 for fitting of each single ply prosthetic of an above-the-knee amputation; and L8485 for fitting of each single ply prosthetic of an upper limb amputation.

L8604

L8604 Injectable bulking agent, dextranomer/hyaluronic acid copolymer implant, urinary tract, 1 ml, includes shipping and necessary supplies

Lay Description

Dextranomer/hyaluronic acid is a bulking agent used to treat vesicoureteral reflux (VUR) in children. VUR occurs when there is a defect in the area where the ureters connect to the bladder. Dextranomer/hyaluronic acid is a biocompatible, biodegradable gel that is injected in the bladder near the opening of each ureter to prevent the flow of urine back into the ureter and kidneys. It is injected with the aid of a cystoscope. HCPCS Level II code L8604 represents 1 ml of dextranomer/hyaluronic acid and it includes shipping and necessary supplies.

M0064

M0064 Brief office visit for the sole purpose of monitoring or changing drug prescriptions used in the treatment of mental psychoneurotic and personality disorders

Lay Description

This code represents an office visit of a very short duration solely for the purpose of monitoring or changing drug prescriptions used for the treatment of mental psychoneurotic and personality disorders. Code M0064 should be used when no other evaluation and management service is provided.

Medicare Information

All psychotherapy services that are covered on an outpatient basis are subject to the outpatient mental health services limitation of 62.5 percent, which is applicable to all therapeutic, follow-up diagnostic, and medical services with a diagnosis of mental, psychoneurotic, or personality disorders. This limitation is not applicable to the following:

- Psychiatric consultations
- Psychiatric testing
- Initial evaluation and management services
- Hospital inpatient therapy
- Services provided for a primary diagnosis of Alzheimer's disease, senility, dementia, or organic brain syndrome

Since outpatient psychiatric services are reimbursed at 62.5 percent of the Medicare fee schedule allowable amount, on nonassigned claims, the patient is responsible up to the limiting charge. On assigned claims, the beneficiary is responsible for the difference in the Medicare payment up to the full allowable amount.

Clinical psychologists may bill for services provided at all place-of-service locations.

Nonclinical psychologists may bill only for services provided in the office (place of service 11).

Clinical social workers may bill for services provided in the office. Inpatient services must be billed by the hospital to Part A, and hospital outpatient services must be billed by the hospital to Part B.

M0075

M0075 Cellular therapy

Lay Description

Cellular therapy is the practice of injecting humans with foreign proteins, such as those derived from the placenta or lungs of unborn lambs. Cellular therapy is currently without scientific or statistical evidence to document its therapeutic efficacy and, in fact, is considered a potentially dangerous practice.

M0076

M0076 Prolotherapy

Lay Description

Prolotherapy is also known as proliferative injection therapy or sclerotherapy. The practice of prolotherapy is used by physicians to treat a number of different types of chronic pain. Prolotherapy consists of a series of trigger point injections of "proliferative" solutions into ligaments and tendons near the pained area to induce the proliferation of new cells. Proponents of this treatment suggest that looseness in the supporting ligaments and tendons around the joints causes the pain, inducing the muscles to contract against the ligament and irritate the nerve endings. Three types of solutions are used to initiate inflammation: chemical irritants (e.g., phenol), osmotic shock agents (e.g., hypertonic dextrose and glycerin), and chemotactic agents (e.g., morrhuate sodium, a fatty acid derivative of cod liver oil). These injections irritate or inflame the area where they are injected and are intended to mimic the natural healing process by causing an influx of fibroblasts that synthesize collagen at the injection site, leading to the formation of new ligament and tendon tissue. The newly produced collagen is intended to support the injured or loosened ligaments, creating a more stable and strong muscle base, in the process, alleviating pain.

M0100

M0100   Intragastric hypothermia using gastric freezing

Lay Description

Intragastric hypothermia using gastric freezing is an obsolete treatment for chronic peptic ulcer disease. The treatment is a non-surgical procedure designed to reduce or eliminate the production of gastric acid by freezing the secretory cells with a supercooled fluid introduced into a balloon positioned in the stomach. The treatment was popular about 20 years ago but now is seldom doneperformed. Gastric freezing provided provides only temporary improvement to most patients. It has been largely abandoned due to a high complication rate and its lack of effectiveness in double-blind, controlled clinical trials.

M0300

M0300   IV chelation therapy (chemical endarterectomy)

Lay Description

Intravenous chelation therapy is infusion of a solution, traditionally a synthetic amino acid called ethylene diamine tetraacetic acid (EDTA). The EDTA binds with metals and minerals, which are then excreted from the body with the EDTA. This therapy, which removes unwanted metal ions from the body purportedly has therapeutic and preventative effects. Chelation therapy, when used as a treatment for atherosclerosis, is sometimes referred to as a chemical endarterectomy. The application of chelation therapy using EDTA for the treatment and prevention of atherosclerosis is controversial. There is no widely accepted rationale to explain the beneficial effects attributed to this therapy. Its safety is questioned and its clinical effectiveness has never been established by well-designed, controlled clinical trials.

M0301

M0301   Fabric wrapping of abdominal aneurysm

Lay Description

Fabric wrapping of an abdominal aneurysm is a treatment where the aneurysm is wrapped with cellophane or fascia lata. No other procedure is performed on the aneurysm or its surrounding tissue. The procedure has not been shown to prevent eventual rupture. In extremely rare instances, external wall reinforcement may be indicated when the current accepted treatment (excision of the aneurysm and reconstruction with synthetic materials) is not a viable alternative, but external wall reinforcement is not fabric wrapping. CMS believes that this treatment is ineffective and it is not covered by Medicare and many other payers.

P2028

P2028   Cephalin floculation, blood

Lay Description

Cephalin ßoculation is a test performed on serum using cephalin or a cephalin-cholesterol emulation. The flocculation or dispersion of the blood into discrete visible particles may indicate the presence of liver cell disease. This test is considered obsolete.

Medicare Information

Services that are investigational, experimental, or not reasonable or necessary are not covered. To bill the patient for procedures and services that are not covered requires an Advance Beneficiary Notice (ABN) to be obtained before the service is rendered. Claims for P2028 will always be reviewed; they must currently be billed with the unlisted CPT procedure code 88299.

P2029

P2029   Congo red, blood

Lay Description

Congo red is an odorless dark red or brown powder which decomposes upon exposure to acid fumes. It is used as a diagnostic aid in amyloidosis. The Congo red dye is injected intravenously. If after one hour more than 60 per cent of the dye has disappeared, amyloidosis is indicated. This test is considered obsolete.

Medicare Information

Services that are investigational, experimental, or not reasonable or necessary are not covered. To bill the patient for procedures and services that are not covered requires an Advance Beneficiary Notice (ABN) to be obtained before the service is rendered. Claims for P2029 will always be reviewed; they must currently be billed with the unlisted CPT procedure code 88299.

P2033

P2033   Thymol turbidity, blood

Lay Description

Thymol turbidity is a test performed on serum using the chemical thymol. The serum precipitates into albumin and globulin, which can then be measured to look for indications of liver disease. Although popular in the past, it has been superseded by quantitative determination of specific proteins and direct measurement of liver enzymes. This test is considered obsolete.

Medicare Information

Services that are investigational, experimental, or not reasonable or necessary are not covered. To bill the patient for procedures and services that are not covered requires an Advance Beneficiary Notice (ABN) to be obtained before the service is rendered. Claims for P2033 will always be reviewed; they must currently be billed with the unlisted CPT procedure code 88299.

P2038

P2038 Mucoprotein, blood (seromucoid) (medical necessity procedure)

Lay Description

Mucoprotein is a general term for a protein-polysaccharide complex, wherein the protein component is the major part of the complex. The compound is present in all connective and supporting tissues. It is sometimes called glycoprotein, although this term usually refers to those mucoproteins that contain less than four percent carbohydrate. This code represents an assay of the mucoproteins contained in a sample of blood. Most testing performed currently are for a more specific component of the complex.

Medicare Information

Services that are investigational, experimental, or not reasonable or necessary are not covered. To bill the patient for procedures and services that are not covered requires an Advance Beneficiary Notice (ABN) to be obtained before the service is rendered. Claims for P2038 will always be reviewed; they must currently be billed with the unlisted CPT procedure code 88299.

P3000-P3001

P3000 Screening Papanicolaou smear, cervical or vaginal, up to 3 smears, by technician under physician supervision
P3001 Screening Papanicolaou smear, cervical or vaginal, up to 3 smears, requiring interpretation by physician

Lay Description

A screening Papanicolaou (commonly referred to as pap) smear, cervical or vaginal, is a microscopic examination of cells scraped from the cervix or vaginal wall. The smears are examined for any cells that appear to be abnormal. It is a screening procedure when no known disease process exists. Report P3000 when the review of the smear is performed by a technician under a physician's supervision. Code P3001 is used when the review is conducted by a physician because of cell abnormalities that require the physician's medical interpretation.

Medicare Information

In P3000, Medicare covers a screening Pap smear every two years or annually if there is a high risk for cervical cancer. The professional component (the interpretation) of abnormal Pap smears furnished to a hospital inpatient by a hospital physician or an independent laboratory is paid according to the physician fee schedule. Payment for Pap smears in all other situations is made under the clinical laboratory fee schedule. The Part B deductible and coinsurance for screening Pap services is not applicable.

In P3001, the professional component (the interpretation) of abnormal Pap smears furnished to a hospital inpatient by a hospital physician or an independent laboratory is paid according to the physician fee schedule. Payment for Pap smears in all other situations is made under the clinical laboratory fee schedule. The Part B deductible and coinsurance for screening Pap services is not applicable.

Unless the advance notice provision is met, the patient is not liable for services denied as not medically necessary. The patient is also not liable for services that are denied as bundled into another service.

P7001

P7001 Culture, bacterial, urine; quantitative, sensitivity study

Lay Description

A culture is the inoculation and incubation of a growth medium. In this case, urine is inoculated onto a growth medium with the intention of determining the types and amounts of bacteria that grow. A sensitivity test follows. The bacteria that have been grown are tested against antibiotics to determine which antibiotic has the greatest effecacy against the bacteria. This code should be used only for urine cultures when both a culture and sensitivity are performed consecutively on the same specimen.

P9010-P9011

P9010 Blood (whole), for transfusion, per unit
P9011 Blood, split unit

Lay Description

Whole blood is blood without any component removed. Whole blood is the liquid medium containing the microscopic elements of erythrocytes (red blood cell), leukocytes (white blood cells), and thrombocytes (blood platelets). Whole blood is drawn from a selected donor under strict aseptic conditions. The blood is usually mixed with a citrate ion or heparin to prevent coagulation. It may be banked and used as a replacement when blood is lost. Blood is classified into four phenotypes based upon the characteristics present: A, B, AB and O. Additionally, an Rh factor of negative or positive is assigned, denoting the absence or presence of an Rh antigen. Before any blood, with the exception of type O negative, can be transfused into a patient, tests must be run to determine the compatibility of the donor blood with the patient's own blood. Type O negative is said to be the universal donor as this type of blood contains no factors that may adversely interact with the blood of the recipient. Due to the variety and number of incompatibilities that may exist, whole blood is used only when absolutely necessary and blood components are more routinely transfused. Report P9010 when one unit of whole blood is transfused; P9011 when a split unit of whole blood is transfused.

Medicare Information

A physician or other supplier who accepts assignment may bill the patient the reasonable charge for unreplaced blood (e.g., any of the first three units in a calendar year) but may not charge for replaced blood. Whenever a supplier accepts blood donated in advance, in anticipation of need by a specific patient as an autologous donation, or blood donated by another individual or blood assurance group, these donations are considered replacements for units that are subsequently provided to the patient.

Payment for all blood administration charges and blood charges after the patient has received the first three units in a calendar year are subject to the annual cash deductible and coinsurance provisions.

Charges for the administration of whole blood or packed cells are not subject to the blood deductible. This means the charge for the blood and for the administration must be considered separately by the carrier. Make sure the charges for each service are broken down separately on the claim form.

P9012

P9012 Cryoprecipitate, each unit

Lay Description

Cryoprecipitate is the cold insoluble portion of plasma that precipitates (settles into solid particles) when fresh frozen plasma is thawed at 1-6 oC. The supernatant (or liquid plasma) is removed and the residual cryoprecipitate (approximately 15 ml) is refrozen and stored at -18 oC. A single unit of cryoprecipitate contains an average of 80-100 units of factor VIII and von Willebrand factor, 150-250 mg of fibrinogen and some factor XIII and fibronectin. No compatibility testing is required and typing is not necessary. When cryoprecipitate is ordered, units are thawed, suspended in sterile, normal saline (20ml/bag) and pooled. Cryoprecipitate is the only fibrinogen concentrate available for intravenous use. In the past, cryoprecipitate had been used as a treatment for von Willebrand's disease and hemophilia A. However, newer products are the treatment of choice now. Cryoprecipitate may also be used in the preparation of fibrin glue. This glue is used in neurosurgery, orthopedic, and other surgeries. Although widespread, such use is not FDA-approved. Autologous (the patient's own blood) units can be collected prior to surgery and processed into fibrin glue. This code represents one unit of cryoprecipitate.

P9016

P9016 Red blood cells, leukocytes reduced, each unit

Lay Description

Red blood cells (RBCs) are a singular component of whole blood. RBCs are prepared from whole blood by the removal of most of the plasma, or by apheresis collection. RBCs are stored in one of several saline-based anticoagulant/ preservative solutions, yielding a hematocrit (Hct) between 55-80 percent. Leukocytes (or WBCs) are reduced or removed from the unit as the leukocytes may provoke an adverse reaction or antibody formation when they interact with the patient's own blood. RBC transfusions increase the oxygen-carrying capacity of blood. Transfusions may also treat chronic anemia when pharmacologic therapy is not effective or available, active bleeding, Sickle cell disease, or other conditions. RBCs require compatibility testing. Transfusions should be completed within four hours per unit. A unit may be divided by the blood bank in advance and administered in two or more aliquots. This code represents one unit of RBCs.

P9017

P9017 Fresh frozen plasma (single donor), frozen within 8 hours of collection, each unit

Lay Description

Plasma is the liquid portion of whole blood. Plasma is prepared by separating it from whole blood using a centrifuge, or by hemapheresis using centrifugation or filtration. The volume of plasma varies and appears on the label. One unit of fresh frozen plasma contains the plasma from one unit of whole blood, approximately 250 ml, separated and frozen within eight hours of collection. While plasma may be pooled (multiple units of whole blood are separated and combined), this code represents plasma obtained from a single donor. Plasma contains all soluble clotting factors, though some may be substantially reduced, such as Factors V and VIII. Units of plasma transfused should be ABO compatible with the recipient, but crossmatching and Rh compatibility are not required. Plasma may be indicated in the treatment of thrombotic thrombocytopenic purpura and related syndromes, congenital or acquired coagulation factor deficiency when no concentrate is available, and for specific plasma protein deficiencies such as an anti-thrombin III or C-1 esterase deficiency. Plasma may also be indicated for bleeding, preoperative, or massively transfused patients with a deficiency of multiple coagulation factors, or for patients on warfarin therapy who are bleeding and/or who are facing urgent invasive procedures. This code should be used for one unit of fresh frozen plasma that was frozen within eight hours of its collection from a single donor.

P9019-P9020

P9019 Platelets, each unit
P9020 Platelet rich plasma, each unit

Lay Description

Platelets are thrombocyte cells removed from whole blood. Platelets may be separated from the whole blood of many different donors by the use of a centrifuge or may be harvested from a single donor by hemapheresis. Pooled random donor platelets are typically prepared from four to six units of random donor platelets. Platelet rich plasma contains pooled amounts of platelets. Platelets may be suspended in donor plasma. Volume is specified on the label. Compatibility testing is not required but units of platelets transfused should be ABO compatible when possible. Transfusion of large quantities of ABO incompatible plasma may lead to a positive direct antiglobulin test and, rarely, clinically significant red cell destruction. Rh compatibility is important but not always possible. Platelets may be indicated for the prevention and treatment of non-surgical bleeding due to thrombocytopenia, for patients with accelerated platelet destruction with significant bleeding (such as autoimmune or drug-induced thrombocytopenia), for patients with documented low level platelet counts who are bleeding or who face major invasive procedures, and for patients with diffuse microvascular bleeding following cardiopulmonary bypass or massive transfusions. Use code P9019 for one unit of platelet. Report P9020 for one unit of platelet rich plasma.

P9021

P9021 Red blood cells, each unit

Lay Description

This code reports each unit of red blood cells. Whole blood is run through centrifugation where plasma (liquid portion of the whole blood) and red blood cells are separated. Red blood cells contain hemoglobin. Hemoglobin is a complex iron containing protein that carries oxygen through the body and gives blood its red coloring. There are approximately one billion red blood cells in two to three drops of blood. Red blood cells are manufactured in the bone marrow.

Medicare Information

A physician or other supplier who accepts assignment may bill the patient the reasonable charge for unreplaced blood (e.g., any of the first three units in a calendar year) but may not charge for replaced blood. Whenever a supplier accepts blood donated in advance, in anticipation of need by a specific patient as an autologous donation, or blood donated by another individual or blood assurance group, these donations are considered replacements for units that are subsequently provided to the patient.

Payment for all blood administration charges and blood charges after the patient has received the first three units in a calendar year are subject to the annual cash deductible and coinsurance provisions.

Charges for the administration of whole blood or packed cells are not subject to the blood deductible. This means the charge for the blood and for the administration must be considered separately by the carrier. Make sure the charges for each service are broken down separately on the claim form.

P9022

P9022 Red blood cells, washed, each unit

Lay Description

Whole blood is ran through centrifugation where the plasma (liquid portion of the whole blood) and what is left is the red blood cells. Red blood cells contain hemoglobin. Hemoglobin is a complex iron containing protein taht carries oxygen through the body and gives blood, its red coloring. There are approximately one billion red blood cells in two to three drops of blood. Red blood cells are manufactured in the bone marrow. These red blood cells are washed with normal saline.

P9023-P9024

P9023 Plasma, pooled multiple donor, solvent/detergent treated, frozen, each unit

Lay Description

Plasma is the liquid portion of whole blood. Plasma is prepared by separating it from whole blood using a centrifuge, or by hemapheresis using centrifugation or filtration. The volume of plasma varies and appears on the label. One unit of fresh frozen plasma contains the plasma from one unit of whole blood, approximately 250 ml, separated and frozen within eight hours of collection. While plasma may be obtained from a single donor, this code represents plasma that has been pooled (multiple units of whole blood separated and combined). Plasma contains all soluble clotting factors, though some may be substantially reduced, such as Factors V and VIII. Plasma may be "washed" or treated with a solvent or detergent to destroy any lipid bound viruses, including HIV1 and 2, hepatitis B and C, and HTLVI and II. The process does not destroy non-enveloped viruses or prion particles. Units of plasma transfused should be ABO compatible, but crossmatching and Rh compatibility are not required. Plasma may be indicated in the treatment of thrombotic thrombocytopenic purpura and related syndromes, congenital or acquired coagulation factor deficiency when no concentrate is available, and specific plasma protein deficiencies such as an anti-thrombin III or C-1 esterase deficiency. Plasma may also be indicated for bleeding, preoperative, or massively transfused patients with a deficiency of multiple coagulation factors, or for patients on warfarin therapy who are bleeding and/or who are facing urgent invasive procedures. This code should be used for one unit of plasma that has been pooled from multiple donors, solvent or detergent treated, and frozen.

P9031-P9037

P9031 Platelets, leukocytes reduced, each unit
P9032 Platelets, irradiated, each unit
P9033 Platelets, leukocytes reduced, irradiated, each unit
P9034 Platelets, pheresis, each unit
P9035 Platelets, pheresis, leukocytes reduced, each unit
P9036 Platelets, pheresis, irradiated, each unit
P9037 Platelets, pheresis, leukocytes reduced, irradiated, each unit

Lay Description

Platelets are the thrombocyte cells removed from whole blood. Platelets may be separated from the whole blood of many different donors by the use of a centrifuge, or may be harvested from a single donor by hemapheresis. Pooled random donor platelets are typically prepared from four to six units of random donor platelets. Platelet rich plasma contains pooled amounts of platelets. Platelets may be suspended in donor plasma. Volume is specified on the label. Compatibility testing is not required, but units of platelets transfused should be ABO compatible when possible. Rh compatibility is important but not always possible. Platelets may be leukocyte (white blood cell) reduced, which is the filtered removal of contaminating leukocytes. Platelets may be irradiated using gamma radiation to destroy the ability of lymphocytes (a type of leukocyte) to respond to foreign antigens, such as those in the recipient's blood. Leukocytes may provoke an adverse reaction or antibody formation in the patient's blood. They may also transmit certain viruses, including cytomegalovirus (CMV) and human T-cell lymphotropic virus (HTLV-I/II). Pheresis (apheresis) is a targeted removal of blood component from whole blood with the return of the remaining blood components to the donor. Pheresis uses a centrifuge device to separate blood components. Plasma, platelet, and leukocytes are the components that may be removed using pheresis.

The designated component (in this case platelets) is removed and the remaining blood components are retransfused into the donor. Platelets are indicated for the prevention and treatment of non-surgical bleeding due to thrombocytopenia, for patients with accelerated platelet destruction with significant bleeding (such as autoimmune or drug-induced thrombocytopenia), for patients with documented low level platelet counts who are bleeding or who face major invasive procedures, and for patients with diffuse microvascular bleeding following cardiopulmonary bypass or massive transfusions. Use code P9031 for one unit of platelets that have been leukocyte reduced. Report P9032 for one unit of platelets that have been irradiated. Use P9033 for one unit of platelets that has been both leukocyte reduced and irradiated. Use P9034 for one unit of platelets that have been obtained using pheresis. Report P9035 for platelets that have been obtained using pheresis that have been leukocyte reduced. Use P9036 for one unit of platelets that have been obtained using pheresis that have been irradiated. Use P9036 for one unit of platelets that have been obtained using pheresis and that have been both leukocyte reduced and irradiated.

P9038-P9040

P9038 Red blood cells, irradiated, each unit
P9039 Red blood cells, deglycerolized, each unit
P9040 Red blood cells, leukocytes reduced, irradiated, each unit

Lay Description

Red blood cells (RBCs) are a singular component of whole blood. RBCs are prepared from whole blood by the removal of most of the plasma, or by apheresis collection. RBCs are stored in one of several saline-based anticoagulant/ preservative solutions, yielding a hematocrit (Hct) between 55-80percent. RBCs may be leukocyte (or white blood cell) reduced, which is the filter removal of contaminating leukocytes. RBCs may be irradiated using gamma radiation to destroy the ability of lymphocytes (a type of leukocyte) to respond to foreign antigens in the recipient's blood. Leukocytes may provoke an adverse reaction or antibody formation when they interact with the patient's own blood. They may also transmit certain viruses, including cytomegalovirus (CMV) and human T-cell lymphotropic virus (HTLV-I/II). Prior to freezing, glycerol may be added to the RBCs. When this glycerol is removed upon thawing, the RBCs are termed "deglycerolized." A major indication for RBC transfusions is prevention or treatment of symptoms of tissue hypoxia by increasing the oxygen-carrying capacity of blood. RBCs may also be indicated in the treatment of symptomatic chronic anemia when pharmacologic therapy is not effective or available, active bleeding with signs and symptoms of hypovolemia, preoperative anemia with impending major blood loss, Sickle cell disease, and anemia due to renal failure/hemodialysis. RBCs require compatibility testing and should be ABO and Rh compatible. The initial transfusion period may be carefully monitored with a slow transfusion rate to allow tearly detection of a reaction. Transfusions should be completed within four hours per unit. Alternatively, the unit may be divided by the blood bank in advance and administered in two or more aliquots. Report P9038 for one unit of RBCs that has been irradiated; P9039 for a unit of RBCs that has been deglycerolized; P9040 for one unit of RBCs that has been leukocyte reduced and irradiated.

P9041

P9041   Infusion, albumin (human), 5%, 50 ml

Lay Description

Albumin is a protein manufactured by the liver and carried throughout the body by plasma and is the most prevalent protein found in blood plasma. Plasma is collected and pooled, then fractionated to separate the albumin. Unlike other plasma proteins, albumin has several essential physiologic functions in the human body and is an important therapeutic agent. Albumin maintains the osmotic pressure that causes fluid to remain within the blood stream instead of leaking out into the tissues. It also transports thyroid hormone, drugs, and bilirubin. It increases total blood volume by drawing fluid from body tissues. Albumin may be indicated as a treatment for shock, hypovolemia, acute liver failure, burns and other thermal injuries, hypoproteinemia, adult respiratory distress syndrome, cardiopulmonary bypass, neonatal hemolytic disease, renal dialysis, acute nephrosis, erythrocyte, acute peritonitis, pancreatitis, and cellulitis. Albumin is available with varying concentrations of protein: 5 percent, 20 percent, and 25 percent. The recommended concentration and dosage depends upon the patient and reason for administration. It is administered by intravenous infusion. HCPCS Level II code P9041 represents 50 ml of 5 percent concentration of albumin.

P9043

P9043   Infusion, plasma protein fraction (human), 5%, 50 ml

Lay Description

Plasma protein fraction is a sterile solution of selected proteins derived from the blood plasma of adult human donors. It typically contains 4.5 to 5.5 grams of protein per 100 ml. This protein consists of 83 to 90 percent albumin, with the remainder alpha-and beta-globulins. Plasma Protein Fraction is the solution remaining once cryoprecipitate, fibrinogen, and immunoglobulins have been removed. Plasma protein faction is usually heat treated to destroy viruses. Indications for its use are similar to those for albumin. Administered intravenously, it increases total blood volume by drawing fluid from body tissues. Other indications include shock, hypovolemia, acute liver failure, burns and other thermal injuires, hypoproteinemia, adult respiratory distress syndrome, cardiopulmonary bypass, neonatal hemolytic disease, renal dialysis, acute nephrosis, erythrocyte resuspension, acute peritonitis, pancreatitis, mediastinitis and cellulitis. This code represents 50 ml of a 5 percent concentration of plasma protein fraction.

P9044

P9044   Plasma, cryoprecipitate reduced, each unit

Lay Description

Cyroprecipitate reduced plasma is the solution remaining once the cold insoluble portion has been removed. Cryoprecipitate settles into solid particles when fresh frozen plasma is thawed at 1-6 oC. The liquid plasma removed is the cyroprecipitate-reduced plasma. Cyroprecipitate reduced plasma is deficient in Von Willebrand factor, Factor VIII, Factor XIII, fibrinogen, and fibronectin. It may be indicated for the treatment of thrombotic thrombocytopenic purpura. This code represents one unit.

P9045-P9047

P9045   Infusion, albumin (human), 5%, 250 ml
P9046   Infusion, albumin (human), 25%, 20 ml
P9047   Infusion, albumin (human), 25%, 50 ml

Lay Description

Albumin is a protein manufactured by the liver and carried throughout the body by plasma and is the most prevalent protein found in blood plasma. Plasma is collected and pooled, then fractionated to separate the albumin. Unlike other plasma proteins, albumin has several essential physiologic functions in the human body and is an important therapeutic agent. Albumin maintains the osmotic pressure that causes fluid to remain within the blood stream instead of leaking out into the tissues. It also transports thyroid hormone, drugs, and bilirubin. It increases total blood volume by drawing fluid from body tissues. Albumin may be indicated as a treatment for shock, hypovolemia, acute liver failure, burns and other thermal injuries, hypoproteinemia, adult respiratory distress syndrome, cardiopulmonary bypass, neonatal hemolytic disease, renal dialysis, acute nephrosis, erythrocyte, acute peritonitis, pancreatitis, and cellulitis. Albumin is available with varying concentrations of protein: 5 percent, 20 percent, and 25 percent. The recommended concentration and dosage depends upon the patient and reason for administration. It is administered by intravenous infusion. HCPCS Level II code P9045 represents 250 ml of 5% concentration of albumin. HCPCS Level II code P9046 represents 20 ml of 25 percent concentration of albumin with P9047 representing 50 ml of the same.

P9048

P9048   Infusion, plasma protein fraction (human), 5%, 250 ml

Lay Description

Plasma protein fraction is a sterile solution of selected proteins derived from the blood plasma of adult human donors. It contains 4.5 to 5.5 grams of protein per 100 ml. This protein consists of 83 to 90 percent albumin with the remainder alpha-and beta-globulins. Plasma Protein Fraction is the solution remaining once cryoprecipitate, fibrinogen, and immunoglobulins have been removed from plasma. Plasma protein faction is usually heat treated to destroy HIV, hepatitis viruses, and CMV. Indications for its use are similar to those for albumin. Administered intravenously, it increases total blood volume by drawing fluid from body tissues. Other indications include shock, hypovolemia, acute liver failure, burns and other thermal injuries, hypoproteinemia, adult respiratory distress syndrome, cardiopulmonary bypass, neonatal hemolytic disease, renal dialysis, acute nephrosis, erythrocyte resuspension, acute peritonitis, pancreatitis, mediastinitis, and cellulitis. This code represents 250 ml of a 5 percent concentration of plasma protein fraction.

P9050

P9050   Granulocytes, pheresis, each unit

Lay Description

Granulocytes are types of leukocytes (white blood cells) consisting of neutrophils, basophils, or eosinophils. They are distinguished by the granules (insoluble nonmembranous particles) found within their cytoplasm. Granulocytes surround and destroy microorganisms. These granules within each cell are filled with chemicals, which upon their release, help to degrade the microorganism that the granulocyte surrounds. The cells are named for the way they stain in the laboratory. For example, eosinophils, absorb acidic dyes such as eosin. Pheresis (apheresis) is a targeted removal of blood component from whole blood with the return of the remaining blood components to the donor. Pheresis uses a a centrifuge to separate blood components. Plasma, platelet, and leukocytes are the components that may be removed using pheresis. The designated component (in this case granulocytes) is removed and the remaining blood components are retransfused into the donor. A standard adult concentrate contains approximately 20-50x10^9 granulocytes, 20-50 ml red blood cells, and 200-400 ml plasma. Granulocyte concentrates for neonates contain approximately 5x10^9 granulocytes in 30 µl plasma. Prior to the collection of granulocytes, donors are given G-CSF to stimulate their production. Granulocytes must be ABO and RH compatible with the recipient as there are large numbers of red cells in granulocyte concentrates. Granulocyte concentrates are always irradiated using gamma radiation to destroy the ability of lymphocytes to respond to foreign antigens, such as those in the recipient's blood. Granulocytes may be indicated as a treatment for infections that are unresponsive to antibiotic therapy.

P9051

P9051   Whole blood or red blood cells, leukocytes reduced, CMV-negative, each unit

Lay Description

Whole blood is blood without any component removed. Blood consists of plasma, or the liquid medium containing the microscopic elements of erythrocytes (red blood cells), leukocytes (white blood cells), and thrombocytes (blood platelets). Red blood cells (RBCs) are a singular component of whole blood. RBCs are prepared from whole blood by the removal of most of the plasma, or by apheresis collection. RBCs are stored in one of several saline-based anticoagulant/ preservative solutions, yielding a hematocrit (Hct) between 55-80 percent. Both whole blood and RBCs require compatibility testing and should be ABO and Rh compatible. Leukocytes (or white blood cells) are reduced or removed from the unit as the leukocytes may provoke an adverse reaction or antibody formation when they interact with the patient's own blood. Cytomegalovirus (CMV) is a herpes type virus that is found universally throughout all geographic locations and socioeconomic groups, and infects between 50 and 85 percent of adults in the United States by 40 years of age. For most healthy persons who acquire CMV, there are few symptoms and no long-term health consequences. For the vast majority of people, CMV infection is not a serious problem. However, CMV infection is important to certain high-risk groups. These groups include pregnant women, people who work with children, and immunocompromised people, such as organ transplant recipients and persons infected with human immunodeficiency virus (HIV). Blood products intended for people in a high-risk group are usually tested for CMV. The major indication for RBC transfusions is prevention or treatment of symptoms of tissue hypoxia by increasing the oxygen-carrying capacity of blood. RBCs may also be indicated in the treatment of symptomatic chronic anemia when pharmacologic therapy is not effective or available, active bleeding, with signs and symptoms of hypovolemia, preoperative anemia with impending major blood loss, Sickle cell disease, and anemia due to renal failure/hemodialysis refractory to erythropoietin therapy. Due to the variety and number of incompatibilities that may exist, whole blood is used only when absolutely necessary and blood components are more routinely transfused. This code represents one unit of either whole body or RBCs that has been leukocyte reduced and has tested negative for the presence of the CMV virus.

P9052-P9053

P9052 Platelets, HLA-matched leukocytes reduced, apheresis/pheresis, each unit
P9053 Platelets, pheresis, leukocytes reduced, CMV-negative, irradiated, each unit

Lay Description

Platelets are the thrombocyte cells removed from whole blood. They may be separated from the whole blood of many different donors by the use of a centrifuge or may be harvested from a single donor by hemapheresis. Platelets may be suspended in donor plasma. Volume is specified on the label. Human leukocyte antigens (HLAs) are proteins located on the surface of white blood cells (WBCs) and certain tissues within the body. HLAs are inherited. There are three groups of HLA: HLA-A, HLA-B and HLA-DR. Each group contains many specific proteins, each labeled with a number (e.g., HLA-A1). Not every person possesses every type of protein (e.g., one person may be HLA-A1 and another HLA-A2). HLA testing determines the compatibility between the donor and recipient blood at the level of the A and B antigens. HLA-matched blood products are then crossmatched. HLA platelets are irradiated. Leukocytes (or WBCs) are reduced or removed from the unit, as the leukocytes may provoke an adverse reaction or antibody formation when they interact with the patient's own blood. Leukocytes may also transmit certain viruses, including cytomegalovirus (CMV) and human T-cell lymphotropic virus (HTLV-I/II). Pheresis (apheresis) is a targeted removal of blood component from whole blood with the return of the remaining blood components to the donor. Essentially, the blood is centrifuged to separate components, in this case the platelets. The remaining blood components are retransfused into the donor. Cytomegalovirus (CMV) is a herpes-type virus that is found universally throughout all geographic locations and socioeconomic groups, and infects between 50 and 85 percent of adults in the United States by 40 years of age. Most healthy persons who acquire CMV exhibit few symptoms and no long-term health consequences. Some persons may experience a mononucleosis-like syndrome with prolonged fever, and mild hepatitis. Once a person is infected, the virus remains alive, but usually dormant within that person's body for life. Recurrent disease rarely occurs unless the person's immune system is suppressed due to therapeutic drugs or disease. Blood products intended for people in high-risk groups are usually tested for CMV. HLA-matched platelets may be indicated for patients who have become refractory to random donor platelets. Use code P9052 for one unit of HLA-matched, leukocyte reduced platelets obtained via pheresis (apheresis).Use code P9053 for one unit of leukocyte reduced platelets that has been irradiated, has tested negative for CMV, and has been obtained via pheresis (apheresis).

P9054

P9054 Whole blood or red blood cells, leukocytes reduced, frozen, deglycerol, washed, each unit

Lay Description

Whole blood is blood without any component removed. Whole blood contains the microscopic elements of erythrocytes (red blood cells), leukocytes (white blood cells), and thrombocytes (blood platelets). Red blood cells (RBCs) are a singular component of whole blood. RBCs are prepared from whole blood by the removal of most of the plasma, or by apheresis collection. RBCs are stored in one of several saline-based anticoagulant/ preservative solutions, yielding a hematocrit (Hct) between 55-80 percent. Both whole blood and RBCs require compatibility testing. Leukocytes (or WBCs) are reduced or removed from the unit as the leukocytes may provoke an adverse reaction or antibody formation when they interact with the recipient blood. Glycerol may be added to the RBCs prior to freezing. When this glycerol is removed after thawing, the RBCs are termed "deglycerolized." Both whole blood and RBCs may be "washed" or treated with solvent to destroy any lipid bound viruses including HIV and hepatitis B and C. RBC transfusions increase the oxygen-carrying capacity of blood. Transfusions may also treat chronic anemia when pharmacologic therapy is not effective or available, active bleeding, Sickle cell disease, and other conditions. Due to the variety and number of incompatibilities that may exist, whole blood is used only when absolutely necessary and blood components are more routinely transfused. This code represents a unit of either whole body or RBCs that has been leukocyte reduced, frozen, deglycerolized, and washed.

P9055

P9055 Platelets, leukocytes reduced, CMV-negative, apheresis/pheresis, each unit

Lay Description

Platelets are the thrombocyte cells removed from whole blood. Platelets may be separated from the whole blood of many different donors by the use of a centrifuge or may be harvested from a single donor by hemapheresis. Pooled random donor platelets are typically prepared from four to six units of random donor platelets. Platelet rich plasma is plasma which contains pooled amounts of platelets. Platelets may be suspended in donor plasma. Volume is specified on the label. Compatibility type testing is not generally required. . Rh compatibility is important but not always possible. Platelets may be leukocyte (or white blood cell) reduced, which is the filter removal of contaminating leukocytes. Leukocytes may provoke an adverse reaction or antibody formation when they interact with the patient's own blood. They may also transmit certain viruses, including cytomegalovirus (CMV) and human T-cell lymphotropic virus (HTLV-I/II). Blood products intended for people in a high-risk group are usually tested for CMV. Pheresis (apheresis) is a targeted removal of blood component from whole blood with the return of the remaining blood components to the donor. Essentially, the blood is centrifuged to separate components. Plasma, platelets, and leukocytes are components that may be removed by pheresis. The designated component, in this case platelets, is removed and the remaining blood components are retransfused into the donor. Use code P9052 for one unit of platelets that have been leukocyte reduced, obtained via pheresis, and that has tested negative for CMV.

P9056

P9056 Whole blood, leukocytes reduced, irradiated, each unit

Lay Description

Whole blood is blood without any component removed. Blood consists of plasma or the liquid medium containing the microscopic elements of erythrocytes (red blood cell), leukocytes (white blood cells) and thrombocytes (blood platelets). Whole blood is drawn from a selected donor under strict aseptic conditions. The whole blood is usually mixed with a citrate ion or heparin to prevent coagulation. It is typically used as a replacement for blood loss. Blood is classified into four phenotypes based upon the characteristics present: A, B, AB and O. Additionally, a Rh factor of negative or positive is assigned denoting the absence or presence of an Rh antigen. Tests are run to determine compatibility of the donor blood with the patient's own blood. Type O negative is said to be the universal donor, as this blood type contains no factors which may adversely affect or interact with the blood of the recipient. Whole blood may be leukocyte (white blood cell) reduced using a filter. Whole blood may be gamma irradiated to destroy the ability of lymphocytes (a type of leukocyte) to respond to foreign antigens, such as those in the recipient's blood. Leukocytes may provoke an adverse reaction or antibody formation when they interact with the patient's own blood. Due to the variety and number of incompatibilities that may exist, whole blood is used only when absolutely necessary and blood components are more routinely transfused. Use P9056 for one unit of whole blood that has been leukocyte reduced and irradiated.

P9057-P9058

P9057 Red blood cells, frozen/deglycerolized/washed, leukocytes reduced, irradiated, each unit

P9058 Red blood cells, leukocytes reduced, CMV-negative, irradiated, each unit

Lay Description

Red blood cells (RBCs) are a singular component of whole blood. RBCs are prepared from whole blood by the removal of most of the plasma, or by apheresis collection. RBCs are stored in one of several saline-based anticoagulant/preservative solutions, yielding a hematocrit (Hct) between 55-80 percent. RBCs require ABO and Rh compatibility testing. Leukocytes (white blood cells) are reduced or removed from the unit, as the leukocytes may provoke an adverse reaction or antibody formation when they interact with the patient's own blood. RBCs may also be gamma irradiated to destroy the ability of lymphocytes (a type of leukocyte) to respond to foreign antigens, such as those in the recipient's blood. Glycerol may be added to the RBCs prior to freezing. When this glycerol is removed after thawing, the RBCs are termed "deglycerolized." RBCs may be "washed" or treated with solvent to destroy any lipid bound viruses. Blood products intended for people in a high-risk group are usually tested for cytomegalovirus (CMV). RBC transfusions increase the oxygen-carrying capacity of blood. RBCs transfusion may be indicated for symptomatic chronic anemia when pharmacologic therapy is not effective or available, active bleeding, preoperative anemia with impending major blood loss, Sickle cell disease, among other conditions. Due to the variety and number of incompatibilities that may exist, whole blood is used only when absolutely necessary and blood components are more routinely transfused. Code P9057 represents one unit of RBCs that has been leukocyte reduced, frozen, deglycerolized and washed and irradiated; P9058 for one unit of RBCs that have been leukocyte reduced, irradiated and has tested negative for CMV.

P9059-P9060

P9059 Fresh frozen plasma between 8-24 hours of collection, each unit
P9060 Fresh frozen plasma, donor retested, each unit

Lay Description
Plasma is the liquid portion of whole blood. Plasma is prepared by separating it from whole blood by centrifuge, or by hemapheresis using centrifugation or filtration. The volume of plasma varies and appears on the label. One unit of fresh frozen plasma contains the plasma from one unit of whole blood, approximately 250 ml, separated and frozen. Plasma may be pooled (multiple units of whole blood separated and combined). Plasma contains all soluble clotting factors, though some may be substantially reduced, such as Factors V and VIII. Units of plasma transfused should be ABO compatible with the recipient, but crossmatching and Rh compatibility are not typically required. Donors may be tested and retested for communicable diseases. Plasma may be indicated for a number of conditions and syndromes. Plasma may also be indicated for preoperative or massively transfused patients with a deficiency of multiple coagulation factors. Report P9059 for one unit of fresh frozen plasma that has frozen more than 8 but less than 24 hours from its collection; P9060 is reported for one unit of fresh frozen plasma that indicates that the donor has been retested.

P9603-P9604

P9603 Travel allowance, one way in connection with medically necessary laboratory specimen collection drawn from homebound or nursing homebound patient; prorated miles actually travelled.
P9604 Travel allowance, one way in connection with medically necessary laboratory specimen collection drawn from homebound or nursing homebound patient; prorated trip charge

Lay Description
Some laboratories will send technicians to a person's home or to a nursing home to collect the specimens necessary to perform a physician-ordered test. The patient must be unable to travel to the laboratory. The laboratory may have a set travel fee that is charged for such collections, or it may charge by the number of miles traveled. HCPCS Level II code P9603 is used to report the actual number of one-way miles traveled. This mileage must be prorated or divided between all the patients that had specimen collection performed during one specific trip. Report P9604 when the laboratory has a set fee charged for each trip. This fee must also be prorated among the patients that had specimen collection performed during the trip.

Medicare Information
Medicare covers a per-mile travel allowance for laboratory technicians to travel to the patient in order to gather a specimen. Separate payment may be made for the drawing or collecting of laboratory specimens when it involves venipuncture for drawing blood or collection of a urine sample by catheterization.

A per-mile travel allowance has been established based on the federal mileage rate of 36 cents per mile and an additional 45 cents per mile to cover the technician's time and travel costs.

Only one collection fee is allowed for each type of specimen for each patient encounter, regardless of the number of specimens drawn. When a series of tests is required to complete a single test (such as a glucose tolerance test), the series is treated as a single encounter.

P9612-P9615

P9612 Catheterization for collection of specimen, single patient, all places of service
P9615 Catheterization for collection of specimen(s) (multiple patients)

Lay Description
Patients who cannot produce a urine specimen when required for physician ordered testing may need to be catherized. Catherization is the insertion of a small tube through the urethra to the bladder. Urine ordinarily flows freely through the tube, allowing for collection and testing. Catherizations may be performed in hospitals, physician's offices, nursing homes, or the patient's home. P9612 is used when a single patient has been catherized to collect a specimen and may be reported for any site of service. P9615 is used when multiple patients are catherized during a single trip or visit (e.g., a trip to a nursing home when two or more patients are catherized to obtain specimens.

Q0035

Q0035 Cardiokymography

Lay Description
Cardiokymography involves the use of a noninvasive device to record the anterior left ventricle segmental wall motion. The device typically consists of a 5cm diameter capacitive plate transducer as part of a high frequency, low-power oscillator with recording probe. Changes in wall motion affect the magnetic field and thus the oscillatory frequency, which is then recorded on a multichannel analog waveform polygraph. Medicare and most payers cover this type

of test only as an adjunct to electrocardiographic stress testing to evaluate coronary artery disease and only when specific clinical indications are present. For male patients there must be atypical angina pectoris or nonischemic chest pain. For female patients, there must be angina, either typical or atypical.

Medicare Information

Medicare only covers cardiokymography in conjunction with electrocardiographic stress testing in male patients with atypical angina or nonischemic chest pain. Medicare will cover female patients with angina.

Q0081

Q0081 Infusion therapy, using other than chemotherapeutic drugs, per visit

Lay Description

Intravenous infusion is the administration of a liquid through the patient's veins for therapeutic or diagnostic purposes. This code should not be used for the infusion of any chemotherapeutic drug (see Q0084 for chemotherapeutic infusions). This code should be reported only once per visit.

Medicare Information

Medicare covers the administration charges for IV therapy. Coverage varies depending on the type of drug involved and the patient's diagnosis. Check with your local carrier for a determination.

Q0083

Q0083 Chemotherapy administration by other than infusion technique only (e.g., subcutaneous, intramuscular, push), per visit

Lay Description

This code is used for the administration of chemotherapy by any technique other than infusion. Chemotherapy administration may include intramuscular or subcutaneous injection or a "push." A push is the direct intravenous injection of a drug slowly over one to two minutes. Typically drugs that are pushed are not diluted with any type of intravenous solution (e.g., D5W, saline). Chemotherapy is the treatment of any disease with chemical agents, but commonly refers to the administration of anti-neoplastic drugs. This code should be reported only once per visit.

Q0084

Q0084 Chemotherapy administration by infusion technique only, per visit

Lay Description

This code is used for the administration of chemotherapy through the patient's vascular system for therapeutic purposes. Chemotherapy is the treatment of any disease with chemical agents, but commonly refers to the administration of anti-neoplastic drugs. This code should be reported only once per visit.

Q0085

Q0085 Chemotherapy administration by both infusion technique and other technique(s) (e.g. subcutaneous, intramuscular, push), per visit

Lay Description

This code is used for the administration of chemotherapy by both infusion and other techniques. Chemotherapy is the treatment of any disease with chemical agents, but commonly refers to the administration of anti-neoplastic drugs. This code should be reported only once per visit.

Q0091

Q0091 Screening Papanicolaou smear; obtaining, preparing and conveyance of cervical or vaginal smear to laboratory

Lay Description

A screening Papanicolaou (commonly referred to as pap) smear, cervical or vaginal, is a microscopic examination of cells scraped from the cervix or vaginal wall. The smears are examined for any abnormal appearing cells. It is a screening procedure when no known disease process currently exists and the test is looking for any possible abnormalities. Code Q0091 reports the collection and preparation of a screening vaginal or cervical pap smear. This code includes the conveyance or transportation of the smear to the laboratory.

Medicare Information

Medicare covers a screening Pap smear every two years or annually if there is a high risk for cervical cancer. Medicare also covers the obtaining, preparing, and conveyance of a cervical or vaginal smear to the laboratory.

The professional component (the interpretation) of abnormal Pap smears furnished to a hospital inpatient by a hospital physician or an independent laboratory is paid according to the physician fee schedule. Payment for Pap smears in all other situations is made under the clinical laboratory fee schedule. The Part B deductible and coinsurance for screening Pap services is not applicable.

Unless the advance notice provision is met, the patient is not liable for services denied as not medically necessary. The patient is also not liable for services that are denied as bundled into another service.

Q0092
Q0092 Set-up portable x-ray equipment

Lay Description
The set-up of portable x-ray equipment is the procedure of unpacking and readying portable radiologic devices for use. Use R0070 or R0075 to report the transportation of this equipment. This code should only be used by portable x-ray suppliers when the equipment is transported and set-up in a place of residence used as the patient's home (such as a nursing home) or in a nonparticipating institution. Portable x-ray services and their set-up must be performed under the general supervision of a physician and certain health and safety conditions must be met. Portable studies should be performed only when there is true medical necessity and when the patient cannot access or otherwise be examined on fixed conventional x-ray equipment. These studies should not be performed for "routine" purposes or for reasons of minor convenience. A set-up component can be paid for each radiological procedure (other than retakes of the same procedure) during both single patient and multiple patient trips. This code should not be used when the portable x-ray supplier performs an EKG.

Q0111
Q0111 Wet mounts, including preparations of vaginal, cervical or skin specimens

Lay Description
A wet mount is the placement of a specimen on a microscope slide with the addition of a liquid. The liquid helps support the specimen and fills space between the cover slip and slide, which allows more light to pass and better visualization of the specimen. Wet mounts may be used for cervical, vaginal, and prostate smears, and examination of skin or feces specimens.

Q0112
Q0112 All potassium hydroxide (KOH) preparations

Lay Description
Potassium hydroxide (KOH) preparations are wet mounted slides where the added liquid is potassium hydroxide. The KOH dissolves cellular elements, such as skin cells, leaving only fungus and yeast visible.

Q0113
Q0113 Pinworm examinations

Lay Description
Pinworms are nematodes or round worms that live in the perianal area and migrate from the bowel to the skin to lay eggs. The eggs are very resistant to dehydration and can easily be dispersed into the air. Pinworm examinations involve the application of a special tape or swab at different times. The tape or swab is then examined for the presence of the pinworm or its eggs.

Q0114
Q0114 Fern test

Lay Description
A fern test is named for the pattern that the fluid takes when viewed under a microscope. The liquid crystallizes into a fern pattern. Cervical fluids may be analyzed in this manner to detect estrogen activity. As ovulation approaches, the pattern features more ferning. The test may also be used to detect amniotic fluid leakage in a pregnant uterus. A slide of vaginal fluid is allowed to dry. Amniotic fluid crystallizes to form a fern-like pattern due to its concentrations of sodium chloride, proteins, and carbohydrates.

Q0115
Q0115 Postcoital direct, qualitative examinations of vaginal or cervical mucous

Lay Description
The microscopic analysis of cervical mucus may be performed within hours of timed intercourse in order to observe and evaluate the interaction of sperm, semen, and cervical mucus. A small sample is obtained and examined under a microscope to determine the quality of sperm and its interaction with the cervical mucosa.

Q0138-Q0139
Q0138 Injection, ferumoxytol, for treatment of iron deficiency anemia, 1 mg (non-ESRD use)

Q0139 Injection, ferumoxytol, for treatment of iron deficiency anemia, 1 mg (for ESRD on dialysis)

Lay Description
Ferumoxytol is an iron oxide used to treat low iron in patients with chronic kidney disease. It is coated with a carbohydrate layer that helps surrounds the iron from the plasma until can be used for

hemoglobin. The recommended dose starts with 510 mg with a follow-up injection three to eight days later. Ferumoxytol is administered as an IV injection. Report Q0138 per mg for non-ESRD patients and Q0139 per mg for patients with ESRD.

Q0144

Q0144   Azithromycin dihydrate, oral, capsules/powder, 1 g

Lay Description

Azithromycin dehydrate is an antibiotic indicated for use in patient's with mild to moderate infections caused by susceptible strains of various microorganisms. Indications include pneumonia, pharyngitis and tonsillitis, staph and strep skin infections, cervicitis and urethritis due to gonorrhea and chlamydia, and genital ulcers. This code represents one gram of the oral tablets or powder.

Q0163

Q0163   Diphenhydramine HCl, 50 mg, oral, FDA approved prescription antiemetic, for use as a complete therapeutic substitute for an IV antiemetic at time of chemotherapy treatment not to exceed a 48-hour dosage regimen

Lay Description

Diphenhydramine hydrochloride is an antihistamine, a histamine receptor antagonist that has anticholinergic, antitussive, antiemetic, antivertigo, antipruritic, antidyskinetic, and sedative effects. It blocks the effects of histamine on the smooth muscle of the bronchial tubes, GI tract, uterus, and blood vessels. It also acts as a local anesthetic by preventing transmission of nerve impulses. Diphenhydramine hydrochloride is indicated for the treatment of anaphylaxis, Parkinsonism when the patient cannot tolerate other medications, drug-induced extrapyramidal disorders, motion sickness, allergies, vertigo, insomnia, and to suppress nausea and prevent vomiting. Its antiemetic effects allow it to be prescribed to treat nausea and vomiting associated with chemotherapy. Diphenhydramine hydrochloride is available in self-administrable oral forms and in an injectable form. The injectable form is administered by intramuscular or intravenous injection. HCPCS Level II code J1200 represents up to 50 mg of injectable diphenhydramine hydrochloride. HCPCS Level II code Q0163 represents 50 mg of the oral version of diphenhydramine hydrochloride for use as a complete substitute for an IV antiemetic at the time of chemotherapy treatment not to exceed a 48-hour dosage regimen.

Documentation Standards

A narrative diagnosis and/or ICD-9-CM diagnosis code describing the patient's cancer must be entered on the order by the provider. There must also be a statement on the order that indicates that the oral antiemetic drug is a full therapeutic replacement for an intravenous antiemetic drug and is used as part of a cancer chemotherapy regimen. This order must be available to the DME MAC on request. The supplier may bill using Q0163–Q0180 only if it has a written order with this specific attestation.

Claims for Q0180 must be accompanied by the name of the drug, the NDC code, the manufacturer, the dosage strength dispensed, the number of tablets, and frequency of administration during the covered time period (24–48 hours) as specified on the order.

Medicare Information

See the chapter titled "Medicare Guidelines," under "Drugs, Biologicals, and Radiopharmaceuticals," for Medicare information.

Q0164-Q0165

Q0164   Prochlorperazine maleate, 5 mg, oral, FDA approved prescription antiemetic, for use as a complete therapeutic substitute for an IV antiemetic at the time of chemotherapy treatment, not to exceed a 48-hour dosage regimen

Q0165   Prochlorperazine maleate, 10 mg, oral, FDA approved prescription antiemetic, for use as a complete therapeutic substitute for an IV antiemetic at the time of chemotherapy treatment, not to exceed a 48-hour dosage regimen

Lay Description

Prochlorperazine/prochlorperazine maleate is an antiemetic used for severe nausea and vomiting, such as that associated with the administration of chemotherapy and prior to induction of anesthesia to control nausea and vomiting during and after surgery. The drug inhibits nausea and vomiting by acting on the chemoreceptor trigger zone and partially depresses the vomiting center. Prochlorperazine is also indicated for treating adult psychiatric illnesses including schizophrenia, non-psychotic anxiety, and mild psychotic disorders. Prochlorperazine is available in injection form for intramuscular (IM) and intravenous (IV) use, in tablets, extended release capsules and syrup for oral administration, and in suppository form. The dosage, route of administration, and frequency of administration depends on the patient's diagnosis, the severity of symptoms, and, in the injectable form, by the patient's weight. Parenteral adult doses range from 2.5 to 10 mg at no more than 5 mg/minute IV for adults or 5 to 20 mg IM. The maximum parenteral adult dose is 40 mg a day. The drug should be injected or infused slowly. For children, 0.132 mg/kg may be administered IM. Oral doses range from 5 to 10 mg three or four times a day for tablets, or for extended-release capsules, 15 mg daily or 10 mg every 12 hours. HCPCS Level II codes Q0164 and Q0165 represent 5 mg and 10 mg, respectively, of oral prochlorperazine maleate for which benefits are provided when used as a complete therapeutic substitute for an IV antiemetic when chemotherapy is provided, not to exceed 48 hours of therapy.

Q0166

Q0166   Granisetron HCl, 1 mg, oral, FDA approved prescription antiemetic, for use as a complete therapeutic substitute for an IV antiemetic at the time of chemotherapy treatment, not to exceed a 24-hour dosage regimen

Lay Description

An anti-emetic is a drug given to suppress nausea and prevent vomiting. Patients receiving chemotherapy treatment have to contend with a great deal of nausea and vomiting as a side effect and are given an anti-emetic at the time of treatment. These codes all report FDA approved prescription anti-emetics to be taken orally, for use as a complete therapeutic substitute for an anti-emetic given by IV injection at the time of therapy, not to exceed a 48-hour dosage regimen. Report Q0163 for diphenhydramine HCL 50 mg, Q0164 for prochlorperazine maleate 5 mg, Q0165 for prochlorperazine maleate 10 mg, Q0167 for dronabinol 2.5 mg, and Q0168 for dronabinol 5 mg. Report Q0166 for granisetron HCL 1 mg, oral, not to exceed a 24-hour dosage regimen. HCPCS Level II code Q0166 represents 1 mg of oral granisetron hydrochloride for use as a complete therapeutic substitute for an IV antiemetic at the time of chemotherapy treatment, not to exceed a 24-hour dosage regimen.

Q0167-Q0168

Q0167   Dronabinol, 2.5 mg, oral, FDA approved prescription antiemetic, for use as a complete therapeutic substitute for an IV antiemetic at the time of chemotherapy treatment, not to exceed a 48-hour dosage regimen
Q0168   Dronabinol, 5 mg, oral, FDA approved prescription antiemetic, for use as a complete therapeutic substitute for an IV antiemetic at the time of chemotherapy treatment, not to exceed a 48-hour dosage regimen

Lay Description

Dronabinal is a cannabinoid with an active ingredient that is found in marijuana. It is used to treat anorexia associated with weight loss in patients with AIDS and nausea and vomiting for patients on chemotherapy. Dronabinol may be used as a complete therapeutic substitute for intravenous antiemetic therapy at the time of a chemotherapy treatment. When used to treat anorexia associated with AIDS or as a prolonged treatment for nausea and vomiting for patients on chemotherapy, an initial dose of 2.5 mg of dronabinal is administered before lunch and dinner. This can be gradually increased to 20 mg per day. Dronabinal is administered orally. HCPCS Level II code Q0167 represents 2.5 mg and Q0168 represents 5 mg of oral dronabinal for use as a complete therapeutic replacement for an IV antiemetic at the time of chemotherapy.

Q0169-Q0170

Q0169   Promethazine HCl, 12.5 mg, oral, FDA approved prescription antiemetic, for use as a complete therapeutic substitute for an IV antiemetic at the time of chemotherapy treatment, not to exceed a 48-hour dosage regimen
Q0170   Promethazine HCl, 25 mg, oral, FDA approved prescription antiemetic, for use as a complete therapeutic substitute for an IV antiemetic at the time of chemotherapy treatment, not to exceed a 48-hour dosage regimen

Lay Description

Promethazine hydrochloride is a phenothiazine derivative with antihistamine, sedative, antiemetic, and anticholinergic properties. The drug binds to histamine receptors preventing the histamine from dilating capillaries, constricting the bronchial smooth muscles, and increasing gastric secretions. Promethazine hydrochloride is indicated as an antiemetic, a sedative in anesthesia, as a treatment for motion sickness, and for allergic reactions, including rhinitis and pruritic skin reactions. The drug may be combined with other drugs in cough and cold preparations. Promethazine hydrochloride is available in injectable, oral, and rectal suppository forms. The injectable form is administered by intramuscular or intravenous injection. Dosage varies from 25 to 50 mg. HCPCS Level II code Q0169 represents 12.5 mg of oral promethazine hydrochloride and Q0170 represents 25 mg of oral promethazine hydrochloride used as a complete therapeutic substitute for an IV anti-emetic at the time of chemotherapy treatment.

Q0171-Q0172

Q0171   Chlorpromazine HCl, 10 mg, oral, FDA approved prescription antiemetic, for use as a complete therapeutic substitute for an IV antiemetic at the time of chemotherapy treatment, not to exceed a 48-hour dosage regimen

Q0172   Chlorpromazine HCl, 25 mg, oral, FDA approved prescription antiemetic, for use as a complete therapeutic substitute for an IV antiemetic at the time of chemotherapy treatment, not to exceed a 48-hour dosage regimen

Lay Description

Chlorpromazine hydrochloride (HCl) is used in the treatment of manic psychosis, preoperative sedation, acute intermittent porphyria, an adjunct treatment for tetanus, intractable hiccups, some behavior problems in children, and nausea and vomiting. The main pharmacological actions are psychotropic. The mechanism of action is not known. It has a sedative and antiemetic effect. HCPCS Level II code Q0171 represents 10 mg of oral chlorpromazine HCl for use as a complete therapeutic substitute for an IV antiemetic at the time of chemotherapy; and Q0172 represents 25 mg of oral chlorpromazine HCl for use as a complete therapeutic substitute for an IV antiemetic at the time of chemotherapy.

Q0173

Q0173   Trimethobenzamide HCl, 250 mg, oral, FDA approved prescription antiemetic, for use as a complete therapeutic substitute for an IV antiemetic at the time of chemotherapy treatment, not to exceed a 48-hour dosage regimen

Lay Description

Trimethobenzamide hydrochloride (HCl) is an antiemetic used to alleviate nausea and vomiting. The mechanism of action is not known but it appears to act on the chemoreceptor trigger zone (CTZ) in the brain where vomiting impulses are transmitted. It can be administered via intramuscular injection. Trimethobenzamide HCl also comes in capsule and suppository forms. HCPCS Level II code Q0173 represents 250 mg of oral trimethobenzamide HCl for use as a complete therapeutic substitute for an IV antiemetic at the time of chemotherapy treatment.

Q0174

Q0174   Thiethylperazine maleate, 10 mg, oral, FDA approved prescription antiemetic, for use as a complete therapeutic substitute for an IV antiemetic at the time of chemotherapy treatment, not to exceed a 48-hour dosage regimen

Lay Description

Thiethylperazine maleate is indicated for the relief of nausea and vomiting. The exact mechanism of action is not known. However, it appears to have an effect on the vomiting center and the chemoreceptor trigger zone (CTZ) of the brain. Recommended oral dose is 10 to 30 mg a day. Thiethylperazine maleate can be administered orally or by intramuscular injection. Recommended intramuscular injection dose is 10 mg one to three times a day. HCPCS Level II code Q0174 represents 10 mg of oral trimethobenzamide HCl for use as a complete therapeutic substitute for an IV antiemetic at the time of chemotherapy treatment.

Q0175-Q0176

Q0175   Perphenazine, 4 mg, oral, FDA approved prescription antiemetic, for use as a complete therapeutic substitute for an IV antiemetic at the time of chemotherapy treatment, not to exceed a 48 hour dosage regimen

Q0176   Perphenazine, 8 mg, oral, FDA approved prescription antiemetic, for use as a complete therapeutic substitute for an IV antiemetic at the time of chemotherapy treatment, not to exceed a 48 hour dosage regimen

Lay Description

Perphenazine is used in treating psychosis and severe nausea and vomiting. The mechanism of action is not known. However, it does have an effect on the entire central nervous system particularly the hypothalamus. Dose is based on the condition and response of the patient. Perphenazine is administered orally. Q0175 represents 4 mg of oral perphenazine for use as a complete therapeutic substitute for an IV antiemetic at the time of chemotherapy treatment; and Q0176 represents 8 mg of oral perphenazine for use as a complete therapeutic substitute for an IV antiemetic at the time of chemotherapy treatment.

Q0177-Q0178

Q0177 Hydroxyzine pamoate, 25 mg, oral, FDA approved prescription antiemetic, for use as a complete therapeutic substitute for an IV antiemetic at the time of chemotherapy treatment, not to exceed a 48-hour dosage regimen

Q0178 Hydroxyzine pamoate, 50 mg, oral, FDA approved prescription antiemetic, for use as a complete therapeutic substitute for an IV antiemetic at the time of chemotherapy treatment, not to exceed a 48-hour dosage regimen

Lay Description

Hydroxyzine is a piperazine derivative that has central nervous system depressant, antispasmodic, antihistamine, and antifibrillatory properties. It is used to treat a variety of conditions such as anxiety, pruritus from allergies, psychiatric and emotional emergencies, and nausea and vomiting. Hydroxyzine may be used as a complete therapeutic substitute for intravenous antiemetic therapy at the time of a chemotherapy treatment. It is often used as a preoperative medication. It tends to increase the effect of meperidine and barbiturates. It can be administered via intravenous push, intramuscular injection, or orally. Hydroxyzine hydrochloride is used to treat anxiety, manifestations of allergic dermatoses, as an antiemetic, and as a preoperative medication. It is administered by intramuscular injection or orally. Hydroxyzine pamoate has uses similar to the hydrochloride version. The pamoate version is administered orally. HCPCS Level II codes Q0177 and Q0178 represent 25 mg and 50 mg of oral hydroxyzine pamoate respectively, to be used as a complete therapeutic replacement for an IV antiemetic at the time of chemotherapy.

Q0179

Q0179 Ondansetron HCl 8 mg, oral, FDA approved prescription antiemetic, for use as a complete therapeutic substitute for an IV antiemetic at the time of chemotherapy treatment, not to exceed a 48-hour dosage regimen

Lay Description

Ondansetron hydrochloride is a chemical compound that is a selective blocker of serotonin 5-HT3 receptors. It is an antiemetic drug available in oral and injectable forms. Serotonin 5-HT3 receptors are present on the vagal nerve and at sensory nerve endings. Cytotoxic chemotherapy appears to trigger the release of serotonin in the small intestine, which may trigger the 5-HT3 receptors and initiate the vomiting reflex. Ondansetron hydrochloride is indicated for the prevention of nausea and vomiting associated with surgery and antineoplastic drugs. The oral version is also indicated for the prevention of nausea and vomiting associated with radiation therapy. The drug is available in oral and injectable versions. The injectable version is administered by intravenous injection. When administered in conjunction with antineoplastic drugs, ondansetron hydrochloride should be diluted. The recommended dosage for this indication is a single 32 mg or three doses at 0.15 mg/kg of body weight infused over 15 minutes. Subsequent dosages may be infused at four and eight hours after the initial dose. When used to suppress postoperative vomiting, the drug does not need to be diluted. The recommended dose is 4 mg or 0.1 mg/kg of body weight administered by intravenous or intramuscular injection. Dosages for the oral version vary from 8 to 24 mg depending on the indication and patient. HCPCS Level II code Q0179 represents 8 mg of the oral version of ondansetron hydrochloride for use as a complete therapeutic substitute for an IV anti-emetic at the time of chemotherapy.

Q0180

Q0180 Dolasetron mesylate, 100 mg, oral, FDA approved prescription antiemetic, for use as a complete therapeutic substitute for an IV antiemetic at the time of chemotherapy treatment, not to exceed a 24-hour dosage regimen

Lay Description

Dolasetron mesylate is an antiemetic drug with a chemical compound that is a selective blocker of serotonin 5-HT3 receptors. Serotonin 5-HT3 receptors are present on the vagal nerve and at sensory nerve endings. Cytotoxic chemotherapy appears to trigger the release of serotonin in the small intestine, which may trigger the 5-HT3 receptors and initiate the vomiting reflex. It is indicated to prevent and treat nausea and vomiting associated with chemotherapy or surgery. HCPCS Level II code Q0180 represents 100 mg of the oral version of dolasetron mesylate used as a complete therapeutic substitute for an IV antiemetic at the time of chemotherapy treatment, not to exceed a 24-hour dosage regimen.

Q0181

Q0181   Unspecified oral dosage form, FDA approved prescription antiemetic, for use as a complete therapeutic substitute for an IV antiemetic at the time of chemotherapy treatment, not to exceed a 48-hour dosage regimen

Lay Description

Oral antiemetic drugs are a therapeutic substitute for intravenous antiemetic drugs. Oral antiemetic drugs help patients better tolerate the effects of chemotherapy. Report Q0181 for an unspecified oral dosage of an antiemetic drug used as a complete therapeutic substitute for an IV antiemetic at the time of chemotherapy treatment.

Q0478-Q0506

Q0478   Power adapter for use with electric or electric/pneumatic ventricular assist device, vehicle type
Q0479   Power module for use with electric or electric/pneumatic ventricular assist device, replacement only
Q0480   Driver for use with pneumatic ventricular assist device, replacement only
Q0481   Microprocessor control unit for use with electric ventricular assist device, replacement only
Q0482   Microprocessor control unit for use with electric/pneumatic combination ventricular assist device, replacement only
Q0483   Monitor/display module for use with electric ventricular assist device, replacement only
Q0484   Monitor/display module for use with electric or electric/pneumatic ventricular assist device, replacement only
Q0485   Monitor control cable for use with electric ventricular assist device, replacement only
Q0486   Monitor control cable for use with electric/pneumatic ventricular assist device, replacement only
Q0487   Leads (pneumatic/electrical) for use with any type electric/pneumatic ventricular assist device, replacement only
Q0488   Power pack base for use with electric ventricular assist device, replacement only
Q0489   Power pack base for use with electric/pneumatic ventricular assist device, replacement only
Q0490   Emergency power source for use with electric ventricular assist device, replacement only
Q0491   Emergency power source for use with electric/pneumatic ventricular assist device, replacement only
Q0492   Emergency power supply cable for use with electric ventricular assist device, replacement only
Q0493   Emergency power supply cable for use with electric/pneumatic ventricular assist device, replacement only
Q0494   Emergency hand pump for use with electric or electric/pneumatic ventricular assist device, replacement only
Q0495   Battery/power pack charger for use with electric or electric/pneumatic ventricular assist device, replacement only
Q0496   Battery, other than lithium-ion, for use with electric or electric/pneumatic ventricular assist device, replacement only
Q0497   Battery clips for use with electric or electric/pneumatic ventricular assist device, replacement only
Q0498   Holster for use with electric or electric/pneumatic ventricular assist device, replacement only
Q0499   Belt/vest/bag for use to carry external peripheral components of any type ventricular assist device, replacement only
Q0500   Filters for use with electric or electric/pneumatic ventricular assist device, replacement only
Q0501   Shower cover for use with electric or electric/pneumatic ventricular assist device, replacement only
Q0502   Mobility cart for pneumatic ventricular assist device, replacement only
Q0503   Battery for pneumatic ventricular assist device, replacement only, each
Q0504   Power adapter for pneumatic ventricular assist device, replacement only, vehicle type
Q0505   Miscellaneous supply or accessory for use with ventricular assist device
Q0506   Battery, lithium-ion, for use with electric or electric/pneumatic ventricular assist device, replacement only

Lay Description

A ventricular assist device (VAD) is a mechanical device that compresses the heart to aid pumping function in patients with heart failure. The device is implanted into the chest and connects to an external controlling mechanism. The codes listed above are used to report replacement of various components of the VAD.

Q0510-Q0512

Q0510 Pharmacy supply fee for initial immunosuppressive drug(s), first month following transplant
Q0511 Pharmacy supply fee for oral anticancer, oral antiemetic, or immunosuppressive drug(s); for the first prescription in a 30-day period
Q0512 Pharmacy supply fee for oral anticancer, oral antiemetic, or immunosuppressive drug(s); for a subsequent prescription in a 30-day period

Lay Description

Medicare pays a dispensing or supplying fee for immunosuppressive drugs, oral anti-cancer chemotherapeutic drugs, and oral anti-emetic drugs used as part of an anti-cancer chemotherapeutic regimen. These fees are payable to a pharmacy, dialysis facility in the state of Washington, or any hospital outpatient department not subject to the OPPS for each supplied prescription of the above-mentioned drugs. Medicare also pays a separately billable supplying fee of $50 for the initial supplied prescription of immunosuppressive drugs during the first month following a patient?s transplant. When multiple prescriptions are supplied in a 30-day period, Medicare will pay $24 for the first prescription of the above-mentioned drugs, and $16 for each subsequent prescription. A pharmacy will be limited to one $24 fee per 30-day period even if the pharmacy supplies drugs from more than one of the above-mentioned categories to a beneficiary (e.g., an oral-anticancer drug and an oral anti-emetic drug). Supply fees and dispensing fees must be billed on the same claim as the drug. Report Q0510 for the first immunosuppressive prescription after a transplant. Report Q0511 for the supplying fee for immunosuppressive, oral-anti-cancer, and oral anti-emetic drugs, first prescription in a 30-day period. Report Q0512 for the supplying fee for each subsequent prescription of these drugs in a 30-day period.

Q0513-Q0514

Q0513 Pharmacy dispensing fee for inhalation drug(s); per 30 days
Q0514 Pharmacy dispensing fee for inhalation drug(s); per 90 days

Lay Description

Medicare pays a dispensing or supplying fee for inhalation drugs furnished through durable medical equipment. Medicare will pay a dispensing fee of $57 to a pharmacy for the initial 30-day period of inhalation drugs furnished through DME, regardless of the number of shipments or drugs dispensed or the number of pharmacies used by a beneficiary during that time. This is a one-time fee applicable only to someone who is using inhalation drugs for the first time as a Medicare beneficiary. Subsequently, Medicare will pay a dispensing fee of $33 to a pharmacy/supplier for each 30-day supply of inhalation drugs furnished through DME, regardless of the number of shipments or drugs dispensed during the 30-day period. Medicare will pay a dispensing fee of $66 to a pharmacy/supplier for each 90-day period of inhalation drugs furnished through DME, regardless of the number of shipments or drugs dispensed during the 90 days. Only one 30-day dispensing fee will be payable per 30-day period, and only one 90-day dispensing fee will be payable per 90-day period, regardless of the number of suppliers used. A 30-day and 90-day supplying fee cannot be applied to drugs supplied for the same month. Medicare will not pay separately for compounding drugs; this cost is in the dispensing fees. Supply fees and dispensing fees must be billed on the same claim as the drug. Report Q0513 for the 30-day pharmacy dispensing fee for inhalation drugs, and Q0514 for the 90-day pharmacy dispensing fee for inhalation drugs.

Q0515

Q0515 Injection, sermorelin acetate, 1 mcg

Lay Description

Sermorelin acetate is a synthetic peptide that contains a portion of the 191 amino acids that compromise natural human growth hormone (HGH). The drug stimulates the pituitary gland to produce HGH. HGH has a direct effect on the metabolism of protein, carbohydrates, and fat and controls skeletal and visceral growth. Sermorelin acetate is used in the diagnosis of HGH deficiencies and is indicated for the treatment of idiopathic HGH deficiency in children with growth failure. Treatment with sermorelin acetate should begin at a bone age of younger than 7.5 years for females and younger than 8 years for males and should be discontinued when the epiphyses are fused. The drug is administered subcutaneously daily at a dosage of 30 mcg per kg body weight and may be self-administered. HCPCS Level II code Q0515 represents 1 mcg of sermorelin acetate.

Q1003-Q1005

Q1003 New technology, intraocular lens, category 3 (reduced spherical aberration)

Q1004 New technology intraocular lens category 4 as defined in Federal Register notice

Q1005 New technology intraocular lens category 5 as defined in Federal Register notice

Lay Description

Cataracts are the clouding of the crystalline lens of the eye, which obstructs vision. An intraocular lens (IOL) is usually placed during or subsequent to cataract extraction. New technology intraocular lenses (NTIOL) are FDA-approved prosthetic implants that demonstrate clinical advantages and superiority over existing intraocular lenses. The FDA, based upon published clinical data, determines if a lens has clinical advantages and superiority over existing IOLs with regard to reduced risk of intraoperative or postoperative complication or trauma, accelerated postoperative recovery, reduced induced astigmatism, improved postoperative visual acuity, more stable postoperative vision, or other comparable clinical advantages. Each subset or category of NTIOLs are separated into groups that meet the criteria for being treated as NTIOLs and share a common feature that distinguishes them from other IOLs. For example, all new technology IOLs that are made of a particular bioengineered material could comprise one subset, while all that rely on a particular optical innovation would encompass another. Code Q1003 is currently in use for a category 3 NTIOL that reduces spherical aberration. Codes Q1004, and Q1005 are reserved for future definitions of NTIOLs. Any assignment and definition of the categories of four and five will be announced in a *Federal Register* notice prior to their use.

Medicare Information

FDA-approved intraocular lens implantation services following cataract surgery or congenital absence of a lens, as well as the lens itself, may be covered if reasonable and necessary for the individual. Implantation services may include hospital, surgical, and other medical services, including preimplantation ultrasound (A-scan) eye measurement of one or both eyes. For patients with a dense cataract, an ultrasound (B-scan) may be used.

Q2004

Q2004 Irrigation solution for treatment of bladder calculi, for example renacidin, per 500 ml

Lay Description

Irrigation solution for treatment of bladder calculi is a liquid containing various minerals and weak acids that is used to irrigate or wash calculi from the bladder. The solution acts upon the stones by dissolving portions of or the entire calculi, depending on its size. Report Q2004 for 500 ml of irrigation solution, such as Renacidin.

Q2009

Q2009 Injection, fosphenytoin, 50 mg phenytoin equivalent

Lay Description

Fosphenytoin is a prodrug that is converted within the body to the anticonvulsant phenytoin. It is indicated for the control of status epilepticus, the prevention or control of seizures during neurosurgery, and for short-term parenteral administration when other means of phenytoin administration are unavailable, inappropriate, or less advantageous. It is thought to alter the sodium channels and block the calcium flow across the neuronal membranes, modulate the voltage-dependent calcium channels of neurons, and enhance the sodium-potassium ATPase activity of neurons and glial cells. Fosphenytoin may be administered by intravenous injection, intravenous infusion, or intramuscular.

Q2017

Q2017 Injection, teniposide, 50 mg

Lay Description

Teniposide is a semisynthetic derivative of podophyllotoxin, a toxic compound found in the rhizomes and roots of the mandrake plant. Teniposide is closely related to etoposide. It is an antineoplastic drug used in combination with other approved antineoplastic agents for induction therapy in patients with refractory childhood acute lymphoblastic leukemia. It acts on cells by preventing them from entering mitosis. Teniposide is administered via intravenous infusion over 30 to 60 minutes. HCPCS Level II code Q2017 represents 50 mg of teniposide.

Q2026

Q2026 Injection, Radiesse, 0.1ML

Lay Description

Radiesse is an injectable implant placed under the skin for treatment of defects such as moderate to severe wrinkles, and folds such as as nasolabial folds and facial lipoatrophy in patients with human immunodeficiency virus (HIV). It is also used to treat certain dental defects, as a tissue marker, and for treatment of vocal fold insufficiency. Radiesse contains a synthetic calcium hydroxylapatite in an injectable gel. It provides temporary filling and helps stimulate the body's collagen formation. The treatment can last up to one year or more. The recommended dose varies based on location and severity of the defect.

Q2027

Q2027 Injection, Sculptra, 0.1ML

Lay Description

Sculptra is an injectable implant placed under the skin for treatment of facial lipoatrophy in patients with human immunodeficiency virus (HIV). Sculptra contains microparticles of poly-L-lactic acid, a biodegradable, biocompatible synthetic polymer from the alpha-hydroxy-acid family. It provides temporary fullness to improve the sunken appearance from the fat loss that may accompany HIV therapy. Sculptra treatments can last up to two years. The recommended dose varies based on location and size of the treatment area.

Q3025-Q3026

Q3025 Injection, interferon beta-1a, 11 mcg for intramuscular use
Q3026 Injection, interferon beta-1a, 11 mcg for subcutaneous use

Lay Description

Interferon beta-1a is a synthetic version of natural interferon beta-1a produced by recombinant DNA technology from Chinese hamster ovaries. Interferons are small naturally occurring proteins that bind to specific cell membranes and initiate a series of events that include the inhibition of virus replication and the enhancement of macrophage and lymphocyte destruction of foreign cells. There are several types of interferons. Interferon beta-1a has been shown to control symptoms of muscular sclerosis, but its exact mechanism of action if unknown. Interferon beta-1a is indicated for the treatment of patients with relapsing forms of multiple sclerosis to decrease the frequency of clinical exacerbations and delay the onset of the physical disabilities associated with the disease. The drug may be self-administered as a subcutaneous injection. Interferon beta-1a is also available as an intramuscular injection. HCPCS Level II code Q3025 represents 11 mcg of the intramuscular version of interferon beta-1a. HCPCS Level II code Q3026 represents 11 mcg of the subcutaneous version of interferon beta-1a.

Q3025-Q3026

Q3025 Injection, interferon beta-1a, 11 mcg for intramuscular use
Q3026 Injection, interferon beta-1a, 11 mcg for subcutaneous use

Lay Description

Interferon beta-1a, injection, is a biological response modifier given to patients with multiple sclerosis to decrease the times that clinical symptoms are exacerbated and to delay levels of permanent disability. Side effects include headache, dizziness, nausea, diarrhea, trouble digesting, muscle aches and flu-like symptoms, and possible upper respiratory infection. Depression and suicidal thoughts may become apparent upon taking this drug. Interferon beta-1a is given as an intramuscular or subcutaneous injection.

Q3031

Q3031 Collagen skin test

Lay Description

This code reports the kit supplied for performing a collagen skin test. A collagen skin test is done to test for delayed hypersensitivity before any collagen procedure is carried out. The test is given as a small injection into and just under the skin, where a small lump is formed and watched for redness or irritation in the days following.

Q4001-Q4051

Q4001 Casting supplies, body cast adult, with or without head, plaster
Q4002 Cast supplies, body cast adult, with or without head, fiberglass
Q4003 Cast supplies, shoulder cast, adult (11 years +), plaster
Q4004 Cast supplies, shoulder cast, adult (11 years +), fiberglass
Q4005 Cast supplies, long arm cast, adult (11 years +), plaster
Q4006 Cast supplies, long arm cast, adult (11 years +), fiberglass
Q4007 Cast supplies, long arm cast, pediatric (0–10 years), plaster
Q4008 Cast supplies, long arm cast, pediatric (0–10 years), fiberglass
Q4009 Cast supplies, short arm cast, adult (11 years +), plaster
Q4010 Cast supplies, short arm cast, adult (11 years +), fiberglass
Q4011 Cast supplies, short arm cast, pediatric (0–10 years), plaster
Q4012 Cast supplies, short arm cast, pediatric (0–10 years), fiberglass
Q4013 Cast supplies, gauntlet cast (includes lower forearm and hand), adult (11 years +), plaster

Q4014	Cast supplies, gauntlet cast (includes lower forearm and hand), adult (11 years +), fiberglass
Q4015	Cast supplies, gauntlet cast (includes lower forearm and hand), pediatric (0–10 years), plaster
Q4016	Cast supplies, gauntlet cast (includes lower forearm and hand), pediatric (0–10 years), fiberglass
Q4017	Cast supplies, long arm splint, adult (11 years +), plaster
Q4018	Cast supplies, long arm splint, adult (11 years +), fiberglass
Q4019	Cast supplies, long arm splint, pediatric (0–10 years), plaster
Q4020	Cast supplies, long arm splint, pediatric (0–10 years), fiberglass
Q4021	Cast supplies, short arm splint, adult (11 years +), plaster
Q4022	Cast supplies, short arm splint, adult (11 years +), fiberglass
Q4023	Cast supplies, short arm splint, pediatric (0–10 years), plaster
Q4024	Cast supplies, short arm splint, pediatric (0–10 years), fiberglass
Q4025	Cast supplies, hip spica (one or both legs), adult (11 years +), plaster
Q4026	Cast supplies, hip spica (one or both legs), adult (11 years +), fiberglass
Q4027	Cast supplies, hip spica (one or both legs), pediatric (0–10 years), plaster
Q4028	Cast supplies, hip spica (one or both legs), pediatric (0–10 years), fiberglass
Q4029	Cast supplies, long leg cast, adult (11 years +), plaster
Q4030	Cast supplies, long leg cast, adult (11 years +), fiberglass
Q4031	Cast supplies, long leg cast, pediatric (0–10 years), plaster
Q4032	Cast supplies, long leg cast, pediatric (0–10 years), fiberglass
Q4033	Cast supplies, long leg cylinder cast, adult (11 years +), plaster
Q4034	Cast supplies, long leg cylinder cast, adult (11 years +), fiberglass
Q4035	Cast supplies, long leg cylinder cast, pediatric (0–10 years), plaster
Q4036	Cast supplies, long leg cylinder cast, pediatric (0–10 years), fiberglass
Q4037	Cast supplies, short leg cast, adult (11 years +), plaster
Q4038	Cast supplies, short leg cast, adult (11 years +), fiberglass
Q4039	Cast supplies, short leg cast, pediatric (0–10 years), plaster
Q4040	Cast supplies, short leg cast, pediatric (0–10 years), fiberglass
Q4041	Cast supplies, long leg splint, adult (11 years +), plaster
Q4042	Cast supplies, long leg splint, adult (11 years +), fiberglass
Q4043	Cast supplies, long leg splint, pediatric (0–10 years), plaster
Q4044	Cast supplies, long leg splint, pediatric (0–10 years), fiberglass
Q4045	Cast supplies, short leg splint, adult (11 years +), plaster
Q4046	Cast supplies, short leg splint, adult (11 years +), fiberglass
Q4047	Cast supplies, short leg splint, pediatric (0–10 years), plaster
Q4048	Cast supplies, short leg splint, pediatric (0–10 years), fiberglass
Q4049	Finger splint, static
Q4050	Cast supplies, for unlisted types and materials of casts
Q4051	Splint supplies, miscellaneous (includes thermoplastics, strapping, fasteners, padding and other supplies)

Lay Description

Casting materials are made of plaster-imbedded strips or bandages or fiberglass wraps or strips, available in varieties pertinent to the type of fracture or post-surgical state requiring the support and protection of a cast. Some of these materials are initially dry and are water-activated, while others come premoistened for immediate application. Plaster varieties can be imbedded with strength-adding chemical compounds such as polyurethane. Splints are used when a cast is not necessary but the injury or condition requires immobilization. Casts and casting materials support and protect fractured or strained extremities or other body areas. They hold manipulated (set) fractures in place or can assist other devices (pins, wires, screws) in doing so and protect against reinjury. Codes Q4001-Q4051 identify the different casting materials (e.g., fiberglass or plaster), the type of immobilization provided such splint or cast for adult or pediatric patients, and the length or shape of casts for the different types of injuries or conditions (e.g., shoulder or body cast, long or short leg or arm).

Documentation Standards

If the item is furnished secondary to a fracture, a copy of the x-ray study that confirmed the fracture should be easily accessible within the medical record.

Medicare Information

Under MPFS, casting supplies were removed from the practice expenses for all HCPCS codes, including CPT codes for fracture management and for casts and splints in the Medicare fee schedule that began in 2001. In settings where CPT codes are used to pay for services that include the provision of a cast or splint, the temporary codes are established to pay providers and other practitioners for the supplies

HCPCS Lay Descriptions

used in creating casts. The work and practice expenses involved with the creation of the cast or splint should be coded using the appropriate CPT code.

Previous codes used to report cast and splint supplies were invalid for Medicare use on or after July 1, 2001 for carrier-processed claims, and October 2001 for intermediary processed claims. The previous codes have been replaced by the Q codes.

Cast Supply Codes Crosswalk-HCPCS Level I to HCPCS Level II Codes:

HCPCS Level I (CPT)	HCPCS Level II
29000	Q4001 or Q4002
29058	Q4003
29345	Q4029–Q4032
29010	Q4001 or Q4002
29065	Q4005 Q4008
29355	Q4029–Q4032
29015	Q4001 or Q4002
29075	Q4009–Q4012
29365	Q4033–Q4036
29020	Q4001 or Q4002
29085	Q4013–Q4016
29405	Q4037–Q4040
29025	Q4001 or Q4002
29105	Q4017–Q4020
29425	Q4037–Q4040
29035	Q4001 or Q4002
29125	Q4021–Q4024
29435	Q4037–Q4040
29040	Q4001 or Q4002
29126	Q4021–Q4024
29440	Q4050
29044	Q4001 or Q4002
29130	Q4049
29445	Q4037–Q4040
29046	Q4001 or Q4002
29131	Q4051
29450	Q4035, Q4036, Q4039, Q4040
29049	Q4050
29305	Q4025–Q4028
29505	Q4041–Q4044
29055	Q4003 or Q4004
29325	Q4025–Q4028
29515	Q0445–Q4048

These codes should not be used by facilities.

Q4074

Q4074 Iloprost, inhalation solution, FDA-approved final product, noncompounded, administered through DME, unit dose form, up to 20 mcg

Lay Description

Iloprost is an inhaled form of prostacyclin, an analogue of prostaglandin. Prostaglandin is a naturally occurring, long-chain fatty acid that regulates smooth muscle contractions, is a vasodilator, lowers blood, and affects other hormones. It is an orphan drug indicated for use in pulmonary arterial hypertension (WHO group I) patients who have New York Heart Association (NYHA) Class III or IV symptoms. The NYHA classification system identifies Class II patients as those patients with marked limitation of activity, who are comfortable only at rest. NYHA Class IV patients are those patients who should be at complete rest, for whom any physical activity brings on discomfort. The drug is administered via a pulmonary drug delivery device with an initial inhaled dose of 2.5 mcg increasing to 5.0 mcg if tolerated. Iloprost should be inhaled six to nine times a day during waking hours, no more than once every two hours.

Q4081

Q4081 Injection, epoetin alfa, 100 units (for ESRD on dialysis)

Lay Description

Epoetin alfa (EPO) is a biologically engineered protein that stimulates the bone marrow to make new red blood cells. EPO is administered to treat anemia in patients with end-stage renal disease (ESRD) on a regular course of dialysis, as well as patients with other primary and secondary anemias. EPO is administered by subcutaneous or intravenous injection. This code is specific to patients with ESRD on dialysis and reports 100 units of EPO.

Q4101

Q4101 Apligraf, per sq cm

Lay Description

Apligraf is a skin substitute created from biological ingredients found in healthy human skin. It contains an outer layer of protective skin cells and an inner layer to aid in wound healing. It looks like a round piece of skin but does not include hair follicles, sweat glands, or blood vessels. When healthy skin cells get damaged, proteins and growth factors in the skin trigger the body to regenerate new skin. In certain conditions, such as diabetes or circulatory problems, the triggers are missing and wounds do not heal. Apligraf contains fresh cells, nutrients, and proteins that are applied directly to the wound and initiate the healing process. It is used to heal sores such as diabetic foot and venous leg ulcers that are not healing after three to four weeks, despite treatment with conventional therapies. After debriding the wound of necrotic, damaged, or infected tissue, the physician applies the Apligraf and covers it with a nonadhering dressing and an outer wrap. HCPCS Level II code Q4101 should be reported per square centimeter.

Q4102-Q4103
Q4102 Oasis wound matrix, per sq cm
Q4103 Oasis burn matrix, per sq cm

Lay Description
Oasis is a skin substitute created from a biomaterial found in porcine small intestine. The material is processed to remove all cells and then dehydrated. This leaves a matrix or scaffold material that the body uses to surround cells, binding it to tissue and replacing extracellular matrix (ECM). ECM is a necessary component in wound healing. Oasis is used to treat nonhealing wounds such as diabetic, venous, and pressure ulcers, as well as second-degree burns. After debriding the wound of necrotic, damaged, or infected tissue, the physician applies Oasis to the wound and a small area of surrounding tissue. The dehydrated sheet is fixed into place using Steri-strips, sutures, or staples and rehydrated with sterile saline. The wound is covered with a nonadherent dressing, an absorptive dressing for wet wounds, or a moist dressing for dry wounds, and covered with a secure dressing. Oasis is absorbed and forms a gel leaving ECM material. Oasis may be reapplied every seven days over the top of the ECM gel. HCPCS Level II code Q4102 is reported for wounds other than burns and Q4103 is reported for second-degree burns. Both are reported per square centimeter.

Q4104
Q4104 Integra bilayer matrix wound dressing (BMWD), per sq cm

Lay Description
Integra bilayer wound matrix is a biologic matrix that provides coverage for partial and full-thickness wounds. It is used to treat chronic and traumatic wounds including pressure ulcers, venous ulcers, diabetic ulcers, chronic and vascular ulcers, surgical wounds, traumatic wound abrasions, lacerations, and draining wounds. It is a two-layer material created from three-dimensional porous material made from the fibers of a cross-linked bovine tendon collagen and a glycosaminoglycan. This provides the framework for dermal tissue and capillary growth. As the tissue is repaired, the matrix dissolves. For large wounds, an epidermal autograft may also be used. The outer layer is made of silicone and provides moisture control and a bacteria barrier. When the Integra bilayer wound matrix is applied, fluid is quickly adhered to the wound and is conforms to the shape of the wound. It can also be adhered with sutures, staples, or other materials. About 21 days after application, the outer silicone layer is removed, which allows further healing of the epidermis. The bilayer wound matrix may be used in conjunction with Integra matrix wound dressing. HCPCS Level II code Q4104 represents 1 square centimeter.

Q4105
Q4105 Integra dermal regeneration template (DRT), per sq cm

Lay Description
Integra dermal regeneration template is a bilayer matrix or scaffold for dermal regeneration. It is a two-layer material created from the fibers of a cross-linked bovine tendon collagen and a glycosaminoglycan. The outer layer is made of silicone and provides moisture control and bacteria barrier of the wound. The dermal layer is a collagen that provides a scaffold for dermal tissue and blood vessels. This provides a viable surface for autografting. This product is used for the immediate treatment of partial or full-thickness burns. It can also be used to treat scar contractures when there are not adequate donor sites or the patient's condition prohibits immediate grafting. As skin cells grow into the matrix, the collagen is slowly absorbed into the body and replaced with protein that the skin naturally produces. In about 14 to 21 days, new dermal skin is produced and the outer layer can be removed. The physician can then perform an autograft of the patient's epidermis. HCPCS Level II code Q4105 should be reported per square centimeter.

Q4106
Q4106 Dermagraft, per sq cm

Lay Description
Dermagraft is a human dermal substitute manufactured from newborn foreskin tissue. It is made of fibroblasts, extracellular matrix, and a bioabsorbable scaffold. The fibroblasts reproduce and infiltrate the scaffold and secrete human dermal collagen, matrix proteins, growth factors, and cytokines to create a three-dimensional human skin substitute. Dermagraft does not contain macrophages, lymphocytes, blood vessels, or hair follicles. Dermagraft is approved for use in the treatment of full-thickness diabetic foot ulcers lasting longer than six weeks but without exposure of the tendon, muscle, joint capsule, or bone. The physician prepares the wound bed, thaws and rinses the Dermagraft, and applies it to the site. The wound

is dressed and left undisturbed for 72 hours. HCPCS Level II code Q4106 represents 1 square centimeter.

Q4107

Q4107 GRAFTJACKET, per sq cm

Lay Description

GRAFTJACKET is a three-dimensional, freeze dried biologic tissue matrix that forms a tissue scaffold used for diabetic foot ulcers. The material is derived from donated human skin. The epidermal and dermal cells are removed. The result is a matrix of preserved human dermal tissue, including its native protein, collagen structure, blood vessel channels, and essential biochemical composition to allow repair and revascularization. There are two distinct sides to the GRAFTJACKET. The dermal or vascular side is placed down, closest to the wound bed. The basement membrane side is exposed to the secondary dressing. The wound is prepared to receive the graft, and the graft is cut to size and rehydrated. Two or more sheets can be sewn together for larger wounds. The matrix is applied and fixed into place with sutures or staples and a moist dressing is applied. HCPCS Level II code Q4107 represents 1 square centimeter.

Q4108

Q4108 Integra matrix, per sq cm

Lay Description

Integra matrix is a biologic matrix that provides coverage for partial and full-thickness wounds. It is used to treat chronic and traumatic wounds including pressure ulcers, venous ulcers, diabetic ulcers, chronic and vascular ulcers, tunneled or undermined wounds, surgical wounds, traumatic wounds abrasions, lacerations, and draining wounds. It is a single layer material created of three-dimensional porous material made from the fibers of a cross-linked bovine tendon collagen. This provides the framework for tissue and capillary growth. Within seven to 14 days, the tissues and blood vessels invade the scaffold and the matrix is absorbed. For deeper wounds, Integra matrix can be used in conjunction with Integra bilayer wound dressing. An epidermal autograft can be performed 21 to 56 days later if necessary. HCPCS Level II code Q4108 represents 1 square centimeter.

Q4110

Q4110 PriMatrix, per sq cm

Lay Description

PriMatrix is an acellular collagen matrix that provides the framework for tissue and vascular growth. It is used to treat partial- and full-thickness wounds, pressure ulcers, diabetic ulcers, venous ulcers, second-degree burns, surgical wounds, skin tears, and tunneled or undermined wounds. It is derived from fetal bovine dermal tissue and consists of type I and type III collagen. It delivers collagen to the wound, which stimulates tissue growth and collagen production. The physician debrides the wound as appropriate. The PriMatrix is cut to size, rehydrated, and applied to the wound. It is affixed with a surgical closure and covered with a nonadherent dressing. Hydrogel is applied and the wound is dressed. HCPCS Level II code Q4100 represents 1 square centimeter.

Q4111

Q4111 GammaGraft, per sq cm

Lay Description

GammaGraft is a skin substitute derived from human cadaver tissue. It contains a dermal and epidermal layer of human skin that is irradiated. GammaGraft is used as a temporary covering when the patient's own skin is not available and provides a protection from bacteria and reduces fluid loss. It is used to treat burns, chronic wounds, and partial- and full-thickness wounds. The physician debrides the wound of infected or necrotic tissue. The GammaGraft is applied and affixed with sutures or other means. The wound is covered by a nonadherent dressing and covered with gauze. HCPCS Level II code Q4111 represents 1 square centimeter.

Q4112

Q4112 Cymetra, injectable, 1 cc

Lay Description

Cymetra is a small, particulate substance derived from donated human tissue. It contains collagens, elastin, proteins, and proteoglycans. It provides a structure for cell regrowth and helps the body produce tissue growth and vascularization. It is used as a substitute for the patient's own tissue to correct soft tissue defects and laryngoplasty. HCPCS Level II code Q4112 represents 1 cc.

Q4113

Q4113 GRAFTJACKET Express, injectable, 1 cc

Lay Description

GRAFTJACKET express is a micronized substance derived from human dermis. This substance contains biologic components and structure of the dermal matrix. It forms a tissue scaffold and is used for damaged or inadequate integumentary tissue, such as deep dermal wounds. The freeze-dried powder is rehydrated and injected as appropriate. HCPCS Level II code Q4113 represents 1 cc.

Q4114

Q4114 Integra flowable wound matrix, injectable, 1 cc

Lay Description

Integra flowable wound matrix is a biologic gel that provides coverage for partial- and full-thickness wounds. It is used to treat chronic and traumatic wounds including pressure ulcers, venous ulcers, diabetic ulcers, chronic and vascular ulcers, tunneled or undermined wounds, surgical wounds, traumatic wound abrasions, lacerations, and draining wounds. This product is not used for third-degree burns. Since the wound matrix needs to be in contact with the wound bed, the flowable matrix is used for tunneled or irregular shaped defects. It is a single layer material created of three-dimensional porous material made from the fibers of a cross-linked bovine tendon collagen and mixed with sterile saline to form a gel. This provides the framework for tissue and capillary growth. The wound is debrided and probed for depth and tracking. The powdered product is mixed with sterile saline and injected into the site. A dressing is applied to ensure adherence and protect the wound. HCPCS Level II code Q4114 represents 1 cc of Integra flowable wound matrix.

Q4115

Q4115 AlloSkin, per sq cm

Lay Description

AlloSkin is an allograft made from donated human skin used for partial and full thickness wounds. It has two layers, both epidermal and dermal. It provides protection from infection by covering exposed tissue and allowing time for the wound to heal. HCPCS Level II code Q4115 is for one square centimeter of AlloSkin.

Q4116

Q4116 AlloDerm, per sq cm

Lay Description

AlloDerm is a regenerative tissue matrix used to repair hernias and in postmastectomy reconstruction. The matrix is derived from donated human skin in which all the dermal and epidermal cells are removed. This provides a scaffold of accellar biological components that encourages revascularization, cell migration, and regeneration.

HCPCS Level II code Q4116 represents oe square centimeter of AlloDerm.

Q5001

Q5001 Hospice care provided in patient's home/residence

Lay Description

Hospice care services are designed to address the physical, mental, emotional, and spiritual needs of terminally ill patients and their families. Hospice care is a palliative service that is provided when a cure is not possible. Services focus on keeping the patient comfortable by relieving pain and other symptoms and supporting the family during the terminal phase of the patient's illness. Hospice services also include bereavement counseling following the patient's death. Hospice care is typically delivered by an interdisciplinary health care team of physicians, nurses, social workers, counselors, home health aides, clergy, therapists, and trained volunteers. When hospice care is provided in a home-care setting, much of the responsibility for the daily care of the patient falls to the primary care giver. The interdisciplinary team provides some medical and nursing care services, and also provides training, support, and respite services to the primary care giver. Report Q5001 for hospice care provided in the patient's home.

Q5002-Q5004, Q5010

Q5002 Hospice care provided in assisted living facility
Q5003 Hospice care provided in nursing long-term care facility (LTC) or nonskilled nursing facility (NF)
Q5004 Hospice care provided in skilled nursing facility (SNF)
Q5010 Hospice home care provided in a hospice facility

Lay Description

Hospice care services are designed to address the physical, mental, emotional, and spiritual needs of terminally ill patients and their families. Hospice care is a palliative service that is provided when a cure is not possible. Services focus on keeping the patient comfortable by relieving pain and other symptoms and supporting the family during the terminal phase of the patient's illness. Hospice services also include bereavement counseling following the patient's death. Hospice care is typically delivered by an interdisciplinary health care team of physicians, nurses, social workers, counselors, home health aides, clergy, therapists, and trained volunteers. Hospice care is most often provided in a home-care setting, but may be provided in other settings if the patient's condition is such that more intensive professional services are required. When services are provided in an assisted living center, long-term care facility, non-skilled nursing facility, or skilled nursing facility, members of the hospice team provide professional services and support to the patient, as well as support, education, and counseling to the family members, staff, and other residents of the facility.

Q5005-Q5009

Q5005 Hospice care provided in inpatient hospital
Q5006 Hospice care provided in inpatient hospice facility
Q5007 Hospice care provided in long-term care facility
Q5008 Hospice care provided in inpatient psychiatric facility
Q5009 Hospice care provided in place not otherwise specified (NOS)

Lay Description

Hospice care services are designed to address the physical, mental, emotional, and spiritual needs of terminally ill patients and their families. Hospice care is a palliative service that is provided when a cure is not possible. Services focus on keeping the patient comfortable by relieving pain and other symptoms and supporting the family during the terminal phase of the patient's illness. Hospice services also include bereavement counseling following the patient's death. Hospice care is typically delivered by an interdisciplinary health care team of physicians, nurses, social workers, counselors, home health aides, clergy, therapists, and trained volunteers. Hospice care is most often provided in a home-care setting, but may be provided in other settings if the patient's condition is such that more intensive professional services are required. Hospitals often have inpatient hospice programs. These programs may consist of a separate hospice unit or of a hospice team that provides care to terminally ill patients throughout the hospital. There are also freestanding inpatient hospice facilities that specialize in the care of the terminally ill patient. Other facilities such as long-term acute care facilities and inpatient psychiatric facilities may also provide hospice services. Report Q5005 for hospice care provided in an inpatient hospital, Q5006 for care provided in an inpatient hospice facility, Q5007 for hospice care provided in a long-term acute care facility, Q5008 for hospice care provided in an inpatient psychiatric facility, and Q5009 for hospice care provided in a facility that is not otherwise specified (NOS).

Q9951, Q9965-Q9967

Q9951 Low osmolar contrast material, 400 or greater mg/ml iodine concentration, per ml
Q9965 Low osmolar contrast material, 100–199 mg/ml iodine concentration, per ml
Q9966 Low osmolar contrast material, 200–299 mg/ml iodine concentration, per ml
Q9967 Low osmolar contrast material, 300–399 mg/ml iodine concentration, per ml

Lay Description

Low osmolar contrast material (LOCM) is a type of iodinated radiology contrast media that has a substantially lower concentration of particles contained in solution than high osmolar contrast material at the same iodine concentration. LOCM is supplied in radiological diagnostic procedures when the patient is known to have sensitivity to standard high osmolar contrast material or when other sensitivities or medical conditions exist that can increase the chances of a reaction in the patient. Contrast material is the dye that physicians use in diagnostic procedures to enable them to visualize the best picture possible and hence help to diagnose a patient's illness/disease, locate the point of the abnormality, or to assist in determining the extent of disease. LOCM is reported per ml based on the iodine concentration.

Q9953

Q9953 Injection, iron-based magnetic resonance contrast agent, per ml

Lay Description

Magnetic resonance imaging (MRI) is a radiation-free, noninvasive technique to produce high-quality sectional images of the inside of the body in multiple planes. MRI uses the natural magnetic properties of the hydrogen atoms in our bodies that emit radiofrequency signals when exposed to radio waves within a strong electromagnetic field. These signals are then processed and converted by the computer into high-resolution, three-dimensional, tomographic images. Iron is a common metal with strong magnetic properties. Various forms of the metal are used to enhance an MRI. The iron is administered intravenously and is taken up by reticuloendothelial cells, allowing greater detail to be captured by the MRI. The iron-based solution congregates in the spleen and liver allowing for the detection and evaluation of lesions. Dosage depends on patient body weight with a recommended dose of 0.05 ml per kg. HCPCS Level II code Q9953 represents 1 milliliter of an iron-based MRI contrast.

Q9954

Q9954 Oral magnetic resonance contrast agent, per 100 ml

Lay Description

Magnetic resonance imaging (MRI) is a radiation-free, noninvasive technique to produce high-quality sectional images of the inside of the body in multiple planes. MRI uses the natural magnetic properties of the hydrogen atoms in our bodies that emit radiofrequency signals when exposed to radio waves within a strong electromagnetic field. These signals are then processed and converted by the computer into high-resolution, three-dimensional, tomographic images. Oral MRI contrast may be composed of several paramagnetic metals including magnetite, gadolinium, or iron. The contrast is administered orally and is distributed through the gastrointestinal system enhancing its delineation from other adjacent organs and tissues. Recommended dose is 600 ml. HCPCS Level II code Q9954 represents 1 milliliters of an oral MRI contrast.

Q9955

Q9955 Injection, perflexane lipid microspheres, per ml

Lay Description

Perflexane lipid microspheres are microscopic spheres of perflexane gas surrounded by a semi-synthetic phospholipid membrane that enhance echocardiogram imaging. Perflexane lipid microspheres are indicated in suboptimal echocardiograms to opacify the left ventricular chamber and enhance delineation of the left ventricular endocardial border. The drug is administered as a single intravenous bolus with a recommended dose of 0.00625 ml per kg of patient body weight. HCPCS Level II code Q9955 represents 1 milliliter of perflexane lipid microspheres.

Q9956

Q9956 Injection, octafluoropropane microspheres, per ml

Lay Description

Octafluorpropane is a gas used in contrast material to help enhance ultrasound images of the heart.

Q9958-Q9964

Q9958 High osmolar contrast material, up to 149 mg/ml iodine concentration, per ml
Q9959 High osmolar contrast material, 150–199 mg/ml iodine concentration, per ml
Q9960 High osmolar contrast material, 200–249 mg/ml iodine concentration, per ml
Q9961 High osmolar contrast material, 250–299 mg/ml iodine concentration, per ml
Q9962 High osmolar contrast material, 300–349 mg/ml iodine concentration, per ml
Q9963 High osmolar contrast material, 350–399 mg/ml iodine concentration, per ml
Q9964 High osmolar contrast material, 400 or greater mg/ml iodine concentration, per ml

Lay Description

High osmolar contrast material (HOCM) refers to a water-soluble, iodinated, monomeric, ionic radiology contrast material. Contrast material is the dye that physicians use in diagnostic procedures to enable them to visualize the best picture possible and hence help to diagnose a patient's illness/disease, locate the point of the abnormality, or to assist in determining the extent of disease. HOCM is a type of iodinated radiology contrast media that has a higher concentration of particles contained in solution than low osmolar contrast material at the same iodine concentration. HOCM is supplied in radiological diagnostic procedures when the patient does not have sensitivity to standard high osmolar contrast material or other medical conditions that would preclude the use of the higher particle concentration. HOCM is reported per ml based on the iodine concentration. High osmolar contrast is administered via intravenous push. HCPCS Level II code Q9958 represents up to 149 mg/ml; Q9959 represents 150-199 mg/ml; Q9960 represents 200-249 mg/ml; Q9961 represents 250-299 mg/ml; Q9962 represents 300-349 mg/ml; Q9963 represents 350-399 mg/ml; and Q9964 represents 400 or greater mg/ml of high osmolar contrast material.

Medicare Information

HOCM is covered. Payment for HOCM is included in the payment for the procedure.

Q9965-Q9967

Q9965 Low osmolar contrast material, 100–199 mg/ml iodine concentration, per ml
Q9966 Low osmolar contrast material, 200–299 mg/ml iodine concentration, per ml
Q9967 Low osmolar contrast material, 300–399 mg/ml iodine concentration, per ml

Lay Description

Please refer to code Q9951 for the description, coding, and billing information.

S0014

S0014 Tacrine HCl, 10 mg

Lay Description

Tacrine hydrochloride is a reversible cholinesterase inhibitor. Cholinesterase is an enzyme that catalyzes the breakdown of acetylcholine, a neurotransmitter. Early changes in the brain of Alzheimer's patients result in a deficiency of acetylcholine. This deficiency is thought to account for some of the mild to moderate dementia characteristic of Alzheimer's disease. Tacrine hydrochloride inhibits the breakdown of and increases the concentration of acetylcholine in the cerebral cortex. The drug is indicated as a treatment for mild to moderate dementia of Alzheimer's disease. Tacrine hydrochloride is self-administered orally in dosages ranging from 10 to 40 mg four times a day. HCPCS Level II code S0014 represents 10 mg of tacrine hydrochloride.

S0017

S0017 Injection, aminocaproic acid, 5 g

Lay Description

Aminocarproic acid is a an amino acid that inhibits fibrinolysis. After long-term use, this medication distributes throughout extravascular and intravascular compartments of the body, penetrating red blood cells and other tissue cells. It is used to treat fibrinolytic bleeding that may frequently be associated with surgical complications following heart surgery and portacaval shunt; hematological disorders such as aplastic anemia; abruptio placentae; hepatic cirrhosis; and neoplastic disease such as carcinoma of the prostate, lung, stomach, and cervix. It may also be used to treat urinary fibrinolysis associated with complications following severe trauma, anoxia, shock, complications following prostatectomy, nephrectomy, or nonsurgical hematuria accompanying polycystic or neoplastic diseases of the genitourinary system. Aminocarproic acid can be administered via intravenous infusion or orally. HCPCS Level II code S0017 represents 5 grams of aminocaproic acid.

S0020

S0020 Injection, bupivicaine HCl, 30 ml

Lay Description

Bupivacaine hydrochloride (HCl) is a local anesthetic that blocks the feeling of pain by inhibiting the conduction of nerve impulses. The order of loss of nerve function is pain, temperature, touch, proprioception, and skeletal muscle tone. It is often used for dental procedures and during labor and delivery. Bupivacaine can be administered by infiltration, caudal injection, lumbar epidural injection, peripheral nerve block, retrobulbar block, or sympathetic block. Bupivacaine is not recommended for intravenous or regional anesthesia (Bier Block). HCPCS Level II code S0020 represents 30 milliliters of bupivacaine HCl.

S0021

S0021 Injection, cefoperazone sodium, 1 g

Lay Description

Cefoperazone sodium is a broad spectrum antibiotic. It is used to treat respiratory tract infections, skin infections, and urinary tract infections. Susceptible bacteria include S. pneumoniae, H. influenzae, S. aureus, S. pyogenes, P. aeruginosa, Klebsiella pneumoniae, E. coli, Proteus mirabilis, Enterobacter species; anaerobic gram-negative bacilli, Pseudomonas aeruginosa, Klebsiella, Clostridium; anaerobic gram-positive cocci, N. gonorrhoeae, and S. epidermidis. The usual dose is two to four grams per day administered at 12-hour intervals in equally divided doses. Cefoperazone is administered via intramuscular injection or intravenous infusion. HCPCS Level II code S0021 represents 1 gram of cefoperazone sodium

S0023

S0023 Injection, cimetidine HCl, 300 mg

Lay Description

Cimetidine is a histamine H2 receptor antagonist that inhibits the action of histamine at the histamine H2 receptors of the parietal cells. It inhibits gastric acid secretions. It is used in treatment and maintenance therapy for duodenal ulcers, short-term treatment of gastric ulcers, gastroesophageal reflux disease (GERD), prevention of upper gastrointestinal bleeding in critically ill patients, and for the treatment of pathological hypersecretory conditions (i.e., Zollinger-Ellison syndrome, systemic mastocytosis, multiple endocrine adenomas). HCPCS Level II code S0023 represents 300 mg of cimetidine.

S0028
S0028 Injection, famotidine, 20 mg

Lay Description
Famotidine is a histamine H2 receptor antagonist that inhibits the action of histamine at the histamine H2 receptors of the parietal cells. It inhibits gastric acid secretions. It is used for treatment and maintenance therapy for duodenal ulcers, short-term treatment of gastric ulcers, gastroesophageal reflux disease (GERD), prevention of upper gastrointestinal bleeding in critically ill patients, and for the treatment of pathological hypersecretory conditions (i.e., Zollinger-Ellison syndrome, systemic mastocytosis, multiple endocrine adenomas). Famotidine can be administered orally and via intravenous infusion. HCPCS Level II code S0128 represents 20 mg of famotidine.

S0030
S0030 Injection, metronidazole, 500 mg

Lay Description
Metronidazole is an antibacterial and anti-protozoal. It is thought to work in an anaerobic environment by entering the organism, and being reduced by intracellular electron transport proteins. Because of this alteration to the metronidazole molecule, a concentration gradient is maintained that promotes the drug's intracellular transport. Presumably, free radicals are formed which, in turn, react with cellular components resulting in death of the microorganism. It is effective against the following bacteria and protozoa: Clostridium species, Eubacterium species, Peptococcus niger, Peptostreptococcus species, Bacteroides fragilis group (B. fragilis, B. distasonis, B. ovatus, B. thetaiotaomicron, B. vulgatus), Fusobacterium species, Entamoeba histolytica, and Trichomonas vaginalis. Metronidazole is used to treat symptomatic trichomoniasis; asymptomatic trichomoniasis, when the organism is associated with endocervicitis, cervicitis, or cervical erosion; asymptomatic consorts; T. vaginalis infection; acute intestinal amebiasis (amebic dysentery) and amebic liver abscess; serious infections caused by susceptible anaerobic bacteria, peritonitis, intra-abdominal abscess, and liver abscess; skin infections; inflammatory lesions of rosacea; endometritis; endomyometritis; tubo-ovarian abscess and postsurgical vaginal cuff infection; bacterial septicemia; bone and joint infections; meningitis and brain abscess; pneumonia; empyema; lung abscess; and endocarditis. Metronidazole can be administered topically, orally, or via intravenous infusion. The loading dose is 15 mg/kg of body weight or about 1 gram infused over one hour. Following that 500 mg is infused over one hour and administered every six hours. HCPCS Level II code S0030 represents 500 mg of metronidazole.

S0032
S0032 Injection, nafcillin sodium, 2 g

Lay Description
Nafcillin sodium is a semisynthetic antibiotic substance derived from 6-amino-penicillanic acid. This is a penicillinase-resistant penicillin and is used to treat infections caused by penicillinase-producing staphylococci that have shown to be susceptible to the drug. The drug can be administered orally or via intramuscular injection, intravenous push, or intravenous infusion. HCPCS Level II code S0032 represents 2 grams of nafcillin sodium.

S0034
S0034 Injection, ofloxacin, 400 mg

Lay Description
Ofloxacin is a broad spectrum antibiotic of the quinolone class. It inhibits the DNA enzymes in bacteria that are required for the DNA to replicate. This drug is chemically different than aminoglycosides, macrolides, and beta-lactam antibiotics, including penicillins, and therefore may be used to treat bacteria resistant to these antibacterials. Ofloxacin is effective against the following bacteria: Staphylococcus aureus (methicillin-susceptible strains), Staphylococcus epidermidis, Enterobacter cloacae, Streptococcus pneumoniae (penicillin-susceptible strains), Streptococcus pyogenes, Citrobacter (diversus) koseri, Enterobacter aerogenes, Proplonol bacterium acnes, Escherichia coli, Haemophilus influenzae, Serratia marcescens, Proteus mirabilis, Klebsiella pneumoniae, Neisseria gonorrhoeae, Proteus mirabilis, Chlamydia trachomatis, Gardnerella vaginalis, Legionella pneumophila, Mycoplasma hominis, Mycoplasma pneumonia, Ureaplasma urealyticum, and Pseudomonas aeruginosa. Some strains of Pseudomonas aeruginosa may quickly develop a resistance to ofloxacin during treatment. It is used to treat acute bacterial exacerbations of chronic bronchitis, community-acquired pneumonia, uncomplicated skin infections, conjunctivitis, corneal ulcers, acute uncomplicated urethral and cervical gonorrhea, nongonococcal urethritis and cervicitis, mixed infections of the urethra and cervix, acute pelvic inflammatory disease, uncomplicated cystitis, complicated urinary tract infections, and prostatitis. Ofloxacin can be administered orally, by ophthalmic drops, and via slow intravenous infusion over 60 minutes. It should not be administered via intramuscular injection, subcutaneous injection, or intravenous push. HCPCS Level II code S0034 represents 400 mg of ofloxacin.

S0039

S0039 Injection, sulfamethoxazole and trimethoprim, 10 ml

Lay Description

Sulfamethoxazole and trimethoprim is an antibiotic that blocks two necessary steps in the biosynthesis of nucleic acids and proteins that are critical to many bacteria. It is effective against the following bacteria: Streptococcus pneumoniae, Haemophilus influenzae, Shigella flexneri, Shigella sonnei, Escherichia coli, Klebsiella species, Enterobacter species, Morganella morganii, Proteus mirabilis, and Proteus vulgaris. Sulfamethoxazole and trimethoprim is indicated in the treatment of Pneumocystis carinii pneumonia, enteritis, urinary tract infections, acute otitis media, acute exacerbations of chronic bronchitis, traveler's diarrhea, and for prophylaxis against Pneumocystis carinii pneumonia in individuals who are immunosuppressed and considered to be at an increased risk of developing Pneumocystis carinii pneumonia. Sulfamethoxazole and trimethoprim is administered orally or via intravenous infusion over 60 to 90 minutes. This drug should not be given via rapid intravenous infusion or by intramuscular injection. HCPCS Level II code S0039 represents 10 ml of sulfamethoxazole and trimethoprim.

S0040

S0040 Injection, ticarcillin disodium and clavulanate potassium, 3.1 g

Lay Description

Ticarcillin disodium and clavulanate is a combination drug consisting of a semisynthetic form of penicillin and clavulanate. Penicillins block the actions of transpeptidase, an enzyme needed to create the cell wall. This weakens the bacterial cell wall causing cellular death. Many bacteria have developed a resistance to penicillin. Resistant bacteria produce an enzyme, penicillinase or beta-lactamase, that protects it from the effects of penicillin. Clavulanic acid or clavulanate binds to the penicillinase and inhibits it from blocking the actions of penicillin. Ticarcillin disodium is indicated for the treatment of infections with susceptible anaerobic, gram-negative, and positive bacteria. Specific conditions and susceptible bacteria include Septicemia/bacteremia caused by Staphylococcus aureus, Escherichia coli, Pseudomonas aeruginosa, and other Pseudomonas species; lower respiratory infections caused by Staphylococcus aureus, haemophilus influenza, Klebsiella species; bone and joint infections caused by Staphylococcus aureus; skin and skin-structure infections caused by Staphylococcus aureus, Escherichia coli, Klebsiella species; urinary tract infections caused by Escherichia coli, Klebsiella species, Pseudomonas aeruginosa and other Pseudomonas species, Citrobacter species, Enterobacter cloacae, Staphylococcus aureus, Serratia marcescens; gynecological infections caused by Prevotella melaninogenicus, Enterobacter species, Escherichia coli, Klebsiella pneumoniae, Staphylococcus aureus, Staphylococcus epidermidis; and intra-abdominal infections caused by Escherichia coli, Klebsiella pneumoniae, and Bacteroides fragilis. The drug is administered via an intravenous infusion. HCPCS Level II code S0040 represents a 3.1 gram dose of ticarcillin disodium and clavulante.

S0074

S0074 Injection, cefotetan disodium, 500 mg

Lay Description

Cefotetan disodium is an antibiotic that inhibits the cell wall synthesis in bacteria. It is effective against the following bacteria: Escherichia coli, Haemophilus influenzae, Klebsiella species, Morganella morganii, Neisseria gonorrhoeae, Proteus mirabilis, Proteus vulgaris, Providencia rettgeri, Serratia marcescens, Staphylococcus aureus, Staphylococcus epidermidis, Streptococcus agalactiae, Streptococcus pneumoniae, Streptococcus pyogenes, Prevotella bivia, Prevotella disiens, Bacteroides fragilis, Prevotella melaninogenica, Bacteroides vulgatus, Fusobacterium species, Gram-positive bacilli, Peptococcus niger, and Peptostreptococcus species. Cefotetan is indicated in the treatment of urinary tract infections, lower respiratory infections, skin infections, gynecological infections, intra-abdominal infections, bone and joint infections, and may be used as a preventive treatment prior to surgery. This drug can be administered via intramuscular injection, intravenous push, or intravenous infusion, usually less than one hour. HCPCS Level II code S0074 represents 500 mg of cefotetan disodium.

S0077

S0077 Injection, clindamycin phosphate, 300 mg

Lay Description

Clindamycin phosphate is an antibiotic used to treat serious, susceptible strains of streptococci, pneumococci, and staphylococci infections. It is used for patients who are allergic to penicillin or for whom penicillin treatment is inappropriate. It is effective against the following bacteria: Staphylococcus aureus, Staphylococcus epidermidis, Streptococci, (except Enterococcus faecalis), Pneumococci, Bacteroides species (including Bacteroides fragilis group and Bacteroides melaninogenicus group), Fusobacterium species, Propionibacterium, Eubacterium, Actinomyces species, Peptococcus species, Peptostreptococcus species, Microaerophilic streptococci, and

Clostridium perfringens. The injectable form is administered by intramuscular or intravenous injection followed by an intravenous infusion over 30 minutes. The usual dose is 600 to 1,200 mg per day in two, three, or four equal doses or for more severe infections 1,200 to 2,700 mg per day in two, three, or four equal doses. HCPCS Level II code S0077 represents 300 mg of clindamycin phosphate.

S0081

S0081 Injection, piperacillin sodium, 500 mg

Lay Description

Piperacillin is a broad-spectrum antibiotic that works by inhibiting septum and cell wall synthesis in bacteria. It is effective against the following bacteria: Enterococci, including Enterococcus faecalis, Streptococcus pneumoniae, Streptococcus pyogenes, Acinetobacter species, Enterobacter species, Escherichia coli, Haemophilus influenzae (non-lactamase-producing strains), Klebsiella species, Morganella morganii, Neisseria gonorrhoeae, Proteus mirabilis, Proteus vulgaris, Providencia rettgeri, Pseudomonas aeruginosa, Serratia species, Anaerobic cocci, Clostridium species, Bacteroides species including Bacteroides fragilis, Streptococcus agalactiae, Streptococcus bovis, Viridans group streptococci, Burkholderia cepacia, Citrobacter diversus, Citrobacter freundii, Pseudomonas fluorescens, Stenotrophomonas maltophilia, Yersinia enterocolitica, Actinomyces species, Eubacterium species, Fusobacterium necrophorum, Fusobacterium nucleatum, Porphyromonas asaccharolytica, Prevotella melaninogenica, and Veillonella species. Piperacillin is indicated in the treatment of intra-abdominal infections including hepatobiliary and surgical infections, urinary tract infections, endometritis, pelvic inflammatory disease, pelvic cellulitis, septicemia, lower respiratory tract infections, skin infections, bone and joint infections, uncomplicated gonococcal urethritis, and may be used as a preventive treatment prior to surgery. It is also effective for treatment of mixed infections and is used to treat infections prior to identification. Piperacillin can be administered via intramuscular injection, intravenous push, or intravenous infusion over 30 minutes. The maximum intramuscular dose is two grams per injection site. HCPCS Level II code S0081 represents 500 mg of piperacillin sodium.

S0088

S0088 Imatinib, 100 mg

Lay Description

Imatinib is an antineoplastic drug that inhibits the bcr abl tyrosine kinase, the constitutive abnormal tyrosine kinase created by the Philadelphia chromosome abnormality in chronic myeloid leukemia (CML). It inhibits production and induces apoptosis in bcr-abl positive cell lines, as well as fresh leukemic cells from Philadelphia chromosome positive CML. It is also an inhibitor of the receptor tyrosine kinases for platelet-derived growth factor (PDGF) and stem cell factor (SCF), c-kit, and inhibits PDGF- and SCF-mediated cellular events. It is used to treat adults with newly diagnosed Philadelphia chromosome positive chronic myeloid leukemia in chronic phase. It is also indicated for the treatment of patients with Philadelphia chromosome (CML) in blast crisis, accelerated phase, or in chronic phase after failure of interferon-alpha therapy and patients with Kit (CD117) positive unresectable and/or metastatic malignant gastrointestinal stromal tumors (GIST). Imatinib can be used for children with Ph+ chronic phase CML whose disease has recurred after stem cell transplant or who are resistant to interferon-alpha therapy. Adult dose is 400 to 800 mg per day. Imatinib is administered orally. HCPCS Level II code S0088 represents 100 mg of imatinib.

S0090

S0090 Sildenafil citrate, 25 mg

Lay Description

Sildenafil citrate is a selective inhibitor of an enzyme that controls cyclic guanosine monophosphate. The drug is used to treat erectile dysfunction. Penile erection is a hemodynamic process that involves the release of nitric acid by the corpus cavernosum during sexual stimulation. The nitric acid activates the enzyme cyclic guanosine monophosphate, which produces smooth muscle relaxation in the corpus cavernosum and allows the inflow of blood. Another enzyme, phosphodiesterase type 5, controls the tissue concentration of the cyclic guanosine monophosphate. Sildenafil citrate inhibits the neutralizing effect of the phosphodiesterase type 5. Since the local release of nitric acid is initiated by sexual stimulation and the erectile process is catalyzed by nitric acid, this drug has no effect in the absence of sexual stimulation. The drug is self-administered orally in dosages ranging from 25 to 100 mg. The drug may be taken at anywhere from one-half hour to four hours prior to sexual activity. HCPCS Level II code S0090 represents 25 mg of sildenafil citrate.

S0092

S0092 Injection, hydromorphone HCl, 250 mg (loading dose for infusion pump)

Lay Description

Hydromorphone is a narcotic and opioid analgesic classified as a schedule II controlled substance. This drug binds to opiate nerve center receptors and alters the human pain response, as well as suppressing the cough reflex. It is available in oral and injectable forms. The injectable form can be administered by intramuscular, subcutaneous, and intravenous injection, or by intravenous infusion. Hydromorphone hydrochloride is indicated for the relief of moderate to severe pain. HCPCS Level II code S0092 represents 250 mg of hydromorphone hydrochloride to be used only for a loading dose for an infusion pump.

S0108

S0108   Mercaptopurine, oral, 50 mg

Lay Description

Mercaptopurine is a potent chemotherapeutic drug belonging to a class of drugs known as antimetabolites. Antimetabolites resemble nutrients required for cancer cell growth. The cancer cells take up mercaptopurine, which interfere with cancer cell nucleic acid biosynthesis. Specifically, mercaptopurine inhibits the first enzyme unique to the de novo pathway for purine ribonucleotide synthesis. It is not known exactly which of the biochemical effects of mercaptopurine is responsible for cell death. Mercaptopurine is used to treat acute lymphatic and acute myelogenous leukemia. It has also been shown to be effective in the treatment of some chronic myelogenous leukemias and some acute undifferentiated leukemias. Efficacy depends on the particular subclassification of the leukemia. Mercaptopurine may be used in combination with other chemotherapy drugs as an initial treatment to induce remission. It may also be used as maintenance therapy for lymphatic (lymphocytic, lymphoblastic) leukemia. The induction dose varies; however, the usual dose for both children and adults is 2.5 mg/kg of body weight. The maintenance dose is 1.5 to 2.5 mg/kg per day once the patient is in remission. This medication is administered orally. HCPCS Level II code S0108 represents 50 mg of mercaptopurine.

S0122

S0122   Injection, menotropins, 75 IU

Lay Description

Menotropins is a purified preparation of gonadotropins extracted from the urine of postmenopausal women. It contains follicle-stimulating hormone (FSH) activity and luteinizing hormone (LH) activity. Menotropins is used to treat infertility in women. The medication is administered for seven to 12 days to stimulate follicular growth in women who do not have primary ovarian failure. Menotropins treatment results in follicular growth and maturation. An additional drug has to be given to induce ovulation. Menotropins is administered by subcutaneous or intramuscular injection. HCPCS Level II code S0122 represents 75 IU of menotropins.

S0126

S0126   Injection, follitropin alfa, 75 IU

Lay Description

Follitropin alfa contains a human follicle stimulating hormone (FSH) preparation of recombinant DNA origin. FSH, the active component of follitropin alfa, is responsible for follicular growth, maturation, and gonadal steroid production. It is found in genetically modified Chinese hamster ovary (CHO) cells cultured in bioreactors. Follitropin alfa contains no luteinizing hormone (LH) activity. Based on available data derived from physico-chemical tests and bioassays, follitropin alfa and follitropin beta are indistinguishable. Follitropin is used to treat infertility in women and to induce spermatogenesis in men with hypogonadotropic hypogonadism. Follitropin alfa stimulates ovarian follicular growth in women who do not have primary ovarian failure. In order to continue final phase of follicle maturation, resumption of meiosis and rupture of the follicle in the absence of an endogenous LH surge, human chorionic gonadotropin (hCG) must be given following the administration of follitropin when patient monitoring indicates that appropriate follicular development has occurred. Follitropin alfa is administered with hCG to men with hypogonadotropic hypogonadism to stimulate spermatogenesis. FSH is the primary hormone responsible for spermatogenesis. Follitropin alfa can be administered via subcutaneous injection. HCPCS Level II code S0126 represents 75 IU of follitropin alfa.

S0128

S0128   Injection, follitropin beta, 75 IU

Lay Description

Follitropin beta contains a human follicle stimulating hormone (FSH) preparation of recombinant DNA origin. FSH, the active component of follitropin alfa, is responsible for follicular growth, maturation, and gonadal steroid production. It is found in genetically modified Chinese hamster ovary (CHO) cells cultured in bioreactors. Follitropin beta has a dimeric structure containing two glycoprotein subunits (alpha and beta). Follitropin beta contains no luteinizing hormone (LH) activity. Based on available data derived from physico-chemical tests and bioassays, follitropin alfa and follitropin beta are indistinguishable. Follitropin is used to treat infertility in women and to induce spermatogenesis in men with hypogonadotropic hypogonadism. Follitropin alfa stimulates ovarian follicular growth in women who do not have primary ovarian failure. In order to continue final phase of follicle maturation, resumption of meiosis and rupture of the follicle in the absence of an endogenous LH surge, human chorionic gonadotropin (hCG) must be given following the administration of follitropin when patient monitoring indicates that appropriate follicular development has occurred. Follitropin alfa is administered with hCG to men with hypogonadotropic hypogonadism to stimulate spermatogenesis. FSH is the primary hormone responsible for spermatogenesis. Follitropin beta can be administered via subcutaneous or intramuscular injection for women and only by subcutaneous injection for men. HCPCS Level II code S0128 represents 75 IU of follitropin beta.

S0132

S0132   Injection, ganirelix acetate, 250 mcg

Lay Description

Ganirelix acetate is a synthetic decapeptide with high antagonistic activity against naturally occurring gonadotropin-releasing hormone (GnRH). The pulsatile release of GnRH stimulates the synthesis and secretion of luteinizing hormone (LH) and follicle-stimulating hormone (FSH). The large increase of GnRH at mid-cycle results in an LH surge. This results in ovulation, resumption of meiosis in the oocyte, and luteinization. Ganirelix is given to women undergoing fertility treatment to prevent the eggs from being released prematurely. The usual dose is 250 micrograms once a day. It is administered via subcutaneous injection during the mid to late portion of the follicular phase. HCPCS Level II code S0132 represents 250 micrograms of ganirelix acetate.

S0136

S0136   Clozapine, 25 mg

Lay Description

Clozapine is an atypical antipsychotic medication used to treat severely ill schizophrenic patients who do not respond effectively to standard drug treatment. It is considered an atypical antipsychotic medication because its profile of binding to dopamine receptors and its effects on various dopamine-mediated behaviors differ from those exhibited by more typical antipsychotic drug products. Specifically, although it does interfere with the binding of dopamine at D1, D2, D3, and D5 receptors and has a high affinity for the D4 receptor, it does not induce catalepsy nor inhibit apomorphine-induced stereotypy. It is a tricyclic dibenzodiazepine derivative. Doses can vary from 600 to 900 mg a day. Patients are started on small doses and the amount is gradually increased to obtain a therapeutic dose. Clozapine is administered orally. HCPCS Level II code S0136 represents 25 mg of clozapine.

S0137

S0137   Didanosine (ddI), 25 mg

Lay Description

Didanosine (ddI) is an antiviral used in combination with other drugs to treat human immunodeficiency virus (HIV). It is a synthetic nucleoside analogue of the naturally occurring nucleoside deoxyadenosine in which the 3-hydroxyl group is replaced by hydrogen. In the cell, didanosine is converted by cellular enzymes to, the active metabolite, dideoxyadenosine 5'- triphosphate, which inhibits the activity of HIV-1 reverse transcriptase both by competing with the natural substrate, deoxyadenosine 5'-triphosphate, and by its incorporation into viral DNA. This causes failure of viral DNA chain elongation. The usual dose is 400 mg for patients weighing $\geq$ 60 kg and 250 mg for patients weighing $\leq$ 60 kg. Didanosine is administered orally and should be taken on an empty stomach. HCPCS Level II code S0137 represents 25 mg of didanosine.

S0139

S0139   Minoxidil, 10 mg

Lay Description

Minoxidil is a peripheral vasodilator used to treat hypertension by decreasing peripheral vascular resistance. It is usually used on patients who do not respond adequately to maximum doses of other hypertensive medications and diuretics. It is usually given in conjunction with beta-blockers and diuretics. The recommended dose for adults older than age 12 is 5 mg a day but can be increased to a maximum of 100 mg a day. The recommended dose for children age 12 and younger is 0.2 mg per kg with a maximum dose of 50 mg per day. Minoxidil used in the treatment of hypertension is administered orally. Minoxidil is also available in topical form. The topical form is used as a hair restorer for men and women with certain types of hair loss. HCPCS Level II code S0139 represents 10 mg of oral minoxidil.

S0140

S0140   Saquinavir, 200 mg

Lay Description

Saquinavir is a chemical complex that is an HIV protease inhibitor. HIV protease is an enzyme required for replication of the HIV virus. Saquinavir binds to the protease active site and inhibits the activity of the enzyme, which prevents cleavage of the virus polypeptides and results in the formation of immature noninfectious virus particles. Saquinavir in combination with ritonavir and other antiretroviral agents is indicated for the treatment of HIV infection. Saquinavir is administered orally and is available in

200 and 500 mg capsules. The recommended dose of saquinavir is 1,000 mg per day to be used in combination with ritonavir and other antiretroviral agents. HCPCS Level II code S0140 represents 200 mg of Saquinavir.

S0145

S0145 Injection, pegylated interferon alfa-2a, 180 mcg per ml

Lay Description

Interferon alfa-2a pegylated is a covalent conjugate of interferon alfa-2a recombinant. It is a drug that uses a genetically engineered Escherichia coli bacterium containing DNA that codes for the human protein. In the pegylated form, a special strand (commonly called a PEG) is attached to the interferon molecule that helps to protect the interferon from being destroyed by the immune system. Interferon alfa-2a pegylated is used to treat chronic hepatitis C with compensated liver disease and HBeAg positive and HBeAg negative chronic hepatitis B with evidence of viral replication and liver inflammation. The recommended dose is 180 micrograms once a week. Interferon alfa-2a is administered via subcutaneous injection. HCPCS Level II code S0145 represents 180 micrograms per ml of pegylated interferon alfa-2a.

S0148

S0148 Injection, pegylated interferon alfa-2B, 10 mcg

Lay Description

Interferon alfa-2b pegylated is a covalent conjugate of interferon alfa-2b recombinant. It is a drug that uses a genetically engineered *Escherichia coli* bacterium containing DNA that codes for the human protein. In the pegylated form, a special strand (commonly called a PEG) is attached to the interferon molecule that helps protect the interferon from being destroyed by the immune system. Interferon alfa-2b is used to treat chronic hepatitis C with compensated liver disease. The recommended dose is 1 microgram per kg on the same day each week for one year. Interferon alfa-2b is administered via subcutaneous injection.

S0155

S0155 Sterile dilutant for epoprostenol, 50 ml

Lay Description

Epoprostenol is a prostaglandin that acts as a direct vasodilator of pulmonary and systemic arteries and an inhibitor of platelet aggregation. It is usually administered parenterally through a permanent indwelling central venous catheter as a long-term medication to treat primary pulmonary hypertension and pulmonary hypertension secondary to scleroderma in NYHA Class III and IV patients. Initial administration may be through a peripheral intravenous infusion until a central venous catheter is established. It is manufactured as a powder that must be reconstituted with sterile diluent specific to the epoprostenol. Dosages vary dependent upon body weight and response. Once a regimen of epoprostenol has been established, it should never be stopped suddenly. HCPCS Level II code S0155 represents the 50 ml of the sterile diluent for eporprostenol.

S0156

S0156 Exemestane, 25 mg

Lay Description

Exemestane is an irreversible, steroidal aromatase inactivator. It acts as a false substrate to the aromatase enzyme and binds to the active site of this enzyme in postmenopausal women to cause its inactivation. Exemestane lowers the circulating concentration in postmenopausal women. Many breast cancers have estrogen receptors and growth of these tumors can be stimulated by estrogen. It is used in adjuvant treatment of postmenopausal women with estrogen receptor positive early breast cancer who have received two to three years of tamoxifen and are switched to exemestane to finish a total of five consecutive years of adjuvant hormonal therapy. Exemestane has proven effective for the treatment of advanced breast cancer in postmenopausal women whose disease has progressed following tamoxifen therapy. The recommended dose is 25 mg once per day after a meal. Exemestane is administered orally. HCPCS Level II code S0156 represents 25 mg of exemestane.

S0157

S0157 Becaplermin gel 0.01%, 0.5 gm

Lay Description

Becaplermin gel is a human platelet-derived growth factor (PDGF), a substance naturally produced by the body, that helps to promote wound healing. Becaplermin is available as a gel that is applied to the skin, usually once per day. The amount of gel applied depends on the size of the ulcer and may be changed every one to two weeks as the ulcer heals. It is supplied in a 15 gram tube. Becaplermin gel is used to treat ulcers of the foot, ankle, or leg in patients with diabetes. When used in combination with standard ulcer care that includes cleaning, pressure relief, and infection control, it works by bringing the cells that the body uses to repair wounds to the site of the ulcer. The gel may cause localized skin rash. HCPCS Level II code S0157 represents 0.5 grams of becaplermin gel.

S0160

S0160 Dextroamphetamine sulfate, 5 mg

Lay Description

Dextroamphetamine sulfate is an amphetamine. Amphetamines are noncatecholamine, sympathomimetic amines with central nervous system (CNS) stimulant activity. They elevate blood pressure and stimulate respirations and are highly addictive. Dextroamphetamine is used to treat narcolepsy and as part of a treatment regimen in attention deficit disorder with hyperactivity in children ages 3 to 6. The recommended dose is 5 to 60 mg per day depending on the patient. Dextroamphetamine is administered orally. HCPCS Level II code S0160 represents 5 mg of dextroamphetamine sulfate.

S0164

S0164 Injection, pantoprazole sodium, 40 mg

Lay Description

Pantoprazole sodium is a compound that inhibits gastric secretions. Pantoprazole is a proton pump inhibitor (PPI) that suppresses the final step in gastric acid production by forming a covalent bond to two sites of the ATPase enzyme system at the secretory surface of the gastric parietal cell. This effect is dose-related and leads to inhibition of both basal and stimulated gastric acid secretion irrespective of the stimulus. This binding results in a period of antisecretory effect that persists longer than 24 hours for all doses tested. This drug is indicated for short-term treatment (seven to 10 days) for patients with gastroesophageal reflux disease (GERD) and a history of erosive esophagitis, and the hypersecretory conditions that may be associated with Zollinger-Ellison syndrome or other neoplastic conditions. HCPCS Level II code S0164 represents 40 mg of pantoprazole sodium.

S0166

S0166 Injection, olanzapine, 2.5 mg

Lay Description

Olanzapine is a psychotropic agent that belongs to the thienobenzodiazepine class. It is used to treat schizophrenia, acute mixed or manic episodes associated with bipolar disorder, agitation associated with schizophrenia, and bipolar disorder. HCPCS Level II code S0166 represents 2.5 mg of olanzapine.

S0170

S0170 Anastrozole, oral, 1 mg

Lay Description

Anastrozole is a non-steroidal aromatase inhibitor. Anastrozole is converted to estrone in adipose tissue of the breast. The estrone is further converted to estradiol, which is the primary source of estrogen in postmenopausal women. Many breast cancers have estrogen receptors and growth of these tumors can be stimulated by estrogen. Anastrozole is used to treat postmenopausal women with hormone receptor positive early breast cancer and for the first-line treatment of postmenopausal women with hormone receptor positive or hormone receptor unknown locally advanced or metastatic breast cancer. Recommended dose is 1 mg per day. Anastrozole is administered orally. HCPCS Level II code S0170 represents 1 mg of anastrozole.

S0171

S0171 Injection, bumetanide, 0.5 mg

Lay Description

Bumetanide is a potent diuretic that is in the class of loop diuretics. It blocks fluid and sodium reabsorbsion from the kidney's tubules. This medication is used to treat mild to moderate hypertension, edema associated with heart failure, renal disease, and cirrhosis of the liver. HCPCS Level II code S0171 represents 0.5 mg of bumetanide.

S0172

S0172 Chlorambucil, oral, 2 mg

Lay Description

Chlorambucil is a nitrogen mustard type of antineoplastic drug. It is used as palliative treatment for chronic lymphatic (lymphocytic) leukemia and malignant lymphomas, including lymphosarcoma, giant follicular lymphoma, and Hodgkin's disease. The usual oral dosage is 0.1 to 0.2 mg per kg body weight daily for three to six weeks. Chlorambucil is administered orally. HCPCS Level II code S0172 represents 2 mg of chlorambucil.

S0176

S0176 Hydroxyurea, oral, 500 mg

Lay Description

Hydroxyurea is an antineoplastic drug used to treat melanoma, resistant chronic myelocytic leukemia, and recurrent, metastatic, or inoperable carcinoma of the ovary, and in conjunction with radiation therapy for primary squamous cell (epidermoid) carcinomas of the head and neck, excluding the lip. Hydroxyurea is administered orally. HCPCS Level II code S0176 represents 500 mg of hydroxyurea.

S0177

S0177 Levamisole HCl, oral, 50 mg

Lay Description

Levamisole is an antineoplastic drug used as an adjuvant therapy in conjunction with 5-fluorouracil after surgical resection to treat patients with Dukes' Stage C colon cancer. The initial dose is 50 mg every eight hours beginning seven to 30 days after surgery for three days. The maintenance dose is 50 mg every eight hours for three days every two weeks. Levamisole is administered orally. HCPCS Level II code S0177 represents 50 mg of levamisole.

S0178

S0178 Lomustine, oral, 10 mg

Lay Description

Lomustine is used to treat primary and metastatic brain tumors in patients who have already undergone surgical or radiation therapy, and as secondary therapy in Hodgkin's disease for patients who relapse while being treated with other medications or do not respond to primary therapy. Lomustine is administered orally. HCPCS Level II code S0178 represents 10 mg of lomustine.

S0179

S0179 Megestrol acetate, oral, 20 mg

Lay Description

Megestrol acetate is an antineoplastic medication used as palliative treatment for advanced carcinoma of the breast or endometrium. Megestrol acetate has a direct cytoxic effect on tumors in the breast. In metastatic cancer, hormone receptors may be present in some tissues but not others. The receptor mechanism is a cyclic process whereby estrogen produced by the ovaries enters the target cell, forms a complex with cytoplasmic receptor, and is transported into the cell nucleus. Inside the cell nucleus it alters the normal cell function. This medication decreases the number of hormone-dependent human breast cancer cells and can change or eliminate the way estrogen acts upon these cells. It is not known how megestrol acetate acts on endometrial cancer. Recommended dose for breast cancer is 40 mg four times a day. Recommended dose for endometrial cancer is 40 to 320 mg per day in divided doses. The usual treatment lasts two months. Megestrol acetate is administered orally. HCPCS Level II code S0179 represents 20 mg of megestrol acetate.

S0182

S0182 Procarbazine HCl, oral, 50 mg

Lay Description

Procarbazine hydrochloride is used to treat stage III and stage IV Hodgkin's disease. It is used in combination with other antineoplastic drugs. The recommended dose is 50 mg per m2 of body surface per day for the first week. After that 100 mg per m2 of body surface per day should be given until the maximum response is obtained or until thrombocytopenia or leukopenia occurs. When the maximum response is attained, the dose may be maintained at 50 mg per m^2 of body surface per day. Procarbazine is administered orally. HCPCS Level II code S0182 represents 50 mg of procarbazine hydrochloride.

S0187

S0187 Tamoxifen citrate, oral, 10 mg

Lay Description

Tamoxifen citrate is a nonsteroidal antiestrogen used to treat metastatic breast cancer in men and women, ductal carcinoma in situ, and women at high risk to develop breast cancer. High risk is defined as women at least 35 years of age with a five-year predicted risk of breast cancer $\geq$ 1.67%, as calculated by the Gail Model. In premenopausal women with metastatic breast cancer, tamoxifen citrate is an alternative to oophorectomy or ovarian irradiation. It is believed that patients whose tumors are estrogen receptor positive are more likely to benefit from tamoxifen citrate therapy. It is recommended for postmenopausal women with node positive breast cancer who have undergone mastectomy, axillary dissection, and radiation therapy. Recommended dose is 20 to 40 mg per day. Tamoxifen citrate is administered orally. HCPCS Level II code S0187 represents 10 mg of tamoxifen citrate.

S0189

S0189 Testosterone pellet, 75 mg

Lay Description

Testosterone is an anabolic steroid used primarily to treat male hypogonadism. It stimulates targeted tissues to develop normally in androgen-deficient men. Testosterone may also have some anti-estrogen properties, making it useful in treating certain estrogen-dependent breast cancers. This drug is used to treat male hypogonadism, unusually late sexual maturity, myotonia congenita, inflammation and rotation of the testes, undescended testicle, absence of testicles, Klinefelter syndrome, anemia, and in the prevention of breast pain and engorgement in postpartum women. HCPCS Level II code S0189 represents a 75 mg testosterone pellet.

S0191

S0191 Misoprostol, oral, 200 mcg

Lay Description

Misoprostol is a synthetic prostaglandin E1 analog. It is used to reduce the risk of gastric ulcers in patients undergoing NSAID treatment who may be at high risk for complications of ulcers, including elderly patients, those with a history of gastric ulcers, and patients with a concomitant debilitating disease. Misoprostol inhibits gastric acid secretion and may have mucosal protective properties. NSAIDs reduce prostaglandin synthesis, and a lack of prostaglandins within the gastric mucosa may lead to diminishing bicarbonate and mucus secretion and may contribute to the mucosal damage caused by these agents. Recommended dose is 200 mcg four times a day with food with the last dose at bedtime. Misoprostol is administered orally. HCPCS Level II code S0191 represents 200 mcg of misoprostol.

S0194

S0194 Dialysis/stress vitamin supplement, oral, 100 capsules

Lay Description

Vitamins and minerals are organic compounds that are necessary for the metabolic functioning of the body. Multivitamins are combined forms of vitamins and may include minerals. Multivitamins are usually oral tablets. Pregnant patients, patients on dialysis, patients with malabsorption diseases, and those with deficient diets may need exogenous sources of multiple vitamins. Liquid forms may be added to TPN solutions. Multivitamins are sold over-the-counter and are self-administered orally. HCPCS Level II code S0194 may be reported for 100 capsules of dialysis or stress vitamins.

S0195

S0195 Pneumococcal conjugate vaccine, polyvalent, intramuscular, for children from 5 years to 9 years of age who have not previously received the vaccine

Lay Description

Vaccines are suspensions of weakened, altered, or killed microorganisms or of the antigen proteins derived from the microorganism administered for the prevention, improvement, or treatment of an infectious disease. The microorganism or the antigen proteins within the vaccine stimulate the immune system to produce antibodies to the specific microorganism. Pneumococcal infections are caused by the bacterium Streptococcus pneumoniae. There are more than 80 distinct types of polysaccharides associated with the capsule of the bacterium. Pneumococcus most commonly causes lobar pneumonia, but may also cause meningitis, septicemia, empyema, and peritonitis. There are currently two different types of pneumococcal vaccines. One is a heptavalent conjugate vaccine containing purified polysaccharides of the capsular antigens of the bacterium types 4, 6B, 9V, 14, 18C, 19F, and 23F. In the conjugate vaccine, the polysaccharides are coupled with a nontoxic purified diphtheria protein. The conjugate vaccine is administered as an intramuscular injection to children younger than 23 months and children ages 24 to 59 months who are at high risk for pneumococcal infection, including those with sickle cell disease, HIV infection, those immunocompromised, and those with chronic illness, such as cardiac or pulmonary disease or diabetes mellitus. The second type of vaccine is a polyvalent, 23-valent vaccine containing the capsular polysaccharide of the bacterium, types 1-5, 8, 9, 12, 14, 17, 19, 20, 22, 23, 26, 34, 43, 51, 54, 56, 57, 68, and 70, which are responsible for about 90 percent of pneumococcal disease in the U.S. The polyvalent vaccine is administered intramuscularly to individuals older than 2 years of age who are at increased risk for the disease or its complications, such as those with chronic illnesses. The polyvalent vaccine is also administered to individuals age 65 years and older and persons residing in nursing homes or other institutions. HCPCS Level II code S0195 represents a pneumococcal conjugate vaccine, polyvalent, for children five to nine years of age who have not previously received the vaccine.

S0197

S0197 Prenatal vitamins, 30-day supply

Lay Description

Vitamins and minerals are organic compounds that are necessary for the metabolic functioning of the body. Multivitamins are combined forms of vitamins and may include minerals. Multivitamins are usually oral tablets. Pregnant patients, patients on dialysis, patients with malabsorption diseases, and those with deficient diets may need exogenous sources of multiple vitamins. Liquid forms may be added to TPN solutions. Multivitamins are sold over-the-counter and are self-administered orally. HCPCS Level II code S0197 represents a 30-day supply of prenatal vitamins.

S0250

S0250 Comprehensive geriatric assessment and treatment planning performed by assessment team

Lay Description

A comprehensive geriatric assessment involves evaluation and treatment planning designed to optimize an elderly person's ability to maintain good health, improve quality of life, reduce the need for hospital and long-term care services, and enable independent living. Because of the comprehensive scope of this exam, it must be performed by a multi-disciplinary team of experts that may include physicians, geriatric nurse practitioners, ancillary personnel, social workers, psychologists, physical/occupational therapists, dieticians, and pharmacists. The assessment begins with an examination of the elderly person's current status including physical, mental, and psycho-social health status. The ability to function independently and perform basic activities of daily living are assessed including dressing, bathing, meal preparation, and medication management. The individual's living arrangement, social network, and access to support services is evaluated. Next, current problems related to the status assessment are identified and evaluated as to their potential to cause future problems. Based on these findings a comprehensive care plan is developed that addresses all current and potential problems. Specific interventions are proposed, including recommendations regarding necessary resources and support services. Management of resources is initiated with the elderly person and family to assure that the necessary services will be provided. A plan for ongoing monitoring is provided so modifications to the care plan can be initiated as required.

S0265

S0265   Genetic counseling, under physician supervision, each 15 minutes

Lay Description

Individuals who have a family history of certain genetic diseases or disorders, such as cystic fibrosis, sickle cell anemia, Tay-Sachs disease, or other diseases may be referred for genetic counseling. Genetic counseling is a service that includes evaluating family history and medical records, ordering genetic tests, evaluating the test results, and helping the individuals understand the test results and reach decisions based on the results of the testing. Before meeting with a genetic counselor, information about family history, including relatives with genetic disorders, multiple miscarriages, or early or unexplained deaths, should be gathered. A personal history and medical record information related to ultrasounds, prenatal test results, past pregnancies, and medications should also be provided The counselor will review the family and personal history information, determine if additional tests are necessary, assist the individuals in obtaining the necessary tests, and conduct follow-up when the results of testing are available. During the follow-up, the genetic counselor will help the patient understand options and make any necessary referrals to other health care professionals. Code S0265 is reported for each 15 minutes of genetic counseling provided under physician supervision.

S0302

S0302   Completed early periodic screening diagnosis and treatment (EPSDT) service (list in addition to code for appropriate evaluation and management service)

Lay Description

Early periodic screening diagnosis and treatment (EPSDT) is a free service provided to children ages birth through 21 who are eligible for Medicaid. EPSDT enables children to get medical exams, check-ups, follow-up care, and any special care needed to ensure optimum health. EPSDT legislation requires states to provide Medicaid-eligible children with periodic screening, vision, dental, and hearing services. States are required to assess a child's health needs through initial and periodic examinations and evaluations to assure that health problems are diagnosed and treated early, before they become more complex. States must perform the required evaluations according to a standardized schedule, called a periodicity schedule. At a minimum, these screenings must include comprehensive health and developmental history, including assessment of both physical and mental health development; comprehensive unclothed physical exam; appropriate immunizations according to age and health history; laboratory tests, including a lead toxicity screening; health education, including anticipatory guidance; vision and hearing screens; and dental screens. In addition, EPSDT legislation requires states provide any medically necessary inter-periodic health screens and care, even if the service is not available under the state's Medicaid plan to adults. Code S0260 reports completion of an EPSDT service and is reported in addition to the appropriate evaluation and management service.

S0310

S0310   Hospitalist services (list separately in addition to code for appropriate evaluation and management service)

Lay Description

A hospitalist is a board-certified physician specializing in the care of hospitalized patients. The hospitalist is a single point person who oversees each patient's care throughout the hospital stay. The hospitalist makes daily rounds, checks on each patient as needed throughout the day, monitors the patient's in-hospital care, tracks nursing care, and works to coordinate care between the patient's primary care physician and other physician specialists. In addition, the hospitalist coordinates scheduling of tests and procedures that may be required and follows up to make sure test results are reported and reviewed by the appropriate person. Code S0310 reports hospitalist services and should be listed separately in addition to the code for the appropriate evaluation and management service.

S0400

S0400 Global fee for extracorporeal shock wave lithotripsy treatment of kidney stone(s)

Lay Description

The physician pulverizes a kidney stone (renal calculus) by directing shock waves through a liquid medium. Two different methods are currently available to accomplish this procedure. The physician first uses radiological guidance to determine the location and size of the renal calculus. In the first method, the patient is then immersed in a liquid medium (degassed, deionized water) with shock waves directed through the liquid to the kidney stone. In the second method, the one most often used, the patient is placed on a specially designed treatment table. A series of shock waves are directed through a water-cushion or bellow that is placed against the patient's body at the location of the kidney stone. Each shock wave is directed to the stone for only a fraction of a second, and the entire procedure generally takes from 30 to 50 minutes. The treatment table is equipped with video x-ray so the physician can view the pulverization process. Over several days or weeks, the tiny stone fragments pass harmlessly through the patient's urinary system and are discharged during urination. Code S0400 reports the global fee for the extracorporeal shock wave lithotripsy treatment of the renal calculus.

S0620-S0621

S0620 Routine ophthalmological examination including refraction; new patient

S0621 Routine ophthalmological examination including refraction; established patient

Lay Description

The ophthalmologist or optometrist performs a routine eye (ophthalmological) examination including refraction. A complete eye examination involves a series of tests to evaluate vision and check for eye diseases. A visual exam is performed on the external eye to check the pupils' response to light, the clarity and shininess of the cornea and iris, and the position and movement of the eyes, eyelids, and eyelashes. The provider checks the eye muscles to ensure they are functioning properly. Tests on the eye muscles involve following movement of an object up-and-down and side-to-side to detect any eye muscle weakness or uncontrolled movement. A visual acuity test is performed using an eye chart. Following the visual acuity test, a refraction assessment is performed on individuals who need corrective lenses to determine the prescription required. The provider may use a computerized refractor to estimate the prescription or alternatively a retinoscopy may be performed. A retinoscopy involves shining a light into the eye and measuring the refractive error by evaluating the movement of the light that is reflected by the retina. These results are verified and fine-tuned using a Phoroptor, which consists of a series of lenses through which the patient views an eye chart and indicates which lens provides the clearest vision. The provider checks peripheral vision by means of a visual field (perimetry) test. A slit lamp exam is performed. A slit lamp uses an intense line of light to examine the cornea, iris, lens, and anterior eye chamber. The provider performs a glaucoma test, which checks intraocular pressure. The pupils are dilated and the retina is examined. Report S0620 for a routine ophthalmological examination with refraction on a new patient and S0621 for an established patient.

S0625

S0625 Retinal telescreening by digital imaging of multiple different fundus areas to screen for vision-threatening conditions, including imaging, interpretation and report

Lay Description

Retinal telescreening by digital imaging of multiple different fundus areas is performed to screen for vision threatening conditions such as diabetic retinopathy. A trained photographer located in or near the primary care physician's office administers drops to dilate the patient's pupils. The trained photographer uses a retinal telescreening system to obtain seven standard field, stereoscopic, 30-degree digital fundus photographs. These photographs are transmitted to a reading center for examination and grading by a trained non-physician technician. Selected samples are reread for quality assurance. Any image sets with questionable pathology or non-typical findings are referred to an ophthalmologist for secondary evaluation. Code S0625 reports the complete procedure including imaging, interpretation, and report.

S0630

S0630 Removal of sutures; by a physician other than the physician who originally closed the wound

Lay Description

The physician removes sutures that have been placed by another physician. When a laceration or an incision for a surgical procedure has required suturing, any non-absorbable stitches must by removed. The area is cleansed with an antiseptic cleanser to remove any dried blood and loosen any scar tissue. Sterile forceps are used to lift the suture at the knot. The suture material is then clipped as close to the skin as possible using sterile forceps and removed. When all the sutures are removed, the area is cleaned again with antiseptic. Adhesive strips and a dry dressing may be applied as needed.

S1040

S1040 Cranial remolding orthotic, pediatric, rigid, with soft interface material, custom fabricated, includes fitting and adjustment(s)

Lay Description

This code reports the supply of a special cranial remolding orthosis used to treat plagiocephaly. Plagiocephaly refers to misshapen or flattened skull bones and a variety of causes are noted, including premature closure of cranial sutures, birth trauma, torticollis, or repetitive sleeping positions. This type of cranial remolding orthosis consists of a custom-fabricated, helmet-like device structured to address the specific cranial malformation of the infant. The orthosis has a soft interface material for comfort, as many are worn up to 23 hours per day. Some models consist of broad bands with mild elastic properties, while others are fabricated by molding to the patient's skull. The cranial remolding orthosis is designed to address plagiocephaly and manipulate skull development toward a more normal shape, or to maintain skull structure. This code reports the supply, fitting, and any required adjustments of the custom-fabricated, rigid, pediatric, cranial orthosis.

S2066

S2066 Breast reconstruction with gluteal artery perforator (GAP) flap, including harvesting of the flap, microvascular transfer, closure of donor site and shaping the flap into a breast, unilateral

Lay Description

Gluteal artery perforator (GAP) is breast reconstruction using the gluteal artery perforator flap, which includes harvesting the flap, the microvascular transfer, closure of the donor site, and shaping the flap into a breast. HCPCS Level II code S2066 is a unilateral procedure.

S2067

S2067 Breast reconstruction of a single breast with "stacked" deep inferior epigastric perforator (DIEP) flap(s) and/or gluteal artery perforator (GAP) flap(s), including harvesting of the flap(s), microvascular transfer, closure of donor site(s) and shaping the flap into a breast, unilateral

Lay Description

Deep inferior epigastric perforator/gluteal artery perforator (DIEP/GAP) is breast reconstruction of a single breast with a stacked deep inferior epigastric perforator or superficial inferior epigastric artery (SIEA) flap. This procedure includes harvesting of the flap, microvascular transfer, closure of the donor site, and shaping the new flap into a breast.

S2070

S2070 Cystourethroscopy, with ureteroscopy and/or pyeloscopy; with endoscopic laser treatment of ureteral calculi (includes ureteral catheterization)

Lay Description

S2325

S2325 Hip core decompression

Lay Description

The physician performs a hip core decompression of the femoral head. Hip core decompression is used in the treatment of osteonecrosis in patients with small-sized to medium-sized precollapse lesions of the femoral head. Hip core decompression relieves pressure within the rigid structure of the femoral head, thereby relieving joint pain. An incision is made over the femoral head. The soft tissues are divided. Next, one of two techniques may be used to perform the hip core decompression, which involves drilling a small hole or holes in the diseased bone. Using the more traditional technique, a hole is drilled in line with the axis of the femoral neck at the point where the lateral cortex begins to thicken. An 8 to 10 mm wide reamer is used to over-ream the drill hole. A second, newer technique utilizes a 3 mm Steinman pin to create multiple small drill holes in the diseased bone of the femoral head. Surgical instruments are then removed. The surgical area is flushed with normal saline and the incision is closed.

S3860

S3860 Genetic testing, comprehensive cardiac ion channel analysis, for variants in 5 major cardiac ion channel genes for individuals with high index of suspicion for familial long QT syndrome (LQTS) or related syndromes

Lay Description

Genetic testing is used to determine mutations or variances in genes that may be responsible for certain conditions or diseases. Genetic testing for cardial icon channel analysis involves examination of the DNA taken from the patient's blood for identification of mutations in five cardiac ion channel genes that have been associated with cardiac channel disorders (channelopathies), such as long QT syndrome (LQTS). Congenital long QT syndrome is an inherited condition. It is described as the lengthening of the repolarization phase of the ventricular action potential (an abnormally long QT interval seen on EKG tracings). This condition may put the patient at risk for arrhythmic episodes, and may result in syncope (fainting episodes) and sudden cardiac death (SCD). Many instances of sudden unexpected deaths in children can be attributed to long QT syndrome. This can occur with strenuous physical activities or emotional excitement. Diagnostic criteria for long QT syndrome have been established, which focus on EKG findings, as well as clinical and family history.

S3866

S3866 Genetic analysis for a specific gene mutation for hypertrophic cardiomyopathy (HCM) in an individual with a known HCM mutation in the family

Lay Description

A genetic disorder is a disease caused in whole or in part by a mutation of a gene. Genetic disorders can be passed on to family members who inherit the genetic abnormality. A small number of rare disorders are caused by a mistake in a single gene. Genetic testing can be predictive, used to confirm a diagnosis or used to determine if a person is a carrier for the disease. Genetic tests attempt to identify abnormalities in an individual's genes, which include the presence or absence of key proteins whose production is directed by specific genes. These abnormalities in either the presence or absence of proteins could indicate an inherited disposition for a disorder.

S3870

S3870 Comparative genomic hybrization (CGH) microarray testing for developmental delay, autism spectrum disorder and/or mental retardation

Lay Description

Genetic variations are often seen with developmental delay and other disorders. Standard cytogenetic analysis detects visible chromosomal alterations, such as an extra chromosome band, but smaller defects could not be reliably found. Improvements in molecular cytogenetics have enabled new more accurate and sensitive tests. Array CGH (comparative genome hybridization) is designed to detect cytogenetic imbalances that are smaller than what can be detected through routine chromosome analysis. Probes are used on glass slides as arrays to hybridize a differentially labed patient and normal DNA. The result is an identification of changes throughout the genome. They are arranged to correspond to genes that are known to affect development. The test will detect loss or duplication of chromosomes on the array.

T4531-T4532

T4531 Pediatric sized disposable incontinence product, protective underwear/pull-on, small/medium size, each

T4532 Pediatric sized disposable incontinence product, protective underwear/pull-on, large size, each

Lay Description

These codes report individual pediatric-size disposable pull-on underwear used for leakage protection and incontinence. This underwear is used by patients with the inability to voluntarily control bladder or bowel functions, or who are unable to use toilet facilities. Report T4531 for each small/medium size pediatric pull-on and T4532 for large.

T4533-T4534

T4533 Youth sized disposable incontinence product, brief/diaper, each

T4534 Youth sized disposable incontinence product, protective underwear/pull-on, each

Lay Description

These codes report individual youth-sized disposable incontinence products for leakage protection, for use by patients with the inability to voluntarily control bladder and/or bowel functions. Report T4533 for each youth-size brief/diaper and T4534 for each protective underwear or pull-on.

T4535

T4535 Disposable liner/shield/guard/pad/undergarment, for incontinence, each

Lay Description

This code reports an individual disposable liner, shield, guard, pad, or undergarment for use by patients with bladder or bowel incontinence, the inability to voluntarily control bladder and/or bowel excretory functions.

T4536

T4536 Incontinence product, protective underwear/pull-on, reusable, any size, each

Lay Description

This code reports an individual, reusable, protective pull-on or underwear of any size for use by patients with bladder or bowel incontinence, the inability to voluntarily control bladder and/or bowel excretory functions.

T4537, T4540

T4537 Incontinence product, protective underpad, reusable, bed size, each
T4540 Incontinence product, protective underpad, reusable, chair size, each

Lay Description

These codes report an individual protective, reusable underpad for use by patients with incontinence, the inability to voluntarily control bladder and/or bowel excretory functions. Report T4537 for each bed size underpad and T4540 for each chair size.

T4538-T4539

T4538 Diaper service, reusable diaper, each diaper
T4539 Incontinence product, diaper/brief, reusable, any size, each

Lay Description

Code T4538 reports each reusable diaper provided by a diaper service. T4539 reports each reusable diaper or brief of any size for use by patients with incontinence, the inability to voluntarily control bladder, and/or bowel excretory functions.

T4540

T4540 Incontinence product, protective underpad, reusable, chair size, each

Lay Description

Please refer to code T4537 for the description, coding, and billing information.

T4541-T4542

T4541 Incontinence product, disposable underpad, large, each
T4542 Incontinence product, disposable underpad, small size, each

Lay Description

Disposable underpads are used by patients with incontinence, the inability to voluntarily control bladder and/or bowel excretory functions. Report T4541 for each large underpad and T4542 for each small underpad.

T4543

T4543 Disposable incontinence product, brief/diaper, bariatric, each

Lay Description

This code reports individual disposable pull-on underwear or diapers used for leakage protection and incontinence. These products are used by patients with the inability to voluntarily control bladder or bowel functions, or who are unable to use toilet facilities. This code represents briefs or diapers specifically made for patients who have undergone bariatric surgery.

V2100-V2102

V2100 Sphere, single vision, plano to plus or minus 4.00, per lens
V2101 Sphere, single vision, plus or minus 4.12 to plus or minus 7.00d, per lens
V2102 Sphere, single vision, plus or minus 7.12 to plus or minus 20.00d, per lens

Lay Description

A single vision lens provides one viewing surface in the lens that is concave on the back surface. This concave shape follows the shape of the eye and allows the back of the lens to stay at the same distance when the eye moves. It is used to treat refractive errors that cause the patient to have trouble seeing near or far distances. The sphere is the strength of the long or short sightedness and its value is in diopters. A plus sign (+) in front of the sphere reading indicates the amount of correction for near sight or reading whereas the minus sign (-) indicates the power of correction for far distance correction. If there is not a correction one way or another, it will be listed as plano, 0.00, or P.

V2101-V2102

V2101 Sphere, single vision, plus or minus 4.12 to plus or minus 7.00d, per lens
V2102 Sphere, single vision, plus or minus 7.12 to plus or minus 20.00d, per lens

Lay Description

Single vision eyeglass lenses address the correction of one focal power such as nearsightedness or farsightedness. Lenses are made from glass or plastic to the specific level of correction required to improve vision. Report V2101 for plus or minus 4.12 to plus or minus 7.00d, per lens; V2102 for plus or minus 7.12 to 20.00d, per lens.

V2103-V2114

V2103 Spherocylinder, single vision, plano to plus or minus 4.00d sphere, 0.12 to 2.00d cylinder, per lens
V2104 Spherocylinder, single vision, plano to plus or minus 4.00d sphere, 2.12 to 4.00d cylinder, per lens
V2105 Spherocylinder, single vision, plano to plus or minus 4.00d sphere, 4.25 to 6.00d cylinder, per lens
V2106 Spherocylinder, single vision, plano to plus or minus 4.00d sphere, over 6.00d cylinder, per lens
V2107 Spherocylinder, single vision, plus or minus 4.25 to plus or minus 7.00 sphere, 0.12 to 2.00d cylinder, per lens
V2108 Spherocylinder, single vision, plus or minus 4.25d to plus or minus 7.00d sphere, 2.12 to 4.00d cylinder, per lens
V2109 Spherocylinder, single vision, plus or minus 4.25 to plus or minus 7.00d sphere, 4.25 to 6.00d cylinder, per lens
V2110 Spherocylinder, single vision, plus or minus 4.25 to 7.00d sphere, over 6.00d cylinder, per lens
V2111 Spherocylinder, single vision, plus or minus 7.25 to plus or minus 12.00d sphere, 0.25 to 2.25d cylinder, per lens
V2112 Spherocylinder, single vision, plus or minus 7.25 to plus or minus 12.00d sphere, 2.25d to 4.00d cylinder, per lens
V2113 Spherocylinder, single vision, plus or minus 7.25 to plus or minus 12.00d sphere, 4.25 to 6.00d cylinder, per lens
V2114 Spherocylinder, single vision, sphere over plus or minus 12.00d, per lens

Lay Description

A single vision lens provides one viewing surface in the lens that is concave on the back surface. This concave shape follows the shape of the eye and allows the back of the lens to stay at the same distance when the eye moves. Spherocylinder single vision eyeglass lenses address the correction of one focal power such as nearsightedness or farsightedness, and astigmatism. The sphere is the strength of the long or short sightedness and its value is in diopters. A plus sign (+) in front of the sphere reading indicates the amount of correction for near sight or reading whereas the minus sign (-) indicates the power of correction for far distance correction. If there is not a correction one way or another, it will be listed as plano, 0.00, or P. The cylinder, also measured in + or -, is the measurement for astigmatism.

V2107-V2110

V2107 Spherocylinder, single vision, plus or minus 4.25 to plus or minus 7.00 sphere, 0.12 to 2.00d cylinder, per lens
V2108 Spherocylinder, single vision, plus or minus 4.25d to plus or minus 7.00d sphere, 2.12 to 4.00d cylinder, per lens
V2109 Spherocylinder, single vision, plus or minus 4.25 to plus or minus 7.00d sphere, 4.25 to 6.00d cylinder, per lens
V2110 Spherocylinder, single vision, plus or minus 4.25 to 7.00d sphere, over 6.00d cylinder, per lens

Lay Description

Spherocylinder single vision eyeglass lenses address the correction of one focal power such as nearsightedness or farsightedness, and astigmatism. Lenses are made from glass or plastic to the specific level of correction required to improve vision. These codes report plus or minus 7.00d sphere and the specific level of astigmatism per lens. Report V2107 for 0.12 to 2.00d cylinder; V2108 for 2.12 to 4.00d cylinder; V2109 for 4.25 to 6.00d cylinder; and V2110 for more than 6.00d cylinder.

Medicare Information

See chapter titled "Medicare Guidelines," under "Lens," for Medicare billing and documentation information.

V2111-V2113

V2111 Spherocylinder, single vision, plus or minus 7.25 to plus or minus 12.00d sphere, 0.25 to 2.25d cylinder, per lens
V2112 Spherocylinder, single vision, plus or minus 7.25 to plus or minus 12.00d sphere, 2.25d to 4.00d cylinder, per lens
V2113 Spherocylinder, single vision, plus or minus 7.25 to plus or minus 12.00d sphere, 4.25 to 6.00d cylinder, per lens

Lay Description

Spherocylinder single vision eyeglass lenses address the correction of one focal power such as nearsightedness or farsightedness, and astigmatism. Lenses are made from glass or plastic to the specific level of correction required to improve vision. These codes report plus or minus 7.25d to plus or minus 12.00d sphere and the specific level of astigmatism per lens. Report V2111 for 0.25 to 2.25d cylinder; V2112 for 2.25 to 4.00d cylinder; V2113 for 4.25 to 6.00d cylinder; and V2113 for more than 6.00d cylinder.

Medicare Information

See chapter titled "Medicare Guidelines," under "Lens," for Medicare billing and documentation information.

V2114

V2114 Spherocylinder, single vision, sphere over plus or minus 12.00d, per lens

Lay Description

Spherocylinder single vision eyeglass lenses address the correction of one focal power such as nearsightedness or farsightedness, and astigmatism. Lenses are made from glass or plastic to the specific level of correction required to improve vision. This code reports plus or minus 12.00d.

Medicare Information

See chapter titled "Medicare Guidelines," under "Lens," for Medicare billing and documentation information.

V2115

V2115 Lenticular (myodisc), per lens, single vision

Lay Description

Lenticular lenses are designed for very strong prescriptions generally requiring plus or minus 10.00d or higher. The specified prescription power is found in the center of the lens and the edges are ground down to reduce the weight and thickness of the lens. Report V2115 for myodisc.

V2118

V2118 Aniseikonic lens, single vision

Lay Description

Aniseikonic lenses are for correction in cases where patients report unequal visual images. This commonly occurs with a cataract, corneal surgical corrections, radial keratotomy, photoreactive keratectomy, laser surgeries, and scleral buckling. The football shaped lenses have several aspects for correction including base curve and lens thickness, refractive index, and the difference of magnification between lenses.

Medicare Information

See chapter titled "Medicare Guidelines," under "Lens," for Medicare billing and documentation information.

V2121, V2215, V2221, V2321

V2121 Lenticular lens, per lens, single
V2215 Lenticular (myodisc), per lens, bifocal
V2221 Lenticular lens, per lens, bifocal
V2321 Lenticular lens, per lens, trifocal

Lay Description

A lenticular lens changes the magnification depending on the viewing angle. They may be thick in the center and thin at the edges or very thick at the edge and thinner in the center. The lenses were used to treat patients after cataract surgery when lenses weren't implanted. They may still be used occasionally to treat patients who need prescriptions of minus 10 diopters or higher.

V2200-V2202

V2200 Sphere, bifocal, plano to plus or minus 4.00d, per lens
V2201 Sphere, bifocal, plus or minus 4.12 to plus or minus 7.00d, per lens
V2202 Sphere, bifocal, plus or minus 7.12 to plus or minus 20.00d, per lens

Lay Description

Bifocal vision eyeglass lenses address the correction of two focal powers for distance and work such as reading that requires a close up focus. Lenses are made from glass or plastic to the specific level of correction required to improve vision. The lens provides two viewing surfaces in the lens that is concave on the back surface. This concave shape follows the shape of the eye and allows the back of the lens to stay at the same distance when the eye moves. The sphere is the strength of the long or short sightedness and its value is in diopters. A plus sign (+) in front of the sphere reading indicates the amount of correction for near sight or reading whereas the minus sign (-) indicates the power of correction for far distance correction. If there is not a correction one way or another, it will be listed as plano, 0.00, or P.

Medicare Information

For patients who are aphakic who do not have an intraocular lens (IOL) (ICD-9-CM diagnosis codes 379.31, 743.35), the following lenses are covered when determined to be medically necessary:

- Bifocal lenses in frames

Note: See chapter titled "Medicare Guidelines," under "Lens," for additional Medicare billing and documentation information.

V2203-V2214

V2203 Spherocylinder, bifocal, plano to plus or minus 4.00d sphere, 0.12 to 2.00d cylinder, per lens
V2204 Spherocylinder, bifocal, plano to plus or minus 4.00d sphere, 2.12 to 4.00d cylinder, per lens
V2205 Spherocylinder, bifocal, plano to plus or minus 4.00d sphere, 4.25 to 6.00d cylinder, per lens
V2206 Spherocylinder, bifocal, plano to plus or minus 4.00d sphere, over 6.00d cylinder, per lens
V2207 Spherocylinder, bifocal, plus or minus 4.25 to plus or minus 7.00d sphere, 0.12 to 2.00d cylinder, per lens
V2208 Spherocylinder, bifocal, plus or minus 4.25 to plus or minus 7.00d sphere, 2.12 to 4.00d cylinder, per lens
V2209 Spherocylinder, bifocal, plus or minus 4.25 to plus or minus 7.00d sphere, 4.25 to 6.00d cylinder, per lens
V2210 Spherocylinder, bifocal, plus or minus 4.25 to plus or minus 7.00d sphere, over 6.00d cylinder, per lens
V2211 Spherocylinder, bifocal, plus or minus 7.25 to plus or minus 12.00d sphere, 0.25 to 2.25d cylinder, per lens
V2212 Spherocylinder, bifocal, plus or minus 7.25 to plus or minus 12.00d sphere, 2.25 to 4.00d cylinder, per lens
V2213 Spherocylinder, bifocal, plus or minus 7.25 to plus or minus 12.00d sphere, 4.25 to 6.00d cylinder, per lens
V2214 Spherocylinder, bifocal, sphere over plus or minus 12.00d, per lens

Lay Description
Bifocal vision eyeglass lenses address the correction of two focal powers for distance and work such as reading that requires a close up focus. Lenses are made from glass or plastic to the specific level of correction required to improve vision. The lens provides two viewing surfaces in the lens that is concave on the back surface. This concave shape follows the shape of the eye and allows the back of the lens to stay at the same distance when the eye moves. The sphere is the strength of the long or short sightedness and its value is in diopters. A plus sign (+) in front of the sphere reading indicates the amount of correction for near sight or reading whereas the minus sign (-) indicates the power of correction for far distance correction. If there is not a correction one way or another, it will be listed as plano, 0.00, or P. The cylinder, also measured in + or -, is the measurement for astigmatism.

V2215

V2215 Lenticular (myodisc), per lens, bifocal

Lay Description
See description for V2121.

V2221

V2221 Lenticular lens, per lens, bifocal

Lay Description
See description for V2121.

V2300-V2302

V2300 Sphere, trifocal, plano to plus or minus 4.00d, per lens
V2301 Sphere, trifocal, plus or minus 4.12 to plus or minus 7.00d per lens
V2302 Sphere, trifocal, plus or minus 7.12 to plus or minus 20.00, per lens

Lay Description
Trifocal lenses have three visibly identifiable zones of vision divided by two segment lines of variable widths. Trifocal lenses offer three fixed fields of focus (near/intermediate/distant) for patients with higher levels of presbyopia. The lens provides three viewing surface in the lens that is concave on the back surface. This concave shape follows the shape of the eye and allows the back of the lens to stay at the same distance when the eye moves. It is used to treat refractive errors that cause the patient to have trouble seeing near or far distances. The sphere is the strength of the long or short sightedness and its value is in diopters. A plus sign (+) in front of the sphere reading indicates the amount of correction for near sight or reading whereas the minus sign (-) indicates the power of correction for far distance correction. If there is not a correction one way or another, it will be listed as plano, 0.00, or P.

Medicare Information
See chapter titled "Medicare Guidelines," under "Lens," for Medicare billing and documentation information.

V2303-V2314

V2303 Spherocylinder, trifocal, plano to plus or minus 4.00d sphere, 0.12 to 2.00d cylinder, per lens
V2304 Spherocylinder, trifocal, plano to plus or minus 4.00d sphere, 2.25 to 4.00d cylinder, per lens
V2305 Spherocylinder, trifocal, plano to plus or minus 4.00d sphere, 4.25 to 6.00 cylinder, per lens
V2306 Spherocylinder, trifocal, plano to plus or minus 4.00d sphere, over 6.00d cylinder, per lens
V2307 Spherocylinder, trifocal, plus or minus 4.25 to plus or minus 7.00d sphere, 0.12 to 2.00d cylinder, per lens
V2308 Spherocylinder, trifocal, plus or minus 4.25 to plus or minus 7.00d sphere, 2.12 to 4.00d cylinder, per lens
V2309 Spherocylinder, trifocal, plus or minus 4.25 to plus or minus 7.00d sphere, 4.25 to 6.00d cylinder, per lens
V2310 Spherocylinder, trifocal, plus or minus 4.25 to plus or minus 7.00d sphere, over 6.00d cylinder, per lens
V2311 Spherocylinder, trifocal, plus or minus 7.25 to plus or minus 12.00d sphere, 0.25 to 2.25d cylinder, per lens
V2312 Spherocylinder, trifocal, plus or minus 7.25 to plus or minus 12.00d sphere, 2.25 to 4.00d cylinder, per lens
V2313 Spherocylinder, trifocal, plus or minus 7.25 to plus or minus 12.00d sphere, 4.25 to 6.00d cylinder, per lens
V2314 Spherocylinder, trifocal, sphere over plus or minus 12.00d, per lens

Lay Description

Spherocylinder trifocal vision eyeglass lenses address the correction of focal power such as nearsightedness or farsightedness, and/or astigmatism. Trifocal lenses have three visibly identifiable zones of vision divided by two segment lines of variable widths. Trifocal lenses offer three fixed fields of focus (near/intermediate/distant) for patients with higher levels of presbyopia. Lenses are made from glass or plastic to the specific level of correction required to improve vision. The lens provides three viewing surfaces in the lens that is concave on the back surface. This concave shape follows the shape of the eye and allows the back of the lens to stay at the same distance when the eye moves. The sphere is the strength of the long or short sightedness and its value is in diopters. A plus sign (+) in front of the sphere reading indicates the amount of correction for near sight or reading whereas the minus sign (-) indicates the power of correction for far distance correction. If there is not a correction one way or another, it will be listed as plano, 0.00, or P. The cylinder, also measured in + or -, is the measurement for astigmatism.

Medicare Information

See chapter titled "Medicare Guidelines," under "Lens," for Medicare billing and documentation information.

V2311-V2314

V2311 Spherocylinder, trifocal, plus or minus 7.25 to plus or minus 12.00d sphere, 0.25 to 2.25d cylinder, per lens
V2312 Spherocylinder, trifocal, plus or minus 7.25 to plus or minus 12.00d sphere, 2.25 to 4.00d cylinder, per lens
V2313 Spherocylinder, trifocal, plus or minus 7.25 to plus or minus 12.00d sphere, 4.25 to 6.00d cylinder, per lens
V2314 Spherocylinder, trifocal, sphere over plus or minus 12.00d, per lens

Lay Description

Spherocylinder trifocal vision eyeglass lenses address the correction of focal power such as nearsightedness or farsightedness, and/or astigmatism. Trifocal lenses have three visibly identifiable zones of vision divided by two segment lines of variable widths. Trifocal lenses offer three fixed fields of focus (near/intermediate/distant) for patients with higher levels of presbyopia. Lenses are made from glass or plastic to the specific level of correction required to improve vision. Report V2311 for a spherocylinder trifocal lens, plus or minus 7.25 to plus or minus 12.00d sphere, 0.25 to 2.25d cylinder; V2312 for plus or minus 7.25 to plus or minus 12.00d sphere, 2.25 to 4.00d cylinder; V2313 for plus or minus 7.25 to plus or minus 12.00d sphere, 4.25 to 6.00d cylinder; and V2314 for a spherocylinder trifocal lens, sphere higher than plus or minus 12.00d. Each is reported per lens.

Medicare Information

See chapter titled "Medicare Guidelines," under "Lens," for Medicare billing and documentation information.

V2315

V2315 Lenticular, (myodisc), per lens, trifocal

Lay Description

Lenticular lenses are designed for very strong prescriptions generally requiring plus or minus 10.00d and higher. The specified prescription power is found in the center of the lens and the edges are ground down to reduce the weight and thickness of the lens. Trifocal lenses have three visibly identifiable zones of vision divided by two segment lines of variable widths. Trifocal lenses offer three fixed fields of focus (near/intermediate/distant) for patients with higher levels of presbyopia. Report V2315 for a lenticular (myodisc) trifocal lens.

Medicare Information

See chapter titled "Medicare Guidelines," under "Lens," for Medicare billing and documentation information.

V2318

V2318 Aniseikonic lens, trifocal

Lay Description

Aniseikonic lenses are for correction in cases where patients report unequal visual images. This commonly occurs with a cataract, corneal surgical corrections, radial keratotomy, photoreactive keratectomy, laser surgeries, and scleral buckling. The football shaped lenses have several aspects for vision correction including base curve and lens thickness, refractive index, and the difference of magnification between lenses. Trifocal lenses have three visibly identifiable zones of vision divided by two segment lines of variable widths. Trifocal lenses offer three fixed fields of focus (near/intermediate/distant) for patients with higher levels of presbyopia. Code V2318 is reported for a trifocal aniseikonic lens.

Medicare Information

See chapter titled "Medicare Guidelines," under "Lens," for Medicare billing and documentation information.

V2321

V2321 Lenticular lens, per lens, trifocal

Lay Description

See description for V2121.

V2410

V2410 Variable asphericity lens, single vision, full field, glass or plastic, per lens

Lay Description

Aspheric single vision lenses address the correction of one focal power such as nearsightedness or farsightedness. They are also a higher quality premium lens, used for patients with slight astigmatism and at the early stages of development of presbyopia. Lenses are made from glass or plastic to the specific level of correction required to improve vision. Report this code for a full field, variable asphericity, single vision lens.

Medicare Information

For patients who are aphakic who do not have an intraocular lens (IOL) (ICD-9-CM diagnosis codes 379.31, 743.35), the following lenses are covered when determined to be medically necessary:

- Bifocal lenses in frames

Note: See chapter titled "Medicare Guidelines," under "Lens," for additional Medicare billing and documentation information.

V2430

V2430 Variable asphericity lens, bifocal, full field, glass or plastic, per lens

Lay Description

Aspherical bifocal vision lenses address the correction of two focal powers for distance and work, such as reading, which requires a close up focus. They are also a higher quality premium lens, used for patients with slight astigmatism and at the early stages of development of presbyopia. Lenses are made from glass or plastic to the specific level of correction required to improve vision. Report this code for a full field, variable asphericity, bifocal lens.

Medicare Information

For patients who are aphakic who do not have an intraocular lens (IOL) (ICD-9-CM diagnosis codes 379.31, 743.35), the following lenses are covered when determined to be medically necessary:

- Bifocal lenses in frames

Note: See chapter titled "Medicare Guidelines," under "Lens," for additional Medicare billing and documentation information.

V2500

V2500 Contact lens, PMMA, spherical, per lens

Lay Description

Polymethyl methacrylate (PMMA) spherical contact lenses are rigid lenses worn directly on the cornea to correct vision and have a spherical anterior (convex) surface and spherical posterior optical zone that approximates the curvature of the sclera. Spherical contact lenses have the same corrective power at each part of the lens, which allows the eye to focus and have clear vision. This code is reported per lens.

Medicare Information

See chapter titled "Medicare Guidelines," under "Lens," for Medicare billing and documentation information.

V2501

V2501 Contact lens, PMMA, toric or prism ballast, per lens

Lay Description

Polymethyl methacrylate (PMMA) toric or prism ballast contact lenses are rigid lenses worn directly on the cornea to correct vision and have a special curvature designed to correct astigmatism. Astigmatism is a visual defect in which the cornea is not perfectly round. Toric lenses are used when conventional soft or rigid lenses do not correct the defect. This code is reported per lens.

V2502

V2502 Contact lens PMMA, bifocal, per lens

Lay Description

Polymethyl methacrylate (PMMA) bifocal contact lenses are rigid lenses worn directly on the cornea to correct vision. Bifocal contact lenses address the correction of two focal powers for distance and work, such as reading, which requires a close up focus. This code is reported per lens.

V2510

V2510 Contact lens, gas permeable, spherical, per lens

Lay Description

A spherical gas permeable contact lens is generally a rigid lens worn directly on the cornea to correct vision and has a spherical anterior (convex) surface and spherical posterior optical zone that approximates the curvature of the sclera. Spherical contact lenses have the same corrective power at each part of the lens, which allows the eye to focus and have clear vision. This lens also allows for oxygen exchange. It consists of materials, such as cellulose acetate butyrate, polyacrylate-silicone, or silicone elastomers, which typically do not attract water. Code V2510 is reported per lens.

Medicare Information

See chapter titled "Medicare Guidelines," under "Lens," for Medicare billing and documentation information.

V2511

V2511 Contact lens, gas permeable, toric, prism ballast, per lens

Lay Description

A gas permeable toric contact lens is generally a rigid lens worn directly on the cornea to correct vision and has a special curvature designed to correct for astigmatism (a visual defect in which the cornea is not perfectly round). This lens also allows for oxygen exchange. It consists of materials, such as cellulose acetate butyrate, polyacrylate-silicone, or silicone elastomers, that typically do not attract water and are used when conventional soft or rigid lenses do not correct the defect. Code V2511 is reported per lens.

Medicare Information

See chapter titled "Medicare Guidelines," under "Lens," for Medicare billing and documentation information.

V2512

V2512 Contact lens, gas permeable, bifocal, per lens

Lay Description

A gas permeable bifocal contact lens is generally a rigid lens worn directly on the cornea to correct vision and address the correction of two focal powers for distance and work, such as reading, which requires a close up focus. This lens also allows for oxygen exchange. It consists of materials, such as cellulose acetate butyrate, polyacrylate-silicone, or silicone elastomers, that typically do not attract water. Code V2512 is reported per lens.

Medicare Information

See chapter titled "Medicare Guidelines," under "Lens," for Medicare billing and documentation information.

V2513

V2513 Contact lens, gas permeable, extended wear, per lens

Lay Description

A gas permeable extended wear contact lens is generally a rigid lens intended to be worn directly on the cornea to correct vision and may be worn for an extended period of time (does not have to be taken out of the eye on a daily basis). This lens also allows for oxygen exchange. It consists of materials, such as cellulose acetate butyrate, polyacrylate-silicone, or silicone elastomers, that typically do not attract water. Code V2513 is reported per lens.

Medicare Information

See chapter titled "Medicare Guidelines," under "Lens," for Medicare billing and documentation information.

V2520

V2520 Contact lens, hydrophilic, spherical, per lens

Lay Description

A spherical hydrophilic (soft) contact lens is worn directly on the cornea to correct vision and has a spherical anterior (convex) surface and spherical posterior optical zone that approximates the curvature of the sclera. Spherical contact lenses have the same corrective power at each part of the lens, which allows the eye to focus and have clear vision. This lens consists of a variety of polymer materials that absorb or attract a certain amount of water and are used when conventional soft or rigid lenses do not correct the defect.

Medicare Information

See chapter titled "Medicare Guidelines," under "Lens," for Medicare billing and documentation information.

V2521

V2521 Contact lens, hydrophilic, toric, or prism ballast, per lens

Lay Description

A hydrophilic toric contact lens is worn directly on the cornea to correct vision and has a special curvature designed to correct for astigmatism (a visual defect in which the cornea is not perfectly round). This lens consists of a variety of polymer materials that absorb or attract a certain amount of water and are used when conventional soft or rigid lenses do not correct the defect.

Medicare Information

See chapter titled "Medicare Guidelines," under "Lens," for Medicare billing and documentation information.

V2522

V2522 Contact lens, hydrophilic, bifocal, per lens

Lay Description

A hydrophilic bifocal contact lens is worn directly on the cornea to correct vision and address the correction of two focal powers for distance and work, such as reading, which requires a close up focus. This lens consists of a variety of polymer materials that absorb or attract a certain amount of water, making it more comfortable for the wearer. Code V2522 is reported per lens.

V2523

V2523 Contact lens, hydrophilic, extended wear, per lens

Lay Description

A hydrophilic extended wear contact lens is worn directly on the cornea to correct vision and may be worn for an extended period of time (does not have to be taken out of the eye on a daily basis). This lens consists of a variety of polymer materials that absorb

or attract a certain amount of water. Code V2523 is reported per lens.

Medicare Information

See chapter titled "Medicare Guidelines," under "Lens," for Medicare billing and documentation information.

V2530-V2531

V2530 Contact lens, scleral, gas impermeable, per lens (for contact lens modification, see 92325)

V2531 Contact lens, scleral, gas permeable, per lens (for contact lens modification, see 92325)

Lay Description

A scleral contact lens is generally a rigid lens worn directly on the sclera that fits underneath the top and bottom eyelids. These lenses are used for patients who have problems wearing conventional lenses, patients with high refractive errors, or for patients with ocular surface disease. It consists of materials, such as cellulose acetate butyrate, polyacrylate-silicone, or silicone elastomers, that typically do not attract water. Report V2530 for each scleral, gas impermeable lens and V2531 for one that allows for oxygen exchange.

Medicare Information

See chapter titled "Medicare Guidelines," under "Lens," for Medicare billing and documentation information.

V2600

V2600 Hand held low vision aids and other nonspectacle mounted aids

Lay Description

A low vision aid or magnifier is a type of magnifying lens used by patients who have impaired vision. This magnifier is hand held or may be used with another piece of equipment, but is not mounted onto glasses.

Medicare Information

See chapter titled "Medicare Guidelines," under "Lens," for Medicare billing and documentation information.

V2610

V2610 Single lens spectacle mounted low vision aids

Lay Description

A low vision aid or magnifier is a type of magnifying lens used by patients who have impaired vision. This magnifying aid is used on a single lens and mounted onto glasses.

Medicare Information

See chapter titled "Medicare Guidelines," under "Lens," for Medicare billing and documentation information.

V2623

V2623   Prosthetic eye, plastic, custom

Lay Description

An eye prosthesis is created for a patient with absence or shrinkage of an eye due to a birth defect, trauma, or surgical removal. Eye prostheses assist in maintaining the internal orbital eye structures by filling in the void created by the missing natural eye. A byproduct of the prosthesis allows for a cosmetic enhancement by allowing the patient to appear to have two eyes. Code V2623 reports a custom prosthetic eye that is made out of plastic.

Medicare Information

Replacement is covered every five years, with exceptions allowed when documentation supports medical necessity for more frequent replacement.

When ocular prostheses are provided bilaterally and the same code is used for both prostheses, bill both on the same claim line using modifiers LT and RT and 2 units of service.

V2627

V2627   Scleral cover shell

Lay Description

A scleral cover shell is a device made out of glass or plastic and placed over the cornea and sclera to be worn for a short period of time for cosmetic or reconstructive reasons. It is typically not implanted in the eye.

V2744

V2744   Tint, photochromatic, per lens

Lay Description

Photochromatic tinted lenses are those in which the degree of tint changes in response to changes in ambient light. Report this code for photochromatic tint per lens.

V2745

V2745   Addition to lens; tint, any color, solid, gradient or equal, excludes photochromatic, any lens material, per lens

Lay Description

Tinted lenses are made by putting coatings on the lens material to reduce the amount of light entering the eye. Report this code for the addition of tint to a lens, any color, solid, gradient or equal, excluding photochromatic.

V2750

V2750   Antireflective coating, per lens

Lay Description

Antireflective coating reduces glare on the surface of a lens and also reduces the reflected glare of headlights to improve nighttime driving. Report this code for antireflective coating, per lens.

V2755

V2755   U-V lens, per lens

Lay Description

UV lenses protect eyes from the potentially harmful ultraviolet rays generated from the sun or other light sources by blocking them from penetrating the lens material and reaching the eye. Report this code per lens.

V2760

V2760   Scratch resistant coating, per lens

Lay Description

Scratch resistant coating is a protective coating applied directly to the lens that reduces the potential for normal scratching or scraping of the lens material, reducing potential lens distortion. Report this code per lens.

V2770

V2770   Occluder lens, per lens

Lay Description

An occluder lens typically is a soft lens that can be worn for up to seven days (extended wear) and is blackened out, blocking vision in the eye wearing it. This type of prosthetic lens in used for treating patients, generally children, with amblyopia, or "lazy eye." The occluder lens forces the development of the amblyopic eye by blocking out all vision in the other eye. This type of lens may also be used in aphakic infants, where patch therapy has failed. This code is reported per lens.

V2781

V2781   Progressive lens, per lens

Lay Description

No-line multifocal lenses that provide the needed correction for multiple focal lengths, but do not have a visible seam or line in the lenses are called progressive lenses. Report this code per progressive lens.

V5008

V5008 Hearing screening

Lay Description

A hearing screening is a unilateral or bilateral test consisting of the patient's case history, a visual inspection of the ear, pure tone screening within a range of 1000-4000 Hz, speech audiometry, and a self-assessed judgment of hearing difficulty. The screening is conducted by a certified audiologist, speech-language pathologist, or other personnel under the supervision of an audiologist.

V5010-V5020

V5010 Assessment for hearing aid
V5011 Fitting/orientation/checking of hearing aid
V5014 Repair/modification of a hearing aid
V5020 Conformity evaluation

Lay Description

During an assessment for a hearing aid, an audiologist reviews the results of the initial hearing screening with the patient, discusses the type and degree of hearing loss including the configuration of the loss (whether unilateral or bilateral), the options available based on the information gathered, and costs. The audiologist also obtains audiometric measurements and an impression of the ear canal. The hearing aid is fitted during an orientation in which the audiologist explains how to operate the hearing aid. At this fitting, internal controls of the hearing aid are set or programmed. The patient is scheduled for a conformity evaluation to confirm that the hearing aid is meeting the needs of the patient. Report V5010 for the hearing aid assessment, and V5011 for the fitting/orientation/checking of the hearing aid. Repairs and modifications to the hearing aid are reported with V5014. Report V5020 for the conformity evaluation.

V5030-V5040

V5030 Hearing aid, monaural, body worn, air conduction
V5040 Hearing aid, monaural, body worn, bone conduction

Lay Description

A body worn monaural (one ear), air conduction hearing aid (V5030) is specifically designed with bigger controls for patients who have less dexterity and have a problem with feedback. It consists of a small box that is clipped to clothing or slips inside a pocket. This connects to a lead to an earphone and attaches to the ear-mould. The bone conduction hearing aid (V5040) is designed for patients who have an abnormality of the ear canal. Due to drainage, a narrow canal, or no canal at all, the patient is precluded from using an air conduction device. The bone conductor is held onto the mastoid bone by an implanted screw or by using a headband. It works by transmitting vibrations through the skull to the inner ear.

V5050-V5060, V5241

V5050 Hearing aid, monaural, in the ear
V5060 Hearing aid, monaural, behind the ear
V5241 Dispensing fee, monaural hearing aid, any type

Lay Description

There are two types of in the ear (ITE) monaural hearing aids available. The full shell aid is for mild to severe hearing loss and is the largest and least expensive available. It covers the entire ear opening and is the most versatile of all the hearing aids. The half-shell/conch aid is for mild to moderately severe hearing loss and is the most popular model. Smaller than the full shell, it covers only the bowl portion of the ear. The behind the ear (BTE) model is connected to the ear by an ear-mold and is used mostly by patients with severe hearing loss, although it can be used for any and all forms of hearing loss. This type is more durable and less flexible than the ITE model. Report V5050 for a monaural ITE hearing aid and V5060 for a monaural BTE hearing aid. Report V5241 for the dispensing fee of a monaural hearing aid, any type.

V5241

V5241 Dispensing fee, monaural hearing aid, any type

Lay Description

Please refer to codes V5050-V5060 for the description, coding, and billing information.

V5242-V5243, V5248-V5249

V5242 Hearing aid, analog, monaural, CIC (completely in the ear canal)
V5243 Hearing aid, analog, monaural, ITC (in the canal)
V5248 Hearing aid, analog, binaural, CIC
V5249 Hearing aid, analog, binaural, ITC

Lay Description

The analog hearing aid has a volume control that is adjusted by the patient. It is battery operated and works by converting sound waves to an electronic signal. When the volume is adjusted, all of the sounds are uniformly adjusted. Report V5242 for an analog, monaural (one ear) CIC (completely in the ear canal) hearing aid and V5243 for one ITC (in the canal) hearing aid. For an analog, binaural (both ears) CIC hearing aid, report V5248 and report V5249 for an analog, binaural ITC hearing aid.

V5244-V5247, V5250-V5253

V5244 Hearing aid, digitally programmable analog, monaural, CIC
V5245 Hearing aid, digitally programmable, analog, monaural, ITC
V5246 Hearing aid, digitally programmable analog, monaural, ITE (in the ear)
V5247 Hearing aid, digitally programmable analog, monaural, BTE (behind the ear)
V5250 Hearing aid, digitally programmable analog, binaural, CIC
V5251 Hearing aid, digitally programmable analog, binaural, ITC
V5252 Hearing aid, digitally programmable, binaural, ITE
V5253 Hearing aid, digitally programmable, binaural, BTE

Lay Description

Digitally programmable analog hearing aids are battery operated and work by making sound waves larger and breaking them into distinct units. This digital signal is free from distortion and treats soft sounds differently than loud sounds, thus allowing for more clarity of sound, rather than only allowing more volume. The sound waves are converted from an electronic signal and then passed through an A/D converter. These codes all represent digitally programmable analog monaural hearing aids. Report V5244 for the CIC (completely in the canal) model; V5245 for the ITC (in the canal) model; V5246 for the ITE (in the ear) model; and V5247 for the BTE (behind the ear) model. For digitally programmable analog binaural hearing aids, report V5250 for the CIC model; V5251 for the ITC model; V5252 for the ITE model; and V5253 for BTE model.

V5248-V5249

V5248 Hearing aid, analog, binaural, CIC
V5249 Hearing aid, analog, binaural, ITC

Lay Description

Please refer to codes V5242-V5243 for the description, coding, and billing information.

V5250-V5253

V5250 Hearing aid, digitally programmable analog, binaural, CIC
V5251 Hearing aid, digitally programmable analog, binaural, ITC
V5252 Hearing aid, digitally programmable, binaural, ITE
V5253 Hearing aid, digitally programmable, binaural, BTE

Lay Description

Please refer to codes V5244-V5247 for the description, coding, and billing information.

V5262-V5263

V5262 Hearing aid, disposable, any type, monaural
V5263 Hearing aid, disposable, any type, binaural

Lay Description

Disposable hearing aids are made of a soft material that is intended to last the user approximately 40 days. A disposable hearing aid has a mushroom-shaped tip that fits in the ear canal and can be fitted to most adults. Report V5262 for any type of monaural, disposable hearing aid, and V5263 for any type binaural.

Medicare Information

Medicare has a quantity limit for V5262.

V5266

V5266 Battery for use in hearing device

Lay Description

Hearing devices require select batteries to provide power to the listening device. Batteries are available in different brands, sizes, and quantity packs depending on the requirements of the device. This code reports a battery for use in a hearing device.

V5268

V5268 Assistive listening device, telephone amplifier, any type

Lay Description

Telephone assistive listening devices are used to amplify sound for the hearing impaired. Some of the telephone assistive listening devices available are portable phones, in-line amplifiers, ring signalers, and super phone ringers. This code is reported for any type of telephone amplifier assistive listening device for the telephone.

V5269

V5269 Assistive listening device, alerting, any type

Lay Description

There are two types of alerting assistive listening devices: visual and vibration. The visual alert includes a flashing light, or strobe light, to assist the hearing impaired user in becoming aware of an event such as ringing smoke alarms, doorbells, baby monitors, or alarm clocks. Some patients find that vibrating devices such as pillow shakers or wrist shakers are more effective. This code is used for an alerting assistive listening device of either type.

V5270-V5271

V5270 Assistive listening device, television amplifier, any type
V5271 Assistive listening device, television caption decoder

Lay Description

An assistive listening device used with a television amplifies the audio signal from the television and is generally transmitted through infrared to a headset. Closed captioning decoders are also available for older models of televisions in which a decoder is not built into the system. Report V5270 for any type of television amplifier and V5271 for a caption decoder.

V5272

V5272 Assistive listening device, TDD

Lay Description

A TDD is a telecommunication device for the deaf. These include text telephones and teletype machines. These assistive listening devices allow a person with hearing impairment to use the telephone. The device is connected to a small keyboard that allows the user to type the message to be sent. If both the caller and receiver have TDDs, a printed message is read on a screen. However, if the receiver does not have a TDD, the messages are relayed through an operator.

V5273

V5273 Assistive listening device, for use with cochlear implant

Lay Description

An assistive listening device for use with a cochlear implant is designed to amplify the voice in a setting such as a classroom or boardroom directly to the person with the implant without amplifying background noise. These systems include an infrared system with a jack.

V5275

V5275 Ear impression, each

Lay Description

Impressions are made of the ear to obtain a hearing device specifically for the individual. The ear canal is visualized through an otoscope to check for wax build up, anomalies, and to check the tympanic membrane. A plug made of soft cotton is inserted just beyond the canal to provide a "wall" for the mold and to ease the removal of debris. The impression material is mixed according to the manufacturer's specifications and loaded into a syringe. The tip of the syringe is placed in the canal and then emptied to fill the ear canal, the pinna, concha, and helix. After the material has set for the time indicated, the impression and cotton wall are removed. The audiologist visualizes the canal with the otoscope to be certain all debris has been removed. Use this code for each impression.

V5362

V5362 Speech screening

Lay Description

Speech screenings focus on testing the repetitive oral movements of articulation, laryngeal functions of voice, and velopharyngeal function of resonance. The patient is asked to read or repeat a variety of sounds to determine and compare the developmental level or degree of speech impairment.

V5364

V5364 Dysphagia screening

Lay Description

Dysphagia screenings test the difficulty a patient has with the swallowing reflex. There are three phases that are observed: the oral phase, pharyngeal phase, and esophageal phase. The patient is given a small amount of water that is swallowed while the practitioner feels for the swallow above and below the larynx. The patient is observed for delayed swallow, cough on swallowing, drooling, and dysphonia.